Complications in Pediatric Otolaryngology

Edited by
Gary D. Josephson, M.D.
Daniel L. Wohl, M.D.

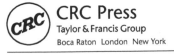

CRC Press
Taylor & Francis Group
Boca Raton London New York

CRC Press is an imprint of the
Taylor & Francis Group, an **informa** business

CRC Press
Taylor & Francis Group
6000 Broken Sound Parkway NW, Suite 300
Boca Raton, FL 33487-2742

First issued in paperback 2019

© 2007 by Taylor & Francis Group, LLC
CRC Press is an imprint of Taylor & Francis Group, an Informa business

No claim to original U.S. Government works

ISBN-13: 978-0-8247-2437-5 (hbk)
ISBN-13: 978-0-367-39268-0 (pbk)

Library of Congress Cataloging-in-Publication Data

Complications in pediatric otolaryngology /
   edited by Gary Josephson, Daniel Wohl.
     p. ; cm.
   Includes bibliographical references and index.
   ISBN-13: 978-0-8247-2437-5 (hardcover : alk. paper)
   ISBN-10: 0-8247-2437-2 (hardcover : alk. paper)
   1. Pediatric otolaryngology.
   2. Children--Surgery--Complications. I. Josephson, Gary.
  II. Wohl, Daniel.

RF47.C4C665 2004
618.92'09751--dc22
                                    2004058210

Visit the Taylor & Francis Web site at
http://www.taylorandfrancis.com

and the CRC Press Web site at
http://www.crcpress.com

In Memoriam

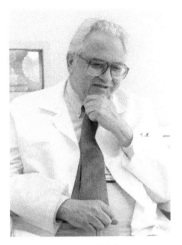

1925–2004
Sylvan Stool, M.D.

Dedication

_____

To my wife, whose love and friendship are treasured every single day.
To my two children, who have helped me appreciate life's wonderful diversity.
To my family, who have led by example.
To my patients, who continue to inspire me to do my very best.

Daniel L. Wohl, M.D.

This book is dedicated to my wife Patricia, who has supported all my ideas and ambitions, and who has brought meaning to my life.
To my children Samantha and Grayson, who have taught me the depth to which a child could be loved.
To my parents Stanley and Sheila, who have provided me with love and the resources to attain my goals.
To my brother Jordan, who introduced and laid the foundation for my career as an otolaryngologist.
To my brother Mark and sister Amy, who have always been a source of support.
To my teachers and mentors, who have given me the education and skills to care for my patients.
And to my patients and their parents, who have given me permission, the opportunity, and the privilege to perform my trade and care for them the best way I know how.
I am forever grateful.

Gary D. Josephson, M.D.

American Academy of Otolaryngology–Head and Neck Surgery Foundation Code of Ethics

The Physician–Patient Relationship

Each patient must be treated with respect, dignity, compassion, and honesty. The patient's right to participate in the treatment process must be recognized and promulgated by the otolaryngologist. Discrimination against a patient on the basis of race, color, gender, age, sexual orientation, socioeconimic status, religion or national origin is inappropriate. The otolaryngologist must establish and maintain appropriate relational boundaries, avoiding exploitation of patient vulnerability.

Colleague Interactions

Interactions with colleagues should be based on mutual respect and a desire to improve patient care. Communication with colleagues must be truthful and forthright. Disparagement of any kind is to be discouraged.

Commercial Interests

This Code of Ethics does not seek to restrict legal trade practices. However, a physician's commercial or financial interests should never be placed ahead of the interests and welfare of patients. Conflicts that develop between a physician's financial interests and the physician's responsiblities to the patient should be resolved to the benefit of the patient.

Referral Practices

All decisions regarding patient referral should be based primarily upon consideration of the needs and best interests of the patient. A physician's referral practice should never lead to exploitation of patients or third party payors.

Prescribing Practices

Financial interests that the physician might have in the company supplying the product should not influence a physician in the prescribing of drugs, devices, appliances, or treatments. Neither should a physician's referral or admission patterns be constructed so as to enhance the physician's financial interest in any health facility.

Patents

Physicians should be allowed to patent devices, but the use of these devices must be in accordance with the patient's best medical interests, without regard to the physician's financial interests. Medical and surgical procedures contribute to a universal body of medical knowledge. Unrestricted access to that knowledge is one of the defining characteristics of the medical and surgical profession. Enforcing patent restrictions on medical and surgial procedures limits access to medical knowledge, denies potential benefit to patients, and thus is unethical.

Advertising

It is not unethical for otolaryngologists to advertise their services. Advertisements must be truthful and not misleading. An otolaryngologist should not misrepresent his/her qualifications and/or training, and should not exaggerate the efficacy or uniqueness of treatments rendered.

Research

Otolaryngologist–head and neck surgeons must conduct biomedical research according to ethical, moral, medical, and legal guidelines. All research should respect the dignity and sanctity of human life. The goal of research should be the betterment of mankind, the alleviation of suffering, and the ultimate improvement of medical practice. Research that knowingly and unnecessarily jeopardizes the health, safety, or longevity of human subjects is unethical.

Character Issues

Patients and society at large place a high level of trust in physicians. Physicians are held to the highest moral standards in the community. This level of trust is based on an assumption that the physican maintains a high degree of personal integrity and adheres to a professional code of ethics. Otolaryngologists should conduct themselves morally and ethically so as to merit the confidence placed in them. Otolaryngologists have an obligation to their colleagues to assist them in avoiding or eliminating behavior which is not conducive to maintaining personal integrity.

Impairment

Physician impairment represents a potential hazard to patients and to the affected physician. Otolaryngologists should make every effort to recognize the signs of impairment in themselves and in their colleagues. The otolarygologist who suspects impairment in a colleague has an ethical obligation to the impaired physician and his/her patients. Self-referral for appropriate treatment should be advised and encouraged. Physicians who have completed rehabilitation for impairment should not be restricted from practice, provided that proper post-rehabilitation monitoring shows no evidence of relapse.

Illegal Activity

Otolaryngologists should realize that they are subject to all civil and criminal statutes appli-cable to the region in which they practice. They are further subject to federal regulations governing medical practice. Otolaryngologists who knowingly participate in illegal or fraudulent behavior should be reported to the appropriate local authorities.

Fees

Fees must be commensurate with the service(s) rendered. It is unethical for a physician to charge an illegal or excessive fee. Fee collection efforts should take into acount the ability of the patient to pay. Physicians should not withhold vital or emergent treatment to patients because of their inability to pay. Physicans should not abandon a patient in a postoperative period because of that patient's inability to pay.

Community Relations

Physicians have been bestowed by society with trust and respect that no other profession can claim. Physicians in turn have a responsibility to their communities that goes beyond that of other commercial enterprises. Physicians must preserve their role as health advocates within the community. Otolaryngologists should not abandon the underprivileged segments of our society and should be encouraged to devote some time in caring for patients who are unable to pay.

Disciplinary Actions

Otolaryngologists have an ethical duty to report colleagues to state licensing authorities when documentary evidence exists of illegal activity. The American Academy of Otolaryngology–Head and Neck Surgery will not act as an enforcement agency but as an education vehicle regarding acceptable physician behavior.

May 1, 2000

American Society of Pediatric Otolaryngology Code of Ethics

1. The member should provide appropriate services to all patients with full respect for human dignity, respecting trust and confidence and rendering to each a full measure of service and dedication.
2. Members should strive to improve patient care through clinical knowledge and skill.
3. Members should seek to safeguard their patients from harm.
4. Members should provide care to all persons without regard to race, religion, ethnicity or gender.
5. Members should respect patient autonomy while exercising sound clinical judgment and skill.
6. Patient confidentiality should be respected unless otherwise required by law.
7. Members should honestly and accurately represent their professional qualifications and services to the public.
8. Profession advertisement should not be false, dishonest or misleading.
9. The member will not engage in inaccurate or dishonest solicitation of patients.
10. Members should not receive or pay a commission for patient referral.
11. Research, clinical presentations, and published articles are to be based on scientific principles and conducted in an ethical manner. Financial interests of any type are to be clearly stated in the publication and presentation.
12. Disclosure of professionally-related commercial interests and other interests that may influence decision-making is required in communications to patients, public, and colleagues.

Foreword

Every surgical procedure has the possibility of complications; although many of these can be predicted, a number cannot be anticipated. Surgery is a complex organizational effort in which the surgeon may be compared with an orchestra conductor who relies on a number of participants as well as a score. The surgeon may encounter unsuspected difficulties. For example, a patient may have cryptic abnormalities that may lead to complications not previously anticipated. This is especially true in children, in whom the ultimate outcome depends on growth and development.

The knowledge of complications that have occurred is one way of avoiding them in the future. The editors of this book have assembled an excellent group of experienced surgeons who have shared their experiences and those of their mentors in discussing the complications inherent in the practice of pediatric otolaryngology. They have also supplemented the surgeons' points of view with those from an outstanding group of pediatric subspecialists and from such fields as nursing, anesthesia, and law.

Otolaryngologists have cared for diseases of the ear, nose, and throat in children since the specialty developed, and most of this type of care is still rendered by general otolaryngologists. However, in the past 40 years, significant changes have taken place, such as the increased survival of premature infants, development of cardiac surgery, and improved survival of children with malignancies. Each of these advances has been accompanied by new potential complications. In his book of complications — published less than 30 years ago, John Conley did not mention many of the subjects found in this book.

This text is unique in the field because it details not only complications that can occur with specific operative procedures, but also more comprehensive issues. The initial chapters on education, stress management, and risk management are especially helpful for workers entering the field. The importance of the hospital experience is important because many of the difficulties involve this aspect, over which the surgeon may have little control. The child with systemic disorders may have complications related to these conditions of which the surgeon and even the parents are not aware and that may be instrumental in an unfortunate outcome.

Specific procedures such as tonsillectomies, which are commonly performed, account for many total complications and are important to discuss — in part, because of the large number performed. Airway problems constitute a large percentage of cases in pediatric otolaryngology, and these are treated extensively within the text. These procedures are frequently performed as emergencies and the anticipation of complications is important in their prevention and redemption. Otology is a major effort in pediatrics; the avoidance of complications is important from functional and cosmetic points of view, as are the treatment of cleft palate and plastic procedures.

This new textbook will be of value to general as well as pediatric subspecialists as a readily available text that can address the needs of the child patient and the parent.

Sylvan Stool

Preface

The field of pediatric otolaryngology has significantly evolved as a distinct subspecialty within the field of otolaryngology–head and neck surgery over the past two decades. Otolaryngologists with a strong interest in caring for infants and children have led to the expansion of the field in managing airway anomalies, cleft lip and palate, cochlear implantation, head and neck masses and more. With such growth, specialty societies in pediatric otolaryngology have been introduced. The American Society of Pediatric Otolaryngology (ASPO), the Society of Ear, Nose and Throat Advances in Children (SENTAC), and the Section of Otolaryngology and Bronchoesophagology of the American Academy of Pediatrics (AAP), to name a few, advocate for treating children with ear, nose, and throat, head and neck, and communication disorders. These organizations bring together otolaryngologists, primary care and pediatric specialty physicians, physician extenders, and related healthcare providers such as audiologists and speech/language pathologists, providing an ongoing forum for communication and education about the diagnosis, medical and surgical treatment, and sequelae of these diseases and their therapies.

Advancing technologies and practices have led to an increasing survival of preterm infants, as well as the survival of infants and children with complicated diseases. Despite these advances, tolerance by society and the medical–legal community has decreased with respect to patient outcomes. Unfortunately, complications and adverse sequelae of disease processes and their therapies can occur even in the best of hands. It is unrealistic to think that perfection ought to be the standard of care in medicine. It should be our *objective*, and we should always strive to perform our utmost to the best of our capabilities. However, humans are not perfect and Mother Nature works in mysterious ways. Medicine is not — and will not ever be — an exact science. It is a collaborative process and we should be prepared to learn from all of our results. We do not live in an ideal world, but we believe society would be comforted to know that greater lengths and honorable efforts are being undertaken continually by clinicians to provide the best treatments and obtain the best outcomes.

This textbook represents the first pediatric-focused compilation of the subject matter. We have gathered numerous accomplished otolaryngologists, specialists, and providers with expertise in a diverse array of assigned subjects. Our primary goal is to provide a resource for physicians and other healthcare providers who manage pediatric patients in the prevention, early identification, and management of complications in the field of pediatric otolaryngology. A secondary goal is to contribute to the current intellectual dialogue on error management in medicine. Certainly, discussing complications can be an emotionally difficult proposition. But, in the best interest of serving our patients, and for the continued growth in our field toward better outcomes, education in this area is our best resource. We hope that all of us who have been given the privilege of providing medical and surgical care to children will remain humble, and share, learn and educate from the experiences we have encountered so we may continue to strive for perfection while working on our most precious asset, our children.

We thank the contributors to this new textbook for their excellent efforts and look forward to ongoing dialogue with them, as well as with you — our colleagues — in this noble pursuit.

Gary D. Josephson, M.D.
Daniel L. Wohl, M.D.

Contributors

Ellis M. Arjmand, M.D., Ph.D.
Associate Professor, University of
  Cincinnati
Pediatric Otolaryngology
Cincinnati Children's Hospital Medical
  Center
Cincinnati, Ohio

James E. Arnold, M.D.
Professor & Chair, Otolaryngology-Head
  and Neck Surgery
University Hospitals of Cleveland
Rainbow Babies Children's Hospital
Cleveland, Ohio

Benjamin F. Asher, M.D.
Private Practice, Restorative ENT
Assistant Professor of Otolaryngology
SUNY Downstate Medical Center
New York, New York

Thomas J. Balkany, M.D.
Hotchkiss Professor and Chair
Department of Otolaryngology
Professor of Neuro-Otologic Surgery and
  Pediatrics
University of Miami Miller School of
  Medicine
Miami, Florida

Judith M. Barnes, M.S., CCC-SLP
Supervisor, Communication Sciences
Division of Pediatric Otolaryngology–HNS
Nemours Children's Clinic
Jacksonville, Florida

Walter M. Belenky, M.D.
Chief Emeritus, Department of Pediatric
  Otolaryngology
Children's Hospital of Michigan
Detroit, Michigan

John P. Bent III, M.D.
New York Otolaryngology Institute
Assistant Professor
Albert Einstein School of Medicine
New York, New York

Joann N. Bodurtha, M.D., M.P.H.
Professor, Human Genetics & Pediatrics
Virginia Commonwealth University
Richmond, Virginia

Charles M. Bower, M.D.
Associate Professor, Department of
  Otolaryngology
University of Arkansas for Medical Sciences
Arkansas Children's Hospital
Little Rock, Arkansas

Linda Miller Calandra, M.S.N., C.P.N.P.
Division of Otolaryngology
Children's Hospital of Philadelphia
Philadelphia, Pennsylvania

Steve V. Collins, M.D.
Department of Pediatric Anesthesiology
Nemours Children's Clinic
Instructor, Mayo Clinic College of Medicine
Jacksonville, Florida

Timothy M. Crombleholme, M.D.
Professor of Surgery, Obstetrics and
  Gynecology and Pediatrics
Director, Fetal Care Center of Cincinnati
Director, Center for Molecular Fetal Therapy
Fetal Care Center of Cincinnati
Cincinnati, Ohio

Michael J. Cunningham, M.D.
Associate Professor of Otology and
  Laryngology
Department of Otolaryngology
Harvard Medical School
Massachusetts Eye and Ear Infirmary
Boston, Massachusetts

David H. Darrow, D.D.S., M.D.
Assistant Professor of Otolaryngology and
  Pediatrics
Eastern Virginia Medical School
Attending Otolaryngologist, Children's
  Hospital of The King's Daughters
Norfolk, Virginia

Joanna A. Davis, M.D.
Associate Professor of Clinical Pediatrics
Division of Pediatric Hematology-Oncology
University of Miami Miller School of
  Medicine
Miami, Florida

Craig S. Derkay, M.D.
Professor of Otolaryngology and Pediatrics
Vice-Chairman, Department of
  Otolaryngology
Eastern Virginia Medical School
Attending Otolaryngologist, Children's
  Hospital of the King's Daughters
Norfolk, Virginia

Ellen S. Deutsch, M.D.
Associate Professor, Otolaryngology, Head
  and Neck Surgery and Pediatrics
Jefferson Medical College
Philadelphia, Pennsylvania
Pediatric Otolaryngology
Alfred I. DuPont Hospital for Children
Wilmington, Delaware

Laurence J. DiNardo, M.D.
Professor & Vice Chairman
Otolaryngology/Head and Neck Surgery
Virginia Commonwealth University
Richmond, Virginia

Jay N. Dolitsky, M.D.
Assistant Professor of Otolaryngology
New York Medical College
New York Eye and Ear Infirmary
New York, New York

Amelia F. Drake, M.D.
Professor of Otolaryngology
Chief, Division of Pediatric Otolaryngology
University of North Carolina
Chapel Hill, North Carolina

Roland Eavey, M.D.
Professor of Otology and Laryngology
Department of Otolaryngology
Harvard Medical School
Massachusetts Eye and Ear Infirmary
Boston, Massachusetts

Tara Eggleston, M.S.
formerly of Department of Audiology
Virginia Commonwealth University Medical
  Center
Richmond, Virgnia

Ronald M. Epstein
Professor of Family Medicine and Psychiatry
Director of Research in Family Medicine
Associate Dean for Education Evaluation and
  Research
University of Rochester
Rochester, New York

Adrien A. Eshraghi, M.D.
Associate Professor of Otolaryngology
Department of Otolaryngology
University of Miami Miller School of Medicine
Miami, Florida

Cynthia A. Gauger, M.D.
Division of Hematology-Oncology
Nemours Children's Clinic
Jacksonville, Florida

William C. Giles, M.D.
Private Practice, Centa Medical Group
Associate Professor, Pediatrics & Surgery
University of South Carolina School of
  Medicine
Columbia, South Carolina

Paul Gluck, M.D.
Associate Clinical Professor, Department of
  Obstetrics and Gynecology
University of Miami Miller School of Medicine
Vice Chair, National Patient Safety Foundation
Miami, Florida

Charles W. Gross, M.D.
Professor, Department of Otolaryngology and
  Pediatrics
University of Virginia Health Sciences Center
Charlottesville, Virginia

Kenneth M. Grundfast, M.D.
Professor and Chair, Department of
  Otolaryngology
Professor of Pediatrics
Boston University School of Medicine
Boston, Massachusetts

Joseph Haddad Jr., M.D.
Lawrence Savetsky Chair and Professor of
  Clinical Otalaryngology/Head and Neck
  Surgery
Vice Chairman, Department of
  Otolaryngology/Head and Neck Surgery
Columbia College of Physicians and Surgeons
Director of Pediatric Otolaryngology/Head and
  Neck Surgery
Children's Hospital of New York-Presbyterian
New York, New York

Earl H. Harley, M.D.
Associate Professor, Otolaryngology
Georgetown University Medical Center
Washington, D.C.

Linda Harvey, M.S., L.H.R.M.
Nemours Children's Clinic
Jacksonville, Florida

Suzanne Hasenstab, Ph.D.
Professor and Director of Audiology
Virginia Commonwealth University Medical
  Center
Richmond, Virginia

Andrew J. Hotaling, M.D.
Professor, Department of Otolaryngology and
  Pediatrics
Loyola University Medical Center
Maywood, Illinois

Gregory F. Hulka, M.D.
Associate Professor, Division of
  Otolaryngology, Head and Neck Surgery
Duke Medical Center
Durham, North Carolina

Chandra M. Ivey, M.D.
Resident, Department of Otolaryngology
University of Cincinnati
Cincinnati, Ohio

Ian N. Jacobs, M.D.
Attending Surgeon
Director, Pediatric Airway Program
Children's Hospital of Philadelphia
Philadelphia, Pennsylvania

Jacqueline E. Jones, M.D.
Associate Professor of Clinical
  Otolaryngology
Weill-Cornell Medical School
New York, New York

Gary D. Josephson, M.D.
Chief, Division of Pediatric Otolaryngology-
  HNS
Nemours Children's Clinic
Associate Professor, Mayo Clinic College of
  Medicine
Jacksonville, Florida

Jordan S. Josephson, M.D.
Director, New York Nasal and Sinus Institute
Attending Physician, Manhattan Eye, Ear &
  Throat Hospital, Lenox Hill Hospital and
  Roosevelt Hospital
New York, New York

Bernadette Koch, M.D.
Associate Professor of Radiology
Assistant Professor of Pediatrics
Children's Hospital Medical Center
Cincinnati, Ohio

Melissa G. Kress, D.O.
Division of Pediatric Otolaryngology-HSN
Nemours Children's Clinic
Jacksonville, Florida

Paul Lambert, M.D.
Professor and Chair, Department of
  Otolaryngology-Head and Neck Surgery
Medical University of South Carolina
Charleston, South Carolina

David W. Low, M.D.
Clinical Associate Professor
Division of Plastic Surgery
Children's Hospital of Philadelphia
Philadelphia, Pennsylvania

Jeanne Lusher, M.D.
Department of Hematology/Oncology
Children's Hospital of Michigan
Detroit, Michigan

Rodney P. Lusk, M.D.
Vice Director, Boys Town National Research
  Hospital
Omaha, Nebraska

David N. Madgy, D.O.
Department of Pediatric Otolaryngology
Children's Hospital of Michigan
Detroit, Michigan

Eric A. Mair, M.D.
Director, Pediatric Otolaryngology
Wilford Medical Center
San Antonio, Texas

W. Scott McDonald, M.D.
Associate Professor, Department of Plastic
  Surgery
University of Miami Miller School of
  Medicine
Miami, Florida

William F. McGuirt, M.D.
Private Practice, Pediatric Otolaryngology
Piedmont Ear Nose Throat Associates, PA
Winston-Salem, North Carolina

Louis M. Mendelson, M.D.
Connecticut Asthma and Allergy Center
Clinical Professor of Pediatrics
University of Connecticut Health Center
West Hartford, Connecticut

Samir Midani, M.D.
Chief, Division of Infectious Disease
Nemours Children's Clinic
Jacksonville, Florida

Harlan R. Muntz, M.D.
Pediatric Otolaryngology-Head and Neck
  Surgery
University of Utah, Pediatric Otolaryngology
Primary Children's Medical Center
Salt Lake City, Utah

Charles M. Myers III, M.D.
Professor, Department of Otolaryngology-Head
  and Neck Surgery
Children's Hospital Medical Center
Cincinnati, Ohio

Thomas A. Nakagawa, M.D.
Associate Professor, Director of Pediatric
  Intensive Care Unit
Pediatric Anesthesiology and Pediatric Critical
  Care
Brenner Children's Hospital
Wake Forest University Baptist Medical Center
Winston-Salem, North Carolina

Walter E. Nance, M.D., Ph.D.
Professor and Chair
Department of Human Genetics
Virginia Commonwealth University
Richmond, Virginia

Paul A. Pitel, M.D.
Division of Hematology-Oncology
Chairman, Department of Pediatrics
Nemours Children's Clinic
Jacksonville, Florida

James S. Reilly, M.D.
Chair, Department of Surgery
Division of Pediatric Otolaryngology
Alfred I. DuPont Hospital for Children
Wilmington, Delaware

Jon Robitschek, M.D.
Department of Otolaryngology
Tripler Army Medical Center
Honolulu, Hawaii

Richard M. Rosenfeld, M.D., M.P.H.
Professor of Clinical Otolaryngology
SUNY Downstate Medical Center
Director of Pediatric Otolaryngology
Long Island College Hospital
Brooklyn, New York

Scott R. Schoem, M.D.
Director of Otolaryngology
Connecticut Children's Medical Center
Associate Professor of Clinical Otolaryngology
University of Connecticut Health Center
Hartford, Connecticut

Dale Schrum, M.D.
Division of Pulmonology, Allergy, &
  Immunology
Nemours Children's Clinic
Jacksonville, Florida

Mary Jo Schuh, M.S., CCC-A
Supervisor, Audiology Services
Division of Pediatric Otolaryngology-HNS
Nemours Children's Clinic
Jacksonville, Florida

Nancy Sculerati, M.D.
Associate Professor
Department of Otolaryngology
New York University Medical Center
New York, New York

Robert W. Seibert, M.D.
Professor of Department of Otolaryngology
University of Arkansas for Medical Sciences
Arkansas Children's Hospital
Little Rock, Arkansas

Andrew Shapiro, M.D.
Private Practice, Associated Otolaryngologists
  of Pennsylvania
Clinical Associate Professor
Department of Surgery
Division of Pediatric Otolaryngology
Pennsylvania State University College of
  Medicine
Hershey, Pennsylvania

Lora Lee Sparacino, M.S.N., C.P.N.P.
Private Practice, Rochester Otolaryngology
Rochester, New York

Laura M. Sterni, M.D.
Assistant Professor, Department of
  Pediatrics-Pulmonology
Johns Hopkins University School of
  Medicine
Baltimore, Maryland

Michael G. Stewart, M.D., M.P.H.
Associate Professor
Associate Dean of Clinical Affairs
Chief of Otolaryngology-Head and Neck
  Surgery Service at Ben Taub General Hospital
Director of Resident Education
Baylor College of Medicine
Houston, Texas

Sylvan Stool, M.D. (deceased)
Professor of Otolaryngology and Pediatrics
University of Colorado School of Medicine
Attending Physician, Children's Hospital of
  Denver
Denver, Colorado

David W. Tellez, M.D.
Pediatric Medical Director
Phoenix Children's Hospital
Phoenix, Arizona

David E. Tunkel, M.D.
Associate Professor of Otolaryngology, Head
  and Neck Surgery & Pediatrics
Johns Hopkins University School of Medicine
Director, Pediatric Otolaryngology
Johns Hopkins Hospital
Baltimore, Maryland

Ralph F. Wetmore, M.D.
Attending Surgeon
Director, Pediatric Otolaryngology Fellowship
  Program
Children's Hospital of Philadelphia
Philadelphia, Pennsylvania

Michelle S. Whiteman, M.D.
Department of Radiology
Cleveland Clinic Foundation
Weston, Florida

Daniel L. Wohl, M.D.
Private Practice, Pediatric and Adolescent
  Otolaryngology
Courtesy Associate Professor, Department of
  Otolaryngology
University of Florida
Jacksonville, Florida

Andrew Woods, M.D.
Department of Anesthesiology
University of Virginia Health Sciences Center
Charlottesville, Virginia

Audie L. Woolley, M.D.
Assistant Professor of Otolaryngology and
  Pediatrics
Medical Director of Pediatric Cochlear Implant
  Program
Children's Hospital
Birmingham, Alabama

George H. Zalzal, M.D.
Chair, Otolaryngology
Children's National Medical Center
Washington, D.C.

Contents

SECTION IX   Facial Plastic and Reconstructive Surgery

SECTION X   Epilogue

Section I

Personal Responsibility

1 Risk Management

Daniel L. Wohl and Linda Harvey

A good pilot is compelled to always evaluate what's happened, so that he can apply what he's learned.

Adapted from *Top Gun*

CONTENTS

INTRODUCTION

Society encourages and demands the advancement of medical knowledge. Yet, at the same time, society does not fully entrust the medical profession to create and maintain a safe environment which dissuades physicians from embarking on diagnostic and management pathways that extend their experience. A balance between these often opposing forces must be established while simultaneously managing outcomes and risks.

We have chosen to organize our philosophy around the temporally linked concepts of complication avoidance, complication recognition, and complication management. One must first aspire to maximize the potential for complication avoidance. However, because complications can and do occur, complication recognition becomes sequentially important. Third, if a complication has been identified, the next element to be assessed and addressed is the means by which to manage the resultant clinical, social, and legal issues.

Each of these three elements of risk management — complication avoidance, recognition, and management — requires a sustained reasonable thought process. It is our hope that physicians and society recognize that this triad represents three points along a continuous cycle. Once the management process has been concluded, the lessons learned can and should be used to further minimize the potential for future complications.

AVOIDANCE

Is It Better to Be Lucky than Good?

As author Harold Kushner[1] has pointed out, bad things happen to good people. Although we might prefer not to think about it, bad outcomes do happen to physicians despite the delivery of appropriate care. In many scenarios true complications do occur. This may be a devastating experience for even the most seasoned professional. At the other end of the spectrum, we may also begin to question our own judgment and further question our ability to practice quality medicine simply when a series of positive outcomes is less than optimal. How does a doctor stay out of trouble? Most surgeons would not be described as risk-averse personalities. However, character traits can be modified over time as a result of the cumulative burden of experience. The more appropriately applied terminology might be that successful surgeons have learned to "manage risk" while optimizing patient care to the best of their abilities.

Judgment

How does one teach judgment? Lead by example. However, can one avoid the unavoidable? One may possess a vast degree of knowledge and yet exercise poor judgment when making clinical decisions. Is good judgment an inherent quality or is it something that can be taught? A propensity for good judgment may well be a natural part of one's makeup. However, it is possible to enhance one's judgment and decision-making skills through good mentoring and a keen desire to raise one's consciousness.

Contract with Society

Physicians have an unspoken contract with society when carrying out their duty (Table 1.1), of which *Article One* is *primon non nocere* ("above all, do no harm"). There must be reasonable utilization of limited resources combined with a responsible application of knowledge and experience in order to best avoid risk. *Article Two* of the social contract is "to thy own self be true" — also stated as "know yourself." It is incumbent upon each individual physician to minimize risk by honestly assessing his strengths and limitations and then learning how to stay within his comfort

---

TABLE 1.1
The Physician's Contract with Society

Article One	Above all, do no harm.
Article Two	Know yourself.
Article Three	Educate the patient.
Article Four	Always remain ethical.

---

zone. Simultaneously, each physician must also keep abreast of the current opinions, standards, and specific techniques that pertain to his specialty. Please refer to Chapter 2 about the difficulty and demands of remaining current with continuing education.

KNOWLEDGE

Knowledge, in and of itself, does not have purpose for the clinician without proper application to patient care. The physician must judiciously and continuously apply knowledge throughout each patient encounter as though it were being applied for the first time. Becoming consistent with a systematic approach is helpful to maintain a level of quality; however, at the same time the physician must not become complacent and inured to the routine. One doctor's "shortcut" may be perceived as fallacious by another whose attention to detail requires a more deliberate thought process. Each physician must take responsibility to learn from a wide array of experiences, tempered with a self-awareness of his own relative strengths and weaknesses, and then determine for himself what is true and correct.

CAN I DO THE JOB?

This is a question whose answer should be continuously monitored. In certain rare conditions experience is limited throughout the field. With advances in preventative medicine as well as medical progress, some procedures that were once very common have now become relatively rare. Some older surgeons who have had a great deal of prior experience that has not been recently applied must decide if they are still comfortable embarking on this pathway when it arises. Conversely, in uncommon or highly complex cases, the experienced surgeon may have the appropriate relevant anatomical and physiologic knowledge and can possess enough transferable surgical skills to achieve a satisfactory outcome more than adequately.

TECHNOLOGICAL AND PHARMACOLOGICAL ADVANCES

Otolaryngology is a technology-dependent specialty with diverse use of lasers, microscopes, and microinstrumentation, often in surgical fields with limited lines of sight. Technology can only serve as a tool to enhance the quality of care delivered, however, and does not make the surgeon infallible. In addition, a wide range of pharmacological management is often applied in the interest of patient care in otolaryngology. Although advancements in technology and pharmacology have raised the level of care and are a tremendous asset, they still present a measure of risk. Until a new "clinical tool" becomes a standard of care, each physician is responsible for determining which methodology to choose in the care of his patient.

MANAGED CARE POLICIES

Managed care policies have undergone two decades of implementation resulting in numerous constraints and contractual commitments placed upon physicians. Collectively, this has created what one could deem "nonclinical complications," which are usually in response to such factors as changes in access to care and cost control measures. Examples include recording signs or symptoms that the patient does not actually have in order to assist the patient in obtaining medical benefits, or attempting to secure access to care or reimbursement for medical coverage for patients. Such behavior is not only illegal and unethical but also may place the physician in the avoidable circumstance of exchanging an esteemed career for fraud abuse charges.[2,3]

COMMUNICATION SKILLS

Communication skills play a key role in avoiding complications because many mistakes in health care are a result of failing to notice common mistakes of everyday life.[4] Written communication must be clearly legible and presented in a visual manner designed to minimize misinterpretation. Verbal communications must be understood and confirmed. In medicine, there is often little time or room for error. Accurate communication is as much the responsibility of the person transmitting the information as it is the responsibility of the individual receiving the information. Furthermore, it is often not one person making one mistake. Rather, an error results from several individuals making several consecutive mistakes within a system not designed to prevent those mistakes from doing harm.[4]

RECOGNITION

IF SOMETHING CAN GO WRONG, IT PROBABLY WILL

Complications come in all varieties. Some problems must be handled emergently while others declare themselves over time. Although it may be difficult to admit, initially, the responsible physician may not recognize a complication. At times, one must accept the fact that intervention by others on the medical team — anesthesia, nursing, or other surgeons — may become necessary in order to minimize or avert progressive risk. When complications do occur, more can be learned about a person's character from how he handles stress and duress than during the times when he demonstrates how he handles success.

GENERAL AND SPECIFIC PEDIATRIC COMPLICATIONS

General risks of surgery include bleeding, infection, and scarring, whereas more specific and perhaps more serious complications in otolaryngology head and neck surgery are the result of the affected area of anatomy and may include major motor or sensory deficits as well as life-threatening hemorrhage. Particularly in children, it is important to be aware of the potential impact any treatment or complication may have on cognitive and physical development. When dealing with children, the physician must be cognizant of this potential because of the possible time lag between the event and the negative effect or outcome.

THINK FIRST AND ACT SECOND

When a complication is identified, at the outset it is important to recognize events that may lead to a subsequent cascade of adverse sequelae. It can be argued that one quality common to many of the best doctors is that they know what they do not know. Therefore, it is critically important always to remember that whenever the need is felt, it is acceptable to stop, "do no harm," think, and possibly seek another medical opinion.

HOW MUCH EXPERIENCE IS ENOUGH?

This question defies an easy answer. It is a fair statement to say that clinical acumen among clinicians varies and that a necessary learning curve is applied throughout a clinician's professional career. Some physicians are better in the classroom, develop a great knowledge base initially, but are less adept at applying their knowledge in the field. Others excel in the clinical realm, exhibiting excellent technical skills and/or the ability to execute complex procedures or treatment algorithms. Competency in the classroom *and* the clinical arena is the ideal, but potential differences in these two cognitive capabilities do not mean that one physician is bad and another is good. Rather, each must recognize his strengths and responsibly apply them while continuously developing professional competencies to the best of his ability throughout his professional career.

STAY COMFORTABLE WITH A MOVING TARGET

Physicians conduct an exquisite dance to stay within their comfort zone as the rules and standards of medical practice continuously change. At the very least, the physician must become thoroughly comfortable with what is "normal" so that he can recognize what is "abnormal" when he encounters it. In this fashion, the physician should know what he is looking at and what could adversely compound the situation, thereby improving the odds that a problem will be recognized early.

MANAGEMENT

DEFINITIONS OF COMPLICATIONS

- An *adverse occurrence* is an exceptionally unexpected negative outcome. Unfortunately, examples of adverse occurrences may include unexpected death, morbidity with permanent disfigurement or disability, an incorrect surgical procedure, or a procedure performed on the wrong side of the body or even the wrong patient.
- In contrast, a *negative surgical or medical sequelae* is a relatively common occurrence such as postventilation tube otorrhea or post-tonsillectomy pain. Although sequelae such as these can be anticipated to occur within a wide percentage of patients, the family may still express significant dissatisfaction, even if previously informed of the possibility.
- *Untoward events* are uncommon, but well-recognized negative outcomes. They are often correctable and usually do not present long-term difficulties. Examples include (non life-threatening) medication side effects, wound infections, post-tonsillectomy bleeds requiring a second procedure, and persistent tympanic membrane perforations after ventilation tube extrusion.

Although the level of concern may be higher with more severe complications, to the patient and family all negative or unexpected outcomes are significant. When a complication is recognized, it is important to develop a coordinated and structured approach that addresses the clinical, social, and legal issues.

MANAGEMENT PRINCIPLES OF SURGICAL OR MEDICAL COMPLICATIONS

- *When does it become necessary to marshal other resources?* If we can learn from the study of history, one of the most difficult concepts to learn and subsequently implement is the military principle of a "tactical retreat." It is important for the surgeon to understand that bringing in other specialists, whether in his field or another, does not constitute defeat. Sometimes, it is better to withdraw in order to gather one's resources for a subsequent offensive maneuver.
- *What are the responsibilities of those in the operating room?* The anesthesia team and operating room nurses have a responsibility to record all perceived variances from the anticipated expectations. It is the surgeon's responsibility personally to document in objective terms his observations and impressions without biased opinions or assignment of culpability.

- *Documentation.* State or federal regulatory agencies and/or national accrediting bodies mandate certain reporting requirements. Obligatory requirements for documentation and reporting of adverse incidents may vary from institution to institution. One should be knowledgeable of all of these requirements within one's jurisdiction.
  - One example is the risk of instrument failure, which is regulated by the Food and Drug Administration. The Medical Device Amendment of 1976 regulates medical devices. In its current form, if a medical device is involved in the death, illness, or injury of a patient, the incident must be reported within 10 working days to the appropriate individuals. It is important to become thoroughly familiar with the reporting requirements in your state or jurisdiction.
  - Another risk is *drug mismanagement.* The most common errors involve prescribing, dispensing, or administering medications. A number of circumstances resulting in medication mismanagement, such as hospital staffing or how drugs are stored, labeled, or packaged within the facility, are beyond direct physician control. In order to reduce liability, the physician should make sure that communication is clear and precise by using standard abbreviations, writing legibly, and obtaining accurate patient information before ordering medications.[5]

MANAGEMENT PRINCIPLES OF SOCIAL ISSUES

Family Communication

Enough cannot be said about creating and maintaining an honest, caring physician–patient interrelationship. This requires an effective two-way dialogue. If a well-recognized complication has occurred, then state it. Initially, balance what the family needs to know with what they are able to understand. Doing so will inevitably raise the patient's and family's medical intelligence quotients, which is a necessary responsibility of the clinician. The discussion should stop when the family indicates directly or indirectly that they have had enough information for the time being. The physician should repeatedly encourage the family to request additional information for better understanding.

It is well documented that the single most important factor in initiating malpractice suits stems from patients' dissatisfaction with what they deem as poor quality of care.[6] This does not necessarily reflect an accurate assessment or understanding of the technical procedure or medical management but rather dissatisfaction surrounding the nontechnical aspects of medical care such as communication, bedside manner, or length of appointment.

Communication with Superiors, Colleagues, and Partners

All professionals, no matter how well trained, can benefit from discussing an occurrence with a responsible, intelligent, sounding board. If someone thinks he should inform risk management, then he probably should inform risk management as soon as practically possible. Caution should be exercised when one discusses details of an adverse occurrence with others, including colleagues and superiors. Divulging too much information at the wrong time could be detrimental to one's defense if a lawsuit should arise.

Postcomplication Follow-Up

It is important to complete the necessary reports and follow the policies and procedures as required by the institution, never give a sense of dishonesty, be realistic in personal evaluation of the case, avoid self-denial, and display a genuine concern for the well-being and best interest of the patient, and avoid conveying a sense of concern over the financial aspect of care unless the family initiates dialogue on the topic.

MANAGEMENT PRINCIPLE OF LEGAL ISSUES

Informed Consent

Obtaining informed consent is a process inherent to the physician–patient relationship and involves ongoing, purposeful communication encompassing far more than having the patient or parent sign a consent form.[7]

- *It's not your decision. Article Three* of the contract with society is to "educate the patient." The treating physician has a duty to present information within reasonable bounds of clinical perspective so that an informed decision can be made. It is a good principle to have the patient, parent, or family feel that they made the therapeutic decision.
- *Discuss the benefits and risks* of the recommended treatment as well as alternative treatments and the risks of receiving no treatment. The general risks acknowledged by lay people, such as bleeding, infection, or scarring, are reasonably straightforward concepts; however, concepts such as pain or change in diet or lifestyle are more subjective and often understood to a lesser degree. To assure understanding, spend appropriate time discussing these aspects and the anticipated outcomes of care. The common specific risks of treatment or a procedure should always be covered. The more unusual risks should be detailed as perceived necessary by the practitioner.
- *Document the benefits and risks.* It is impractical for a single informed-consent document to be exhaustively thorough. Frequently performed procedures with commonly recognized potential complications, such as post-tonsillectomy bleed, must be discussed but not necessarily specifically documented if that is part of the physician's usual and customary routine when obtaining informed consent. Documentation of the discussed uncommon or subjective possibilities should be indicated if a physician senses a heightened level of concern over these possibilities. This can be satisfied with common abbreviations and key phrases. To further strengthen the informed-consent process, some physicians routinely provide comprehensive and detailed procedure-specific instruction forms as a supplement to the discussion.

I've Been Sued!

If, despite a physician's best efforts after a complication has occurred, the patient or family seeks legal recourse, the physician must be cognizant of the legalities involved. By what criteria will he be judged? What constitutes malpractice? What should he expect when a lawsuit is filed?

Physician–attorney relationship. It is in the physician's best interest to make the time to educate his attorney and to work together with him in full cooperation, no matter how emotionally difficult this may be. After all, who should better know the literature, what to quote, and who the experts are? Be prepared. Regrettably, too many doctors limit time with their attorney.

Definitions of Legal Language

- *Legal liability* refers to the condition of being legally responsible for a possible or actual loss as it relates to the patient care that may or may not have been rendered.[8] Physicians are legally responsible for their acts, whether by commission or omission, and at times are also responsible for the individuals whom they supervise.
- *Standard of care* is an applied measure of competence of the physician, which requires the practitioner to exercise the same degree of skill, care, or diligence as exercised by members of the same profession or same field of specialty.[8] Potential differences in regional standards are not taken into consideration because medical experts are routinely

obtained throughout North America. If one fails to exercise the degree of skill and expertise generally exercised by a reasonably prudent member of the same profession such that injury, loss, or damage occurs, then he is said to have committed malpractice.

- *Malpractice* implies that one was negligent and/or committed a medical error in the provision of care by not having done what a reasonably prudent person would have done in a similar circumstance.[8] For example, infection, in and of itself as a complication, is an untoward event. However, failure to recognize and properly treat that complication is malpractice.
- *Negligence* includes departure from the expected conduct of a reasonably prudent person under similar circumstances. To determine whether negligence has occurred, the answer to *all* of the following questions must be "yes":
  - Was a legal or moral obligation owed to the patient because of an established patient–physician relationship?
  - Was there neglect or failure to fulfill this obligation or could care be deemed as not meeting the prevailing standard of care?
  - As a result, did harm, injury, or damage occur from something that one did or did not do, thus resulting in an adverse outcome?
  - Is the alleged harm, injury, or damage causally related to the breach of obligation with failure to adhere to the standard of care, which caused injury to the patient?
  Bear in mind that it is the patient/plaintiff who has the burden of proof that these elements existed. If this is not done, then the plaintiff probably will not prevail in a court of law.[9]
- *Litigation* refers to the legal proceedings of a lawsuit. This sequence of events may be grouped into three phases: *pretrial*, *trial,* and *post-trial.* Although the filing of a formal complaint by a patient marks the beginning of a lawsuit, one should be prepared to wait. The timetable for the following legal proceedings is based on the need to fulfill the requirements of the law. Litigating attorneys are most comfortable with slow, deliberate actions — in contrast to the otolaryngologist, who is often most comfortable giving immediate or at least prompt responses.
  - The filing of a *formal complaint* marks the beginning of a lawsuit. The hospital and treating physicians who have had a documented role in the care of the patient are often routinely included, but some or all of the individuals named as defendants may be dropped over the course of the litigation process. When a physician is served a formal complaint, he must respond within a set time frame. Thus, it is imperative that risk management and legal counsel be involved from the beginning.
  - The complaint triggers the pretrial activities, which include the *discovery process.* The purpose of the discovery process is to gather all the facts, documents, and additional medical records necessary to defend the case. The physician defendant is likely to be directly involved in a deposition, a formal, legally binding process. This phase may last only a few months or as long as several years, depending upon the parties involved.
  - A *settlement* may be reached at any time during these proceedings or the trial.[10] Although a defendant physician may see settlement as "backing down," a defendant law firm is more likely to view the entire matter from a financial perspective. To them, the outcome of the court case is what counts, regardless of the medical facts. If the defendant attorneys are concerned that the plaintiff's case, as presented, stands a good chance of persuading a jury, their position will often be to encourage settlement before a defense is even performed.
  - *The trial.* Once the pretrial phase is complete, a trial date is set. During jury selection, each party questions prospective jurors in an attempt to select a jury that will be most favorable to its position. After the jury has been selected, the trial begins. Each side presents its opening statements, then proceeds to present witnesses, directly exam-

ining and cross-examining. Finally, the jury retires to consider the evidence and reach a verdict.

- *The appeal process*. Even though a verdict may be reached and the trial is concluded, the physician may choose to appeal if the verdict is unfavorable. When a verdict is appealed, it is brought before an appellate court for review. This court does not retry the case; rather, its purpose is to determine if any reversible error occurred. If the appellate court does not conclude in the defendant's favor, he must comply with the original judgment.

WHAT IS PUBLIC INFORMATION?

If a physician loses a verdict or an insurance carrier pays any settlement on his behalf, this must be reported to the National Practitioner's Data Bank (NPDB) in addition to the required state agencies. Established in 1990, the NPDB serves as a central clearinghouse of information on physicians and dentists and, in some cases, other health care practitioners. The NPDB contains information on medical malpractice payments, adverse licensure actions, adverse clinical privilege actions, and adverse professional society membership actions.[11]

It is reasonable to argue that malpractice *settlements* should not be singularly used to judge a physician's abilities or to assign guilt. While it is true that the decision for a settlement payment is often made for financial or emotional reasons and may not indicate negligence or gross incompetency,[12] it is equally true that a pattern of legal activity surrounding a physician supports the increased plausibility that the claims are legitimately incriminating. Whether the physician feels this is fair or not, he should be prepared for the court of public opinion to come to its own conclusion.

CONCLUSION

WHY BAD THINGS HAPPEN TO GOOD DOCTORS

Sandy Koufax, the Hall of Fame, left-handed baseball pitcher, once said that he *tried* to throw a no-hitter every time he pitched, but that he did not *expect* to do so.[13] As the story is told, if he truly expected that level of success every time he pitched, then he would also have expected to have been asked to see the team psychiatrist!

It is ennobling to believe that every physician entered the profession of medicine solely to serve society for the highest of altruistic reasons. The spectrum of reality, however, is far different. No one can really know the true motivation behind another person's actions. What we do know, however, is that being perfect all of the time is not humanly possible. Although the goal is to aspire to provide excellent care consistently, the understanding is that to expect total excellence is unrealistic. We cannot guarantee a perfect result, *but we can guarantee that we will endeavor to do our best at all times*. It is incumbent, therefore, upon all physicians to establish reasonable expectations first within themselves and then for their patients.

This leads to *Article Four*, the final component in the unwritten contract with society. Simply stated, it is to "remain ethical." Each physician must always be prepared to respond ethically to the external and internal forces that may come to bear upon them as they assume a measure of responsibility for the well-being of another human life.

REFERENCES

1. Kushner, H.S. *When Bad Things Happen to Good People*. Boston, MA: G.K. Hall, 1982.
2. Bloche, M.G. Fidelity and deceit at the bedside. *JAMA*, 2000, 283(14), 1881–1884.

3. O'Neal, L.W. Should physicians manipulate reimbursement rules to benefit patients? *JAMA*, 2000, 282(11), 1382.

4. Steinhauer, J. So, the tumor is on the left, is that right? *The New York Times*, April 1, 2001, Sect. L (Metro Section).

5. Channing, B.L. Medication errors — how you can prevent them. South Deerfield, MA: Channing L. Bete Co., Inc., 2000.

6. Levinson, W. Physician-patient communication. A key to malpractice prevention. *JAMA*, 1994, 272(20), 1619–1620.

7. Devlin, M.M. Medical legal highlights. The doctrine of informed consent. *JAMA*, 1996, 11(5): 244–245.

8. Black, H. *Black's Law Dictionary with Pronunciations*. Abridged 6th ed. St. Paul, MN: West Publishing Co., 1991.

9. Showers, J.L. Protection from negligence lawsuits. *Nursing Manage.*, 1999, 30(9), 23–27.

10. Mandell, M. What to expect from your malpractice attorney. *Am. J. Nursing*, 1995, 95(11): 29–31.

11. U.S. Department of Health and Human Services. Introduction. In *National Practitioner Data Bank Guidebook*. 1999, A1–A6. Available from <http://www.npdb-hipdb.org/npdbguidebook.html>.

12. Davis, R. Data on disciplined docs flawed. *USA Today*, December 1, 2000.

13. Koufax, S. *Koufax*. New York, NY: Viking Press, 1966.

2 Continuing Education

*Michael G. Stewart, Richard M. Rosenfeld,
and Melissa G. Kress*

...the physician should illustrate the truth of Plato's saying, "...education is a lifelong process."[1]

Sir William Osler, 1890

CONTENTS

INTRODUCTION

As new medications, procedures, and technologies become available, it can be difficult for the busy clinician to stay up to date on the latest advances in an always changing field. Failure to do so, however, will inevitably result in gradual erosion of one's ability to deliver a consistently high level of care. Fortunately, there are many options, such as medical journals, literature searches, evidence-based medicine reviews, and review of consensus statements or guidelines, for obtaining and sustaining continuing medical education. Physicians should remain aware of the potential advantages and disadvantages of each method when developing a personal continuing education strategy.

WHAT IS CONTINUING MEDICAL EDUCATION AND WHY IS IT IMPORTANT?

Optimal continuing medical education is a highly self-directed curriculum. The content, learning methods, and learning resources are selected specifically for the purpose of improving the knowledge, skills, and attributes required by physicians in their daily professional lives that lead to improved patient outcomes.[2] In the realm of providing and improving the quality of health care to children, three dimensions of outcomes are frequently measured: mortality, morbidity, and functional status.

The only incorrect strategy for continuing medical education is to have no strategy at all, or to rely solely on what others say. Advances in medicine will certainly continue and many will likely reflect groundbreaking progress that should be incorporated into the practice of enlightened clinicians. Other advances, however, should be scrutinized and viewed with healthy skepticism until proven effective through clinical trials. Using appropriate techniques of continuing education, the wise clinician should be able to avoid pitfalls such as embracing the early introduction of new technology subsequently shown to be cost ineffective. Similarly, regarding new medications, clinicians should review the data from clinical effectiveness studies in order to make their own conclusions, rather than taking the recommendations of sales personnel.

Officially accredited continuing medical education (CME) comes in many shapes and sizes — from study-at-your-own-pace individual reading material with self-assessment tests to large organized formal instructional courses. Sir William Osler has described two types of practicing physicians: the "routinist" and the "rationalist." The routinist is a physician who falls into a routine or rut of usual practice and, in Osler's words, falls prey to the "vice of intellectual idleness."[1] In contrast, Osler's rationalist considers patient care as a problem to be solved continuously. Osler further noted that continuing education was important for practicing general physicians as well as specialists and teachers: "We teachers and consultants are in constant need of postgraduate study as an antidote against premature senility. Daily contact with the bright young minds of our associates and assistants, the mental friction of medical societies, and travel are important aids ... to counteract the benumbing influence of isolation."[1]

Stages of Self-Assessment

Studies of adult education by physician educators have defined the stages of self-assessment that motivate physicians to improve their levels of competence:[3]

- Estimate where one ought to be in terms of knowledge, skill, and performance related to the change.
- Estimate what one presently knows or does in terms of the image of change.
- Estimate the discrepancy between what one ought to know or do and what one currently knows or does.
- Experience a level of anxiety because what one knows or does is not a match with what one ought to know or do.

Accreditation and Certification

The process of accreditation for CME activities has been only recently formalized with the establishment of the Accreditation Council for Continuing Medical Education (ACCME) in 1981. The ACCME is made up of seven member organizations: American Medical Association, Association of American Medical Colleges, Association of Hospital Medical Education, American Board of Medical Specialties, Council of Medical Specialty Societies, American Hospital Association, and Federation of State Medical Boards. The Federal Department of Health and the public are represented as well. The ACCME assures that accredited providers of CME are meeting the goals of successful medical education: assessment of educational need, stating of educational objectives, quality design of educational activities, and evaluation of the educational process.

Accreditation and certification are distinct activities.[4] *Accreditation* is granted by the ACCME for a specific period of time if providers meet the accepted standards for accreditation. *Certification* of specific activities is then granted by CME providers so that individual participants can receive credit for the stated number of hours of participation.

Although the ideal of continuing medical education throughout the career of all practicing physicians is a laudable goal, most state licensing boards, an increasing number of hospital credentials committees, and other governing bodies are requiring satisfactory completion of a certain number of CME hours in order to maintain membership, licensure, or other privileges. These

- Reading medical journals that are certified for continuing medical education

- Subscribing to individual study courses, available in different formats (i.e., written, audiotape, computer-based, on-line, etc.)

- Attending Grand Rounds or other regular educational lectures organized by medical school or hospital departments

- Attending local or national education courses

- Attending national medical society meetings, and either taking specific instructional courses or attending lecture sessions

FIGURE 2.1 Sources of certified continuing medical education credit hours.

requirements are likely to increase and become more uniformly enforced in the future. Therefore, it is important that all clinicians understand the goals and opportunities available for completion of CME. Certified CME hours are available from many organizations, including medical schools, hospitals, medical societies, and national organizations. Certified CME hours may typically be obtained through several mechanisms (Figure 2.1) with accumulation on an actual per-hour basis.

The American Medical Association (AMA) established the Physician's Recognition Award (PRA) in 1968 to recognize physicians who participate in CME and to encourage participation in CME. For AMA PRA credit, there are two types of CME activity: Category 1 and Category 2 credits. *Category 1* credit requires that the CME activity be based on demonstrated needs with educational objectives stated; be content level appropriate for physicians; have performance of an evaluation by the physician; and have documentation of physician participation by the sponsor. Medical educational activities that are merely verified by the physician-participant (i.e., not by the sponsor) are designated as *Category 2* hours. These activities include reading authoritative literature, teaching activities, medical writing or presentation of papers, and attendance at sponsor-designated Category 2 courses. As of 1999, the requirements for the AMA PRA standard certificate were 50 hours of CME activity during a year, with at least 20 hours of AMA PRA Category 1 and the remaining 30 hours of Category 1 or Category 2 activity.

READING AND EVALUATING THE LITERATURE

The enlightened clinician should regularly use the medical literature for two purposes: routine browsing or surveillance and problem-oriented searches.[5] For browsing, choosing the best journals to read can be difficult; in general, authors try to publish studies of potential significance in journals with the largest circulation. Thus, those journals are a good place to start for regular surveillance. In addition, journal subscriptions are a benefit of membership in many professional societies. Although yearly subscriptions are not inexpensive, most would argue that the benefit is well worth the cost. Furthermore, a single journal subscription can be shared by several members of a group practice or study group.

Regular browsing can be facilitated by reading article abstracts for content, followed by critical reading of articles of interest. Although "browsing" implies only a cursory review, articles with potential clinical significance should be reviewed carefully before the authors' conclusions are implemented into practice. Although a detailed description of critical literature review is beyond the scope of this chapter, several principles deserve emphasis. A cursory review of the article's main sections should immediately alert the reader to "signs of decadence or grandeur" as outlined in Table 2.1. Articles that appear worthy of further scrutiny should be subjected to the five basic questions listed in Table 2.2. Last, readers should never take statements in the abstract or discussion sections at face value unless they are supported by appropriate methods and results.

TABLE 2.1
Signs of Grandeur and Decadence in Journal Articles

Section	Signs of grandeur	Signs of decadence
Abstract	Structured summary of goals, methods, results, and significance	Unstructured qualitative overview of study; contains more wish than reality
Introduction	Clear, concise, and logical; ends with study rationale or purpose	Rambling, verbose literature review; no critical argument or hypothesis
Methods	Specific enough for the reader to reproduce the study; offers too much detail rather than too little	Vague or incomplete description of subjects, sampling, outcome criteria; no mention of statistical analysis
Results	Logical blend of numbers and narrative with supporting tables and figures	Difficult to read, with overuse or underuse of statistical tests; no tables
Discussion	Main results put in context; review of supporting and conflicting literature; discussion of strengths and weaknesses	Full of fantasy and speculation; rambling and biased literature review; weaknesses are not acknowledged
References	Clear demonstration that work of others has been systematically considered; original research from peer-reviewed journals emphasized	Key articles are conspicuously absent; excessively brief; review articles, book chapters, and lower quality journals emphasized

TABLE 2.2
Five Basic Questions for Interpreting Journal Articles

Question	Why it is important	Underlying principles
What type of study produced the data?	Study design has a profound impact on interpretation; the data collection, degree of investigator control, use of control groups, and direction of inquiry must be scrutinized	Bias, research design, placebo effect, control groups, causality
What are the results?	Results should be summarized with appropriate descriptive statistics; positive results must be qualified by the chance of being wrong, and negative results by the chance of having missed a true difference	Measurement scale, association, p-value, power, effect size, clinical importance
Are the results valid within the study?	Proper statistical analysis and data collection ensures valid results for the subjects studied; measurements must be accurate and reproducible	Internal validity, accuracy, statistical tests
Are the results valid outside the study?	Results can be generalized when the sampling method is sound, subjects are representative of the target population, and sample size is large enough for adequate precision	External validity, sampling, confidence intervals, precision
Are the results strong and consistent?	A single study is rarely definitive; results must be viewed relative to their plausibility, consistency with past efforts, and by the strength of the study methodology	Research integration, level of evidence, systematic review

Other issues to keep in mind when reviewing journal articles are

- Was the study prospective or retrospective (i.e., attempting to measure causality) or cross-sectional (i.e., attempting to measure only association)?
- Was the study performed specifically for research (i.e., using an experimental design) or were data collected during routine clinical care (i.e., an observational study)?
- Was a control or comparison group used?

TABLE 2.3
Explanations for Favorable Outcomes in Treatment Studies

Explanation	Definition	Solution
Bias	Systematic variation of measurements from their true values; may be intentional or unintentional	Accurate, protocol-driven data collection
Chance	Random variation without apparent relation to other measurements or variables; e.g., getting lucky	Control or comparison group
Natural history	Course of a disease from onset to resolution; may include relapse, remission, and spontaneous recovery	Control or comparison group
Regression to the mean	Symptom improvement independent of therapy, as sick patients return to a mean level after seeking care	Control or comparison group
Placebo effect	Beneficial effect caused by the expectation that the regimen will have an effect; e.g., power of suggestion	Control or comparison group with placebo
Halo effect	Beneficial effect caused by the manner, attention, and caring of a provider during a medical encounter	Control or comparison group treated similarly
Confounding	Distortion of an effect by other prognostic factors or variables for which adjustments have not been made	Randomization or multivariate analysis
Allocation (susceptibility) bias	Beneficial effect caused by allocating subjects with less severe disease or better prognosis to treatment group	Randomization or comorbidity analysis
Ascertainment (detection) bias	Favoring the treatment group during outcome analysis; e.g., rounding up for treated subjects, down for controls	Masked (blinded) outcome assessment

Answers to the preceding questions have a critical impact on the investigator's ability to draw meaningful conclusions about the impact of medical or surgical treatments on clinical outcomes. In addition to a "real" treatment effect, numerous explanations exist for favorable outcomes (Table 2.3). Many of these biases can be avoided only with randomized controlled trials of adequate sample size.

Clinical vs. Statistical Significance

The enlightened reader should ask whether the results show *clinical* significance as well as *statistical* significance. For instance, a prospective research study may show that the use of antibiotics improves the treatment success rate in otitis media over placebo with a p-value of 0.02. Therefore, the difference between antibiotic and placebo treatment outcomes is statistically significant, or likely not due to chance. The authors may conclude that the data demonstrate a significant improvement in outcomes after treatment with antibiotics. However, further review of data from the study may show that the actual cure rates were 92% for placebo and 96% for antibiotics. Therefore, the actual difference in treatment outcome is very small, and a large number of children would need to be treated with antibiotics to improve the outcome of only a few children, compared with treating all children with placebo or observation. Based on this, are these findings clinically significant? Should they cause changes in routine clinical management? These are questions that clinicians should ask when reviewing the literature.

Classification of Articles

There is a wide range of published material to read, of which even the most minor may have a relative degree of clinical merit. These include "professional evidence reports" such as case reports, "how I do it" reports, and case series, in addition to retrospective studies, prospective studies, and basic science reports and narrative review articles.

TABLE 2.4

Comparison of Narrative (Traditional) Reviews and Systematic Reviews (Meta-Analyses)

	Narrative review	Meta-analysis
Research design	Free form	*A priori* protocol
Literature search	Convenience sample	Systematic sample
Focus	Broad; summarizes a large body of information	Narrow; tests one or two specific hypotheses
Emphasis	Narrative	Numbers
Validity	Variable; high potential for bias in article selection	Good, provided articles are of adequate quality and combinability
Bottom line	Broad recommendations, often based on personal opinion	Estimates of effect size, based on statistical pooling of data
Utility	Provides quick overview of a subject area	Provides summary estimates for decision analysis, cost effectiveness studies, and practice guidelines

Excessive reliance on "review" articles is fraught with potential problems. A *review article* is only appropriate if all applicable studies — even those that may show results different from the mainstream or the opinion of the review article author — are included, and if all studies are discussed and presented in a fair and impartial light. If the author presents all available studies accurately, review articles on a particular subject can be very useful to the interested clinician.

When available, *systematic reviews* (or "meta-analyses") can be very helpful because they typically utilize rigorous inclusion criteria (Table 2.4). In a meta-analysis, the authors combine the statistics from individual studies and perform a single analysis of the large pooled database to assess for statistical significance and confidence intervals.[6] When performed using appropriate methodology (Table 2.5), a meta-analysis can be extremely helpful to the clinician searching for an answer to a clinical question, especially when individual articles may show conflicting or confusing results.

Book chapters can be very concise and educational. However, although the peer-review process used by medical journals has some potential problems, the clinician should remember that book chapters are typically not peer-reviewed. Thus, although finding a book chapter can be much more convenient than conducting a literature search, the reader is cautioned that he may be reading only the opinions of the authors.

Searching the Literature

When confronted with a particular clinical question, it is appropriate to search for published evidence concerning different methods of diagnosis or treatment. In a nutshell, this is the tenet behind evidence-based medicine, which is growing in recognition and importance in modern medicine. Evidence-based medicine is becoming more accessible to the average clinician for two major reasons: the wide availability of computers with Internet access and free access to MEDLINE literature searches from the National Library of Medicine (NLM).

The process of literature searching has improved and grown significantly over the years — from manual searches in printed volumes many years ago to the current Internet-based "point and click" literature searches available from any individual computer. In 1997, the NLM began offering free and unlimited access to their medical databases for all Americans. The NLM maintains several indices of medical articles. The most well-known is MEDLINE, which contains citations to virtually all major biomedical journals; other available databases include AIDSLINE, which contains citations to the AIDS literature, and CANCERLIT, among many others.[7]

TABLE 2.5
Steps in Performing a Systematic Review

Action	Purpose	Comment
Prepare a detailed *a priori* research protocol	Defines study hypothesis and methodology to test it	Quality research rarely occurs by divine revelation
Specify unambiguous selection criteria for inclusion of articles	Ensures that articles are similar enough to be statistically combined	Criteria should define patients, exposures, outcomes, and methodology of interest
Search the literature and document the search strategy	Identifies all potential data sources	Computer search is incomplete without manual cross checks
Determine which articles meet predefined inclusion criteria; keep a log of rejected trials	Limits selection bias, the Achilles heel of traditional narrative review articles	Base decisions on methods section only; reviewers should be blinded to results
Assess the quality of articles to be combined	Provides quality scores for sensitivity analysis (see below)	Use two reviewers and measure interobserver agreement
Extract data from included articles for predetermined treatment endpoints	Obtains accurate and precise numerical data from source articles for pooling	Use two reviewers and measure interobserver agreement
Statistically combine the data to obtain an estimate of the main effect under study	Improves precision and statistical power by increasing overall sample size	95% confidence intervals are mandatory; a statistical test for homogeneity is highly desirable
Perform a sensitivity analysis	Shows how results vary under different assumptions, tests, and criteria	Include adjustments for quality of the papers combined
Consider the effect of publication bias on results	Authors and journal editors may preferentially publish positive studies	More of a problem with small studies showing marginal benefits of therapy
Discuss clinical significance of the statistical findings	Formulates caveats by putting results into proper perspective	Discuss economic impact and future study directions

Because MEDLINE and other NLM databases are free to any American with Internet access, it is wise for all practicing physicians to become proficient in search techniques. Many medical library and medical school Web sites have links to the NLM, sometimes with their own search engine software; the clinician can log on directly to the NLM at www.nlm.nih.gov. Fortunately, the NLM site and most search engines are very user friendly and do not require a sophisticated computer user. However, a few basic suggestions will help the novice searcher.

The entire search process depends on an appropriate formulation of the search query.[7] Articles in MEDLINE are indexed using a common language called *medical subject heading* (MeSH) terms. There are a finite number of these terms, and all articles are classified into MEDLINE using MeSH terms (although as new diseases, concepts, or technologies are developed, new MeSH terms are added to the vocabulary). Therefore, identifying the appropriate MeSH terms to search for a topic is crucial.

An alternative is to use a technique called a *free-text search*. In this case, the search looks for identical words that are used in the title or abstract of an article. However, the match must be exact. For instance, free-text searching for *tracheostomy* will not identify articles containing the word *tracheotomy*. Similarly, words that may appear in singular and plural forms can limit the comprehensiveness of a free-text search.

Once potential articles have been identified, most programs allow the searcher to combine searches, using the Boolean terms AND, OR, and NOT. Similarly, the searcher can often limit the search to a small range of years, only human subjects articles, only English language articles, etc. After the articles have been identified, the program will often display the article's abstract, which will help the searcher identify whether it is an article appropriate for further review.

TABLE 2.6
Levels of Evidence for Treatment Recommendations

Level	Type of evidence
1	Randomized controlled trial or a systematic review (meta-analysis) of randomized controlled trials
2	Prospective (cohort or outcomes) study with an internal control group or a systematic review of prospective controlled studies
3	Retrospective (case-control) study with an internal control group or a systematic review of retrospective controlled studies
4	Case series without an internal control group (retrospective reviews; uncontrolled cohort or outcome studies)
5	Expert opinion without explicit critical appraisal, or recommendation based on physiology or bench research

EVIDENCE-BASED MEDICINE

Otolaryngology has enjoyed a long and rich legacy in clinical research. Over 75% of articles published in major otolaryngology journals involve clinical research, with a steadily increasing volume of publications from 1969 through 1989.[8] Concurrent with the rapid growth of clinical research is a growing consensus that such work, in particular randomized controlled trials (RCTs) and prospective studies, should be a foundation for treatment decisions by health care providers. This concept is called evidence-based medicine (EBM), which means integrating individual clinical expertise with the best available external clinical evidence from systematic research.[9]

Whereas few would contest the wealth of clinical expertise among practicing otolaryngologists, some have questioned whether the published evidence base is of sufficient quality and breadth to facilitate the practice of EBM.[10,11] These objections become less relevant upon realization that EBM does not necessitate or demand a plethora of RCTs for every imaginable condition. In contrast, EBM simply requires that such evidence, when available, be systemically identified and incorporated into patient care recommendations.

Some experts view EBM as a threat to physician autonomy.[12] Such concern stems from the mistaken view of EBM as a form of "cookbook" medicine based solely on research findings. In contrast, EBM requires a bottom-up approach that balances three distinct influences: (1) best available external evidence, (2) individual clinical expertise, and (3) patient preference.[9] As noted by Sackett, "External clinical evidence can inform, but can never replace individual expertise ... any external guideline must be integrated with clinical expertise in deciding whether and how it matches the patient's clinical state, predicament, and preferences, and thus whether it should be applied."[9]

When research evidence is incorporated into clinical decision-making, articles are assigned an appropriate *level of evidence* based on study design.[13] Levels are numbered 1 through 5 (Table 2.6), with higher numbers indicating poorer quality. Levels of evidence can then be grouped into grades of recommendation:

- Grade A recommendation: Level 1 evidence (RCTs)
- Grade B recommendation: Level 2 or 3 evidence (controlled, observational study)
- Grade C recommendation: Level 4 evidence (case series)
- Grade D recommendation: Level 5 (expert opinion)

Under this system, any clinical recommendation can be qualified by level and grade of evidence. This approach ensures that RCTs will be used, when available, but allows lesser grades of evidence to be appropriately incorporated and qualified if randomized studies do not exist. Areas in need of additional research are also highlighted. Readers should be aware of the evidence grade used to

---

TABLE 2.7
Attributes of Good Clinical Practice
Guidelines

Validity	Clarity
Reliability	Multidisciplinary process
Clinical applicability	Schedule review
Clinical flexibility	Documentation

---

support current practice patterns, as well as the accompanying limitations (particularly for Grade C recommendations or lower).

PRACTICE GUIDELINES AND CONSENSUS PANELS

The last several years have seen a proliferation of practice guidelines and consensus statements created by several different organizations. The goals and intentions behind practice guidelines may vary significantly; many guidelines are intended only to reduce costs or health care utilization, while others are intended as guides to assist physicians and patients in evidence-based clinical care.

The clinician should be cautioned that although a "practice guideline" or "referral guideline" (or other clinical care guideline) might look official and might be released from a respected local or national organization, this does not necessarily mean that the guideline is any more than a consensus of expert opinion or a codification of the status quo. Whenever possible, practice guidelines should be developed by a multidisciplinary group of experts, using defined and reproducible methodology and including recommendations based on data from appropriate clinical studies (i.e., evidence based) as much as possible (Table 2.7).[14]

The Agency for Health Research and Quality (formerly the Agency for Healthcare Policy and Research) has made the development and dissemination of appropriate practice guidelines a significant priority. The agency has played an important role in providing funding for the independent multi-specialty development of several practice guidelines for common conditions and has actually funded centers of excellence for the development of evidence-based practice guidelines. The AHRQ has collected a compendium of published guidelines, which is available through its Web page at http://www.ahrq.gov>.

The *consensus of expert opinion* certainly has its place in medicine, and many times consensus panels or symposiums are convened to record the collective expert opinion and experience concerning the diagnosis and treatment of certain diseases. Typically, these diseases are somewhat rare, and significant clinical research or the development of an evidence-based guideline is impossible or impractical. Under these circumstances, recommendations from expert or consensus panels or guidelines may be helpful, but the clinician should carefully consider the source of the guideline, the motivation behind its development, the methodology used (Table 2.8), and the comprehensiveness and inclusion of all pertinent data.[15]

CONCLUSION

SUGGESTED SELF-STUDY GUIDELINES

Continuing medical education is important to every clinician, especially the pediatric otolaryngologist, in order to maintain the level of expertise in caring for the pediatric patient. Many educational formats exist to provide this necessary training. It is self-evident that different educational formats have advantages and disadvantages. Regular reading of the medical literature is an essential part of continuing education; however, this is probably not sufficient alone because the literature is so

TABLE 2.8
Variations in Methodology for Treatment Recommendations

Methodology used in report or publication	Systematic summary of evidence?	Considers all options and outcomes?	Explicit statement of values?
Review article (narrative)	No	No or yes	No
Systematic review (meta-analysis)	Yes	No or yes	No
Professional evidence report	Yes	No	No
Clinical practice guideline	Yes	Yes	Yes

voluminous that even with significant time spent reading, many important advances might be missed. Furthermore, even if all of the appropriate journals could be read regularly, the delay to publication for new advances can be significant.

However, it would be cost- and time-prohibitive to acquire all CME only through out-of-town travel to formal meetings or courses. Moreover, many cities and states contain a large amount of expertise and educational opportunity, so extensive travel may not be required. Therefore, a mixture of self-directed reading and study — preferably with some sort of test or evaluation to encourage completion — and attendance at local as well as national lectures and courses is probably the best combination for adequate continuing education.

REFERENCES

1. Uhl, H.S.M. A brief history. In Rosof, A.B. and Felch, W.C., Eds. *Continuing Medical Education: A Primer.* 2nd ed. Westport, CT: Praeger Publishers, 1992.
2. Bennett, N.L., Davis, D.A., Easterling, W.E. et al. Continuing medical education: a new vision of the professional development of physicians. *Acad. Med.,* 2000, 75, 1167–1172.
3. Fox, R.D. and Bennett, N.L. Continuing medical education: learning and change: implications for continuing medical education. *Br. Med. J.,* 1998, 316, 466–468.
4. Maitland, F.M. Accreditation of sponsors and certification of credit. In Rosof, A.B. and Felch, W.C., Eds. *Continuing Medical Education: A Primer.* 2nd ed. Westport: Praeger Publishers, 1992.
5. Rosenfeld, R.M. Critical evaluation of articles about otitis media. In Rosenfeld, R.M. and Bluestone, C.D., Eds. *Evidence-Based Otitis Media.* Hamilton: B.C. Decker Inc., 1999.
6. Rosenfeld, R.M. How to systematically review the medical literature. *Otolaryngol. Head Neck Surg.* 1996, 115, 53–63.
7. Stewart, M.G. and Moore, A.S. Searching the medical literature. *Otolaryngol. Clin. North Am.,* 1998, 31, 277–287.
8. Rosenfeld, R.M. Clinical research in otolaryngology journals. *Arch. Otolaryngol. Head Neck Surg.,* 1991, 117, 164–170.
9. Sackett, D.L., Rosenberg, W.M.C., Gray, J.A.M. et al. Evidence-based medicine: what it is and what it isn't. *Br. Med. J.,* 1996, 312, 71–72.
10. Maran, A.G., Molony, N.C., Armstrong, M.W.J., and Ah-See, K. Is there an evidence base for the practice of ENT surgery? *Clin. Otolaryngol.,* 1997, 22, 152–157.
11. Gates, G.A. So where's the evidence? *Otolaryngol. Head Neck Surg.,* 1999, 120, 619–620.
12. Tanenbaum, S.J. Evidence and expertise: the challenge of the outcomes movement to medical professionalism. *Acad. Med.,* 1999, 74, 757–763.
13. Center for Evidence-Based Medicine. Levels of evidence and grades of recommendations, last revised 18 November 1999. Available at: http://cebm.jr2.ox.ac.uk/docs/.
14. Agency for Health Care Policy and Research. Using Clinical Practice Guidelines to Evaluate Quality of Care. Rockville, MD: AHCPR, 1995.
15. Guyatt, G.H., Sinclair, J., Cook, D.J. et al. Users' guides to the medical literature XVI. How to use a treatment recommendation. *JAMA,* 1999, 281, 1836–1843.

3 Managing the Stress of Surgical Complications

Benjamin F. Asher and Ronald M. Epstein

When we make mistakes, we cannot turn the clock back and try again. All we can do is use the present well.

Dalai Lama

CONTENTS

THE "STRESS RESPONSE"

In 1976, Selye first associated stress with disease.[1] He defined stress as a generalized nonspecific set of responses to protect the organism from harm. Stress has been further studied and its definition refined by many authors. The term "fight or flight" has been used to define the body's response to stressful stimuli, with increased heart rate, increased blood pressure, and increased oxygen consumption via stimulation of the sympathetic nervous system, for one example. The stress response, however, as it affects the individual, is actually a far more complex and far-reaching physiologic and behavioral response.

The stress response involves not only the hypothalamo-pituitary-adrenocortical (HPA) and the sympatho-thalamo-adrenomedulllary (SAM) systems, but also the immune system and cytokine production. When these two pathways are stimulated by the stress response, numerous neuroendocrine changes are triggered, including elevations in the levels of hormones and proteins including epinepherine, norepinepherine, renin, calcitonin, cortisol, thyroxine, parathyroid hormone, gastrin, insulin, and erythropoietin. The physiologic result of the stress response includes elevation in blood pressure, increase in heart rate and the galvanic skin response, elevation in blood glucose levels, coagulation time, and increased muscle tension.

In the acute situation, these changes are appropriate for the fight for survival.[2] However, chronic stress debilitates the individual. Extensive research implicates chronic stress as a significant factor in a number of common medical conditions, including hypertension, heart disease, asthma, irritable bowel syndrome, and numerous psychiatric problems.[3] From a public health perspective, society pays a high cost for its stress. It has been estimated that $17 billion are lost in productivity each year to stress-related problems.[4] This amount does not include the cost of pharmaceuticals to directly combat the stress response.

IMPACT OF THE STRESS RESPONSE ON THE SURGEON

The practice of surgery is exhilarating as well as humbling. Procedures that go well and have restored a patient to health are extremely gratifying. When complications arise, however, the story is different. Whether or not the surgeon makes a mistake, he or she usually feels awful and may have many self-recriminations. More than one surgeon has made the analogy that the surgical relationship is like a marriage; a commitment or contract is made between the surgeon and the patient to be together "for better or for worse." Some busy surgeons are making this commitment numerous times per day. The responsibility of this contract is weighty but that weight is not always perceived. Even without a complication, this type of commitment and relationship has the potential to be very stressful.

There are other potential causes of stress in a surgeon's life besides surgical complications, including balancing work with family, night call, long working hours, managed care issues, office staff issues, partner disagreements, competition for patients, abusive training programs, bad outcomes, difficult patients, and litigation. In addition to the stress-related diseases mentioned previously, other potential manifestations of stress overload include sleeplessness, depression, quickness to anger, and abusive behavior that can have a negative impact on the surgeon's sense of well-being.

All professions are associated with their own unique challenges. Those challenges, depending upon an individual's reaction, may trigger different stress responses. One of the great challenges of a surgical practice is managing the complications of surgery as well as the medical errors that may contribute to poor outcomes. With each surgical complication, the physician must

- Take full responsibility for the problem
- Provide a technical solution
- Consider how best to handle his or her relationship with the patient
- Handle his or her psychology in such a way as to keep practicing surgery and deal more effectively with subsequent situations

Each of these situations, depending upon the surgeon's state of mind, is potentially very stressful. The tendency to blame someone else for the problem, the knot in the stomach when things are not going right in the operating room, facing a disappointed or angry patient and his or her family, or possibly dealing with an inner voice that questions one's competence are all stressful aspects of the daily life of a surgeon.

DEVELOPING STRATEGIES FOR MANAGING STRESS IN A SURGICAL PRACTICE

The technical handling of complications is part of every surgical training program. "What to do if ..." scenarios are memorized by every surgical resident for multiple types of operations in preparation for the untoward or the unpredicted event. Textbooks such as this one describe the prevention of mistakes, as well as the recognition and management of these outcomes. Other than in the venue of risk management, however, little has been written about complications and the impact on the physician–patient relationship

It is well known that a positive, honest physician–patient relationship remains a major factor in preventing malpractice lawsuits. Although articles have been written about the psychology of medical error,[5] a thorough review of the medical literature reveals little about the effect of complications on the psychology of the surgeon. In fact, experience indicates that few surgeons discuss this issue with others outside their profession, let alone among their colleagues.

Surgeons appear to have difficulty discussing their errors and admitting the effects of fatigue on performance.[6] Physicians, in general, tend to find dysfunctional ways of protecting themselves from their mistakes and complications in the absence of mechanisms for directly dealing with their feelings.[5] In one story, a prominent head and neck surgical oncologist transferred all of his patients with complications to a ward at the end of the hall, which he never visited because it made him feel fallible.

In spite of superb technical training, surgical complications happen to every surgeon. The age-old adage is that "if you don't have complications, you don't do enough surgery." Given the prevalence of complications, in addition to technical management, what else should the surgeon do to handle the stress effectively? Is it possible that the extensive research accumulated over the last 40 years about the deleterious effects of stress on the mind and body and the effectiveness of multiple techniques of stress reduction can be brought to bear on the management of surgical complications? Should surgeons have some tools in their armamentarium to be able to handle the stress of their jobs better?

Adequate preparation is the foundation of surgical practice. Preparedness comes from study and experience. With a sound knowledge base and broad experience, a surgeon will often be able to apply expert clinical judgment in handling a difficult situation. Clinical judgment, however, is based upon adequate development of explicit and tacit knowledge.[7] An example of explicit knowledge is the use evidence-based guidelines. An example of tacit knowledge is personal clinical experience. The ability to integrate these two objectives successfully is essential to the art of medicine.

MINDFULNESS

The practice of surgery and the successful handling of complications in the operating room require not only preparation and thought but also complete and focused awareness. In the midst of a developing complication or attending to the myriad sequelae of bad outcomes and complications, all attention is brought to the here and now. This type of "here and now awareness" may be defined as "mindfulness." Mindful awareness can also be seen in the rock climber who must be focused and aware for each and every move or risk plummeting off the cliff face.

Jon Kabat-Zinn describes mindfulness as a means of paying attention in a particular way: on purpose, in the present moment and nonjudgmentally, nurturing greater awareness and clarity.[8] Epstein describes 11 characteristics of mindfulness:[7]

- Active observation of oneself, the patient, and the problem
- Peripheral vision
- Preattentive processing
- Critical curiosity
- Courage to see the world as it is rather than as one would have it
- Willingness to examine and set aside categories and prejudices
- Adoption of a beginner's mind
- Humility to tolerate awareness of one's areas of incompetence
- Connection between the knower and the known
- Compassion based on insight
- Presence

It almost goes without saying that mindlessness in the operating room — the opposite of mindfulness — has the potential for disaster. However, the operating room environment is full of distractions that take the surgeon's awareness away from the here and now focus on the patient and the surgical task at hand. Long operations are often fatiguing and inadequate nutrition can contribute to lapses of focus. Arrogance can blind an individual to the realities of the moment. Each of these factors can contribute to error and poor judgment, and create the potential for complications and stress.

As a third-year medical student, one of the authors (R.E.) witnessed a renal artery becoming occluded during a retroperitoneal node dissection. He called it to the attention of the attending surgeon but was ignored because of his low status as a student. Complications ensued that could have been prevented if the surgeon had been mindful and willing to recognize an error.

Mindfulness is an excellent tool for handling stress by maintaining the focus on the present moment. One technique of mindful awareness begins with focusing on the breath. Mindfulness can be used to bring present moment awareness to bear on all of one's activities or physiologic processes or sensations. Another aspect of mindfulness practice is meditation. Mindfulness (which is secular) or Vipassana meditation from the Buddhist tradition uses the breath as a focus for the mind while the mind observes without judgment whatever is present in the moment. This is one of many meditation techniques.

Studies have shown that practicing mindfulness reduces anxiety and depression.[4] The theoretical basis of this is that when the present moment is looked at objectively, it is found to be relatively stress free. Whatever is happening "now" is dealt with in a natural and appropriate manner. This process can reduce anxiety, for example, because anxiety is not based upon present moment reality but caused by worrying about the future or agonizing about the past. By focusing on the breath, attention is brought back to the here and now. It is likely many surgeons have experienced the exhilaration of the flow and natural progression of an operation as each anatomic detail falls into view while the attention is focused solely on each step. In those peak moments, the awareness is almost relaxed, thus allowing a broad perspective on the procedure to develop. If something out of the ordinary should occur in these moments, it is handled with grace. This could be defined as the mindful practice of surgery.

Just as the technical aspect of surgical practice must be acquired through study and practice, the tools for handling stress must also be developed and cultivated outside the stressful moment. Then, when the extreme situation such as a surgical complication arises, there will be a natural ability to handle it. Mindful practice is not the only well-studied stress reduction technique, but it remains one of the most applicable to the operating room environment because it requires nothing more than a change in awareness.

STRESS REDUCTION TECHNIQUES

Stress exists throughout our lives, giving an individual plenty of opportunity to practice one or many stress reduction techniques. Meditation, which remains one of the most common stress reduction techniques, comes in many forms. Most styles of meditation establish a sense of calmness that permeates an individual's life even during states of heightened stress. Much research has been done on other meditation practices.[2] Benson used the term "relaxation response" to describe the *hypo*metabolic state associated with meditation. In that state, the body's oxygen consumption and blood pressure drop. This is a state different from sleep in that the mind is alert while the body is resting. Benson noted four requirements to create this state (the last two items are preferable but not mandatory):[9,10]

- The use of a vehicle such as the breath or a mantra (word)
- An attitude of attentive observation
- A comfortable position
- A quiet environment

Meditation techniques from the Vedic traditions of India often use a mantra (a Sanskrit word) instead of the breath as a focus for the mind. In these techniques, the repetition of the mantra quiets the active mind thereby allowing the body to settle down. Transcendental meditation (TM), a popular technique in the West, uses this form. Centering is a Christian meditation technique that uses a prayer as focus for the mind. Many Jewish meditation techniques have recently become quite popular. Not all techniques are associated with a religious tradition, however. Jon Kabat-Zinn and Thich Nhat Hanh have secularized mindfulness meditation. TM is also not associated with a religion. Progressive relaxation, a type of self-hypnosis, is completely secular.

Much research has been done on TM as well as mindfulness practices. TM has been found to lower blood pressure, reduce anxiety, and increase pain tolerance. Mindfulness has been found to reduce anxiety and improve outcomes in psychotherapy.[2,4] Use of the relaxation response has been shown to be extremely effective for patients with chronic pain.[11]

Other stress reducing techniques are available to the results-driven surgeon. Depending upon one's outside interests or other skills, regular physical exercise through gym work or with individual or team sports can provide a tangible outlet for vexed emotions. Similarly, developing talent in an area of creative art, such as music, theater, painting, or sculpture, can provide a soothing tonic for the troubled heart and mind. Reading, whether humor, fiction, or nonfiction, can be a restful exercise. Additionally, when all life priorities are organized, it will come as no surprise that to many individuals, pursuing a deeper spiritual relationship with their families and religions provides great solace.

CONCLUSION

The preparation for handling the stress of complications begins with cultivating and developing personal strategies for dealing with stress, in addition to the development of a healthy, honest physician–patient relationship. Personal strategies for stress management include meditation, yoga, regular exercise, humor, faith, and prayer. A physician–patient relationship based upon service founded in honesty and trust will be the most helpful if a crisis should arise.

The understanding of the negative effects of stress is not new. Over the last 30 years much research has been done establishing the efficacy of stress reduction as a way of promoting physical health and mental well-being. Multiple popular and effective methods of stress reduction are readily available to any individual with an interest in promoting personal health. It only requires a commitment to choose one and to take the time to practice. The question now is not if there is any benefit to these methods but when one will apply them to his or her own life.

GENERAL PRINCIPLES

- Be aware of the acute and chronic physiologic effects of short-term and long-term stress.
- Be aware of the multiple potential sources of stress in a physician's life.
- Be aware of how stress can negatively impact the ability to practice medicine.
- Remember that managing stress is one of the most important life skills to be learned.
- Develop a sense of "mindfulness" in a crisis whereby complete and focused awareness is brought to bear upon the issues at hand in the here and now.
- Develop stress reduction techniques and apply them throughout the workday as well as in home life.

RESOURCES FOR STRESS REDUCTION

Books:

Benson, H. and Klipper M.Z. *The Relaxation Response*. New York, NY: Quill, 2001.
Kabat-Zinn, J. *Wherever You Go, There You Are, Mindfulness Meditation in Everyday Life*. New York: Hyperion, 1994.
LeShan, L. *How to Meditate, A Guide to Self Discovery*. Boston, MA: Little, Brown & Co., 1999.

Instruction:

Courses in transcendental meditation, yoga, and t'ai chi chuan are available in local communities. Religion-based meditation practices are available through local churches and synagogues.

REFERENCES

1. Selye, H. *The Stress of Life.* New York: McGraw-Hill, 1976.
2. Freeman, L. and Lawlis, F. *Complementary and Alternative Medicine.* St. Louis: Mosby, 2001, 532.
3. Glaser, R., Rabin, B., Chesney, M., Cohen, S., and Natelson, B. Stress-induced immunomodulation: implications for infectious diseases? *JAMA*, 1999, 281, 2268–2270.
4. Astin, J.A. Stress reduction through mindfulness meditation. Effects on psychological symptomatology, sense of control, and spiritual experiences. *Psychother. Psychosom.*, 1997, 66, 97–106.
5. Wu, A.W. Medical error: the second victim. The doctor who makes the mistake needs help too [editorial]. *Br. Med. J.*, 2000, 320, 726–727.
6. Sexton, J.B., Thomas, E.J., and Helmreich, R.L. Error, stress, and teamwork in medicine and aviation: cross sectional surveys. *Br. Med. J.*, 2000, 320, 745–749.
7. Epstein, R.M. Mindful practice [see comments]. *JAMA*, 1999, 282, 833–839.
8. Kabat-Zinn, J. *Wherever You Go, There You Are: Mindfulness Meditation in Everyday Life.* New York: Hyperion, 1994.
9. Benson, H. The relaxation response: history, physiological basis and clinical usefulness. *Acta Med. Scand.*, Suppl 1982, 660, 231–237.
10. Benson, H., Beary, J.F., and Carol, M.P. The relaxation response. *Psychiatry*, 1974, 37, 37–46.
11. Caudill, M., Schnable, R., Zuttermeister, P., Benson, H., and Friedman, R. Decreased clinic use by chronic pain patients: response to behavioral medicine intervention. *Clin. J. Pain*, 1991, 7, 305–310.

Section II

The Hospital Experience

4 Perioperative Care: Family-Centered Surgical Care

Linda Miller Calandra, Lora Lee Sparacino, and Gary D. Josephson

It is the human touch after all that counts the most in our relation with our patients.

Robert Tuttle Morris

CONTENTS

INTRODUCTION

Providing comprehensive patient and family care is the key to a quality perioperative experience. Although the skill of the surgeon is important, a prepared child and family increase the odds for a successful postoperative result. This chapter will focus on areas that, although they may elude the busy surgeon, are precisely the things that can prevent postoperative disasters. After the decision has been made between the surgeon and the family to proceed with surgical management, the surgeon may find it more time-efficient to delegate further family discussions to a nurse. The nurse should have pediatric experience to allow for the most comprehensive approach.

PATIENT MANAGEMENT PREOPERATIVELY

Caring for children can be challenging. One must be able to establish a rapport with the child while gaining the confidence of the family. Understanding and applying developmental theory can assist the practitioner with this process (Table 4.1). Some simple yet important fundamentals in dealing with the younger child will allow the physician better communication. For example, small children will do better while sitting on a parent's lap. The clinician should speak to the child directly and use his name. It can be helpful to know if a nickname is used, and it should also be recorded on the chart. The surgeon may engage a slightly older child in social conversation, introducing himself and telling the child what to call him if it is less formal than Dr. (Surname).

With older children, information can be sought directly from the child. Teenagers can be the most challenging. They may seek independence and may not be as informative in front of their parents. Information regarding the use of alcohol, tobacco, or illicit drugs, as well as body piercing and sexual activity may need to be obtained. Privacy and confidentiality should be maintained.

Preoperative preparation of children should be individualized based on the developmental level. Sometimes, as with a baby or toddler, the teaching focuses on the parents. The time to teach often falls between ideal vs. realistic. Ideally, teaching should occur close to the surgical date; however, this may not always be possible. A second preoperative counseling session with the surgeon one week prior to the surgical date may be beneficial if the surgical schedule is months out. Because the family will not always engage in the teaching and the learning process, counseling in the office and encouraging homework is important. Age-appropriate, simple explanations should be given of

TABLE 4.1
Developmental Theory

	Age (in years)				
Stage	**Infancy (birth to 1)**	**Toddler (1–3)**	**Early childhood (3–6)**	**Middle childhood (6–12)**	**Adolescence (13–18)**
Significant relationship	Maternal	Parental	Family	Neighborhood, school	Peers
Psychosexual stages	Oral sensory	Anal, urethral	Phallic-locomotion	Latency	Puberty
Cognitive	Sensorimotor	Preoperational thought	Preoperational thought	Concrete operations	Formal
	Birth to 18 months	Preconceptual phase: 2–4 years	Intuitive phase: 4–7 years	Inductive reasoning beginning logic	Deductive reasoning
Psychosocial stages	Trust vs. mistrust	Autonomy vs. shame	Initiative vs. guilt	Industry vs. inferiority	Identity and repudiation vs. identity-confusion
Central process	Mutuality with caregiver	Imitation	Identification	Education	Peer pressure; role identifications
Social modalities	To get	To hold on	To make (going after)	To make things (completing)	To be oneself or not to be
	To give in return	To let go	To make like (playing)	To make things together	To share being oneself

Source: Based on the developmental theories of Erik Erikson, Jean Piaget, and Sigmund Freud.

what will happen. Children should be informed about what they need to do and what they cannot do. Time should be allotted to answer questions from the child, parents, and other family members.

Each office facility should have prepared material for the family to take home. Teaching modalities may include pamphlets, booklets, coloring books, and videos. Some hospitals offer children preoperation tours and parties. Children can benefit from a hands-on experience of seeing equipment such as ear thermometer, blood pressure cuff, and hospital attire. This information should be present so that the parents can take advantage of the opportunities available to decrease anxiety. Trust the parents to decide what is in the best interest of their child. These programs should be optional; not any one education form alone is ideal.

Children with special needs may require additional preoperative care. Children with Down syndrome, cerebral palsy, sickle cell anemia, diabetes, seizure disorder, and reactive airway disease are among those who may require additional consultation before surgery. Collaboration among the otolaryngologist, the primary care provider, and the other pediatrics subspecialists ensures that any special needs for these children are identified and managed before, during, and after the surgical procedure.

PREOPERATIVE PARENT MANAGEMENT ISSUES

It is essential to establish and maintain parent trust and confidence. With Internet access available, parents are more knowledgeable about their child's illnesses, so their fund of knowledge should be assessed. They may come with preconceived biases, especially in dealing with the "special child." Religious and cultural concerns may also need special consideration in developing the plan of care. The most common religious concern is the issue of potential blood transfusion in a Jehovah's Witness family. The otolaryngologist must be honest. If both sides cannot mutually agree, the otolaryngologist should tell the parents that they cannot agree and decline care.

Communication is key to successful outcomes. Discussion of surgery can increase parental anxiety and stress. Parents need time to learn their role and to establish realistic expectations. Adequate time needs to be provided to disseminate information and to answer questions. The otolaryngology nurse or nurse practitioner is an ideal facilitator as a member of the professional team.

Many parents react negatively to the nothing by mouth (NPO) restriction prior to surgery. There is a wide variance of practice in this country. Some of the children's hospitals have liberalized this to clear fluids up to 2 hours prior while others remain NPO after midnight. Parents need support for whatever the given restrictions are. They need to understand the rationale for NPO status and the implications for potentially life-threatening complications if disregarded. It may be helpful to offer parents some suggestions such as distraction techniques.

The preoperative office visit is a good time to clarify instructions with parents. Postoperative instruction sheets can be provided and reviewed. Written teaching materials should be developed at a fourth-grade reading level. Make sure parents know where to go and what time to arrive for surgery. Reinforce if the parent must call the hospital prior to surgery or if the hospital will contact them. Prescriptions for postoperative management may be provided in advance. It is helpful for parents to have any prescriptions filled and ready. Review with parents what they need to take with them to the hospital including items of importance that can be easily overlooked such as insurance information. Children may select a special transition object — a stuffed animal, doll, or blanket — that will provide a sense of security. These items are often permitted to go with the child into the operating room. Parents should pack travel essentials for the ride home, such as an emesis basin or bag and towels. If possible, two parents or adult family members per child patient should accompany the child to the surgical procedure.

Parents often ask about being present for anesthesia induction. If the facility allows parent participation, the parent needs to be prepared for his or her role. Staff support for the parent should also be provided. The parent needs to know that he or she is to assist the child with induction and encourage the child to go to sleep. If the child decides to fight and cry, it may make the parent feel bad or guilty. If a medical problem develops during induction, the parent may be asked to leave the operating room. This can be very emotional and may not be best for every parent. If the parent is anxious, the child will sense this, which will deter from any positive effect. Parents should not be forced to do this if uncomfortable.

MANAGED CARE DIFFICULTIES

Gaining approval from third-party payers can be stressful on the family as well as the office staff. This arduous task of dealing with insurance carriers should be delegated to a knowledgeable staff person designated to handle authorizations and precertifications. The parent or insured must be made part of the team in dealing with the insurance company to assure maximum benefit for the patient. Although the burden of payment responsibility still lies with the family, many are unaware of how insurance works. A parent can benefit from an account representative who will help answer insurance questions. Available education brochures on insurance issues may be obtained through different insurance companies. Having this available in the surgical education packet for parents to take home and read may be helpful. Successful reimbursement is a product of proper precertification.

The surgeon can help staff by documenting clearly in the patient's chart the procedure to be scheduled. If more than one code is available, such as in the case of middle ear surgery, the surgeon should select the appropriate code and document supporting evidence in the chart for the code selected. This will help staff if the insurance company calls and has questions about the patient history or the selected procedure. The surgeon should be sure to precertify for all possibilities. An example would be to precertify for a facial nerve monitor during ear surgery. It is easier not to bill for something not used during the time of collection than to add something on after the surgery, which will often lead to denial of a claim.

Insurance authorizations, precertifications, and collections have become increasingly difficult in the face of increasing costs of medical care. This has led to the development of courses and workshops for the physician and his or her office staff. Sending personnel to learn appropriate coding, billing, and collecting issues will be rewarded by fewer denials and higher reimbursement. Ultimately, this will lead to greater patient satisfaction.

DAY OF SURGERY ISSUES

Anxiety often increases significantly as the day of surgery draws near. Parents are often nervous about keeping the child relatively healthy, and additional questions may come to mind. Staff must be courteous and kind in the face of family members' experiencing high levels of stress. Helping keep the parent or caretaker organized and abreast of what is to be expected will help make the process run smoothly. Distraction techniques can be beneficial for the child and predominantly will involve play. Teenagers may appreciate the use of a book, music, or videos.

The child's health status must be reviewed on admission. Every institution should have a preoperative checklist to be completed (Figure 4.1). Separation from parents to leave for surgery can be eased with friendly interactions and transition objects such as a stuffed animal or other favorite toy. Parents may have the option of being present for induction in some institutions. They should be prepared for what will happen, how the child will look, and their role. Ideally, a staff person should be available to support the parent as needed and to escort him or her from the operating room once the child is asleep.

It should be clear where parents wait while the child is in surgery. It is best to have them check in at the waiting area and a receptionist should know where they are at all times. This will facilitate easy contact by the surgical team should there be an unusual finding or an update for delays in the procedure. Depending on the length of the surgery, parents may find this a good time to get something to eat. They will need some sustenance and may not have a lot of time once the child returns. For lengthy cases, a staff person should be designated to provide communication updates

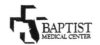

Jacksonville, Florida
PREOPERATIVE CHECKLIST

All blanks must be addressed before the patient is released to the Operating Room.

T	P	R	B/P	Wt	(Kg)	O₂ Sat	%	[ ] N/A

Date:	Allergies				Isolation	[ ] N/A

Initials			
a.	a. IdentaBand Correct	Location:	
b.	b. Allergy Bracelet	Location:	
c.	c. Last Clear Liquids	Time:	
d.	d. Last Solids/Milk	Time:	
e.	e. Face Sheet		
f.	f. Anesthesia Consent		
g.	g. Anesthesia Questionnaire		
h.	h. Surgical Consent		
i.	i. History & Physical		
j.	j. Blood Consent		[ ] N/A
k.	k. Blood Bracelet	Location:	
l.	l. Autologous	Number of Units:	
m.	m. Donor Directed	Number of Units:	
n.	n. Homologous	Number of Units:	
	PRE-OP TEST RESULTS ON CHART		
o.	o. Hgb		[ ] N/A
p.	p. Sickle Cell		[ ] N/A
q.	q. Urine [ ]	[ ]HCG	[ ] N/A
r.	r. Other Labs:		
s.	s. Chest X-Ray		[ ] N/A
t.	t. EKG		[ ] N/A
u.	u. Old Chart [ ] N/A [ ] Current Flow Sheet [ ] MAR		

To Holding: _____ (Time)	Via: [ ] W/C [ ] Parent's Arms	[ ] Ambulatory [ ] Stretcher	[ ] Isolette [ ] Bed/Crib	RN Releasing Patient:
Time Received in Holding:	Transporter:			ID Band Correct?
Medications/Comments:				

Anesthesiologist:	Induction Room: [ ]Yes [ ]No

OR RN: _____ To OR#: _____ at _____	Personal Items: _____ Holding RN: _____

Initials	Signature	
_____	_____	Patient Label

20-443 1/96

FIGURE 4.1 Preoperative checklist used at Wolfson Children's Hospital, Jacksonville, Florida. Printed with permission.

at regular intervals. Once the procedure is complete and the child is stable, the otolaryngologist should speak with the family members about the procedure, findings, and postoperative expectations. Parents greatly appreciate the personal communication. If possible, a second visit with the child and parents before discharge is greatly appreciated and allows the family to ask any additional questions or express afterthoughts. This often will reduce the number of postsurgical calls once the child has left the hospital.

The postanesthesia care unit may or may not be able to accommodate parents. The family should be informed of the approximate length of stay. Once the child has recovered and stabilized, he or she will be transferred to a general postoperative care area as appropriate and reunited with the family. Parents can play an important role in assisting with the child's care. Staff should continue to assess the child and family and provide the appropriate support as needed.

Many pediatric otolaryngic procedures are performed on an ambulatory basis. Discharge instructions and written materials should be clear, concise, and understandable. Parents should have the opportunity to ask questions. They need to know what to watch for and who to call if problems or complications occur. Postoperative follow-up instructions should be clearly delineated. In many cases, the postoperative appointment can be made in advance of surgery. Staff should escort the child and family to the car at discharge. The child should be properly secured in a car seat as required. Recommend that one adult sit in the back with the child to assist as necessary.

HOME MANAGEMENT

Successful postoperative home management requires a thorough preoperative family assessment. Considering the social environment of the child has not traditionally been included in preoperative assessments. Historically, at least one parent or extended family member has been able to care for a postoperative child. However, it is much more common today for nuclear families to have two working parents and live far from relatives. Therefore, the practitioner will want to discuss the impact of surgery on the parents' lives as well as the child's.

PLANNING AHEAD

It is important to give families realistic recovery times and postoperative expectations. This can usually be done with home instruction sheets; however, it is necessary for the surgeon to go over these instructions briefly with the parents. Telling a family that their child has minimal activity restrictions after a tonsillectomy may be misleading and offer them the impression that the child will be well enough to return to school — and thus they to work — within a few days. Preparing families honestly will help reduce postoperative stresses, lead to fewer postoperative phone calls, and eliminate potential complications.

It is important to counsel the family on what to expect at home when caring for the postsurgical child. Parental leave from work, family support, and routine care for pain management may not have been a forethought. Home instruction sheets and time designated to family counseling will help alleviate unexpected social issues. This will be much appreciated by the family and will not go unrecognized. Parents may not want to add additional stresses to their lives around the surgical date and may want to avoid planning such things as

- A vacation
- Selling a house
- Going out of town on business
- Engaging in negotiations in which they are required to be alert
- The birth of a new baby
- Holidays that the child enjoys (e.g., Halloween)
- School trips
- Exam periods for older children

Of course, sometimes surgery cannot be selectively planned. In these situations, it is even more important to help the family plan how they will accommodate changes in their schedules and lives. During this time, the family will be experiencing anxiety and parents may forget important routine activities. Having the family make a list or providing them with a check sheet of items or tasks to remember may be beneficial in allowing them to plan ahead.

- School pick-up and drop-off for other children
- Transportation to after-school or weekend activities for siblings
- Food shopping prior to surgery (including special foods that the patient might like)
- Treats for the siblings so they do not feel left out
- Someone to care for pets while the family is at the hospital
- Stocking up on books/videos/games for the recovery period
- If possible, obtaining postoperative medications prior to surgery
- Clearing work schedules as much as possible from meetings that require a sharp, focused mind if the parents plan to work during the child's recovery period
- Engaging a "helper" (friend, family members) if possible, thus allowing free time for the other children and preventing stress between parent and patient
- Having analgesics such as acetaminophen available in suppository form (in case the child is nauseous) and stocking up on the liquid form
- Checking with employers about the Family Medical Leave Act and filling out necessary paperwork
- Checking with any other specialists that child sees (such as an endocrinologist for diabetes) and getting the name and phone number of a person to help if questions or concerns arise
- Finding out how to contact the surgeon if questions or concerns should arise
- Realizing that this surgical period of time is not a good time to begin toilet training, and being patient because newly acquired developmental skills may regress during this stressful time

Although this list is not all inclusive, it may help families to think of other things that need to be arranged.

HANDLING EMERGENCIES

Instructing families how to handle emergencies before they happen can help prevent disasters. Parents need to have a clear understanding of what the surgeon means. Simply saying, "Call me if your child becomes dehydrated" may mean one thing to the surgeon and another to the parent. Providing clear guidelines of what to look for will allow both to assess the child better. Giving families sheets with explanations is helpful. For example:

- Check your child for signs of dehydration (dryness):
  - Does your child cry with tears?
  - Is your child's mouth moist?
  - How long between bathroom visits?
  - Measure your child's liquid intake if you are unsure how much he or she is drinking.

The surgeon should clearly instruct families about when to be concerned about bleeding and what to do about it. Is it necessary to call and, if so, whom? Should they go to an emergency department and, if so, which one? The surgeon should be sure that families know how to reach him or someone covering for him. If another person, such as a resident or associate, covers calls with the surgeon, he should be sure that families know this and assure them that he will be kept informed by the other person.

If an emergency does arise, the surgeon needs to compliment the family on how they handled it. If the situation could have been handled more smoothly, he should offer suggestions for the future. Making a family feel badly or attempting to place blame for the situation only puts the surgeon at risk for repercussions from an angry family.

EMPOWERING PARENTS TO HANDLE THEIR RECOVERING CHILD

Most parents are frightened not only about surgery but also about the recovery. Often the natural tendency not to "push" an ill child or to "let him do what he wants" is not the most beneficial to the child. An aid to assuring the best recovery of the patient is to educate the parent properly. Helping parents understand the child's natural stages of development will help them to cope better with their sick child. The most important aspect of the recovery is to provide nurturing and comfort while ensuring the child's safety.

INFANTS

In some respects, infants are perhaps the easiest patients with whom to cope. They often continue to feed, even with pain. Parents need to understand the level of pain to be expected with the procedure and which medication to give to ease the pain.

The surgeon should not expect parents to "read the bottle" to figure out a dose; rather, he should accurately calculate the pain medication based on the child's weight. If the surgeon chooses to order medication in cubic centimeters, he should do not expect the parent to know how to convert this to a common household measure. The surgeon can instruct the pharmacist to provide a measuring device and also remind the parent to measure the medication accurately.

If the surgeon suspects feeding might be a problem for the infant, he should tell the parents how much is expected to be ingested to maintain hydration. If he is particularly worried that an infant may not gain weight well postoperatively, a call to the primary care provider would be helpful. The family could arrange to have the child checked and weighed throughout the postoperative course, thus eliminating possible complications. This practice also serves to include the child's primary care provider in the perioperative phase. Primary care physicians will be grateful that they are included in the care of their patients.

TODDLERS

Unfortunately, toddlers do not respond well to bribes. This makes caring for them postoperatively particularly difficult. If a 2-year old chooses not to drink after a tonsillectomy, good luck! Parents need to be told that giving pain medication is important and the use of analgesic suppositories may be necessary. Offering distractions can help during a dressing change or if a child is uncomfortable. Again, preparing parents for alterations in their sleep patterns is helpful. Having a frank discussion with families about postoperative complications such as dehydration is also helpful. Often parents feel they have failed if their child needs to be readmitted for intravenous fluids. Reassurance that this stage of development is often difficult will help ease their guilt or frustrations.

PRESCHOOLERS

Preschool age children are interested in their environments. They are at the stage at which they want to begin asserting their power. Parents can be taught to use this to their advantage. Rather than asking the child if he wants to a have a Popsicle to help his sore throat, they should ask him or her which flavor he wants, thus promoting the behavior they want and at the same time giving the child some control. They can also pretend to role-play with a stuffed animal or doll, acting as a parent to help promote the wanted behavior.

Creating a chart on which the child can put a sticker when he takes his medication may aid with compliance. The surgeon should assure the parents that good parenting means getting tough to ensure compliance and safety while providing choices when possible.

SCHOOL-AGED CHILDREN

School-aged children enjoy increasing levels of independence. Again, tapping into this will help minimize postoperative complications. The surgeon should offer clear explanations about what is happening to the child's body and how he or she can help. Also, bribery works well — for example, "You can watch TV after you take your medicine."

The surgeon should set attainable goals. To tell the child to drink 1 oz every 30 minutes is easier than putting an 8-oz glass in front of the child and saying, "Drink this by noon." Also, it is reasonable to set limits such as "You can watch only 10 more minutes of TV until you have eaten half of your sandwich." Negotiating daily goals of recovery will help the child feel more in control.

OLDER CHILDREN

Appearance is most important in the minds of preteens and teens. Seeing an ear protruding after middle ear surgery may cause them to become withdrawn or upset. Recognizing the difference between emotional pain and true surgical pain can be difficult. Parents should be instructed to offer honest explanations to their child. Explaining the length of the healing process preoperatively can help avoid unrealistic postoperative expectations.

Encouraging participation in activities with friends and school, when the parent feels the child is ready, may help with recovery. Distractions such as a trip to the mall may take a teen's mind temporarily off emotional or physical discomfort. For the most part, children are resilient; however, every surgeon occasionally will face the child who does not recover as expected. To prevent matters from deteriorating further, a few guidelines can be followed.

- Listen carefully to the parent, who knows his or her child best. If a parent thinks the child is not behaving in the expected way, the surgeon should have the patient come in for an exam. Ultimately, this will save everyone time and help recovery. If a parent is anxious, the child will be anxious too.
- Learn to recognize the unusual. It is not unheard of for a child to become clinically depressed after a tonsillectomy and adenoidectomy. If the surgeon does not know if this is the case, the child should be referred to someone for an evaluation. Trying to ignore the situation will not only anger the parent but could be very detrimental to the child.
- Enlist the child's other specialists for help in areas outside the area of expertise. The endocrinologist who knows the child's diabetic needs is in a far better position to help plan the postoperative diet than the surgeon is.
- Be honest with families. If the surgeon believes the child's behavior is a reflection of the parents' lack of control, he should tell them. However, after that, he should be sure to offer helpful suggestions. Helping the patient's family learn to parent the sick child will increase their satisfaction and assure a safe recovery for the child. A happy parent is a satisfied customer.

CONCLUSIONS

Safe perioperative care depends on communication with families and recognition of childhood developmental stages. Astute practitioners will utilize in their practice those who have expertise in various areas to guide families through the perioperative phase. Preparation of the family with appropriate reading materials and availability of the surgeon and staff to answer questions will provide a smooth transition for the child, parents, and family. The information age has led to the availability of material for patients and families through the Internet. Dr. Robert A. Catania from Brown University Medical School has prepared a Website for gathering information regarding perioperative care. This can be offered to patients at www.preopguide.com.

SUGGESTED READING

Lancaster, K.A. Care of the pediatric patient in ambulatory surgery. *Ambulat. Surg.* 1997, 32(2), 441–455.
Noble, R.R., Micheli, A.J., Hensley, M.A., and McKay, N. Perioperative considerations for the pediatric patient. *Adv. Emerg. Top. Perioperat. Nurs.,* 1997, 32(1), 1–16.
Reid, J.H. Literature review. Preoperative information-giving: an essential element of perioperative practice. *Br. J. Theatre Nurs.,* 1998, 8(6), 27–31.

5 Issues in Anesthesia

Andrew Woods and Steven V. Collins

The mistake itself was not as serious as the failure to catch it.

NASA Review Board opinion on the failure of a contractor to convert measurements into metric units resulting in the loss of the $125 million Climate Orbitor probe, which incinerated upon entering the Mars atmosphere

CONTENTS

INTRODUCTION

SIZE MATTERS

The rise of the specialty of pediatric anesthesia over the past two decades has been based in part on the recognition by surgeons who provide care for children that *size matters*. This awareness was the result of the individual and cumulative experiences of surgeons observing complications in the operating room (OR) resulting from the interaction of anesthetic agents, anesthetic equipment, anesthesiologists, and small patients. What was most dramatic was the seemingly exponential increase in complications in inverse relationship to the size of the patient.

ENTER MODERN ANESTHETIC TECHNOLOGY

In the field of otolaryngology, the great Dr. Chevalier Jackson (1844–1945) revolutionized a specialty in which the intraoperative mortality for one procedure (airway foreign body removal in children) approached 25%. Dr. Jackson quickly recognized that general anesthesia (ether, in his day) in a toddler with an airway foreign body was often lethal. For half a century, Jackson and the physicians whom he trained and influenced avoided using general anesthesia in children. He was skillful in the use of topical local anesthesia and judicious morphine sedation (which provided some analgesia as well as depression of airway reflexes), plus several strong orderlies. Arguably, Jackson's greatest accomplishments were in designing anatomically appropriate endoscopic equipment customized for adults and children and the development of teachable technical skills to minimize the duration and morbidity of airway trespass.

INFANTS FEEL PAIN, TOO

Compared with Jackson, surgeons in other disciplines took a somewhat more barbaric approach to the problems associated with general anesthesia in children. As recently as 1980, infants underwent chest surgery at major medical centers in the United States with pancuronium, fentanyl, and oxygen for anesthesia.[1] Pancuronium is a long-acting muscle relaxant that paralyzes the patient without any depression of consciousness or suppression of pain. This is the nightmare of many an adult patient ("Will I be awake and unable to let you know it?"), and it was knowingly inflicted on babies.

This was not done out of malice, of course, but was a result of the legacy of the complications associated with general anesthetics and potent analgesics in infants. Surgeons, anesthesiologists, and neonatologists of this earlier era had convinced each other, their students, and nurses that babies did not really feel pain. Fortunately, investigations that established the fact that newborns and infants feel pain occurred at a time when advances in technology, pharmacology, and the understanding of neonatal physiology allowed for a much greater margin of safety in the administration of general anesthesia in the OR and reasonable analgesia in the postoperative period.

ENTER MODERN TECHNOLOGY

There is a fault line in the surgical specialties between physicians who trained before mid-1980 and those whose training was predominantly after this time. It is defined by the introduction of the pulse oximeter into clinical practice; nowhere was the impact felt more than in pediatric airway cases. Prior to oximetry use, a "STAT" page to an OR where one encountered a cyanotic and severely bradycardic infant was routine (i.e., at least once or twice a week in a busy pediatric operating suite). The best that can be said for this experience is that at least some anesthesia residents finally learned that the initial treatment for severe cyanosis with profound bradycardia was not atropine but an airway, oxygen, ventilation, epinephrine, and, if needed, chest compressions.

Otolaryngologists who trained prior to the introduction of oximetry have a collective awareness of how rapidly disaster can strike. The newer generation of pediatric otolaryngologists benefit from working with predominantly skilled anesthesia practitioners using modern monitoring devices and modern anesthetic equipment. What was previously life-threatening has become routine. The problem with this is that it breeds complacency and lowered vigilance, and it encourages less experienced practitioners (surgeons and anesthesiologists alike) to undertake ever challenging procedures. In this situation, the likelihood of significant complications increases.[2]

CHILDREN ARE DIFFERENT

Over the past two decades, the rate of perioperative complications related to pediatric anesthesia has decreased significantly. What has allowed this great safety advance? The simple answer is recognition of the cliché that "children are different." For many, this conjures up images of developmental stages and emotional issues; however, it is matters of size and physiology that primarily bear upon the increased potential for life-threatening complications. Survival of the human organism depends upon the movement of fluids and gases through tubes. The main fluid is blood (containing oxygen) and the main gas is air (containing oxygen). The main tubes are those of the circulatory system and the airway. Choreographing these flows in order to exchanges gases (oxygen and carbon dioxide) between the blood and air (ventilation/perfusion matching) is the dance of life for each individual being. Anesthesia — local, regional, and general — and surgery can disrupt this dance. It is the goal of this chapter to help all members of the otolaryngology team understand the basis of and setting for many of the complications potentially arising in their patients undergoing anesthesia.

NEONATAL, INFANT, AND CHILD HEMODYNAMIC PHYSIOLOGY

FETAL CIRCULATION

Although this text does not contemplate fetal surgery, an understanding of fetal hemodynamic physiology is important because perioperative events can alter newborn and infant hemodynamics; one of the possible consequences is a reversion to the pattern of fetal circulation.

In utero, the fetus lives in a low-oxygen environment, but with several structural modifications to optimize oxygen delivery to vital organs. Oxygenated blood from the placenta (poorly saturated) returns to the right atrium but mostly bypasses the right ventricle by traversing the foramen ovale into the left atrium. The foramen ovale is a normal and necessary unidirectional pathway between the two fetal atria, an *in utero* "atrial septal defect." From the left atrium, the blood enters the left ventricle and is ejected via the aorta primarily to the cerebral circulation. There is avid uptake of available oxygen by the fetal brain, and the blood that traverses the fetal cerebral circulation returns to the right heart very desaturated. As opposed to partially oxygenated blood from the placenta, the deoxygenated blood from the head and upper body preferentially enters the right ventricle and is ejected into the pulmonary artery. However, pulmonary artery blood flow to the lung is of no benefit in terms of oxygenation *in utero*.

Thus, in the fetus, there is a tubular connection between the pulmonary artery and the descending aorta, the ductus arteriosus, roughly at the level of the left subclavian artery. Because the in utero pulmonary arterial pressures in the fluid-filled lung are higher than the pressures in the aorta, blood bypasses the lung, enters the aorta, and is pumped to the lower body and the placenta for waste elimination and reoxygenation.

NEWBORN CIRCULATION

The ductus arteriosus and the foramen ovale normally close in the immediate newborn period as soon as left-sided (systemic) pressures exceed right-sided (pulmonary) pressures; delayed closure may be noted from 3 months to 1 year. If the ductus arteriosus remains open or reopens (a common condition in premature infants), then the higher pressure in the neonatal aorta relative to the pressures in the pulmonary arteries results in a left-to-right shunt. Blood ejected from the left ventricle traverses the aortic arch and then a portion of it enters the pulmonary circulation via the patent ductus arteriosus (PDA). The ratio of the total blood flow through the pulmonary circulation compared with systemic blood flow may easily be on the order of 4:1 with a large PDA. In spite of the pulmonary congestion and internal hemodynamic derangements that are occurring, newborns with a PDA are typically not cyanotic and may not appear compromised.

The clinical significance of these two fetal pathways is that in situations in which right-side pressures exceed left-side pressures, neonates are at risk for reversal of blood flow and right-to-left shunting, which causes hypoxia and cyanosis. The main factors that contribute to this situation are systemic hypotension and pulmonary hypertension. The former can reflect excessive blood loss, anesthetic overdose, drug reactions, or obstruction of blood return to the heart (e.g., tension pneumothorax). The latter, pulmonary hypertension, is most commonly caused by hypercarbia, hypoxia, and protective airway reflexes. Thus, the maintenance of adequate gas exchange and circulatory stability is much more critical in the newborn than in older patients in whom these fetal pathways are no longer present.

NEWBORN AND INFANT BLOOD VOLUME AND BLOOD PRESSURE

Two items of critical importance in the cardiovascular physiology of newborns are blood volume and blood pressure. Relative to body weight, small premature infants have blood volumes of greater than 100 ml/kg, whereas term infants normally have blood volumes in the range of 85 ml/kg. However, this can be a highly variable factor due to the degree of placenta-to-neonate transfusion at birth. Blood volume as a percent of body weight decreases from newborn levels to 75 to 80 mg/kg by the age of 3 months — values slightly higher than those applicable to adults (70 mg/kg). "Knowing" blood volume (based on age-related estimates) and hemoglobin concentration (from laboratory measurement) allows one to estimate the red blood cell mass in a patient; maintaining an adequate red blood cell mass is essential for maintaining adequate tissue oxygenation.

For an extremely premature newborn (24-week gestation), a systolic blood pressure of 40 to 45 mmHg is considered normal. "Healthy" premature infants at 30 weeks' gestation have systolic blood pressures of 46 to 50 mmHg. A full-term infant should have a blood pressure of 60/40 to 65/55 mmHg.[3,4] Blood pressure steadily increases over the first several months of life and then plateaus at a systolic pressure of approximately 90 to 100 mmHg until puberty, at which time it increases modestly to adult levels.

Hemoglobin Concentration

By 3 to 12 months of age, the circulatory, respiratory, renal, and hepatobiliary systems are all functioning at levels that relative to body mass are not dissimilar to adult values. One major system that does not follow a similar maturation pattern is the hematopoetic system. Newborns have an average hematocrit value of 54% (hemoglobin concentration of approximately 18 g/dl). Hemoglobin concentration decreases rapidly after birth; in sick or premature newborns, the rate of decrease is compounded by iatrogenic blood sampling in the modern neonatal intensive care unit. In normal infants, the physiologic nadir of hemoglobin concentration (10 to 12 g/dl) occurs at approximately 3 months of life; by 6 months of age the hemoglobin concentration is usually increasing and reaches adult concentrations (14 to 16 g/dl) by 1 year of age.

Red Blood Cell Volume: Surgical Concerns

These values have obvious implications for blood loss during surgery. The more severe the degree of anemia (red cell mass as a percentage of total blood volume) in a child undergoing a given procedure, particularly one associated with expected significant blood loss, the greater the likelihood that a blood transfusion will be required. The risk of fatal transfusion errors and infectious complications (contamination, undetected or unknown viruses) will not likely disappear. As head and neck experts, pediatric otolaryngologists should be tuned in to pulling down the lower eyelid to observe the conjunctiva of patients in the clinic. Pale rather than pink tissue should alert one to the possibility of occult anemia. The earlier the diagnosis of the anemia is made and treatment instituted (most often supplemental iron therapy), the more likely the child is to have an adequate volume of red blood cells at the time of surgery. There is no magic number in terms of hematocrit in pediatric patients. Rheology studies indicate that optimal blood flow occurs at a hematocrit value of 30%; however, such studies have little consequence during major bleeding. Optimal or adequate hematocrit values must be always viewed in the context of the procedure, the patient, and what is likely to happen next.

AIRWAY SIZE AND PHYSICS

LAMINAR AND TURBULENT AIRFLOW

Normal flow of air through the airways is laminar. Laminar airflow is silent and proportional to the fourth power of the radius of the tube. Thus, a small decrease in airway caliber causes a dramatic decrease in airflow, at constant pressures. Under laminar flow conditions, flow and pressure are linearly related; that is, once the resistance is determined at a given pressure (by the radius and length of the tube plus the viscosity of the gases flowing through the tube), a twofold increase in that pressure produces a twofold increase in flow (within the limits of the system). In contrast, the disordered state of turbulent airflow exhibits an exponential rather than linear relationship between resistance and flow rate.

ENDOTRACHEAL TUBES AND AIRFLOW

The size of the internal diameter (ID) of endotracheal tube becomes increasingly significant as the size of the patient's trachea becomes smaller. This is because the increase in airflow resistance with a change from a 3.5-mm tube to a 3.0-mm tube is 50%. The smallest endotracheal tube has an internal diameter of 2 mm. This and the 2.5-mm tube are particularly at risk for partial or total occlusion by airway secretions, dried blood, foreign body, or kinking. Small tubes are also the most difficult in terms of passage and function of a suction catheter. Decreasing the length of the tube by cutting off a portion of the proximal end can produce a linear decrease in resistance (Note: never cut the distal end, thereby producing a sharp edge). Particularly with small, thin-walled tubes, the shorter the space is between the point where the tube is anchored to the patient (usually by tape) and the 15-mm connector, the less tolerance there is for changes in positioning of the anesthesia circuit.

BRONCHOSCOPE AND TELESCOPE COMPATIBILITY

With the first generation of modern neonatal bronchoscopes, an imbalance between the rod-lens telescope and bronchoscope sheath existed, especially in the smallest bronchoscopes. The internal diameter of the neonatal bronchoscope (3.2 mm) did not match up well with the provided 2.8-mm telescope.[5,6] When these instruments were used together in neonates, high inspiratory pressures were required to overcome the extremely high resistance of the system.

The small breathing bag on the anesthesia circuit is capable of delivering such pressure. However, the anesthetized neonate is not able to generate correspondingly high pressures for expiration, and this was even more pronounced in the presence of neuromuscular paralysis, during which lung emptying is purely a function of passive recoil of the chest wall and diaphragm. If one is unaware of these high-resistance situations, "stacking" of respirations can occur and intrathoracic pressures may increase dramatically. This increased intrathoracic pressure impedes blood return to the heart and increases the risk for pneumothorax. In such situations, unless the obstructing telescope is removed promptly and effective ventilation and circulation are reestablished, hypoxia, bradycardia, and cardiac arrest can occur.

The resistance profile for the smallest pediatric bronchoscope (4.9 mm ID) and the telescope initially provided for it (4.0 mm ID) was also suboptimal, but not to the degree seen in the neonatal bronchoscopes. Now, 1.9 mm "neonatal" and 2.8 mm "pediatric" telescopes are available that have much better resistance profiles for use with the appropriate neonatal and pediatric bronchoscopes,[5,7] However, the use of additional instruments that partially obstruct the narrow lumen between the telescope and the bronchoscope sheath must always increase one's alertness for expiratory obstruction. As a general rule, one should increase the time allowed for expiration during infant bronchoscopy and remove the telescope whenever possible; monitoring the patient with pulse oximetry and capnography (for CO_2 assessment) during the procedure is now considered standard of care.

"SILENT" AIRWAY OBSTRUCTION DURING BRONCHOSCOPY

Partial airway obstruction in the noninstrumented airway is almost always associated with turbulent flow and a characteristic noise is produced, such as stridor, stertor, rhonchi, or wheezes. However, during infant and child bronchoscopy, partial airway obstruction is usually silent. Most airway sounds are caused by the rapid opening and closing of some segment of the airway in response to rapidly changing pressure relationships on both sides of the airway wall. It is important, therefore, to remember that the rigid metal bronchoscope does not permit such "snapping" and "popping" even though the degree of partial airway obstruction may be severe.

THE NATURE OF ANESTHETIC COMPLICATIONS

Most significant physical complications in pediatric otolaryngology involve airway compromise of some variety, and for the injured it is irrelevant whether the fault lies mainly with the anesthesiologist or the surgeon. The study of anesthetic accidents reveals much similarity to aviation disasters; almost always a series of mistakes and misjudgments occur. When both the surgeon and the anesthesiologist (1) understand the changing nature of airflow dynamics and the effects of size and instrumentation and (2) share this knowledge in a reciprocal manner, continually assessing and reassessing the clinical assumptions of a case in light of the clinical realities as a *standard of practice,* there is the likelihood that the series of errors and misjudgments will be interrupted and corrected.

EMOTIONAL COMPLICATIONS

A practical discussion of complications related to the surgical experience can begin by acknowledging, in addition to physical complications, the potential for significance *emotional* complications as well. These include excess fear, emotional trauma, and postoperative issues such as night terrors, the concerns that *machismo* physicians are most likely to disregard. While physical complications are most often the result of inexperience with the specific situation one is encountering, emotional complications are usually the result of the failure by the responsible medical providers to communicate and execute competence, compassion, and concern.

Preoperative Issues

We Ignore What We Do Not Understand

The subject of emotional complications related to anesthesia and surgery in children is complex and largely subjective because of lack of measuring tools to assess the short- and long-term impact of these events. Adult psychiatry literature and clinical experience reveal that vast numbers of adults had traumatic experiences with *ether* anesthesia. During the ether era, tonsillectomy was the most frequent reason for an inhalational anesthetic induction in a child. Ether was very slow in onset and very pungent, and the induction was typically accomplished by mask-wearing strangers who had taken the child from the arms of terrified parents. How does one assess the long-term impact of a child feeling abandoned to strangers by his parents and of carrying that experience as a conscious and subconscious memory throughout his life? As in many areas of medicine, that which cannot be measured or understood is often ignored.

Pay Attention to Nonverbal Cues and Clues

A child's encounter with the medical system is an area in which a great amount of nonverbal communication takes place among providers, parents, and patient. The child, seemingly engrossed in play, is taking cues from the parents' behavior and level of anxiety. Most parents are seeking the answer to one question, "Can I entrust you with my life's treasure?" The way in which one deals with this seemingly casual but incredibly charged interchange cannot be found in a recipe book; there is no single best approach. It is essential to pay attention to, and search for, emotional clues.

Deliver Essential Information Thoughtfully and Carefully

A child who has a terrifying interaction as part of the operative experience has experienced a significant complication. It is downplayed by the medical system, but not by the parents. Equally, it can be argued that a child who has an experience that violates the standards of family expectation has not received optimal care.

For example, seeing an "intoxicated" child disinhibited by midazolam premedication disturbs a small segment of parents. These are typically people whose religions have strong proscriptions against alcoholic beverages. Similarly, seeing an intoxicated child may not be at all humorous to a mother who was beaten or assaulted as a child by a drunken parent or relative. Explaining the expected effects of midazolam should help reduce any concern from the parents, and descriptors such as "drunk" should be avoided.

A more complex and more crucial interaction is how one deals with the situation in which the patient's parents are Jehovah's Witnesses who are opposed to blood transfusion. It is well established legally that parents do *not* have a right to refuse a blood transfusion for their minor child in a life-threatening situation. However, violation of a deep religious tenet may have significant implications for the treatment of the child once he or she returns to the community. Again, it is a potential emotional complication for which the medical system does not often accept direct responsibility as it does for a physical complication such as a laser burn to the face. This is a situation in which a hurried preoperative discussion with parents in front of a young child is almost guaranteed to increase the anxiety level of the child and does a disservice to all.

One policy to consider in Jehovah's Witness cases gives prime consideration to the emotional maturity of the patient rather than to his chronological age. For children who lack the capacity to make informed and noncoerced choices regarding life and death issues, it is critical to validate the integrity of the parents' religious conviction. This almost always requires a long conversation, but the end result is that the parents do consent by written acknowledgment that they understand that specific blood products may be administered at the point beyond which their child will die if immediate intervention is not provided. Also, the parents, surgeon, and anesthesiologist can make agreements about aborting surgery if bleeding becomes unexpectedly excessive. In all cases, one assures the family that the medical team will endeavor to work as hard as possible to maintain utmost respect for their religious convictions within the limits of the physical safety of their child. Having done this, the OR team must perform in a manner consistent with this agreement.

Presenting Oneself as a Competent and Caring Physician

Although specific techniques of premedication and induction of anesthesia are important, possible adverse emotional reactions are minimized by presenting oneself as a competent and caring physician — a role difficult to impersonate consistently if either facet is truly lacking. This professional presentation, over time, creates trust among members of the operative team; parents and patients sense this trust. Although in some instances the physical safety of the child will dictate the approach taken, in most cases the choices reflect more mundane factors such as "local customs," drug costs, and prior training of the anesthesiologist.

Experience and prior training will affect the projection of caring and competency. A physician recently out of a residency program in which parents were never allowed to be present during pediatric inductions will need mentoring to become comfortable beginning this practice. It can be a difficult adjustment for even a senior anesthesiologist at a new hospital replete with different monitors and new supply routes. On the other hand, the experienced anesthesiologist who has commonly had parents present at the beginning of pediatric inductions will be more likely to identify the terrified parent who may make the situation worse for the child and therefore to choose a different course of action.

Premedication: Assessment

The majority of young pediatric patients receive some type of premedication prior to induction of anesthesia. The need for such drugs, however, is variable and relates mainly to age and developmental stage.

- *Infants under the age of six months.* Infants, in general, have minimal stranger anxiety and will readily separate from a parent or caretaker and accompany the anesthesiologist to the OR. If this assumption is wrong, it is immediately obvious and the plan can be modified.
- *Toddlers* and *preschool children.* Once a child develops stranger anxiety at around six months of age, a normal developmental milestone, fear of parental separation is the greatest concern. There are also age-specific fears and anxieties that can often be elicited in conversations with the parents or the child. A child's imagination has no limits during this age and cannot be argued with, only acknowledged and responding with information that lets the child know that the threat will be taken care of during surgery. An example of this was a fearful (despite midazolam) 3-year-old girl who, prior to be anesthetized for surgery, related her greatest fear: a tiger might escape from the Washington, D.C. zoo (100 miles away) and find her and kill her. The various and extensive security systems that our hospital has to prevent such an event were explained, and her fearfulness receive some These issues persist until the age of reason and this is the age group in which oral midazolam has had to greatest impact.
- *School-aged children.* This period involves the major developmental task of differentiating self from non-self, particularly the parent. Children in this age range develop fears of death or bodily dismemberment. Some may have had an experience with an elderly relative who was hospitalized and died, a loss followed by much parental grief and distraction. Others may have a friend who relates horror stories, real or not, regarding a hospital experience. Premedication in these children is
- *Adolescents.* As children approach puberty (girls earlier than boys) they move into a phase where they are hyperfocused on their own bodies, especially at the time that changes are occurring in the sexual parts. Once this focus begins, it steadily increases into the teenage years. The fear of having their naked bodies exposed to the eyes of strangers is profound for many children and teenagers and, as a group, young girls who are menstruating (very likely in the 10- to 12-year-old age range) tend to be the most distressed. Fortunately vast majority of otolaryngological patients do not require total bodily exposure and can be assured that this will not happen. In particular, they do not need to have their underwear or panties removed and then returned to them afterwards in a clear plastic "baggie"; standard OR protocols that require this should be reevaluated. Addressing this issue, even with those too embarrassed to admit it is a concern, conveys a great deal of understanding and concern on behalf of the surgical team. In this age group, premedication may be helpful but the quality of personal interaction is usually more important, and will be the factor most remembered in making the experience less stressful than expected.

Premedication: Agents and Techniques
Oral/Nasal Premedication

- *Midazalom.* Remarkable anxiolysis and antegrade amnesia can be predictably obtained using oral midazolam (0.5 to .75 mg/kg) in most children if they actually drink all the medication and enough time is allowed (at least 20 minutes to peak effect) before attempted separation or induction. Newer formulations of midazolam have made it less bitter than the original and the medicine taste is easier to disguise. However, medication with original midazolam (an intravenous preparation used orally) mixed in Syrpalta syrup yields more reliable sedation and correspondingly higher plasma levels than an equivalent dose of the commercially formulated and marketed preparation.[6] A few children will refuse to drink anything offered and the effort is often not worth the reward. Intranasal midazolam is commercially available as a concentrated spray as is equally as effective as oral dosing. With midazolam by any route at an anxiolytic dose, the duration of effect is usually not going to last 45 minutes, so appropriate timing is necessary.

- *Fentanyl.* Oral transmucosal fentanyl (OTF) as a lollipop (sweetened solid matrix on a stick) to be sucked and not chewed has been available in the U.S. for over a decade. It has seen limited use, despite proven efficacy in terms of anxiolysis plus significant *analgesia* (not present with midazolam) lasting several hours, in part because it is associated with a significant incidence of *preoperative* nausea and vomiting. This is a side effect of all opiates, is centrally mediated, and is increased by patient motion; no anti-emetic drug has a proven and consistent beneficial effect in such situations. However, selected candidates, particularly non-ambulatory children (i.e., lying still on a bed), may benefit from oral fentanyl, especially if they refuse oral midazolam and sedation is deemed essential. Its speed of onset is similar to that of midazalom but it is a potent respiratory depressant and must be used properly, with reduced dosages in children with impaired liver function.

    In terms of risk/benefit ratios, the likelihood of efficacy approaches 90% and the likelihood of *no vomiting* is about 80%, so there is roughly a 70% chance of an overall successful premedication experience as opposed to about 85% when midazolam is used. Thus, both of these drugs have their place.

- *Tramadol.* Tramadol is an atypical opioid structurally related to codeine that can be viewed as a "partial" opiate. Unfortunately, while it has less respiratory depression than equipotent doses of other opiates, it has the same incidence of nausea and vomiting and is very slow in onset (several hours to peak effect). This is not an ideal profile in children presenting for surgery.

- *Mixtures.* The issue of the use of fentanyl and midazolam has significance for many, many physicians who, until a few years ago, had very little knowledge of these drugs. Now, these drugs are routinely used together in settings all over the hospital and in free-standing clinics—rarely at the hands of an anesthesiologist. The range of use extends from flexible bronchoscopy in the clinic to drainage of a peritonsillar abscess in the ER. Using the right amount of these drugs and obtaining a cooperative child can provide the difference between a smooth rapid procedure and a "thrash." Using too much of these drugs will produce respiratory depression and bradycardia, a potentially lethal combination that is as synergistic on the downside as it is the upside. It is for these reasons that conscious sedation has become a key phrase in almost every hospital in America. The cardinal principle in the use of these drugs is that a person performing a procedure cannot be an appropriate monitor of patient well-being and a person dedicated to that task must be continuous present and documenting vital signs.

- *Intravenous Premedication.* In children with intravenous catheters in place, fentanyl and midazolam alone or in combination provide excellent IV premedication for the OR but carry the same risks as discussed in the previous paragraph, only more rapidly. Fentanyl both slows the heart rate and decreases minute ventilation, as do all narcotics. These two factors, when combined, provide less tissue oxygen delivery and these patients are frequently on the edge of hypoxemia and need to be stimulated and given supplemental oxygen, if not already in use. The additional use of midazolam, which does not have any significant cardiorespiratory effects as usual dosage, enhances the degree of CNS depression and thus these drugs must be respected. Continuous monitoring in such situations is standard of care and airway support/oxygen must be readily available.

Induction of General Anesthesia

The transition from an awake to anesthetized patient carries its own unique set of emotional consequences involving the physician-parent and physician-patient interactions, *plus* the additional risks of serious physical injury that will be discussed in the next section. The emotional issues can be affected by events at all stages of the procedure, from premedication (if any) to induction of anesthesia to emergence, the recovery room and beyond.

Inhalational Induction

The least emotionally traumatic inhalation induction in toddlers and preschool children most likely occurs when (1) the anesthesiologist has taken time to establish rapport with the child and family; (2) a calm and informed parent who understands the upcoming events is present; and (3) the "act" is fast, which requires that the anesthesia circuit be washed out and "primed" with a high anesthetic concentration and that, as soon as the mask contacts the child's face, it stays there with a seal maintained. If this is done, the child will be induced within a few breaths and presumably will have less ability to process the events and store them as a permanent memory.[10] This idea is supported anecdotally by the decrease in traumatic inductions that followed the transition from ether to the more rapid halothane. One can assume that the same benefit of a faster induction will accrue to the patients receiving high concentrations of sevoflurane rather than incremental halothane.

The one variable that cannot be adequately assessed in advance, however, is the emotional response of the parent prior to entering the alien environment of an operation room or an induction room. Thus, someone must always be available to become a caretaker for the parent who faints or otherwise is incapacitated emotionally at a critical juncture during an anesthetic induction.

Intravenous Induction

For school-aged children, it is appropriate to offer the option of an intravenous induction as opposed to use of a mask. Most children of this age are still "needle averse," but many institutions have integrated the use of EMLA cream (eutectic mixture of local anesthetics — lidocaine, prilocaine) into their preoperative regimen. Prior application of EMLA cream under an occlusive dressing 45 to 60 minutes or more before needle insertion will provide an anesthetized area and a painless procedure. Using a mild abrasive to remove the stratum corneum layer of the skin before topical application improves the anesthesia. It is common to place an EMLA patch on two separate sites. For older children it is often a "badge of courage" to be able to have an intravenous catheter placed before surgery; the ability to accomplish this without pain and tears represents a significant medical advance.

Intravenous propofol is associated with pain on injection. This may be minimized with the addition of lidocaine and totally eliminated by injecting into a central venous line or a large antecubital vessel with good blood flow. Intravenous, or intramuscular, induction with ketamine is still routine in many parts of the world due to the low cost of this drug. Ketamine is a dissociative agent and the brain does not "go to sleep." The central nervous system stays very active. Hallucinations are not infrequent and may persist for several hours after emergence; this can be minimized with the concurrent administration of a benzodiazapene. In North America, ketamine injection is selectively utilized by some clinicians in uncooperative patients without an adequate intravenous catheter in place.

Until recently, ketamine for clinical use was a racemic mixture. Now, the S(+) enantiomer of ketamine, with greater analgesic and anesthetic potency and fewer side effects than the R enantiomer, is available in Europe. In cases of hypotensive patients presenting for emergency procedures, etomidate has replaced ketamine as the induction agent of choice because ketamine in the failing heart may further impair contractility.[11]

Emergence

For many children, emergence is the worst part of the surgical experience. Some experience a pervasive sense of ill-being. They are in an altered state, sometimes described as being underwater and struggling to get to the top. They are in an unfamiliar place and can hear voices, but the words are not focused or recognizable. Nausea and possibly vomiting may occur. There may be pain and there is no clear understanding of when and how the suffering will be relieved.

There is a growing awareness of emergence agitation, particularly in preschool-aged children. In this age range, it may be difficult to distinguish between surgical pain and emotional distress. If analgesia is adequate during emergence, then agitation appears to be a function of the speed of emergence from inhalational anesthesia; however, agitation is not seen with the equally rapid emergence from the intravenous agent propofol, used in combination with a narcotic. With short, minimally invasive cases, oral premedication with midazolam,[12] intranasal fentanyl,[13,14] and intravenous ketorolac[15] are among the medications reported to be of benefit in ameliorating emergence agitation.

An adage holds that pediatric patients often "awaken in a similar manner to the way in which they went to sleep" during induction. A group of boys aged 3 to 6 years, anesthetized with halothane, were studied: of 27 boys who were judged to be anxious at induction, 20 had problematic behavior upon emergence; of 79 boys judged calm at induction, only 5 had emergence behavioral problems.[16] Studies that find sevoflurane to have a higher incidence of emergence agitation than halothane may be biased in that the anesthesiologist is rarely blinded to the agent given. Halothane does have a slower onset and requires more time and effort to achieve a calm child — a significant variable to be taken into consideration. However, the agitation is very transient and probably of minimal consequence.

Postoperative Nausea and Vomiting

Nausea and vomiting are, in many cases, more distressing than pain. Postoperative nausea is a pervasive, nonlocalized experience that is probably the most common major "complication" of surgery reported by patients to their anesthesiologist on subsequent surgical encounters. Postoperative nausea and vomiting (PONV) have come under better control because of increased efficacy of prophylactic antiemetic therapy. The oral agent, granisetron, and the intravenous agent, ondansetron, have been shown to be effective in decreasing PONV in high-risk children undergoing tonsillectomies.[17] Concomitant use of nitrous oxide may increase the risk of PONV, possibly due to distension of air pockets within the stomach. Procedures in which blood may be swallowed, such as tonsillectomy or adenoidectomy, have a higher incidence of early PONV that is not affected by gastric suctioning at the end of the case, in part due to the lack of efficacy of standard techniques for gastric suction.

An interesting report from England describes an outpatient protocol that includes strict controls on medications: patients are premedicated with ondansetron and postoperatively receive acetaminophen or a nonsteroidal anti-inflammatory agent within 1 hour and then regularly every 6 hours for a week.[18] Morphine is specifically avoided. Tonsillectomy cases in children are done using a laryngeal mask airway rather than an uncuffed tube because the laryngeal mask has been shown to better prevent blood from entering the esophagus.[19] In a series of over 500 tonsillectomy patients, the rate of PONV averaged 8%. Similar results were seen in children undergoing a wide range of ambulatory surgical procedures; use of rectal acetaminophen at doses of 40 and 60 mg/kg resulted in a decreased need for morphine and less PONV.[20]

One can expect that better antiemetic drugs that can selectively block the emetic effects of potent opioids will become available. Until that time, it must be recognized that a trade-off exists between pain and PONV.

Physical Complications

The key to avoiding anesthetic complications in pediatric otolaryngology is to know at all times what is going on with the procedure, the equipment, and the patient.

Monitoring Devices

Monitors are machines. Patients are people. One must understand what the monitor is actually measuring and realize that the small airway dimensions of infants make them highly susceptible to physiologic variables that in larger children and adults may be clinically inconsequential. Every significant change in a monitor value warrants an immediate mental reaction that asks, "How is the patient?" and not, "Is there something amiss with the monitor?" This involves a rapid reassessment of the patient's color and perfusion status, the activities of the surgeon, the values from other monitors, the integrity of the circuits, etc. Good patient monitoring in the OR is a continual process of integrating data derived from clinical assessment and data derived from monitors. Acting on ominous but erroneous data can in some cases be as disastrous as failing to act in the belief that "the monitor is wrong" when, in fact, the patient has a critical problem.

Pulse Oximetry

All standard pulse oximeters work on a principle that involves shining two light beams through tissue at a target sensor. There is a difference in light absorption between saturated and desaturated hemoglobin and, when this difference is measured, the oximeter is able to use standard nomograms to estimate arterial oxygen saturation.

The fatal mistake associated with use of pulse oximetry is to assume that it equates oxygen saturation with cardiac output. Pulsatile pressure under the sensor can produce "normal" oxygen saturation in the face of minimal forward blood flow. Likewise, a baby can slowly exsanguinate and yet have "normal" oxygen saturation until shortly before cardiac arrest. If one were to draw an arterial blood gas at this time, however, one would find a profound metabolic acidosis and, if blood pressure has been maintained with crystalloid, severe anemia.

In addition to data on oxygen saturation and heart rate, the oximeter may display a plethysmograph that gives insight into stroke volume. The oximeter software can increase the scale of the display as the patient's pulse volume amplitude decreases with decreases in stroke volume; these scale changes are visible when they occur. Repeated scale changes after a period of stability should alert one to the possibility of progressive impairment of cardiac output, which can occur with occult bleeding.

A new type of pulse oximeter probe design is much less susceptible to the artifacts of motion and light that limited earlier oximeter probes.[21,22] Thus, one can expect the credence given to abnormal sounds from the pulse oximeter in the OR, the postanesthesia care unit (PACU), and the ICU to increase.

End-Tidal CO_2

The presence of an end-tidal CO_2 waveform has become the gold standard for verification of endotracheal intubation. However, immediately following intubation of the trachea, there are numerous causes for absent CO_2 measurements, including machine failure and compression or obstruction of the gas sampling tube by someone or something. Absent CO_2 may also result from markedly diminished cardiac output. If the endotracheal tube has been seen to pass through the vocal folds, the chest is moving, breath sounds are appropriate and adequate, and the patient has a good pulse and color, the "crisis" event is most likely not related to the airway. Nonetheless, it is considered good technique to verify the end-tidal CO_2 waveform before proceeding.

The main information one can reliably derive from capnography is that CO_2 is being produced and delivered to the airway; thus, it is a cardiorespiratory monitor of vital importance. The shape and trend of the CO_2 waveform can provide parts of an overall picture of assessment of patient status. A steadily decreasing end-tidal CO_2 observed on the capnograph is most commonly due to overventilation by the anesthesiologist, intentionally or otherwise. Of much greater concern, the same data can reflect hemorrhage and increased dead space ventilation resulting from decreased pulmonary perfusion.[23] A failure of complication recognition arises when one assumes hyperventilation as the cause of a low expired CO_2 and, thus, decreases ventilation, rather than anticipating a hypotensive crisis looming ahead and beginning corrective measures.

A decrease in the slope of the CO_2 upstroke is suggestive of restricted airflow, which can occur in bronchospasm or endotracheal tube partial obstruction. However, this same decrease can also occur with impaired cardiac performance from inadequate volume, excessive anesthesia, or citrate toxicity from rapid blood transfusion.

An animated Web site, <http://www.capnography.com>, contains a wealth of information on the use of capnography.

End-Tidal Nitrogen

Nitrogen monitoring technology is more demanding and, thus, more costly than that associated with most other gas monitoring. Its usefulness is not in question, only its cost/benefit ratio. The presence of a nitrogen spike in a patient breathing enriched oxygen, in which the nitrogen is usually 50% or lower, is indicative of room air reaching the lung. This can happen in three ways:

- A partial or total circuit disconnect
- In a spontaneously breathing patient, entrained air around an endotracheal tube, especially one that is kinked or clogged
- An air embolus from air entrainment from a surgical site or air injected through an intravascular catheter

In cases in which the head is elevated relative to the heart, such as in many head and neck procedures, nitrogen monitoring may alert the anesthesiology team to entrained air accumulating in the pulmonary artery.[24]

Anesthetic Gas Monitoring

Modern anesthetic monitoring systems allow for precise measurement of the concentration of anesthetic gases in inspired and expired gases. However, neither of these truly measures the partial pressure of the gas in the brain, which is what really determines the effect of anesthetic gases. Thus, sophisticated gas monitors have in no way replaced continual monitoring of vital signs and general clinical assessment.

EEG Bispectrum Index

EEG bispectrum index (BIS) is a new technology that is used to assess anesthetic depth and has been marketed as a tool to avoid patient awareness. It has not been standardized for infants and children and is not yet of proven usefulness in this population.[25,26] However, one can expect that the use of such monitors to titrate anesthetic depth more accurately will be strongly marketed to allow more efficient OR utilization.

ANESTHETIC TECHNIQUE IN SHARED AIRWAY CASES

Apneic Oxygenation and Intermittent Ventilation

Even in the absence of ventilation, oxygenation can be maintained for an extended period in any child (not neonate) with normal lung function and no cardiac impairment, as long as one does an initial nitrogen washout with 100% oxygen and then maintains *a patent airway* and a high concentration of oxygen at the glottic opening by a sealed face mask or LMA (laryngeal mask airway). As oxygen molecules are taken up from the alveoli and delivered to the tissues, additional oxygen molecules will move into the alveoli, by simple diffusion, based on the physical laws governing gases. The level of carbon dioxide in the alveoli and body tissues will rise, rather abruptly at first and then at a rate of about 3 torr/min. If the period of apnea has been preceded by moderate hyperventilation, 15 minutes of apnea would likely not result in a PCO_2 much above 80 torr assuming that a deep plane of general anesthesia (and thus decreased cerebral metabolic oxygen need) was well established prior to the period of apnea.

Respiratory acidosis during airway procedures involving apnea can be lessened to the extent that one interrupts the procedure to permit ventilation and thus CO_2 removal. In most cases, this is accomplished by applying a face mask and giving positive pressure breaths until the expired CO_2 concentration is decreased to a satisfactory level before recommencing with another period of apnea. Brief, rapid ventilation will not do a great deal, compared to slower and more sustained efforts, to reverse respiratory acidosis because it is cardiac output that determines the return of excess CO_2 in tissues to the lungs. Intermittent positive pressure ventilation with a face mask is not practical in cases with relatively long set-up times, such as suspension laryngoscopy procedures.

Infants lack the rigid rib cage structure of older children and also have higher metabolic demands. In the absence of ventilation, alveolar collapse is greater due to the weight of the chest wall and high rates of oxygen uptake. Thus, in neonates, apneic oxygenation is not as effective. Furthermore, with this technique, it is important to be mindful that oxygenation may be rapidly impaired if a suction catheter is extensively used in the airway below the point of oxygen delivery.

Insufflation with Spontaneous Ventilation

An alternative technique for airway procedures involves insufflation of inhalational agents while the patient breathes spontaneously. As unobtrusively as possible, a gas and oxygen mixture is delivered into the hypopharynx to be inhaled by the patient. Airway physics results in the anesthetic gas(es) being greatly diluted by entrained room air. In infants, respiratory mechanics (particularly the compliant chest wall) are such that each breath entrains relatively less room air than in older children and adults, thereby diluting anesthetic gas concentration to a lesser degree. Thus, this technique may be quite useful in infant airway procedures.

In practice, insufflation usually involves initial achievement of a sufficient depth of general anesthesia using a mask and a semiclosed system. Complementary use of intravenous anesthesia is often utilized throughout the procedure. In addition, the anesthetic gas not only is insufflated but also can be directed towards the glottic opening with modified use of metal tracheostomy tubes, metal or plastic endotracheal tubes, or a commercial insufflator channel apparatus. Thus, when the vocal folds open with inspiration, the anesthetic agent is delivered with a modest "driving pressure" behind it.

Insufflation with spontaneous ventilation is the prime anesthetic technique for evaluating vocal fold movement and laryngomalacia. With no tube to obstruct or to support the airway, the dynamic movement of the epiglottis and other laryngeal structures can be assessed during spontaneous breathing. Learning to stay within an appropriate level of anesthesia with this technique takes practice; in children with a significant pulmonary history, such as bronchopulmonary dysplasia, it may be more difficult to maintain an adequate depth of anesthesia and spontaneous respiration. Operation room pollution with anesthetic gas that occurs with this technique can be diminished by placement of a scavaging tube under suction just outside the oral cavity.

Jet Ventilation

Jet ventilation takes advantage of the Venturi principle. A jet injector with a small-diameter nozzle is attached to a high-pressure gas source, usually wall oxygen at 50 pounds per square inch (psi). The injector is intermittently open for brief internals (usually a second or so in small children) with the nozzle directed at or through the glottic opening. The force of the injected gas entrains room air, and one can see the chest wall rise reflecting an appropriate tidal volume if the jet is correctly positioned above the open glottis or in the trachea.

One can sample expired gases by attaching a standard CO_2 sampling tube at the nozzle tip. Compared with a simultaneous $PaCO_2$ on an arterial blood gas sample, end tidal CO_2 measured by capnography during supraglottic jet ventilation has been shown to be about 13 mmHg higher, compared with a difference of 6 mmHg during endotracheal intubation.[27] This difference should be anticipated and overventilation avoided.

Anesthesia during the period of jet ventilation is typically maintained with intravenous anesthesia. Propofol–muscle relaxant–opioid and propofol–remifentanil are typical combinations. Remifentanil (a short-acting opioid) is not a muscle relaxant but, when combined with propofol, is able to produce laryngoscopic and intubating conditions comparable with those provided with neuromuscular blockade, e.g., succinylcholine or rocuronium.[28]

The advantage of jet techniques is that the surgeon can have continued access to the airway, and ventilation can be readily maintained. The greatest danger is the presence of a high-pressure gas source so near the airway.[29] The oxygen exits the jet with a very high pressure but a low mass, so the pressure greatly dissipates within a few millimeters of the tip. During jet ventilation, the position (depth of insertion) of the jet stylet should be monitored continuously by the OR team because catheter migration into the trachea may occur. Jet ventilation should be discontinued the moment chest inflation increases or exhalation decreases. In most cases, a rapid rate of jetting (e.g., 10 to 20 jet pulses/min) is unnecessary. One or two jet pulses per 30 to 60 s may be all that is necessary during the entire procedure.

Subglottic Injectors

If a jet nozzle is introduced into the trachea and contacts the tracheal wall, it can cause mucosal damage by shearing forces. Using a device shaped like a four-leaf clover to keep the injector tube in the middle of the trachea may prevent this occurrence.[30] Moreover, if blockage of egress of air from the trachea is significant, lung hyperinflation and resulting pneumothorax/pneumomediastinum can occur with great rapidity and with potentially fatal consequences. Decompressing a tension pneumothrorax and/or evacuating air from the pericardial sac in a small child in full cardiac arrest will challenge even the best pediatric care providers.

Using subglottic jet techniques in patients with a supraglottic mass is usually avoided because of gas egress concerns and the risk for airway obstruction. A review of this issue by Hunsaker describes a subglottic ventilation system using a fluoroplastic, monitored (CO_2 and airway pressure), self-centering, jet ventilation tube (Ben-jet) driven by an automatic ventilator with a shutdown feature in the event of excessive pressure buildup.[31] Although damaged by a high-energy CO_2 laser beam in a test environment, the type of fluoroplastic tubes used did not continue burning even when the laser was used in 100% oxygen.

Supraglottic Injectors

Supraglottic jet ventilation (SGV) techniques, in which the injector tip remains above the trachea, can still cause problems but rarely as catastrophic as those in which the injector tip is below the glottis. A misdirected tip can cause mucosal damage if in very close contact with tissue. If the tip is directed posterior to the glottic opening it may direct air into the esophagus and stomach; this will produce hypoxemia (no lung ventilation) and hypotension (decreased cardiac return due to massive gastric distension). If unrecognized, it may even result in gastric rupture.[32] Gastric distension by a misdirected injector should never challenge competent pediatric care providers, who should recognize and stop the problem, decompress the stomach, ventilate the patient, and get on with the case.

Supraglottic jet ventilation works poorly in patients with decreased lung compliance; premature neonates with lung disease are rarely candidates for SGV. The supraglottic jet cannot generate high airway pressure, and patients with stiff lungs require high airway pressures for ventilation. Such patients can be ventilated with a jet if the injector is placed deep into the trachea, but this is a high-risk technique in these patients. Another concern with jet ventilation techniques is the potential for seeding the distal airway with papillomata or some other tissue or substance at the glottic inlet. This risk increases as the distance between the jet tip and abnormal tissue decreases.

Adding a second injector nozzle to a jet laryngoscope allows for combined high- and low-frequency supraglottic jet ventilation; pressures are monitored at the distal end of the laryngoscope through a third port and connected by a servo mechanism to the ventilator.[33-35] This technique has been described for use during tubeless laryngotracheal surgery in infants and children; children with tracheal stenosis, who require higher inspiratory pressures, could be ventilated as long as expiratory times were increased.[36] Monitoring expired CO_2 via a sample port at the site where the airway pressure is measured can add one more element of safety to this device. As with all new devices, there should be added caution and a dialogue among experts as these tools are introduced into clinical practice. It must be recognized that inserting a machine into the physician–patient interface always adds the element of risk associated with machine failure.

Percutaneous Transtracheal High-Frequency Jet Ventilation

This technique is fraught with danger and cannot be recommended. In Switzerland, experienced practitioners used this technique in 16 infants and children (28 procedures) with severe upper airway lesions; the report indicated three complications: extensive surgical emphysema, bilateral pneumothorax, and severe vagus-induced cardiovascular depression.[37] This experience underlines the critical nature of delivering high inspiratory pressures into the subglottic airway without a confirmed and continuous route of egress.

EQUIPMENT IN THE AIRWAY

Whose Airway Is It, Anyway?

It is the patient's airway. It is the only one that the patient has, and one in which surgeon and anesthesiologist are trusted guests, expected to exercise nothing but the highest levels of respect for all concerned.

The overwhelming majority of inhalation anesthetics in children are delivered through a mask, a laryngeal device or an orotracheal tube. This is well and good except for certain cases that involve the airway. Many airway cases involve the oral cavity only, and nasotracheal intubation allows unimpeded access to the surgical site. Alternatively, standard orotracheal intubation with a device used by the surgeon to stabilize the tube against the tongue provides access to the oral cavity, oropharynx, and hypopharynx while preventing kinking of the endotracheal tube. However, once the surgical site involves the glottic opening and below, these procedures fall into the category of "shared airway" cases.

Shared airway cases typically "end" in terms of the procedure with the patient at a surgical depth of anesthesia. In contrast, the overwhelming majority of other surgical cases end with the skin being cleaned and dressings being applied, which usually occur at a very light plane of anesthesia. Consequently, short-acting *intravenous* anesthetic agents are increasingly used in shared airway cases to minimize operative times by allowing a surgeon continuous and unimpeded access while minimizing patient emergence and recovery times.

Intubation and Endotracheal Tubes

Size

As a general rule, one would prefer to use the largest endotracheal tube (ETT) that the trachea will permit. This has the benefits of maintaining a more "closed" system, thereby limiting environmental gas pollution, decreasing the likelihood of blood or regurgitated/refluxed gastric contents entering the airway, and decreasing the entrainment of room air, thus permitting more reliable gas monitoring.

TABLE 5.1
Suggested Uncuffed Endotracheal
Tube Sizes for Pediatric Patients

Age	Tube size (ID mm)
Premature, <1000 g	2.0
Premature, >1000 g	2.5–3.0
Term neonate — 3 months	3.0–3.5
3–9 months	3.5–4.0
9–18 months	4.0–4.5
>2 years	Age in years ± 16/4

Also, in cases of decreased lung compliance, ventilation is impaired in the presence of a large "leak" between the airway and the ETT.

However, if the ETT is too large in terms of diameter, it may produce ischemia of the tracheal wall. This will occur if the pressure applied to the wall is greater than the capillary pressure, which is usually about 20 to 25 cm H_2O. The same result will occur if a cuffed ETT is used and the inflation pressure in the cuff exceeds the capillary pressure in the tracheal wall at the site of contact. Whether permanent tissue injury results is a function of the duration of the ischemia as well as a number of host factors. These issues are discussed in more detail in a subsequent section.

Many charts and formulas for selecting the correct expected ETT size are available. Age-based guides are the most reliable, but intrapatient variation still warrants the availability of at least one extra tube of one size larger than expected and another one a size smaller. Table 5.1 gives suggested sizes for uncuffed endotracheal tubes in pediatric patients. One commonly used formula for ETT size in children 2 years and older is: (age in years +16) divided by 4. Thus, a 4-year-old would typically require a 5.0 tube (4 + 16 = 20, 20/4 = 5.0). However, regardless of the estimate, the correct size is determined by holding positive airway pressure at a level of 20 cm H_2O and listening for an airway leak once the trachea is intubated. If there is none, a smaller tube should be placed. Some would argue that, if the tube passes easily and the case is expected to be brief, changing the tube is unnecessary. If the leak occurs at less than 10 to 12 cm H_2O and one is using an uncuffed tube, a larger tube may be considered.

Depth

How does one determine how deep to place an ETT? Most pediatric tracheal tubes are marked in centimeters from the distal tip and have a black mark to indicate the recommended positioning at the vocal cords. However, these depths are not uniform among ETT manufacturers. A very simple estimate is that in terms of position at the vocal folds, all 3.0 and 3.5 mm internal diameter tubes may be placed at the 3-cm mark; all 4.0 and 4.5 tubes set at 4 cm; and all 5.0 and 5.5 tubes set at 5 cm. In a study of the 3-4-5 rule, subsequent chest x-rays showed that 79% of the tracheal tubes were in the ideal midtracheal position, one tube was marginally short, and 20% of the tubes were marginally long, without any endobronchial intubations.[38] This simple method can be used to determine tracheal tube length following oral as well as nasal intubation.

Most tiny premature infants that come to the OR will already be intubated, often nasally. It is important to be aware that *extension* of the head and neck, as often occurs during laryngoscopic procedures, tends to move the tip of the tracheal tube more cephalad, increasing the risk for tracheal extubation; flexion moves the ETT tube deeper into the trachea. This is counterintuitive. More movement occurs with oral tubes than with nasal tubes.[39] Table 5.2 provides measurement of the total airway length in premature infants of various weights, as measured from the nares to the carina. What one can derive from these data is that a neonate weighing less than 1000 g who has a nasotracheal tube with the 9-cm mark beyond the nares is at risk for endobronchial intubation.

TABLE 5.2
Length of Airway in Premature Infants from the Nares to the Carina

Body weight (g)	Range (mm)	Mean (mm)
550	72–82	78
700	77–90	82
860	82–95	89
990	87–98	93

Source: Lange, M. et al., *Pediatr. Pulmonol.*, 2002, 34, 455–461.

TABLE 5.3
Suggested Depth of Orotracheal Tubes

Age	Depth from alveolar ridge (cm)
Premature, 1 kg	7.4
Premature, 2 kg	8.2
Newborn	10
6 months	10.5
1 year	11
2 years	12
3 years	13
5 years	15

Probably the safest approach is to place the patient's head in the expected surgical position and then perform direct laryngoscopy to evaluate tube depth; the 2.0 ETT tube should be at a depth of 2 cm below the vocal cords, which means that the 3-4-5 rule can be extended to 2-3-4-5, regardless of whether the intubation is nasal or oral. Alternatively, one may evaluate bilateral breath sounds with the neck in full flexion and extension. In almost all cases, it is easier to deal with an endobronchial intubation than an unintentional extubation during surgery involving a very premature infant.

Table 5.3 gives suggested depth of orotracheal tubes, measured at the teeth or alveolar ridge and intended to provide a midtracheal position for the tip of the ETT. Note that for small children, there is another easy memory relationship: 0, 1, 2, 3, 4, 5 and 10, 11, 12, 13, 14, 15. A newborn (0 years) will usually have an adequate ETT tube placement at 10 cm, a 1-year-old at 11 cm, a 2-year-old at 12 cm, and so on. These are approximations, but if in every case involving small children one did a final check of age compared with ETT depth before incision, it would probably save a certain amount of intraoperative disruption due to improper ETT positioning.

Mechanics of Intubation

Safe and complication-free intubation is best managed with good exposure, light, and suction after a thorough preoperative assessment. In infants and children, the laryngoscope is a fingertip instrument, not a clutched-fist tool. Correct alignment of the various airway axes and gentle finesse with soft tissues, rather than brute force, are essential to minimize the risk of injury. The surgeon should select an appropriate blade shape and length and balance the patient's physical characteristics, retrusive mandible, "short" neck, large tongue, etc., with his comfort level. He should always anticipate the potential for an unexpectedly difficult intubation and remain aware of his options. Advances in instrumentation technology, such as better lighting and improved ergonomics in particular, will always be welcome. More specific information on intubation technique is provided in Chapter 6.

Complications

Intubation complications range from relatively minor to severe. There may be lip lacerations, loosened teeth, palatal lacerations, tonsillar hemorrhage, hypopharyngeal lacerations, arytenoid dislocation, vocal fold trauma, and tracheal lacerations. To minimize complications, the laryngoscope blade should be lifted independently; the upper maxilla (and teeth) should not be used as a fulcrum. The bevel of the endotracheal tube should be oriented and positioned so that the long end advances through the glottis first, with gentle rotation affording ease of passage through the remainder of the tube.

If a nasal approach is used, there is the additional potential for mucosal lacerations, epistaxis, and adenoid hemorrhage. Topical decongestion (with adequate time for efficacy), tube lubrication, and very gentle rotational advancement through the nasopharynx should reduce this risk. Potential bleeding during nasal intubations can be further minimized by using a soft red-rubber catheter as a stylet through the tube, using the largest catheter that will pass. Once the red tube is visualized in the hypopharynx, it provides a guide for the tip of the endotracheal tube that minimizes the risk for shearing injury.

If a cuffed tube is selected (there has been a relative trend to using cuffed tubes in younger children with and without inflation),[40] it is necessary to be certain that the cuff is below the larynx to limit the risk of recurrent laryngeal nerve injury when inflated. Also, if nitrous oxide is used during the case, the cuff must be intermittently checked for overinflation.

Laryngeal Devices

The use of the laryngeal mask airway (LMA) has become routine in modern medical practice.[41,42] Its use avoids the necessity for laryngoscopy and its associated risks. In addition, the LMA can be used to facilitate tracheal intubation in a number of ways, as with the LMA-Fastrack (The Laryngeal Mask Company, Limited, San Diego, CA) or in association with a flexible bronchoscope.

Complications

The two main risks associated with LMA use arise from displacement or overinflation of the device. Displacement during the case can cause partial or total airway obstruction. Use of the LMA in neonates (sizes 1 and 1.5) requires particular attention to stabilizing the device. Rotational torque on the LMA is usually the result of forces generated by the attached anesthesia circuit. Because of the rigidity of the LMA, proximal rotational forces are readily transmitted to the distal cuff unless the tube is securely anchored. Taping the LMA to the upper lip alone is not sufficient because the lip skin is readily stretched and will not prevent proximal rotational torque from being transmitted to the cuff. At a children's hospital, a critical incident rate of almost 10% accompanied the use of a size 1.5 LMA in 10- to 15-kg infants, a smaller than recommended size.[43] Clearly, small patients require a much higher level of vigilance when LMAs are in use and better stabilization systems should be designed.

Overinflation of an LMA cuff may cause pressure injury to the recurrent laryngeal nerve and/or the hypoglossal nerve.[44] It must be assumed that the glossopharyngeal nerve is also at risk, but because it has no motor function, transient injury may go undetected. An overinflated cuff can also cause tissue ischemia if the case is of long duration. Thus, as with a standard endotracheal tube, it is important to assess cuff pressure periodically. Table 5.4 provides recommended LMA sizes and cuff volumes.

Use of Airway Exchange Devices

The most common reasons for ETT changes for airway procedures are to insert a larger tube to facilitate flexible bronchoscopy or because of an excessive "cuff leak." In most of the latter cases,

TABLE 5.4
Suggested Laryngeal Mask Airway Sizes and Cuff Volumes

LMA size	Patient age/weight	Cuff volume (ml)
1	Neonate/infant up to 5 kg	4
1.5	Infant 5–10 kg	7
2	Infant/children 10–20 kg	10
2.5	Children 20–30 kg	14
3	Children, small adolescents >30 kg	20
4	Adolescents/adults 50–80 kg	30
5	Large adolescents/adults >80 kg	40

there is not a cuff leak but a leak at the site of the inflation valve, and cuff pressure can be maintained by simply inflating the cuff and then securely clamping it with a Kelly clamp. One of the most precarious situations one can create is to attempt an ETT exchange in a patient with a severe lung injury requiring very high levels of positive end-expiratory pressure and with a difficult airway. The "crisis moment" most often comes when the physician attempts to pass the new ETT into the glottis over an intubating stylet and meets resistance. If there is a difference between the external diameter of the intubating stylet and the internal diameter of the ETT, it is likely that the tip of the tube has encountered soft tissue, usually lateral and cephalad to the vocal folds.

Positioning the distal tip of the ETT tube against the inner curve of the stylet so that it enters the glottis through the anterior commissure (rotated 90° counterclockwise) can minimize this "hang-up" risk. However, if the ETT tube does not readily pass, even with gentle rotation, it should be immediately withdrawn and a smaller size ETT passed over the stylet. Once the new cuff is inflated and the airway is secure, the patient can be stabilized and further thought given to the risk benefits of the need for a larger ETT.

ENT surgeons may be called to stand by during an endotracheal tube change in a person with a difficult airway. One of the devices used to assist in this procedure is a hollow intubating stylet (Cook Airway Exchange Catheter).[45] In a recent case report, a pneumothorax resulted from the use of jet ventilation through the catheter during the procedure.[46] Haridas followed this report with an excellent discussion of this practice.[47] A healthy individual, after adequate preoxygenation, should be able to maintain acceptable oxygen saturation during changing of an ETT over a stylet. If the patient's ability to maintain oxygen saturation is in doubt, preoxygenation and hyperventilation followed by a trial period of apnea while the original ETT is in place would be useful. Rapid desaturation (within 1 or 2 min) indicates reduced respiratory reserve.

The need to change the ETT should be reviewed. If the ETT does need to be changed, a method of oxygenation during the procedure should be chosen. If the airway exchange catheter (AEC) is inserted until resistance is felt, one cannot assume that the AEC contacted the carina; it might well have abutted a more distal bronchial structure. Distance markings on the ETT and jet stylet should be used to position the stylet at the end of the ETT and in the midtrachea.

INADEQUATE VENTILATION AND PERFUSION

Disorders of gas exchange are the most frequent cause of serious organ injury in pediatric otolaryngology. Failure to appreciate airway obstruction as it is occurring should be viewed as the cardinal sin of pediatric otolaryngology and pediatric anesthesia. Failure to consider ventilation *and* perfusion during anesthesia can result in a cascade of physiologic events with potentially fatal consequences. Until a major anesthetic-related problem is recognized, the severity progressively worsens and the margin for error, as well as the odds of intact survival, decreases. Failed management is less disturbing than failed recognition, for the latter is the first critical misstep. Although thoughtful preparation is, of course, essential to complication avoidance, it is not a foolproof precaution for a patient under anesthesia.

Airway Obstruction

It can be argued that the most common airway complications in pediatric anesthesia are laryngospasm and bronchospasm. These two clinical entities differ in several key ways and thus their accurate diagnosis and management differs.

Laryngospasm. This complication occurs when abrupt and severe spastic contraction of the laryngeal intrinsic striated musculature results in bilateral vocal fold adduction. It is best avoided by not removing an artificial airway (ETT or LMA) in the presence of an inadequate depth (too much or too little) of anesthesia and/or neuromuscular blockade. It is most likely to be encountered during induction and extubation of the trachea when the plane of anesthesia is relatively light and direct pharyngeal, laryngeal, or peripheral painful stimuli are more likely to occur. One of the best clinical indicators that a child is ready for extubation is wrinkling of the skin over the forehead. Coughing and gagging are primitive reflexes; "scrunching" the brow apparently takes somewhat higher cortical functioning. It is important to remember, however, that inspiratory stridor and intercostal and subcostal retractions associated with deteriorating oxygenation can also be consistent with supraglottic obstruction or laryngospasm. When in doubt, the diagnosis of laryngospasm in a flaccid cyanotic patient can be confirmed by directly visualizing the vocal folds while the patient makes inspiratory efforts.

The standard treatment for laryngospasm is to provide gentle positive pressure via a mask seal with 100% oxygen. Thus, when the patient does finally abduct the vocal folds — even briefly — enriched oxygen can be delivered. Manual pressure on a breathing bag cannot always overcome the forces of the powerful laryngeal musculature and may, if persistent and excessive, further complicate the situation by distending the stomach. Patience, therefore, in the presence of a correct diagnosis is usually sufficient therapy.

Short-acting agents such as lidocaine, propofol, and remifentanil can help lessen the risk of laryngospasm and facilitate completion of the transitional planes of anesthesia during induction or extubation. However, particularly in older children and teenagers with pronounced muscular mass, prolonged laryngospasm may lead to postobstructive or posthypoxic pulmonary edema (i.e., so-called negative inspiratory pressure edema, which is most likely hypoxic in etiology). This is best avoided early by the judicious use of muscle relaxants and possible (re)intubation. In adults, a small dose (0.1 mg/kg) of succinylcholine is sufficient to relax the laryngeal muscles; this dose will usually be metabolized so quickly that reintubation is not required.[48]

A brief warning: if a patient has received a recent full dose of a cholinesterase-blocking drug (neostigmine or edrophonium) based on the belief that the airway obstruction was due to inadequate muscle block reversal, one may inadvertently overpotentiate the effect of succinylcholine administered to treat laryngospasm. Succinylcholine is metabolized in the plasma and does not reach the motor end plate. However, in the presence of plasma cholinesterase blockers (reversal drugs), the effective dose of succinylcholine is greatly magnified. A dose of 0.5 mg/kg of succinylcholine should readily reverse severe laryngospasm in a patient who has been exposed to neuromuscular reversal agents.

Bronchospasm. This complication occurs when the nonstriated (smooth) musculature surrounding the lower conductive airway contracts. In most cases, it is a result of direct tracheobronchial stimuli and local reflex arcs. Bronchospasm is typically manifested by expiratory wheezes and prolonged expirations; this is seen as a delayed upstroke on the capnogram. Because a kinked or obstructed endotracheal tube can cause the same effect upon respirations, it is wise to assure patency of the ventilating system before instituting more aggressive therapy.

If the patient is being ventilated by an endotracheal tube, or via a sealed bronchoscopic system, continuous positive pressure and oxygen should allow for adequate ventilation and oxygenation until the episode of bronchospasm has terminated. Fortunately, the commonly used potent inhalational anesthetics are bronchodilators, including sevoflurane;[49] thus, deepening the depth of anesthesia, if ventilation is possible, if usually efficacious. Although childhood asthma has become generally more lethal, for unknown reasons, perioperative anesthetic complications in children with asthma, including bronchospasm, appear to have decreased based upon better understanding of the triggers of the disease and presumably better pre- and perioperative management.[50]

Impaired Alveolar Function

On occasion, a child with a prolonged history of bronchopulmonary dysplasia management will experience hypoxemia during a case with airway instrumentation despite seemingly adequate ventilation. Maintenance of appropriate interventional measures for a longer period of time, as outlined earlier, should result in a return to a more normal respiratory physiological state. This is sometimes referred to as a "BPD bounce" and should be recognized and considered seriously before instituting emergency airway intervention. Recall that these infants, who have often maintained high pulmonary pressures since birth, have the capacity to open right-to-left shunts through the atria, pulmonary (A-V) vessels, aorta-PDA, and/or a ventricular septal defect. Given time, and sometimes a bit of systemic pressure support, as well as desisting from the inciting event until better anesthetic conditions are obtained, cardiorespiratory status can usually be restored.

Endobronchial Intubation

If the end of the endotracheal tube is advanced too far into the left or right main bronchus, one lung is selectively ventilated at the expense of the other. Using an endotracheal tube with a "Murphy eyelet" (a side opening a short distance from the distal tip) may reduce the potential for selective single-bronchus ventilation. The take-off of the right main bronchus is less acute an angle than that of the left main bronchus; therefore, decreased left-sided breath sounds are most frequently observed when the endotracheal tube is placed too deep and enters the right bronchus.

The small size and the compliant chest wall in neonates and infants make it more difficult to distinguish endobronchial intubations (EBI) by auscultation compared with older children. If not recognized and corrected, a drop in oxygen saturation will occur, usually with an increase in airway pressures (if positive pressure is being employed) that may or may not be initially appreciated. Prompt identification of the problem is readily made by assessing the ETT for proper depth. Remember the 3-4-5 rule previously discussed. If a 3 or 3.5 tube is in place, then the 3-cm mark should be visible at the vocal folds.

When EBI is detected, retraction of the tube *tip* to a position above the carina can be expected to promptly reverse the clinically observable changes, most often based on a return to normal oxygen saturation by oximetry. However, the alveoli of the unventilated lung that have collapsed during the period of EBI do not readily re-expand and normal oxygen saturation can coexist with significant areas of atelectasis. Full re-expansion of the collapsed alveoli is a function of the length of time the affected lung was unventilated as well as the presence of concurrent lung disease. Thus, positive pressure ventilation at slightly higher inflation pressures should be continued for 5 to10 minutes following EBI.

Deadspace Ventilation

In the first decade of use of the modern rigid bronchoscopes, it was not unusual for clinicians to use expandable connectors to attach the bulky anesthesia breathing circuit (manufactured for adult use) to the side arm of the bronchoscope in an attempt to minimize interference with the operator. If the volume of the added extension and the "Y" connector of the anesthesia circuit *plus* the volume of the bronchoscope exceeded the lung volume of the infant, which it often did, minimal ventilation took place. The chest would rise normally, breath sounds would be heard, and, in the absence of lung disease or endobronchial intubation, adequate oxygenation was usually maintained. However, the $PaCO_2$ would rise steadily because no CO_2 removal was occurring. All of the expired alveolar gas was rebreathed and thus became dead space ventilation. Dead space gas, by definition, does not participate in oxygen and carbon dioxide exchange.

It is possible to maintain full oxygen saturation during pediatric bronchoscopy without effective ventilation as long as adequate oxygen is present in the conducting airways. However, respiratory acidosis develops and it may be severe with $PaCO_2$ ranging between 80 and 120 mmHg and pH dropping below 7.1.[51] The main physiologic consequence of extreme hypercarbia is pulmonary and systemic hypertension. Although a pure respiratory acidosis is usually well tolerated in healthy older children, pulmonary hypertension can be very problematic in neonates — the patients in whom the problem is most likely to develop and be of critical clinical consequence. Furthermore, the presence of a severe respiratory acidosis, if combined with hypoxemia, decreases the margin of error for the secondary development of metabolic acidosis.

Part of the dead space problem during bronchoscopy has been dealt with by the availability of lightweight pediatric breathing circuits that do not interfere with the "feel" of the rigid bronchoscope and, thus, eliminate the need for flexible extension tubing to separate the endoscopist from the anesthesiologist. However, this is an area in which the original problem tends to be forgotten with time, so if this happens, future clinicians may find ways to repeat the errors of the past.

Decreased Cardiac Output

In most clinical situations, the measuring tools for cardiovascular functions give at least a brief warning of impending disaster, and appropriate cardioresuscitative steps can be initiated. These steps would typically include additional volume, pharmacologic support of cardiac and vascular function (epinephrine, calcium), and removal of inciting agents, if possible. More rare but extremely dangerous situations are cases in which there is no forewarning, and attention is often drawn to the most likely problem, a failure of ventilation.

An example of a situation in which potentially lethal ventilation/perfusion mismatching may occur during anesthetic induction, and in which one's attention is initially and erroneously focused on the ventilation side of the problem, is the case of a child or teenager with a mediastinal mass presenting for cervical node biopsy. The induction of general anesthesia may precipitate what is perceived as an "irreversible" cardiac arrest. Often and properly, management is initially directed at presumed airway obstruction by the chest mass; indeed, in some cases, use of a rigid bronchoscope has been required to maintain airway patency.[52] However, in some of the fatal cases, close observation would have disclosed the early appearance of an ashen color in the child, indicative of a failure of cardiac output rather than abrupt airway obstruction.

Isolated airway obstruction produces hypoxemia and cyanosis; however, cyanosis is associated with clinical signs of perfusion, albeit perfusion of desaturated blood. In contrast, inadequate or absent cardiac output produces poor perfusion, i.e., pallor, the "color of death." If pallor and poor capillary refill are present, one must assume impairment of cardiac output. Profound anemia, in which there is minimal circulating hemoglobin, also results in pallor, but in the illustrative case of a child with a chest mass, this would be a pre-existing state and not one brought on by the induction of anesthesia. It must be remembered that in very low hemoglobin states, even during severe hypoxemia, unsaturated hemoglobin may be insufficient to produce visible cyanosis.

In cases of pediatric patients with mediastinal masses and cardiac arrest on induction of general anesthesia, the etiology sometimes may relate to obstruction of pulmonary venous return to the left heart. The induction of general anesthesia causes changes in chest wall and abdominal tone that can alter anatomic relations in the chest, particularly when a large mediastinal mass is also present. Some of the patients who died on induction might have benefited from prompt position change (lateral, prone) once the airway was secure. The best way to avoid the risk of general anesthesia in such cases is to avoid general anesthesia and perform procedures under local anesthesia with sedation when possible.

Pulmonary Embolus

Pulmonary embolism can occur from air, fat, thrombus, or amniotic fluid. The main physiologic consequence is a decrease or absence of pulmonary blood flow. Regardless of the cause, significant pulmonary embolism is always associated with an abrupt drop in expired carbon dioxide concentration. If continuous monitoring of arterial pressure is available, the blood pressure will also be noted to fall precipitously.

Venous Air Embolism

Any open and noncollapsible vein above the level of the heart can entrain room air. In the OR, *venous* air embolism (VAE) most often occurs during procedures in which the head is elevated relative to the body in order to decrease venous pressure and bleeding in the surgical field. The integrity of intravenous lines must be maintained because a disconnected central venous catheter can convert a collapsible vein into a noncollapsible vein.[53] Furthermore, in patients following wound "cleansing" with hydrogen peroxide there are several reports of VAE, one including a fatality as a result of entrainment of generated gas bubbles.[54]

Early detection is the best medicine. Use of a precordial Doppler ultrasound device for cases with a risk of VAE can be helpful, but this is currently not a universal standard of care.[55–58] Objections to precordial Doppler use focus on the high degree of sensitivity, which allows the detection of even minute, subclinical, amounts of entrained air. The Doppler can serve as an excellent early warning system, however, by alerting the anesthetist to observe carefully for further evidence of a significant embolus.

The treatment for venous air embolism (VAE) is, first, to stop the entry of further air by lowering the head and/or flooding the surgical field with saline or water. The next step is to manage any hemodynamic derangements. The management of a large VAE is controversial. The severity of the problem is related mainly to the amount of air entrained and, to a lesser degree, the hemodynamic state of the child at the time of the insult. Attempting to extract the air via a central venous catheter is of no consistent benefit because the pathophysiologic mechanism of cardiovascular compromise caused by a VAE is air trapping and air locks in the outflow tract of the right heart and pulmonary arteries. Aspirating on a central venous catheter, whose tip is many centimeters proximal to the air collection, will remove blood from the right side of the circulation and further impair cardiac output.

The absence of brisk forward blood flow makes proper advancement of a CVP catheter or a balloon-tipped Swan–Ganz catheter much more problematic than under normal circumstances. Most often, the catheter just makes loops in the right ventricle. It is most likely better to improve cardiac output by giving volume centrally (blood or saline as a rapid bolus) and ionotropes (epinephrine 10 to 100 mcg/kg), depending upon the severity of the event as assessed by the degree of decrease in end tidal CO_2). If there is no immediate improvement, chest compressions should begin and blood continued to be given to elevate right-sided pressures. CPR with the patient's left side down and head lower than the heart may allow the trapped air to be displaced to less obstructive areas of the heart. If available, transesophageal echocardiography (TEE) provides the most sensitive assessment of the location of air bubbles in the heart.[59] TEE can indicate the presence of bubbles in all four heart chambers or the PA. Air in the left heart is indicative of transpulmonary passage (in the absence of a heart defect) and is a positive sign.

Fat Embolus

Recognition and management of fat embolus is primarily a function of the setting and the presentation. Major disruption of the bone marrow is the primary source, particularly from the pelvis and lower extremities following blunt trauma and long-bone fracture.[60] A trauma patient with long-bone fractures who comes to the OR for mandibular surgery several days following his or her injuries is an example of a patient at increased risk for fat embolization to the lung. The main organ of injury is the lung, but cerebral injury is not uncommon as a result of passage of fat across a patent foramen ovale. Hypoxemia is the main presenting symptom, although sudden death is also possible. Symptoms usually develop within 24 hours of the initiating injury, but may appear several days later. Treatment is primarily supportive because no proven therapies are available.

Major Intraoperative Blood Loss

In head and neck surgery, when major blood loss occurs, the failure to give prompt blood and pressor support (epinephrine) in the face of hypovolemic hypotension may be fatal. The anesthetist must remain ever vigilant to accumulating blood loss through communication with the surgical and nursing teams. An accurate accounting of blood loss on sponge pads and absorbable draping, in addition to what is collected in the suction traps, is essential. Waiting for a precipitous monitor change may be too late because "normal" hemodynamic parameters may initially be maintained by an intact autonomic nervous system and shunting of blood flow from nonessential organs. However, in the vast majority of cases involving hemorrhage in which there is a delay in recognition, blood pressure decreases while, in response, the anesthetist decreases the concentration of anesthetic agent — a correct step, but not based upon the correct diagnosis and thus not the essential step.

Re-Emergence of Fetal Blood Flow and Cardiovascular Shunting

Ventilation/perfusion mismatching problems from the re-emergence of fetal blood flow and cardiovascular shunting can be misdiagnosed as isolated airway problems, such as obstruction or bronchospasm. This problem may occur in newborns, particularly during airway procedures such as bronchoscopy. Within the time it takes to read this sentence, a pink baby can become deeply cyanosed and bradycardic because of a rerouting of blood flow in the chest. This re-emergence of the pattern of fetal circulation (i.e., right-to-left shunting) can be precipitated by factors that increase pulmonary artery resistance (mainly hypoxemia or hypercarbia) or by factors that decrease systemic blood pressure such as blood loss, severe myocardial depression from anesthetic drugs or medications, or impaired venous return from, say, a tension pneumothorax. Volume overload can also reopen a closed ductus arteriosus, but this situation is not usually associated with a precipitous change in clinical status.

Reversal of the normal flow pattern can occur with any cardiac lesion that abnormally connects the right heart circulation to the left heart circulation. Because congenital airway lesions have a high association with cardiac lesions, an understanding of the abnormal blood flow associated with a cardiac lesion and the potential for worsening (i.e., becoming more excessive or insufficient, or reversing flow) during anesthesia, endoscopy, and surgery must be appreciated in advance. A brief summary of a fetal and neonatal circulation has been presented earlier in this chapter, but a detailed review of congenital cardiovascular shunting and its management is beyond the scope of this chapter.

A key management principle to remember, however, is that the resulting cardiorespiratory abnormalities may be much more difficult to correct than hypoxemia resulting from transient airway obstruction. Knowledge of the subject matter is critically important in a crisis, however. Therefore, it is incumbent upon the anesthetist, as well as the surgeon, to assure that competent and experienced anesthesia personnel are present and intimately involved or immediately accessible throughout a case with known cardiovascular pathology.

INHALATIONAL ANESTHETICS

During surgery in children, the anesthetic requirement is for lack of pain, lack of awareness, lack of movement, and lack of recall. All of these needs are provided by modern inhalational anesthetics.

Halothane, isoflurane, desflurane, and sevoflurane are organic compounds (the first a polyhalo-genated alkane, the latter three polyhalogenated ethers) that are volatile liquids. The vapors of these compounds, when delivered to the lungs, behave according to physiochemical laws governing gases and their movement in open and contained space and across membranes.

Solubility and Partial Pressures

One of the most clinically important physiochemical properties of an inhalational anesthetic, in addition to nonflammability, is its solubility in blood, referred to as the blood–gas partition coefficient. Insolubility in blood is the factor than separates the currently used gases in terms of speed of onset and offset. Sevoflurane, a "fast" agent, is four times less soluble in blood than halothane, a "slower agent." Because blood carries the inhaled anesthetic gas from the lung to the brain and other organs, the insolubility concept is somewhat counterintuitive. The explanation for this is that it is not solubility but partial pressure (gas tension) that determines anesthesia in the brain. A gas that is highly soluble in a tissue, i.e., brain, muscle, fat, can be present in a large volume in that tissue and yet exert a very low partial pressure.

One simple way to conceptualize the process is that the anesthesiologist can turn a knob on a machine and deliver a very high concentration of a gas to the alveoli. Even though the gas is relatively insoluble in blood, some is taken up and, by virtue of the partial pressure created, unloaded from the blood at the next available area of lower partial pressure, which will be the brain for a large portion of cardiac output. Thus, with each breath and each heartbeat, the partial pressure of the gas in the alveoli and the gas in the brain approaches equilibrium. At the end of the case, when the anesthetic agent is turned off and the partial gas pressure from the pulmonary blood flow is very low, the process is reversed and insoluble agents rapidly exit the brain and tissues of the body.

Anesthetic Concentration

High concentrations of inhalational agents are often used initially to speed induction times. The ability to deliver high concentrations of inhaled anesthetics safely, however, is a function of the agent's degree of airway irritability and degree of myocardial depression. Inhalational induction with the use of high doses of desflurane or isoflurane can be expected to cause coughing and possibly laryngospasm and/or bronchospasm. Compared with these two agents, halothane is less irritating to the airway. However, in high concentrations, sevoflurane is by far the best tolerated of all the inhalational agents during induction.[10] One can begin with the vaporizer set "to the max" (8 vol %) and, with a primed circuit, achieve anesthetic depth as fast as most intravenous agents.

Cardiac Output and Minute Ventilation

The halogenated ethers and alkanes are agents that have vasodilator as well as myocardial depressant properties that can adversely affect cardiac output. Sevoflurane causes less myocardial depression than does halothane in infants[61] and childen.[62] Cardiac index is maintained with sevoflurane and isoflurane, but not with halothane, in children with heart disease.[63] In clinically significant cases of myocardial depression, controlled ventilation may be a greater causative factor than the choice of agent.[2] Because evoflurane and halothane depress respiratory drive, spontaneously breathing patients decrease minute ventilation (due to decreased tidal volume, not respiratory rate) as the depth of anesthesia increases.[64] Thus, this is a built-in safety feature; as anesthetic depth increases, less anesthetic gas is breathed in. However, if the anesthesiologist takes over or greatly augments ventilation, this safety feature is bypassed. Particularly in small patients and those with unappreciated hypovolemia, cardiac arrest can occur with delivered levels of agent that would otherwise seem safe. Controlling ventilation during induction in infants is not contraindicated, but does demand an increased level of vigilance for possible overdose complications.

Ventricular Ectopy

Halothane has the worst profile of all the agents in terms of depressing the myocardium and sensitizing the myocardium to catecholamines, which increases the risk of ventricular ectopy in the event of an increase in either endogenous or exogenously administered catecholamines. This effect is most frequently seen when exogenously administered catecholamines are used for vaso-constrictive purposes prior to and during surgery. The occurrence of ventricular ectopy is increased in the presence of hypercarbia. The ventricular ectopy is readily managed with intravenous lidocaine (1 mg/kg) and augmented ventilation, and it is rarely the sole source of a critical incident.

Halothane-Associated Hepatitis

The incidence of halothane-associated hepatitis (HAH) in children is, fortunately, extraordinarily low. Fulminant hepatic failure after repeated exposure to halothane in children appears to be an immune-mediated hypersensitivity reaction. Sensitization after an earlier exposure produces IgG antibodies, and the majority of children with fulminant HAH have circulating autoantibodies. Common features in most reported cases of HAH include multiple exposures; history of allergy, atopy, or previous adverse reaction to halothane; postoperative fever; and eosinophilia.

Choice of Inhalation Agent

The current "gold standard" inhalational agent (cost aside) for children is sevoflurane. Compared with previous potent inhalation agents, sevoflurane is less pungent (facilitating mask inductions); less irritating to the airway (allowing faster, noncoughing inductions); less depressing of the myo-cardium; and less arrhythmogenic. Thus, it is a safer induction agent than other available options.

Isoflurane is often used in long cases for cost reasons; however, emergence is slower with isoflurane compared with sevoflurane, and tracheal extubation following isoflurane is associated with a higher incidence of undesirable airway events compared with sevoflurane. The dollar cost (OR space and personnel) of 5 or 10 extra minutes in the OR awaiting emergence or managing a case of laryngospasm is almost always greater than the difference in the cost of anesthetic agent. An alternative approach in long cases is to use sevoflurane for induction and isoflurane for main-tenance, and then to discontinue isoflurane approximately 30 minutes before the end of the case and switch to sevoflurane, using gas monitors to confirm the washout of isoflurane.

Nitrous oxide (N_2O) lacks the potency to function as an inhalational anesthetic alone and is used mainly as an adjunct to inhalational, intravenous, regional, or local anesthesia. Like oxygen, nitrous oxide supports combustion and should not be used in the presence of lasers or other high-energy sources capable of igniting flammable material. Also, N_2O occupies a larger volume than nitrogen and in the event of air embolism, the N_2O in the body tissues that hold an enormous volume will move into the trapped air and cause it to expand. Furthermore, nitrous oxide is a "green house" gas; all the nitrous used worldwide is exhausted into the atmosphere with deleterious effects on the ozone layer. Last, there are potential but unproven teratogenic effects. Given all of these factors, one might predict that nitrous oxide will eventually become a once-great drug. However, because of cost and equipment issues, agents already outlawed in the developed world, such as the highly flammable ether, remain in use as staples of anesthesia care in the developing world. Thus, one can expect nitrous oxide to remain in wide use for decades to come.

INTRAVENOUS ANESTHESIA

Total intravenous anesthesia would ideally be accomplished with drugs that

- Are highly potent analgesics and amnestics
- Prevent pain stimuli from affecting the central nervous system

- Have no effect on respiratory drive, pulmonary function, or cardiovascular function
- Have no potential for abuse
- Are short-acting
- Are inexpensive

Although this is still an ideal, newer drugs are becoming available that represent significant advances toward these goals.

Propofol

When used as the primary anesthetic "sleep" agent, intravenous propofol is associated with a sense of well-being upon emergence, in the absence of pain. It is not an airway irritant and has antiemetic properties. The milky white propofol solution has the advantage that it is rarely mistaken for another drug. An earlier formulation was associated with bacterial contamination of the solution when propofol was drawn up in multiple syringes for use in multiple patients over the course of many hours. The new formulation is still not truly bacteriostatic, and proper technique to prevent contamination is essential; once drawn into a syringe, it should be used within 6 hours or discarded. Allergic reactions with propofol can occur to the drug or to its carrier agent, a lipid emulsion made with soy and egg products. Individuals with allergies to those products should not receive propofol.

Opioids: Agonists and Antagonists

The selection of a narcotic agent should be based primarily on the degree and duration of anticipated pain.

Fentanyl

Fentanyl is a potent opioid with an intermediate duration of action. Unlike remifentanil (see following section), large doses result in a prolonged duration of action. This is beneficial toward pain relief but is far less desirable in terms of respiratory depression, a recognized negative side effect of opioids. Of note, clearance of fentanyl is more rapid in neonates when compared with older children and adults, allowing for safe use of seemingly large doses (10 to 40 µg/kg) in longer cases.[65]

Remifentanil

Remfenanil is a potent opioid with very rapid elimination. In low doses, it does not affect cardiac output, or renal or hepatic function. It has an ester linkage that does not depend on plasma cholinesterase for breakdown (as does the well-known ester succinylcholine). The primary metabolite is inactive. A short plasma half-life allows for rapid recovery of central nervous system and respiratory function. In infants less than 2 months of age, remifentanil has been shown to have less depressive effects on postoperative respiratory drive compared with halothane — a potential benefit for expremature infants felt to be at risk for postoperative apnea following general anesthesia.[66] Day-case tonsillectomy and adenoidectomy patients wake up faster following remifentanil-volatile agent than fentanyl-volatile agent, but also with higher pain scores.[67] Thus, remifentanil has no advantage in short cases when pain is longer lasting, unless one has an alternative pain regimen in place.

Remifentanil would appear to be an ideal agent for laryngoscopy and rigid bronchoscopy, procedures with maximal stimulation during the operation and with only a modest degree of postoperative pain. Good clinical studies on the use of remifentanil are forthcoming. As with any newly introduced medication, it is always good advice to proceed with respectful caution during the early days of a supposedly wonderful new drug.[68]

Morphine Sulfate

Morphine sulfate is a potent, long-acting opioid with duration of action of about 4 hours. Its onset is slower than fentanyl or remifentanil, but only by a matter of minutes. Although textbooks give a time to peak brain levels as approximately 20 minutes, 50% of the peak brain level following a bolus intravenous injection of 1 to 2 mg/kg is probably reached within 5 minutes and 85% within 10 minutes. Morphine sulfate should remain popular for clinical use because it is a very inexpensive drug with consistent therapeutic effects. Its well-known side effects are dose-related respiratory depression, nausea (usually motion related), and hypotension related to venodilation.

Naloxone

Nalaxone is a mu-receptor antagonist that reverses the effects of all clinically used opioids. In the immediate postoperative period, reversal of opiate-induced respiratory depression may be desirable, but rapid reversal of analgesia is to be avoided. The typically recommended dosage (0.1 mg/kg/dose in children under 20 kg), except in cases of massive opioid overdose, is almost always vastly in excess of the dose needed to reverse the respiratory depressant effect of narcotics in the OR; 0.001 mg/kg is a more appropriate dose to reverse respiratory depression while minimizing reversal of the analgesic effect of the opiod. Thus, carefully titrated doses of 1 µg/kg (1/100 of the "recommended" dose) are recommended in these cases. The use of naloxone is not without side effects: there is an associated increased risk of postoperative nausea and vomiting.

PREEMPTIVE ANALGESIA

Opioids, when used as part of a general anesthetic, are typically administered before the onset of painful stimuli. Opioids mediate efferent pain signals in the dorsal horn of the spinal cord and can decrease the amount of intraoperative general anesthesia needed as well as possibly decreasing the need for postoperative pain medication. The effects of other intravenous agents, namely, magnesium and lidocaine, appear to affect events similarly within the spinal cord. In the future, it is likely that dorsal horn-specific drugs will be developed that are selective and long-acting; the major benefit of such agents would be an overall decrease in anesthetic and opioid requirement. There has been a resurgence in the use of rectal acetaminophen as a narcotic-sparing adjunctive induction agent, using a rectal suppository after induction at an initial dose of 30 to 60 mg/kg; use of acetaminophen decreases the postoperative opioid requirement and the incidence of post-operative nausea and vomiting.[20,69]

BALANCED ANESTHESIA

"Nitrous-narcotic" was once a popular anesthetic technique. The initial dose of morphine in older children was in the range of 3 to 4 mg/kg; additional analgesia and amnesia were provided with 70% nitrous oxide and 30% oxygen; muscle relaxants were required to keep the patient still. Heavily narcotized patients were able to be extubated relatively smoothly. However, the movement to a stretcher and then subsequent movement to the hospital bed were associated with a high rate of postoperative nausea and vomiting.

Currently, combined intravenous and halogenated inhalational anesthetics are the norm rather than the exception. The basic rationale is that a little of several agents, some intravenous and some inhalational, will provide the optimum balance between satisfactory operating conditions and patient safety in the OR and patient safety and comfort in the postoperative period. These combinations of approaches are referred to by many as "balanced" anesthesia; however, uniform balance is not uniform. In the past, the main anesthetic was an inhalation component and the intravenous agent was usually an induction drug and an intravenous opioid. In the future, one can expect few "pure" inhalational anesthetics for other than brief minor cases such as PE tubes.

What will probably become most common is a combination of techniques with computer monitoring of inhalational agents and infused intravenous drugs coupled with systems far superior to today's practice of having various drugs in little bottles to be mixed and matched and, potentially, confused. These systems will be integrated with even more advanced monitors of vital signs, airway gases, and brain and cardiac function. It is a rosy scenario in which the incidence of complications would be reduced as better systems approaches to reduce sources of error are increasingly implemented.

FLUID AND BLOOD PRODUCT REPLACEMENT

The anesthesiology team is responsible for fluid replacement prior to and throughout the procedure. They establish the routes of administration and the kinds of fluids given while keeping running totals of blood loss and insensible fluid loss. Communication on this matter between the anesthesia and surgery teams is therefore essential. The surgeon has the best perspective on the overall length of the procedure and the potential for significant blood loss. The anesthesiologist is in the best position to monitor losses and to assess clinical impact. Urine output, heart rate, blood pressure, capillary refill, and serial testing of hemoglobin concentration are routinely monitored, with electrolytes and determination of blood gases less commonly employed, to help confirm the visual estimates of lost blood and calculated insensible losses.

All surgical patients come to the OR in a partial state of dehydration because of preoperative restrictions on oral intake. Fluid replacement, therefore, is a combination of "catching up" on the dehydration plus maintenance fluid rates and intraoperative losses during a procedure. It is appropriate not to overstress the hemodynamic system with an inappropriate rate of fluid replacement in a child whose body is already systemically and hormonally stressed by anesthesia and surgery. Therefore, the anesthesia team must be ever vigilant to minimize the potential for a fluid overload state.

Blood and blood product replacement entails its own set of clinical issues. The greatest clinical risk is failing to provide the patient with enough oxygen-carrying capacity (red blood cells). The greatest iatrogenic risk is that of transfusing incompatible blood and causing a catastrophic transfusion reaction. This is almost always the result of clerical error somewhere in the system. Hypotension, flushing, and excessive wound bleeding are sentinel signs of a possible transfusion reaction. These signs, plus confirmed hemoglobinuria, should be considered presumptive evidence of a major transfusion reaction, and progression to shock, disseminated intravascular coagulation, and renal failure may be rapid.

A second issue relates to the composition of transfused blood. Stored red cells will always have time-related elevations in the level of potassium in the media in which they are suspended because intracellular stores leak out. Thus, even though the volume of suspension media is small, the potassium concentration may be quite high. The hypovolemic state that necessitates rapid blood transfusion favors flow to central organs at the exclusion of the vast muscle mass of the body, which is the principal intracellular reservoir for potassium. Thus, elevated potassium levels in transfused red blood cells will be concentrated in the central circulation, and it is possible to produce hyperkalemia in the myocardium. This clinical picture will classically manifest with peaked T-waves on the EKG and possible progression to ventricular tachycardia or ventricular fibrillation. In addition, myocardial contractility can be adversely affected by the binding of citrate, an essential anticoagulant in stored blood, to ionized calcium in the blood.

The treatment for transfusion-related hyperkalemia is calcium chloride (10 mg/kg), preferably through a central catheter, as well as hyperventilation and volume. If available, fresh blood or freshly washed red blood cells should be given at this stage. Glucose/insulin therapy is usually unnecessary. What is required is improved perfusion of the patient to wash the excess potassium out of the heart and allow it to distribute to other tissues of the body.

Packed cells do not contain platelets, and cases requiring a large volume of transfused blood often require platelets to support hemostasis. Fresh frozen plasma is rarely the solution to "oozing" problems in large blood loss cases, although factor deficiencies may become problematic. For most of the clotting factors, a relatively low concentration is required for activity. Also, another item that may initially be underappreciated but can result in later problems is the fact that fresh frozen plasma has four times as much citrate as packed cells. Thus, it can cause a progressive degree of hypocalcemia and exaggerate hypotension.

Early Postoperative Bleeding

A recent bleeding issue has arisen in children who have undergone adenotonsillectomy. Several reports have suggested that children who had received ondansetron as a prophylactic antiemetic and who had major postoperative bleeding may have had a delay in diagnosis because blood was swallowed and not subsequently vomited back up.[70,71] Blood is a gastric irritant and children who swallow significant quantities of blood will typically vomit fresh or clotted blood. Ondansetron, a specific 5-HT$_3$ antagonist, is particularly effective as an antiemetic when the etiology is mediated through the 5-HT$_3$ receptor. It appears that, at least in part, this receptor is involved in emesis following swallowed blood.

Pediatric adenotonsillectomy is a procedure with a risk for postoperative bleeding. Changes in vital signs and clinical appearance following surgery in these children must be responded to promptly, whether or not there is obvious bleeding (emesis or melana). For example, in one case a 10-year-old child had a heart rate of 132 beats/min and a blood pressure of 80/60 mmHg 5 hours after surgery, shortly before she began vomiting 220 ml of fresh blood.[71] In reply to a letter entitled "Ondansetron — Falsely Accused?" the authors acknowledged that early detection of postoperative bleeding "should be achievable with standard postoperative observations performed by a trained staff and a review by the surgical team."[72]

BODY TEMPERATURE

Extreme hypothermia is of benefit when one is deliberately chilling an organ to arrest metabolism; other situations of mild, moderate, and severe hypothermia are almost never of benefit to a child in the OR. They are usually a detriment in parallel with the degree of hypothermia. Conversely, but just as significantly, uncorrected hyperthermia results in a parallel hypermetabolic state that cannot be adequately sustained without the secondary development of systemic complications.

Hypothermia

Body heat is lost through convection, conduction, evaporation, and radiation. All of these methods are usually at play once a child is placed on an operating room table. Pediatric surgeons and OR nurses should be aware of this heat-loss process during prepping and induction and throughout the case. Warm children wake up from anesthesia faster and eliminate residual anesthetic gases and muscle relaxants faster. Warm children bleed less because hypothermia impairs normal clotting mechanisms. The rapid reversal of the anesthetic and/or paralyzed state enhances patient safety and case turnover. This is a win–win situation, but it requires that the entire team have a goal of normothermia in all patients unless specifically intended otherwise. In most ENT cases, once the procedure is fully underway and the child is thermally insulated, room temperatures can be brought down. Experience with forced air heaters, chemically activated warmers, warmed silicone padding, and low fresh gas flow rates have all been positive and contributory to maintenance of core body temperature in babies and children.

Hyperthermia

Pediatric ENT patients are more prone to intraoperative hyperthermia than most other surgical patients because of the limited area of surgical exposure and the need to keep the head, for sterility concerns, as covered as possible. Children under surgical drapes are prone to hyperthermia, but because this hyperthermia is not associated with a metabolic or respiratory acidosis, it is not related to the syndrome of malignant hyperthermia. Furthermore, ENT surgery involves a significant number of "syndromic children" who often have excessive airway secretions. It is beneficial, particularly in airway surgery, to minimize secretions. However, drugs that decrease saliva formation, such as atropine or glycopyrrolate, also decrease sweating, a principal mechanism for heat loss.

Malignant Hyperthermia

True malignant hyperthermia is a relatively rare (1 in 12,000 pediatric surgeries compared with 1 in 40,000 adult surgeries) genetic disorder in which an asymptomatic defect in skeletal muscle calcium metabolism, under certain conditions, may be triggered and result in generalized rigidity, metabolic and respiratory acidosis, and elevated temperature.[73] The best known triggers are halogenated inhalation agents (halothane, sevoflurane) and the muscle relaxant succinylcholine.

Early intraoperative signs of increased metabolic activity are increased carbon dioxide excretion (detectable by respiratory effort and/or capnography) and tachycardia. Temperature elevation is not an early sign. Therefore, when present, marked temperature elevation demands rapid, accurate diagnosis and vigorous interventional therapy. The most rapid diagnostic tool may be a venous blood gas, which may indicate a metabolic acidosis before it is present on an arterial sample.

The first management action when a concern arises for possible malignant hyperthermia intraoperatively is to turn off all halogenated anesthetic agents (and flush the CO_2 absorbent canister). In a child who is receiving or has received a known triggering agent, an unexplained metabolic acidosis (lactate) plus any other sign of hypermetabolism such as tachycardia and hypercapnia should, at a minimum, initiate a hyperthermia protocol. Dantrolene, a calcium channel agent, should be promptly obtained from a well-known storage site and brought to the OR for the process of mixing (which takes a certain amount of time). If the signs and symptoms are still present and are not accounted for by other factors, such as light anesthesia (which may also result in tachypnea and tachycardia), then administration of dantrolene (2 mg/kg IV) is indicated.

If the clinical condition of malignant hyperthermia is more severe at the time of diagnosis, efforts to manage extreme hyperthermia, including cold saline infusion, cold bags of fluid around the patient's body, and cooling blankets, should be implemented. Furthermore, hyperkalemia and potential renal injury from rhabdomyolysis should be managed with glucose and insulin as well as with volume loading and diuresis.

The question of whether to perform surgery in an ambulatory setting in patients with a suspected or proven malignant hyperthermia is, with the availability of safe alternative anesthetic techniques (propofol, short-acting muscle relaxants, regional anesthesia), primarily a function of the comfort level of the providers. Every anesthetizing facility must be prepared to manage unsuspected malignant hyperthermia. An awareness of the condition and a high level of attention to avoid administration of triggering agents, as well as knowledge and experience with alternative anesthetic agents, are of essential importance.

One additional preoperative question should be asked of all children with a suspected family history of malignant hyperthermia. Are they allergic to soy or egg products? If so, then propofol, which uses soy and egg in its carrier, should not be used and another alternative anesthetic regimen should be planned for in advance of surgery.

POSITIONING AND PRESSURE INJURIES

Localized pressure of sufficient force and duration can result in injury to any organ system. Positioning complications can occur by ischemic injury due to compression of blood supply to a region. The likelihood of an ischemic injury is related to

- The amount of pressure relative to the patient's blood pressure at the site of compression
- The pre-existing health of the underlying vascular structures

- The duration of the compression
- The degree of collateral circulation
- Any factor that affects tissue oxygenation such as anemia, hypoxemia, methemoglobin-emia, or cyanide toxicity

For example, during a highly vascular head and neck case in which controlled hypotension is employed, blood loss is excessive, and oxygenation is impaired, the risk of serious pressure injury over a site such as the sacrum or occiput is increased.

Positioning complications may also occur by direct nerve injury due to compression or stretching resulting in neuropraxia or, on occasion, less temporary neural injury. Peripheral nerve injury is typically related to point pressure over a nerve at a place where it crosses a bony structure, such as the ulnar nerve at the elbow or the common peroneal nerve at the knee. Likewise, stretch injuries are frequently related to positions in which a bony structure serves as a fulcrum between the proximal and distal ends of a nerve, e.g., stretching of the nerves of the brachial plexus across the head of the humerus.

Direct pressure injury may also occur in head and neck cases. An assistant using the concealed orbit of a child as support for retraction can cause anterior ischemic optic neuropathy, possibly resulting in permanent blindness. Excessively tight plastic goggles used for patient eye protection during surgery can injure the supraorbital or supratrochlear nerves just above the brow. Excessive anterior infraorbital pressure may result in maxillary nerve injury. A head and neck drape can inadvertently entrap or compress malleable anatomic structures, such as the auricle or the external jugular venous system.

The key to avoiding positioning and pressure injury is awareness. The use of foam rubber and silicon gel padding has done a great deal to decrease pressure injuries, primarily by allowing for redistribution of pressure from sites directly over bony areas, such as the heels and sacrum, to much broader areas so that the pressure per square inch is decreased. Body tissues are adapted to tolerate periods of ischemia; cells can use anaerobic glycolysis for extended periods. Tourniquet ischemia for 1 to 2 hours is a standard part of extremity surgery, for example.

However, in operations of longer duration, and particularly in those involving the risk factors discussed previously, efforts should be made to distribute the pressure that supports the patient maximally and, whenever possible, to allow for tissue reperfusion. Simply lifting the patient's head for several minutes every 2 hours can allow for the high levels of tissue lactate to be washed out and intracellular glycogen stores to be replenished. If possible, the anesthesiologist should lift the arms and legs periodically to make sure that they are lying freely and to allow reperfusion of any areas of excessive pressure. Similarly, the surgical team can release retraction tension in the surgical field throughout long cases.

WEB AND TEXT RESOURCES

Numerous texts and Web sites are available that provide information and discussions related to pediatric anesthesia for otolaryngology — head and neck surgery cases, some dedicated to anesthesia for children specifically with other medical problems.[74] In general, Internet-available information on anesthetic-related complications tends to be embedded in other information and as yet no really efficient filters exist. However, the Harriet Lane WWW Links site at <http://derm.med.jhmi.edu/hll> maintained at Johns Hopkins University provides a reasonable approach at evaluating pediatric information available on the Web. A useful source of information is eMedicine at <http://www.emedicine.com>. There is an online airway atlas at <http://users.rcn.com/jsherry/airwaymap.html>, and the University of Iowa maintains a virtual hospital that has good information for physicians as well as patients at <http://www.vh.org/index.html>. For ENT surgeons who really want to know what is happening on the other side of the surgical drape, the University of Florida has put a virtual anesthesia machine online at <http://www.anest.ufl.edu/~eduweb/vam/VAM.html>.

CONCLUSIONS

Multiple critical knowledge and technical skills pathways require competency in key personnel, anesthesiologists, and surgeons alike to assure safe surgery in children. A truly integrated pediatric surgical team embraces the nonpolitical concepts of open dialogue, free exchange of ideas, professional respect for other specialists, and proactive collaboration with the perioperative nursing and support personnel. Strong interactive leadership is often required to maintain smooth functioning between the disparate surgical and anesthesia talents and egos that may exist within an outwardly successful OR model. Fortunately, for the welfare of children, an institution with coordinated pediatric surgical services tends to attract individuals inclined to work together with multiple specialists in support of a common goal: the safe delivery of highly competent and comprehensive perioperative care for children.

REFERENCES

1. Robinson, S. and Gregory, G. Fentanyl-air-oxygen anesthesia for ligation of patent ductus arteriosus in preterm infants. *Anesthesia Analgesia*, 1981, 60, 331–334.
2. Morray, J.P., Geiduschek, J.M., Ramamoorthy, C. et al. Anesthesia-related cardiac arrest in children: initial findings of the Pediatric Perioperative Cardiac Arrest (POCA) Registry. *Anesthesiology*, 2000, 93, 6–14.
3. Hegyi, T., Anwar, M., Carbone, M.T. et al. Blood pressure ranges in premature infants: II. The first week of life. *Pediatrics*, 1996, 97, 336–342.
4. Anonymous. Systolic blood pressure in babies of less than 32 weeks gestation in the first year of life. Northern Neonatal Nursing Initiative. *Arch. Disease Childhood Fetal Neonatal Ed.*, 1999, 80, F38–42.
5. Woods, A.M. and Gal, T.J. Decreasing airflow resistance during infant and pediatric bronchoscopy. *Anesthesia Analgesia*, 1987, 66, 457–459.
6. Brosius, K.K. and Bannister, C.F. Midazolam premedication in children: a comparison of two oral dosage formulations on sedation score and plasma midazolam levels. *Anesthesia Analgesia*, 2003, 96, 392–395.
7. Marzo, S.J. and Hotaling, A.J. Trade-off between airway resistance and optical resolution in pediatric rigid bronchoscopy. *Ann. Otol., Rhinol. Laryngol.*, 1995, 104, 282–287.
8. Cote, C.J., Cohen, I.T., Suresh, S. et al. A comparison of three doses of a commercially prepared oral midazolam syrup in children. *Anesthesia Analgesia*, 2002, 94, 37–43.
9. Marhofer, P., Freitag, H., Hochtl, A., Greher, M., Erlacher, W., and Semsroth, M. S(+)-ketamine for rectal premedication in children. *Anesthesia Analgesia*, 2001, 92, 62–65.
10. Baum, V.C., Yemen, T.A., and Baum, L.D. Immediate 8% sevoflurane induction in children: a comparison with incremental sevoflurane and incremental halothane. *Anesthesia Analgesia*, 1997, 85, 313–316.
11. Sprung, J., Schuetz, S.M., Stewart, R.W., and Moravec, C.S. Effects of ketamine on the contractility of failing and nonfailing human heart muscles *in vitro*. *Anesthesiology*, 1998, 88, 1202–1210.
12. Ko, Y.P., Huang, C.J., Hung, Y.C. et al. Premedication with low-dose oral midazolam reduces the incidence and severity of emergence agitation in pediatric patients following sevoflurane anesthesia. *Acta Anaesthesiol. Sinica*, 2001, 39, 169–177.
13. Galinkin, J.L., Fazi, L.M., Cuy, R.M. et al. Use of intranasal fentanyl in children undergoing myringotomy and tube placement during halothane and sevoflurane anesthesia. *Anesthesiology*, 2000, 93, 1378–1383.
14. Finkel, J.C., Cohen, I.T., Hannallah, R.S. et al. The effect of intranasal fentanyl on the emergence characteristics after sevoflurane anesthesia in children undergoing surgery for bilateral myringotomy tube placement. *Anesthesia Analgesia,* 2001, 92, 1164–1168.
15. Davis, P.J., Greenberg, J.A., Gendelman, M., and Fertal, K. Recovery characteristics of sevoflurane and halothane in preschool-aged children undergoing bilateral myringotomy and pressure equalization tube insertion. *Anesthesia Analgesia*, 1999, 88, 34–38.
16. Aono, J., Mamiya, K., and Manabe, M. Preoperative anxiety is associated with a high incidence of problematic behavior on emergence after halothane anesthesia in boys. *Acta Anaesthesiol. Scand.*, 1999, 45, 542–544.

17. Fujii, Y. and Tanaka, H. Comparison of granisetron, droperidol, and metoclopramide for prevention of postoperative vomiting in children with a history of motion sickness undergoing tonsillectomy. *J. Pediatr. Surg.*, 2001, 36, 460–462.

18. Church. J. Is postoperative nausea and vomiting following tonsillectomy really a problem? *Anaesthesia*, 2002, 57, 1029–1030.

19. Williams, P. and Bailey, P. Comparison of the reinforced laryngeal mask airway and tracheal intubation for adenotonsillectomy. *Br. J. Anaesthesia,* 1993, 70, 30–33.

20. Korpela, R., Korvenoja, P., and Meretoja, O.A. Morphine-sparing effect of acetaminophen in pediatric day-case surgery. *Anesthesiology,* 1999, 91, 442–447.

21. Bohnhorst, B., Peter, C.S., and Poets, C.F. Pulse oximeters' reliability in detecting hypoxemia and bradycardia: comparison between a conventional and two new generation oximeters. *Crit. Care Med.*, 2000, 28, 1565–1568.

22. Barker, S.J. and Shah, N.K. The effects of motion on the performance of pulse oximeters in volunteers (revised publication). *Anesthesiology,* 1997, 86, 101–108.

23. Benumof, J.L. Respiratory physiology and lung function during anesthesia. In Miller, R.D., Ed. *Miller: Anesthesia,* 5th ed. Philadelphia: Churchill Livingstone, Inc., 2004, 528–618.

24. Sprung, J., Whalley, D., Schoenwald, P.K., O'Hara, P.J., and O'Hara, J. End-tidal nitrogen provides an early warning of slow, ongoing, venous air embolism. *Anesthesiology,* 1996, 85, 1203–1206.

25. Davidson, A.J., McCann, M.E., Devavaram, P. et al. The differences in the bispectral index between infants and children during emergence from anesthesia after circumcision surgery. *Anesthesia Analgesia,* 2001, 93, 326–330.

26. Bannister, C.F., Brosius, K.K., Sigl, J.C., Meyer, B.J., and Sebel, P.S. The effect of bispectral index monitoring on anesthetic use and recovery in children anesthetized with sevoflurane in nitrous oxide. *Anesthesia Analgesia,* 2001, 92, 877–881.

27. Gottschalk, A., Mirza, N., Weinstein, G.S., and Edwards, M.W. Capnography during jet ventilation for laryngoscopy. *Anesthesia Analgesia,* 1997, 85, 155–159.

28. Klemola, U.M. and Hiller, A. Tracheal intubation after induction of anesthesia in children with propofol–remifentanil or propofol–rocuronium. *Can. J. Anaesthesia,* 2000, 47, 854–859.

29. O'Sullivan, T.J. and Healy, G.B. Complications of Venturi jet ventilation during microlaryngeal surgery. *Arch. Otolaryngol.,* 1985, 111, 127–131.

30. Benjamin, B. and Gronow, D. A new tube for microlaryngeal surgery. *Anaesthesia Intensive Care,* 1979, 7, 258–263.

31. Hunsaker, D.H. Anesthesia for microlaryngeal surgery: the case for subglottic jet ventilation. *Laryngoscope,* 1994, 104, 1–30.

32. Gilbert, T.B. Gastric rupture after inadvertent esophageal intubation with a jet ventilation catheter. *Anesthesiology,* 1998, 88, 537–538.

33. Aloy, A., Schachner, M., and Cancura, W. Tubeless translaryngeal superimposed jet ventilation. *Eur. Arch. Oto-Rhino-Laryngol.,* 1991, 248, 475–8.

34. Bacher, A., Pichler, K., and Aloy, A. Supraglottic combined frequency jet ventilation versus subglottic monofrequent jet ventilation in patients undergoing microlaryngeal surgery [comment]. *Anesthesia Analgesia,* 2000, 90, 460–465.

35. Bacher, A., Lang, T., Weber, J., and Aloy, A. Respiratory efficacy of subglottic low-frequency, subglottic combined-frequency, and supraglottic combined-frequency jet ventilation during microlaryngeal surgery [comment]. *Anesthesia Analgesia,* 2000, 91, 1506–1512.

36. Grasl, M.C., Donner, A., Schragl, E., and Aloy, A. Tubeless laryngotracheal surgery in infants and children via jet ventilation laryngoscope. *Laryngoscope,* 1997, 107, 277–281.

37. Depierraz, B., Ravussin, P., Brossard, E., and Monnier, P. Percutaneous transtracheal jet ventilation for paediatric endoscopic laser treatment of laryngeal and subglottic lesions. *Can. J. Anaesthesia,* 1994, 41, 1200–1207.

38. Freeman, J.A., Fredricks, B.J., and Best, C.J. Evaluation of a new method for determining tracheal tube length in children. *Anaesthesia,* 1995, 50, 1050–1052.

39. Lange, M., Jonat, S., and Nikischin, W. Detection and correction of endotracheal-tube position in premature neonates. *Pediatr. Pulmonol.,* 2002, 34, 455–461.

40. Khine, H.H., Corddry, D.H., Kettrick, R.G. et al. Comparison of cuffed and uncuffed endotracheal tubes in young children during general anesthesia. *Anesthesiology,* 1997, 86, 627–631; discussion 27A.

41. Lopez–Gil, M., Brimacombe, J., and Alvarez, M. Safety and efficacy of the laryngeal mask airway. A prospective survey of 1400 children. *Anaesthesia*, 1996, 51, 969–972.

42. Verghese, C. and Brimacombe, J.R. Survey of laryngeal mask airway usage in 11,910 patients: safety and efficacy for conventional and nonconventional usage. *Anesthesia Analgesia*, 1996, 82, 129–133.

43. Bagshaw, O. The size 1.5 laryngeal mask airway (LMA) in paediatric anaesthetic practice. *Paediatr. Anaesthesia*, 2002, 12, 420–423.

44. Dziewas, R. and Ludemann, P. Hypoglossal nerve palsy as complication of oral intubation, bronchoscopy and use of the laryngeal mask airway. *Eur. Neurol.*, 2002, 47, 239–243.

45. Padkin, A. and McIndoe, A. Use of the airway exchange catheter for the patient with a partially obstructed airway [comment]. *Anaesthesia*, 2000, 55, 87–88.

46. Baraka, A.S. Tension pneumothorax complicating jet ventilation via a cook airway exchange catheter [comment]. *Anesthesiology*, 1999, 91, 557–558.

47. Haridas, R.P. Jet ventilation through jet stylets [comment]. *Anesthesiology*, 2000, 93, 295; discussion 297–298.

48. Chung, D.C. and Rowbottom, S.J. A very small dose of suxamethonium relieves laryngospasm. *Anaesthesia*, 1993, 48, 229–430.

49. Hashimoto, Y., Hirota, K., Ohtomo, N., Ishihara, H., and Matsuki, A. *In vivo* direct measurement of the bronchodilating effect of sevoflurane using a superfine fiberoptic bronchoscope: comparison with enflurane and halothane. *J. Cardiothoracic Vascular Anesthesia*, 1996, 10, 213–216.

50. Warner, D.O., Warner, M.A., Barnes, R.D. et al. Perioperative respiratory complications in patients with asthma [comment]. *Anesthesiology*, 1996, 85, 460–467.

51. Rah, K.H., Salzberg, A.M., Boyan, C.P., and Greenfield, L.J. Respiratory acidosis with the small Storz–Hopkins bronchoscopes: occurrence and management. *Ann. Thoracic Surg.*, 1979, 27, 197–202.

52. Ferrari, L.R. and Bedford, R.F. General anesthesia prior to treatment of anterior mediastinal masses in pediatric cancer patients. *Anesthesiology*, 1990, 72, 991–995.

53. Haskal, Z.J. Air embolism during tunneled central catheter placement performed without general anesthesia in children: a potentially lethal complication. *J. Vascular Interventional Radiol.*, 1999, 10, 1416.

54. Donati, S., Barthelemy, A., Boussuges, A. et al. [Severe air embolism after surgical irrigation with hydrogen peroxide]. *Presse Medicale*, 1999, 28, 173–175.

55. Meyer, P.G., Renier, D., Orliaguet, G., Blanot, S., and Carli, P. Venous air embolism in craniosynostosis surgery: what do we want to detect? *Anesthesiology*, 2000, 93, 1157–1158.

56. Coulter, T.D. and Wiedemann, H.P. Gas embolism. *New Engl. J. Med.*, 2000, 342, 2000; discussion 2001–2002.

57. Muth, C.M. and Shank, E.S. Gas embolism. *New Engl. J. Med.*, 2000, 342, 476–482.

58. Palmon, S.C., Moore, L.E., Lundberg, J., and Toung, T. Venous air embolism: a review. *J. Clin. Anesthesia*, 1997, 9, 251–257.

59. Thackray, N.M., Murphy, P.M., McLean, R.F., and deLacy, J.L. Venous air embolism accompanied by echocardiographic evidence of transpulmonary air passage. *Crit. Care Med.*, 1996, 24, 359–361.

60. Fabian, T.C. Unravelling the fat embolism syndrome [comment]. *New Engl. J. Med.*, 1993, 329, 961–963.

61. Wodey, E., Pladys, P., Copin, C. et al. Comparative hemodynamic depression of sevoflurane versus halothane in infants: an echocardiographic study. *Anesthesiology*, 1997, 87, 795–800.

62. Holzman, R.S., van der Velde, M.E., Kaus, S.J. et al. Sevoflurane depresses myocardial contractility less than halothane during induction of anesthesia in children. *Anesthesiology*, 1996, 85, 1260–1267.

63. Rivenes, S.M., Lewin, M.B., Stayer, S.A. et al. Cardiovascular effects of sevoflurane, isoflurane, halothane, and fentanyl–midazolam in children with congenital heart disease: an echocardiographic study of myocardial contractility and hemodynamics. *Anesthesiology*, 2001, 94, 223–229.

64. Walpole, R., Olday, J., Haetzman, M., Drummond, G.B., and Doyle, E. A comparison of the respiratory effects of high concentrations of halothane and sevoflurane. *Paediatr. Anaesthesia*, 2001, 11, 157–160.

65. Gregory, G. Fentanyl-air-oxygen anesthesia for ligation of patent ductus arteriosus in preterm infants. *Anesthesia Analgesia*, 1981, 60(5), 331–334.

66. Galinkin, J.L., Davis, P.J., McGowan, F.X. et al. A randomized multicenter study of remifentanil compared with halothane in neonates and infants undergoing pyloromyotomy. II. Perioperative breathing patterns in neonates and infants with pyloric stenosis. *Anesthesia Analgesia*, 2001, 93, 1387–1392.

67. Davis, P.J., Finkel, J.C., Orr, R.J. et al. A randomized, double-blinded study of remifentanil versus fentanyl for tonsillectomy and adenoidectomy surgery in pediatric ambulatory surgical patients. *Anesthesia Analgesia*, 2000, 90, 863–871.
68. Rothstein, P. Remifentanil for neonates and infants: piano, piano con calma. *Anesthesia Analgesia*, 2001, 93, 1370–1372.
69. van der Marel, C.D., van Lingen, R.A., Pluim, M.A. et al. Analgesic efficacy of rectal versus oral acetaminophen in children after major craniofacial surgery. *Clin. Pharmacol. Thera.*, 2001, 70, 82–90.
70. Blomgren, K., Qvarnberg, Y.H., and Voltonen, H.J. A prospective study on pros and cons of electro-dissection tonsillectomy. *Laryngoscope,* 2001, 111(3), 478–482.
71. Courtman, S.P., Rawlings, E., and Carr, A.S. Masked bleeding posttonsillectomy with ondansetron. *Paediatr. Anaesthesia*, 1999, 9, 467.
72. Hack, H.A. Ondansetron — falsely accused? [letter; comment] *Paediatr. Anaesthesia*, 2000, 10, 343.
73. Pessah, I.N., Lynch, C., III, and Gronert, G.A. Complex pharmacology of malignant hyperthermia. *Anesthesiology*, 1996, 84, 1275–1279.
74. Dsida, R. and Cote, C.J. Nonsteroidal antiinflammatory drugs and hemorrhage following tonsillectomy: do we have the data? [comment]. *Anesthesiology,* 2004, 100(3), 749–751; author reply, Mar. 751–752.

6 Emergency Airway Management and Critical Care Issues for the Child with a Difficult Airway

Thomas A. Nakagawa and David W. Tellez

Physicians are often forced to make critical treatment decisions in states of partial ignorance.

Dr. Jerome Groopman, Chief, Experimental Medicine, Beth Israel Deaconess Medical Center, Boston, Massachusetts, author of *Second Opinions*

CONTENTS

INTRODUCTION

The acutely ill child with a difficult airway problem requires collaboration among pediatric emergency medicine physicians, anesthesiologists, otolaryngologists, and intensivists to prevent or reduce morbidity and mortality. Understanding the anatomic, physiologic, and psychological differences in differently aged children is important to provide appropriate care to this patient population. Care of the critically injured patient begins with airway management. A common theme will be seen throughout this chapter: preparation, planning, and training will minimize the potential for complications related to the care of the intubated infant or child.

This chapter will first discuss pertinent issues regarding emergency management and stabilization of the child with a difficult airway, including identifying the child with respiratory distress and impending respiratory failure, airway control and securing the potentially difficult airway, procedural complications, and care following intubation. The chapter will then review potential management issues when intubated children are in an intensive care unit, including ventilator management, control of pain and sedation, fluids and nutritional support, weaning from mechanical ventilation, and preparation for extubation. The concluding section will review pertinent airway management issues surrounding the transport of a child with an acute airway problem.

EMERGENCY MANAGEMENT AND STABILIZATION OF THE DIFFICULT AIRWAY

AIRWAY AND AIRWAY-RELATED ANATOMY AND PHYSIOLOGY

Developmental Anatomic Differences

Developmental considerations differentiate the child's airway anatomy from that of an adult and the infant's airway from that of an older child. The infant's tongue is proportionally larger in the oral cavity and lies closer to the palate, thus contributing to airway obstruction. The position of the larynx gradually descends within the neck as the child grows, starting out in the infant at the level of the second to third cervical vertebrae and residing at the level of the fifth to sixth cervical vertebrae by mid-childhood. These anatomic differences exaggerate the anterior and more cephalad position of the larynx in children, making visualization of the supraglottic structures more difficult.

The shape and size of the pediatric epiglottis differs from that of the adult epiglottis. The epiglottis of an infant is thicker and shorter, and the omega-shaped epiglottis extends over the glottis and is not as amenable to displacement by vallecular suspension. The vocal folds differ in infants as well. In adults, the vocal folds are thicker and their anterior and posterior attachments are perpendicular to the laryngeal axis; in infants, the anterior vocal fold attachment is inferior to the posterior attachment point. As a result of this angulation, there may be difficulty in advancing an endotracheal tube as it passes through the infant larynx.

The narrowest portion of an adult's or older child's airway is at the level of the glottic opening; in infants, the narrowest point is subglottic, at the level of the cricoid ring. This laryngeal narrowing in infants produces a funnel-shaped structure, unlike the cylindrical shape of an adult larynx. Thus, the narrowed subglottic area ultimately determines the size of an endotracheal tube for children less than 8 years of age. Last, in children with congenital anatomic abnormalities and syndromes, additional anatomic features, such as a short neck, can make intubation more difficult.

Respiratory Physiology Differences

Children also differ from adults in their respiratory physiology. Airflow physics changes dramatically throughout infancy to adulthood. For example, a 1-mm circumferential difference of a 4-mm airway decreasing the diameter to 2 mm will increase resistance 16-fold and decrease the cross-sectional area by 75%. By contrast, in an 8-mm adult airway, this 1 mm of airway edema would result in a fourfold increase in resistance, with only a 44% decrease in cross-sectional area. This increased resistance contributes to decreased airflow and increased work of breathing.

Pulmonary anatomy and physiology are also different in infants and children. The lungs and chest wall are not fully developed at birth, which can contribute to a significant increase in an infant's work of breathing.[1] Infants are born with approximately 70 million alveoli that are underdeveloped with a cross-sectional diameter of about 100 μm compared with the adult with 500 million full-sized alveoli with a cross-sectional diameter of about 200 μm. The lungs of an infant also contain less elastin, thus contributing to increased lung stiffness and decreased compliance. Infants are more dependent on diaphragmatic breathing because their compliant chest wall tends to collapse and reduce the efficiency of ventilation. Additionally, the shape of an infant's chest and insertion of the intercostal muscles reduces the efficiency of chest wall expansion to support ventilation. Finally, exponential growth in the first two years of life correlates with an elevated metabolic rate with a corresponding exponential increase in air-intake needs.

Other Physiologic Differences

Additional physiologic considerations must be taken into account when dealing with infants and children. The infant has a higher resting heart rate in order to maintain cardiac output, and its limited ability to generate a larger stroke volume places it at risk for inadequate cardiac output if bradycardia occurs. Infants are prone to hypothermia due to their increased body surface area, so the health care professional must pay close attention to environmental exposure when dealing with this patient population. Additionally, rapid depletion of glycogen stores places stressed infants at risk for hypoglycemia.

Psychological Differences

It is important to recognize that infants and children also differ psychologically from adults. Their inability to express symptoms, pain, fear, or anxiety verbally needs to be understood and accommodated by health care providers caring for this patient population.

PATIENT ASSESSMENT

Recognition

Recognition of a potentially difficult airway situation in a child with respiratory distress is imperative for those responsible for airway management. Remember the ABCs of basic life support: airway, breathing, and circulation. The caregiver must focus on the patient's airway and ability to provide oxygenation, ventilation, and circulation. Rapid assessment of the airway should determine its stability. The airway may be categorized on one of four levels:

- Stable, requiring no support
- Maintainable
- Compromised, but requiring minimal intervention
- Unstable, requiring immediate intervention such as an artificial airway or airway adjunct to maintain patency

Physical Examination

Assessment of the patient's airway can usually be made by observation without having to complete an examination of the child. Unless immediate intervention is indicated, permit the child to assume a position of comfort; do not force the child into any position, especially supine. The child's level of comfort, respiratory rate, and color can be assessed almost immediately; suprasternal retractions and use of accessory ribcage musculature suggest an increased work of breathing. Careful assessment of air entry by observation or, preferably, by chest and cervical auscultation is critical.

Tachycardia

Tachycardia and tachypnea are ominous signs in a child with respiratory distress. Respiratory distress or impending respiratory failure will result in hypercarbia, which is a potent stimulus for catecholamine release promoting tachycardia.[2] Thus, rapid evaluation of a child with these signs is crucial to determine if emergency intervention is required.

Dysphonia

Dysphonia is one of the first signs of upper airway obstruction in older children, but it is uncommon in infants. This may be associated with progressive airway compromise and increased respiratory effort manifested by the use of accessory muscles. Hoarseness suggests obstruction at the level of the glottis while a muffled vocal quality is often noted in children with a retropharyngeal or peritonsillar abscess. Aphonia, a loss of voice, is a rare sign of airway obstruction and is typically associated with impaired vocal fold adduction. It can also be seen with a laryngeal foreign body.

Stridor

Stridor is caused by turbulent flow across a narrowed airway during inspiration and is indicative of upper airway obstruction. The pitch and duration of stridor indicate the degree of obstruction. High-pitched inspiratory stridor of brief duration suggests a critically compromised airway. Audible, coarse, low-pitched stridor heard throughout the inspiratory cycle is commonly associated with a more patent airway. The acute absence of stridor suggests airway obstruction more often than improvement; such a child should be assessed immediately for respiratory failure and appropriate intervention for airway control.

Wheezing

Wheezing is a higher pitched expiratory sound usually associated with lower airway disease. It is most commonly associated with illnesses causing bronchospasm and can also be associated with tracheomalacia or an airway foreign body. Wheezing results from a dynamic collapse of the airway and is usually associated with a marked prolongation of the expiratory phase.

INTUBATION

Airway stabilization should ideally occur in a well-controlled and prepared environment such as the emergency department, pediatric intensive care unit, or operating suite.

Indications

- Airway protection
- Relief from upper airway obstruction
- Correction of respiratory failure
- Resuscitation for basic and advanced life support
- Cerebral resuscitation
- Airway control during administration of general anesthesia or to permit deep sedation for diagnostic procedures

Intubation Complications

Preparation is essential to minimize the risk of complications from intubation. Prevention of secondary injury, primarily hypoxia, is of greatest concern. Hypoxia can occur from inadequate preoxygenation, airway obstruction or improper placement of the endotracheal tube, failed intubation, and pre-existing lung disease. Cardiovascular compromise from hypoxia resulting in bradycardia or cardiac arrest and dysrhythmias from vagal stimulation or pharmacologic agents such as succinylcholine can occur. Aspiration during intubation can result in pneumonia and alteration of ventilation/perfusion matching, complicating patient care (see the later section on aspiration). Airway trauma may occur in the setting of difficult or repeated attempts at intubation and can result in bleeding, dental trauma and aspiration of teeth, acute supraglottic or subglottic edema, and vocal fold injury.[3] Perforation of the esophagus or trachea is a potentially life-threatening complication that requires immediate intervention.[4,5]

Instrumentation and Equipment Preparation

Prior to intubation, appropriate instruments and equipment should be easily accessible and tested thoroughly to ensure proper functioning.

Endotracheal Tubes

Based on the child's size, an appropriately sized endotracheal tube and selected tubes that are 0.5 mm smaller and larger should be readily available. If a cuffed endotracheal tube is used, a tube 0.5 mm smaller than estimated should be used and the balloon should be tested for an air leak. Stylets should be available and, if used, should not protrude from the distal portion of the endotracheal tube to minimize trauma to the airway. Appropriately sized oral airways and tape cut to secure the endotracheal tube following intubation should be readily available.

Laryngoscopes

The laryngoscope blade should be tested, and the light source should be bright and white. A weak battery or defective bulb will cause a yellowish color. If a blade using a conventional light source and bulb is used, the bulb should be checked and tightened if loose. Newer blades using fiber optic technology eliminate this step. An appropriately sized bag valve mask with supplemental oxygen should be available. If an anesthesia bag using a Mapleson valve or other flow control device is used, the valve should be checked and flow adjusted so that the bag readily fills. The bag should be checked for air leaks that might impair filling it.

Monitors

Intubation and control of the airway should not occur without appropriate cardiac and respiratory monitoring. If rapid sequence intubation (RSI) is contemplated, secure vascular access should be obtained; pharmacologic agents for sedation or short-term paralysis and other adjunctive agents should be drawn up and ready for administration. An end-tidal carbon dioxide (ETCO$_2$) or exhaled CO$_2$ detector to confirm correct endotracheal tube placement is strongly recommended.[6–10] Continuous capnometry monitoring after intubation is helpful for early detection of accidental extubation and is suggested if available.

Support Personnel

Appropriate personnel should be available to assist with the procedure. Personnel will vary depending on the setting. For instance, in the emergency department or intensive care unit, a minimum of three individuals is required: an experienced provider for airway management, a person to administer the appropriate medications, and a person to perform cricoid pressure throughout the procedure and monitor the patient's oxygen saturation and heart rate and rhythm. In the operating suite, this scenario might be different with an anesthesiologist, an operating room nurse, and an otolaryngologist present.

PATIENT PREPARATION

Ideally, prior to medication administration and intubation, spontaneously breathing, adequately ventilating patients are preoxygenated with 100% oxygen delivered through a well-fitted face mask. Preoxygenation creates an oxygen reserve in the lungs and maximizes oxygen-carrying capacity of the blood creating an oxygen reserve.[11,12] Once sedated and paralyzed, the child can remain well oxygenated, thus postponing the need for bag mask ventilation and promoting tolerance for the brief period of apnea associated with the intubation procedure. Positive pressure ventilation should be avoided, if possible, because it can promote gastric distension, thus increasing the risk of aspiration of stomach contents.

TECHNIQUE

Intubation is a commonly performed procedure whose efficiency and success are clearly benefited by practice. Although it may seem easy to pass a small, semiflexible tube through an open channel, one should remain aware of several pitfalls and pointers. Patient positioning can greatly assist ease of intubation if there is a degree of neck flexion and head extension, thereby "opening up" the larynx. Opening the jaw can be problematic in an awake child but should be relatively easy if he or she is sedated, paralyzed, or anesthesitized. Selecting the correct length blade, roughly the length of the child's hand, should allow adequate elevation of the vallecula or epiglottis depending on whether a curved or straight blade is used. The correct line of force with the laryngoscope is "up and away"; a "rocking" motion on the upper alveolus or teeth is to be avoided. Under controlled circumstances, instilling a small, appropriately calculated amount of a topical anesthetic onto the supraglottic and glottic structures can reduce the potential for laryngospasm.

Sometimes, because of an anterior larynx or "short" neck, angulation and positioning are such that only the most posterior aspect of the larynx is seen; there is an epiglottis and a very limited portion of the arytenoid complex. By using one's knowledge of anatomy, the endotracheal tube can be advanced just "under" the epiglottis, feeding the passage of the beveled tip through the glottis; on occasion, rotating or rolling the tube between the fingers facilitates passage into the trachea.

Anterior cricoid pressure is a common maneuver, but it can increase internal laryngeal sensitivity and distort the natural plane of the trachea if pressed too greatly. Using a stylette is also a common adjunct and can be helpful in maintaining the shape and position of the tube tip. However, once the tube has passed through the glottis, it is important to retract the stylette gently as the endotracheal tube is further advanced into the trachea to avoid traumatizing the anterior tracheal wall or placing excess pressure on the posterior glottis.

SUPPORT OF THE CHILD WITH AN ARTIFICIAL AIRWAY

Once the child is successfully intubated, endotracheal tube placement should be confirmed by auscultation, end tidal or exhaled CO_2 ($ETCO_2$) monitoring, and a chest radiograph. The short trachea in children requires precise placement of the endotracheal tube (ETT) to prevent endobronchial intubation or the endotracheal tube's resting on the carina, which results in stimulation of the cough reflex. A routine chest radiograph is strongly recommended if the ETT must be repositioned.[14]

Two useful formulas may be employed to check for proper tube placement:

- The position of the endotracheal tube at the lip in centimeters should be close to three times the millimeter size of the endotracheal tube.[10,11] Thus, a 4.5-mm tube should be approximately 13.5 cm at the lip.
- For children 1 to 12 years of age, one can use 10 plus the age in years to check proper depth placement of the endotracheal tube. Therefore, a 4-year-old should have the endotracheal tube placed approximately 14 cm at the lip.

It cannot be stressed enough, however, that all children are unique and that the decision for tube size and depth of placement should ultimately remain individualized.

The ETT should be secured with tape and the tube should be wrapped in a spiral fashion to prevent it from slipping through the tape from excessive secretions. Appropriate cardiac, respiratory, and $ETCO_2$ monitoring should be initiated. Monitoring of adequate oxygenation and ventilation can be guided by noninvasive monitoring and blood gas analysis. Sedation and pain control to promote tolerance of the endotracheal tube should be administered and neuromuscular blocking agents should be used as needed. Prevention of secondary injury, including hypoxia, barotrauma, infection, nutritional deprivation, and inappropriate fluid balance with resultant edema, is crucial to reduction of morbidity and mortality in this patient population.

TABLE 6.1
Conditions Associated with Difficult Intubation in Children

Micrognathia

Pierre–Robin syndrome	DiGeorge's syndrome
Treacher Collins syndrome	Goldenhar syndrome

Macroglossia

Trisomy 21	Mucopolysaccharidosis (Hunter, Hurler syndromes)
Beckwith Wiedemann syndrome	Glycogen storage disease (Pompe's disease)

Facial anomalies

Mid-face hypoplasia	Facial clefts
Crouzon's syndrome	Facial asymmetry
Apert's syndrome	

Neck anomalies

Rheumatoid arthritis	Cervical spine injury
Ankylosing spondylitis	

Inflammatory/infectious/neoplastic

Hemangiomas	Angioedema
Papillomas	Tempomandibular joint disease
Peritonsillar and retropharyngeal abscess	

Obstructive processes

Foreign body aspiration	Laryngeal web/cyst
Subglottic stenosis	

Miscellaneous

Morbid obesity	Patients in halo traction devices

THE COMPLICATED INTUBATION

The most highly skilled person with pediatric airway experience should perform the intubation for emergent airway stabilization.

General Considerations

Risk factors for some infants and children may be identifiable prior to intubation. Syndromes associated with difficult intubation are listed in Table 6.1. Difficult intubations must be anticipated and an alternative plan for securing the airway should be established before rapid sequence intubation (RSI) and control of the airway are attempted. This plan might include consultation with anesthesia personnel or an otolaryngologist. An alternative means of airway control and ventilation may be considered. Inserting an appropriately sized oral or nasal airway may be followed by bag-mask ventilation.

Appropriate adjunctive equipment such as fiberoptic laryngoscopy, specialized laryngoscopes such as the Bullard scope, light wands, and/or laryngeal mask airways should be readily available. Esophageal combitubes or laryngeal tubes[14] can be considered for the older child. Nasotracheaal intubation in a cooperative, awake, and spontaneously breathing adolescent head and neck trauma patient may be a valid option. Needle cricothyrotomy may provide a life-saving airway when intubation has failed[15] and should only be performed by skilled providers who are familiar with

TABLE 6.2
Agents Commonly Used for RSI

Drug	Dose	Route	Side effects
Cardiovascular adjunct			
Atropine	0.02 mg/kg; min. dose: 0.1 mg; max. dose: 1.0 mg	IV	Paradoxical bradycardia with less than minimal dose; bradycardic response to hypoxemia is blunted
Sedative agents			
Midazolam (Versed®)	0.1–0.2 mg/kg	IV	Hypotension and respiratory depression
Ketamine (Ketalar®)	1–2 mg/kg	IV	Increases secretions and intracranial pressure; laryngospasm
Neuromuscular blocking agents			
Succinylcholine (Anectine®)	Infants: 2 mg/kg; Children: 1 mg/kg	IV	Increase intracranial, intraocular, intragastric pressure; fasciculations; arrhythmias; hyperkalemia
Rocuronium (Zemuron®)	0.6–1.2 mg/kg	IV	Rapid onset of action; duration of action: 20–40 min
Vecuronium (Norcuron®)	0.1–0.2 mg/kg	IV	Slower onset of action (>1 min); duration of action: 30–45 min

Notes: Pharmacologic agents listed are for routine intubation. Other agents are available for intubation with multi-system organ dysfunction. These agents should only be used by skilled providers familiar with doses and side effects.

the anatomy of the pediatric airway. Emergency tracheostomy is rare in a child and is best completed by an otolaryngologist or other surgeon well versed in the anatomy of the pediatric airway.

Rapid Sequence Intubation

Rapid sequence intubation (RSI) should be considered when endotracheal intubation is indicated in the awake or semiconscious pediatric patient. RSI employs pharmacologic agents to facilitate emergent endotracheal intubation and reduce adverse effects, including pain, arrhythmias, airway trauma, gastric regurgitation and aspiration, rise in systemic and intracranial pressure, hypoxemia, psychological trauma, and death.[16] Only properly trained individuals familiar with the pediatric airway and pharmacologic agents used for RSI should utilize this procedure (see Table 6.2).

RSI is not indicated for patients who are in a deep coma or cardiac arrest. Relative contraindications to RSI include: (1) provider concern that intubation or mask ventilation may be unsuccessful; (2) significant facial or laryngeal edema, trauma, or distortion; or (3) a spontaneously breathing, adequately ventilating patient whose airway maintenance is dependent on his own upper airway muscle tone and positioning (e.g., upper airway obstruction, epiglottitis, or mediastinal masses).[16] Inadequately ventilated patients may require preoxygenation via bag mask ventilation prior to RSI.

Rapid Paralysis

Succinylcholine is the only depolarizing agent with rapid onset and short duration; however, it has the potential to produce numerous adverse effects, some potentially fatal. Cardiac dysrhythmias can occur secondarily to hyperkalemia or profound vagal mediated effects. A patient with a history of hyperkalemia, such as renal failure patients, should not receive succinylcholine. Moreover, patients with a history of congenital myotonia, muscular dystrophy, or other muscle disorders are at high risk for malignant hyperthermia and should not receive succinylcholine. Additionally, succinylcholine can raise intragastric and intracranial pressure. Because of these potential detrimental effects, succinylcholine's only remaining indication is for RSI; it should never be used to maintain paralysis after intubation.[17-22]

Atropine can minimize the vagal effects of succinylcholine if administered 1 to 2 minutes prior to intubation. Atropine blocks the bradycardic response to hypoxemia; therefore, pulse oximetry is crucial. In general, atropine should be administered to any child under 1 year of age to prevent excess vagal activation.

Providers choosing to use succinylcholine must be completely familiar with its potential side effects and contraindications and carefully weigh its risk/benefit ratio compared with the available nondepolarizing agents. Newer nondepolarizing agents, such as rocuronium, have a rapid onset of action that approaches succinylcholine and more benign side effect profiles.[23]

Aspiration

Aspiration is a serious complication and should be considered a threat in any emergent operation. Inhalation of contents with a pH of less than 2.5 can cause severe bronchoconstriction and significant injury to the tracheal mucosa. A large volume of fluid may be inhaled or particulate matter may be aspirated; either may cause airway obstruction. Aspirated contents may include pathogenic bacteria or colonic bacilli, which may produce an infection within the lungs. Pulmonary obstruction and atelectasis lead to pulmonary shunting and a widening of the arterial-alveolar oxygen gradient. Life-threatening pulmonary edema and cardiac congestion may occur. Fulminant acute lung injury or acute respiratory distress syndrome (ARDS) may ensue.

Applying cricoid pressure prior to initiation of bag-mask ventilation and maintaining pressure until the child is successfully intubated can reduce aspiration risk during intubation. Administration of a neuromuscular blocking agent as soon as possible after initiation of mask ventilation will make ventilation easier and potentially cause less gastric distension. Placement of an nasogastric tube prior to intubation may cause emesis and promote (additional) aspiration.[22]

If aspiration is suspected, immediate tracheal suctioning is vital; then, rapid intubation should be continued if necessary. The main goal is to clear the airway with saline and suctioning. Although not typically performed, when copious aspiration has occurred, the pH of tracheal secretions can be tested with repeated lavages until they have returned to neutral. If solid material was aspirated, rigid bronchoscopy for foreign body removal may need to be performed. Once the airway is cleared, the patient may benefit from sustained positive end-expiratory pressure (PEEP) ventilation for alveolar recruitment. Antibiotics for bacterial contamination should not be used on a routine basis and should be tailored to tracheal aspirate cultures. Bronchodilators for persistent bronchospasm may be helpful for lower airway obstruction and enhancing mucociliary clearance of secretions and debris.

The Emergency Surgical Airway

Creating a surgical airway in a physically mature patient in a crisis setting in which oral intubation is unreasonable and timing is critical can be a daunting task. Performing this procedure on the far more pliable and smaller cervical structures in the pediatric neck is fraught with even more danger. The most prominent anterior structure in the infant neck is the cricoid ring and not the thyroid cartilage. The interspace between the thyroid and cricoid cartilages is not fully developed until mid-childhood, rendering identification of this surgical landmark problematic. Without an artificial airway in place, the trachea is easily displaced or collapsed with retraction, risking exposure of the carotid sheaths and esophagus. Except in truly life-saving situations, it is far better to continue with alternative means of ventilation through the larynx, however suboptimal, while transporting the patient to a facility where skilled pediatric airway specialists are available.

CRITICAL CARE ISSUES

MECHANICAL VENTILATION

General Considerations

The nature of respiratory support is determined by the underlying pathophysiology. In most cases, ENT emergencies will be primarily related to the upper airway obstruction with minimal or no pulmonary disease. The artificial airway is required primarily to maintain patency of the upper airway; therefore, ventilator management, if needed, is adjusted to maintain adequate gas exchange and prevent ventilator-induced injury. For this section, we will assume normal lung function.

The principles of respiratory support for children are

- Provision and maintenance of a secure airway
- Maintenance of adequate gas exchange
- Reduction of the work of breathing
- Maintenance of airway function including humidification, filtration, conduction, and warming of inspired air

Ventilator Features

Ventilator parameters should be adjusted on an individual basis. Variables that need to be adjusted for mechanical ventilation in children include tidal volume, peak pressure, end-expiratory pressure, and inspiratory time, rate, and oxygen concentration. Initially, it is useful to ventilate the patient manually to assess the child's pulmonary compliance and airway resistance. The magnitude of the tidal breath, defined as the volume of air required to expand the chest adequately by direct observation, usually corresponds to 8 to 10 cc/kg. This value allows for compensation of the ventilator circuit, tubing compliance, and gas compressibility. The lowest possible tidal volume that promotes chest rise is recommended because evidence strongly suggests that high volumes potentiate lung injury.[23]

This optimal tidal volume can be translated into a delivered pressure depending upon the mode of ventilation used. Specifically, patients may be ventilated in volume or pressure modes. The former refers to adjusting the tidal volume and respiratory rate; the latter refers to time-cycled, pressure-limited ventilation. Decisions regarding ventilation strategies are best left to intensivists or anesthesiologists, who routinely provide assisted ventilation to children. PEEP should be provided for all children who are mechanically ventilated to maintain alveolar inflation. The inspiratory time is typically set to provide an inspiratory/expiratory ratio of 1:3 with a rate that is age appropriate. The minimum inspiratory time is 0.5 second. These parameters are adjusted as the patient emerges from sedation and neuromuscular blockade. Further ventilator adjustments will be determined by subsequent blood gas analysis and physical examination.

Many ventilators provide support of spontaneous ventilation. These modes depend on proper adjustment of the ventilator to sense when the patient is making an inspiratory effort. Support is generally provided by increased flow at a fixed pressure for a time period determined by sensing when the patient begins to exhale. These pressure support modes of ventilation are often quite useful in spontaneously breathing children. These modes assist the child by overcoming the work of breathing and provide a modest amount of support with the initiation of each breath.[24] Children who tolerate these support modes will require less sedation. Concentrations of 60 to 100% oxygen are used initially and adjusted based upon pulse oximetry, blood gas analysis, and clinical impression.

MECHANICAL VENTILATION COMPLICATIONS

Endotracheal Tube Complications

Significant injury can result from an endotracheal tube traversing the upper airway. Patients intubated nasally may develop pressure necrosis of the nasal ala or septum.[25–28] Eustachian tube obstruction may result in middle ear effusions,[29] and sinus drainage obstruction by ostial occlusion can result in sinusitis.[28,29] Corneal abrasion, trismus, and infections including laryngitis and sinusitis have been reported.[30,31] Adhesive tape may irritate the sensitive skin of children resulting in skin breakdown on the nose or face.[25] Tissue necrosis can occur at the corners of the mouth in addition to palatal trauma from an oral endotracheal tube. Patients intubated orally may sustain tongue paresis, paralysis, or necrosis; palatal necrosis, clefting, grooving, or asymmetry; alveolar and lip ulceration; primary tooth dilaceration; crossbite; poor speech intelligibility; and enamel hypoplasia.[25–27,32,33]

Laryngeal Trauma

Laryngeal injury — most notably to the vocal folds, aryepiglottic folds, and subglottic region — can occur from intubation.[30,33] A large endotracheal tube resulting in a tight fit can cause edema and major ulceration to the true vocal folds and narrow subglottic space. Eventually, scarring and formation of granulation tissue can result in partial or complete airway obstruction.

Subglottic and Tracheal Trauma

The risk of subglottic and tracheal injury is increased by cuffed endotracheal tubes, tracheal infections, repeated intubations, uncontrolled gastroesophageal reflux disease, cardiovascular instability, suction catheters producing mucosal damage, and prolonged intubation. These injuries can be minimized with close attention to details such as

- Choosing the appropriately sized endotracheal tube
- Careful placement of tape
- Use of soft suction catheters that are not advanced beyond the distal tip of the endotracheal or tracheostomy tube
- Avoidance of cuffed endotracheal tubes in small children unless indicated by their disease process
- Monitoring the air leak around the endotracheal tube
- Appropriate sedation to reduce airway injury
- Good hand-washing to avoid iatrogenic infections

Pulmonary Parenchymal Trauma

Excessive lung distension produced by mechanical ventilation can produce acute lung injury resulting in multiple organ dysfunction or failure.[23] Mechanical ventilation using high peak inspiratory pressure and large tidal volumes can lead to pulmonary edema and diffuse alveolar damage known as volutrauma.[34] The cyclic opening and closing of the distal airways and alveoli with this mode of ventilation can result in progressive injury to the pulmonary parenchyma,[35] which has changed ventilation strategies for children with acute lung injury. Smaller tidal volumes, higher ventilation rates, and permissive hypercapnia limit alveolar stretch, thus reducing the risk of lung injury in this patient population.

Barotrauma is another complication of mechanical ventilation caused by continuous distending pressure of the alveoli and small airways.[36] This all-inclusive term describes pathological changes ranging from pulmonary interstitial emphysema to life-threatening events such as tension pneumothorax. Barotrauma has been associated with high levels of PEEP, in addition to high inflating pressures and prolonged inspiratory times.

Injury to the lungs from barotrauma typically occurs at the broncho-alveolar junction and bronchovascular sheath. Progressive injury can lead to dissection of air toward the hilum and throughout the mediastinum, resulting in subcutaneous air in the mediastinum and peritoneal spaces presenting as pneumomediastinum and pneumoperitoneum, which are relatively benign complications. Life-threatening complications such as tension pneumothorax, pneumopericardium, air embolism, and pulmonary edema can also occur. To minimize the risk of these complications, end expiratory as well as peak inspiratory pressures must be closely monitored.

Secondary Organ System Complications

Mechanical ventilation can also adversely affect other organ systems. Cardiovascular and circulatory depression as a result of decreased venous return to the heart is associated with the use of continuous positive airway pressure (CPAP) or PEEP. Mechanical ventilation has been associated with increased pulmonary vascular resistance, decreased biventricular filling, interventricular displacement from the right to the left ventricle, activation of reflex neurohumoral factors to maintain intravascular volume, and a decrease in left ventricular blood flow.[37–39]

Avoiding controlled modes of ventilation and allowing the patient to breathe spontaneously with positive expiratory pressure while maintaining an adequate intravascular filling pressure can minimize these problems. Neurohumoral responses may be the result of decreased renal blood flow, atrial compression stimulating ADH release, and changes in the distribution of corticomedullary renal perfusion resulting in decreased urine output, creatinine clearance, and renal sodium excretion.[40–42] Decreased cerebral perfusion in head trauma victims and decreased hepatic perfusion have also been described as complications of positive pressure ventilation.

Fluid Overload

Excessive fluid accumulation can result in atrial stretch and release of atrial natriuretic factor (ANF) in an effort to compensate for fluid overload.[42] Most often, however, the net effect of positive pressure ventilation is fluid retention with a risk of generalized tissue edema. The latter can promote pressure necrosis, which is exacerbated in chemically paralyzed children; therefore, frequent turning and positioning are essential to the care of these children. Restricting fluids to 80 to 100% maintenance and/or the use of diuretics can prevent the development of systemic and pulmonary edema. Often, diuretics are used to permit adequate caloric intake, which is accompanied by normal to increased fluid intake, depending on the need for IV fluid administration associated with medication administration.

Atelectasis

Any child with an artificial airway, no matter how healthy, can develop atelectasis. Appropriate use of chest physiotherapy, good suctioning techniques, and frequent turning can minimize these risks. Close attention to chest rise and airway pressures during mechanical or manual ventilation may also be helpful.

Nososcomial Infections

Pneumonia in an intubated child can occur by providing potential pathogens increased access to the trachea and lower airways.[43] The incidence of nosocomial pneumonia can exceed 20% in patients who are mechanically ventilated for more than 48 hours.[44] Common bacterial agents include Gram-negative bacteria aspirated from the gastrointestinal tract or bacteria that colonize the upper airway.

Viruses — most notably respiratory syncytial virus (RSV) — are also common pathogens, especially during outbreaks. Guidelines to minimize this complication have been published.[45]

Intravenous catheter infections may complicate the care of a child requiring airway support in the pediatric intensive care unit. Length of stay in the pediatric intensive care unit (PICU), duration of catheter placement, site of catheter placement, infusion of fluids through the catheter, and underlying illness all contribute to the risk of a catheter-related infection.[43]

PHARMACOTHERAPEUTIC SUPPORT

Neuromuscular Paralysis

Neuromuscular blocking agents and sedatives are often used as adjunctive therapy to promote tolerance to the endotracheal tube and to facilitate mechanical ventilation. Neuromuscular blockade should be used judiciously, but is highly recommended in children with an unstable or extremely critical airway — particularly when movement or dislodgment of the tube poses a threat to the child. Although spontaneous breathing is encouraged as much as possible, on some occasions the use of muscle relaxants is warranted, such as when the patient with severe lung injury requires high volumes and pressures to provide adequate gas exchange. Management of children with severe lung injury extends beyond the scope of this discussion, however; experienced pediatric intensivists or anesthesiologists are best suited to manage their care.

Prolonged Muscle Weakness

Prolonged muscle weakness following use of neuromuscular blocking agents is a known complication[22] that can be exacerbated by the use of steroids or aminoglycoside antibiotics.[46] The optimal approach is to use muscle relaxants only as needed and in the smallest doses possible. It is imperative to remember that neuromuscular blocking agents provide no sedation or analgesic effects. Chemically paralyzed children require adequate sedation and analgesia because their senses remain intact despite their inability to move.[47,48]

Other Risks of Paralysis

Numerous risks are engendered if the child is chemically paralyzed. The physical examination is essentially lost, and the level of sedation and analgesia are difficult to assess. Muscle atrophy can occur with prolonged ventilation. To prevent accumulation of secretions with resultant atelectasis in the lower airways, the child must be turned on a regular basis and routine suctioning of accumulated secretions is essential. If the endotracheal tube becomes dislodged, the patient will be unable to breathe spontaneously until this problem is corrected. Therefore, continuous pulse oximetry and often capnography are important to reduce the risk of these adverse events. Finally, attention to eye and skin care is important to prevent corneal injury and skin breakdown.

Sedation

Continued sedation and intravenous access are two ongoing concerns in children requiring ventilator support. The lack of appropriate pharmacologic sedation or vascular access can have significant consequences if not addressed. Virtually all ventilated children require IV or enteral sedation. Children should be sedated as needed to minimize movement, promote tolerance to the endotracheal tube, facilitate mechanical ventilation, and prevent them from pulling at IV lines or tubes resulting in potential harm to them.

The benzodiazepines are the most useful sedative/hypnotic/anxiolytic drugs in current clinical practice. Administered parenterally or enterally as an infusion or on a routine bolus schedule, they are potent amnestic agents, anticonvulsants, and skeletal muscle relaxants. Although they are generally safe agents, the potential side effects must be considered. In high doses, they can blunt the respiratory response to hypoxia and hypercarbia. This dose-dependent complication is potentiated with the co-administration of any opioid or additional sedative.

Pain

It must be anticipated that pain management will be required in critically ill children for physiologic as well as humanistic reasons. By activating the stress response, pain promotes protein catabolism and a negative nitrogen balance. This stress response can cause fluid and electrolyte derangements via antidiuretic hormone and corticotropin release.[49] Opioids remain the most frequently prescribed analgesics for the critically ill patient. In addition, some opiates such as morphine have sedative effects that are favorable in the patient with pain-induced agitation. They are most commonly given parenterally in the ICU setting but are also effective via enteral, intramuscular, and epidural routes. The potential complications associated with these drugs include muscle rigidity, respiratory depression, histamine-induced hypotension and bronchospasm, prolonged gastric transit times, and urinary retention.

Morphine is an inexpensive, commonly used, and effective opiate for moderate to severe pain. It seems to possess a greater incidence of histamine release, in addition to being more sedating than other opiates. Fentanyl, a synthetic opiate, is 100 times more potent than morphine with a rapid onset and relatively short duration of action, making it an excellent analgesic for short-term or continuous infusion. It does not promote histamine release, has less sedative effect, and is associated with chest wall rigidity when administered rapidly and in high doses. Morphine and fentanyl can be administered as an IV bolus or an infusion.

Codeine is frequently combined with acetaminophen and provides good control of moderate pain when an oral agent is preferred. Other opiates such as meperidine are infrequently used in the ICU setting because of metabolites that can accumulate with repeated dosing and result in seizures.[50] The nonsteroidal anti-inflammatory drugs (NSAIDs) ibuprofen and ketorolac are effective against low to moderate pain and are quite effective when combined with opiates. They work by inhibiting prostaglandin synthesis and thus decreasing the production of inflammatory cytokines. Major side effects associated with NSAIDs are bleeding due to platelet inhibition, renal failure, gastric ulcers, and electrolyte abnormalities.[51] Ketorolac can be administered IM or IV and should be limited to no more than eight doses because of its adverse effects on renal blood flow. Acetaminophen is a widely used analgesic agent that, unlike the NSAIDs, does not possess any anti-inflammatory activity. It is useful for minor to moderate pain and can be administered orally or rectally. The NSAIDs and acetaminophen have antipyretic activity as well.

ICU Psychosis

Additionally, anxiety, fear, and a lack of sleep can potentiate pain and cause psychosis in critically ill children. ICU psychosis is a well-described phenomenon that typically occurs 3 to 5 days after admission to the intensive care unit.[52] A frightening atmosphere, lack of sleep, unusual sounds, and deprivation of day/night cycles contribute to this syndrome. Sedatives help prevent this psychosis by alleviating anxiety and promoting sleep.

Drug Tolerance, Dependence, and Withdrawal

It is not uncommon for children who have been routinely sedated and/or treated with narcotics for several days to require a tapering protocol using methadone (a longer acting opiate) and/or clonidine (a centrally acting alpha-adrenergic agonist) to prevent withdrawal.[53-55] Drug tolerance, dependence, and withdrawal must be anticipated because they cannot always be avoided.[53,54] The dose and duration will determine tolerance to these agents. Signs of withdrawal include excessive central nervous system activation manifested by agitation and diaphoresis, which must be differentiated from respiratory distress and hypoxia.[53,54] Sympathetic nervous system stimulation resulting in tachycardia and hypertension, fever, and piloerection can occur.[54] Irritability, increased wakefulness, tremulousness, hyperactive deep tendon reflexes, pupillary dilation, and hypertonicity may also be noted. Gastrointestinal manifestations include vomiting, watery or diarrheal stools, and feeding intolerance.

Agents such as diphenhydramine (Benadryl® and generics), propofol (Diprivan®), ketamine (Ketalar®), and chloral hydrate also can be used for sedation. In addition to its sedative effects, diphenhydramine can reduce urticaria, which results in discomfort that can occur with morphine sulfate administration. High doses of chloral hydrate can promote dysrhythmias,[56,57] and prolonged infusions of propofol have been associated with metabolic acidosis and sudden death in children.[58,59] Consultation with a pediatric intensivist or anesthesiologist familiar with these drugs should occur if these additional agents are required.

Vascular Access

It is important that all children who require intubation and mechanical ventilation have secure vascular access. Prolonged vascular access, however, can become problematic in this patient population and advanced preparation is appropriate. A central venous line or percutaneous intravenous catheter (PIC) is recommended for children who require long-term ventilation and sedation for more than several days or who may require central hyperalimentation for nutritional support. PICs have a low infection risk due to their peripheral insertion site and can be maintained for long-term use with good catheter and site care.

These specialized catheters can be inserted by the anesthesiologist or surgeon in the operating room at the time of surgery or by the intensivist in the intensive care unit following surgery. Insertion of central venous catheters is associated with complications that need to be recognized. Complications include pneumo- and hemothorax, bleeding, arterial puncture, catheter misplacement, vascular damage including thrombosis, and infection.[60–62]

FLUIDS AND NUTRITION

Fluid Maintenance

Fluid and nutrition physiologic needs complicate the care of children who require assisted ventilation. Normally hydrated children require no more than 80 to 100% maintenance fluids because insensible losses are minimal while ventilated. Even with this relative fluid restriction, diuretic therapy may be required if the child becomes edematous. Mechanical ventilation affects receptors in the lung and alters renal blood flow, resulting in fluid retention due to increased levels of antidiuretic hormone.[39–41]

The simplest method of delivering maintenance fluids is by some form of nutrition. Enteral feedings nourish and stimulate the intestinal tract and can enhance immune function. New information suggests that early enteral feeding is superior to parenteral nutrition by reducing the incidence of intra-abdominal and pulmonary infections following major stress.[63] Parenteral nutrition can have significant complications such as catheter infection, impaired neutrophil function, and worsening metabolic derangement, in addition to increased cost.

The nutritional goal for most sick infants is 115 to 140 kcal/kg/day, and young children (1 to 6 years old) should receive 1300 to 2000 kcal/day.[64] Fluid-restricted patients can achieve these goals by increasing the caloric density of the feeds with additives to reach 30 to 32 cal/oz formula concentrations. Nutrition should not be compromised at the expense of limiting fluids. In many children, liberalizing fluids to meet their nutritional goals and use of diuretics to help maintain fluid balance are ideal.

Enteral Alimentation

When the intestinal tract is functional and there are no contraindications to enteral feeds, it is preferable to use this route. Bacterial translocation resulting in a systemic infection can occur in a bowel that has not been used for a period of time. Opiates may delay gastrointestinal motility, although this is typically limited to gastric emptying and colonic transport. Therefore, sedated patients receiving high-dose opoids will usually tolerate enteral feeds, especially if the feeds are administered directly into the small intestine by nasal/oral feeding tubes. Consultation with a dietitian knowledgeable in pediatric nutrition will assist in proper selection of the many formulas available that can be adjusted for the patient's age and specific needs.

Enteral nutrition can be administered through a feeding tube passed directly into the stomach or duodenum. Gastric feeds can be bolused or administered continuously like duodenal feedings. Though arguably safer and more physiologic than parenteral nutrition, enteral feedings can have complications.

Misplacement of the feeding tube can result in perforation of the esophagus or placement in the trachea delivering feeds directly into the lungs. Therefore, tube placement should be checked by auscultation and radiographic confirmation before initiation of enteral nutrition. Gastroesophageal reflux and aspiration can occur, more commonly with gastric feeds, but can be avoided if the feeding tube is placed distal to the ligament of Treitz. Diarrhea from hyperosmolar formula occurs in some children requiring high caloric density feeds administered by the duodenal route. Feedings delivered into the stomach through a gastric feeding tube act as an osmoregulator and promote a physiologic pancreatic response for better absorption if hyperosmolar formulas are not tolerated. Alternatively, the caloric density of the feeds can be reduced, thus decreasing the osmolarity of the formula. If enteral feedings are not tolerated, parenteral nutrition should be provided for nutritional support.

WEANING FROM MECHANICAL VENTILATION

General Considerations

When the indications for mechanical ventilation are no longer present, the patient should be weaned from ventilator support. This presumes that the underlying disease process has improved and the patient has the ability to assume the greater responsibility of alveolar ventilation without the expenditure of excessive work. Assessment of indices such as tidal volume, minute volume, pulmonary compliance, negative inspiratory force, rapid shallow breathing index, occlusion pressure, work of breathing, and oxygen cost of breathing index can be useful. In addition, newer support modes of ventilation designed to allow reloading of the "respiratory pump" can assist considerably in the weaning process.[65-67] Patients who do not have chronic conditions that mandate a complex weaning protocol can usually tolerate a relatively abrupt discontinuation of mechanical ventilation.

Criteria

The child's ability to respire spontaneously will depend on several factors — easily remembered by the mnemonic CALMS:

"C" is for central nervous system and refers to the general sensorium of the patient. The central nervous system drive to breathe and protect the airway is essential prior to extubation. This can be assessed by testing for a cough and gag, observation for spontaneous respiratory efforts, and possibly a brief trial of CPAP. If the patient is mildly hyperventilated, normalization of the $PaCO_2$ should occur before this trial.

"A" is for airway and refers to the ability to maintain the airway. Determining if sufficient time has elapsed for the airway to heal may be difficult to assess. Bronchoscopy or laryngoscopy may be required. An air leak around the endotracheal tube may indicate decreased edema in the subglottic area but may not be predictive of successful extubation.[68]

"L" refers to lungs and their ability to provide adequate gas exchange without significant work of breathing. The clinical exam, blood gas analysis, cardiac and respiratory monitoring, and chest radiographs provide the useful and necessary information.

"M" refers to musculoskeletal. Muscle strength and nutrition must be assessed. Children who are malnourished or who have received a prolonged course of neuromuscular blockade often require a slower weaning course. Chest wall mechanics need to be intact. Children with chest injuries or impaired diaphragm function will develop respiratory distress if chest expansion cannot occur.

"S" represents secretions, which can be problematic for many small infants or neurologically compromised children. The respiratory therapists and nursing staff can be very helpful in assessing the ability of the patient to handle secretions. The infant must have a strong cough and secretions must be minimal if the child is to maintain lung volume off the ventilator and prevent accumulation of secretions once extubated.

Preparation for Extubation

The intensivist and otolaryngologist should mutually agree on the optimal time for a trial of extubation. The child may be taken to the operating suite for bronchoscopy to evaluate the airway prior to extubation, or fiber optic or direct laryngoscopy can be performed at the bedside. Anticipation of a difficult intubation based upon bronchoscopy or direct laryngoscopy will determine whether anesthesia support or the pediatric otolaryngologist will need to be present during the extubation trial. In addition, specialized airway equipment such as a fiber optic bronchoscope, Bullard laryngoscope, laryngeal mask airway, or laryngeal tubes may be needed if a difficult intubation is anticipated.

As mechanical ventilation is being weaned, anticipation and preparation for extubation is crucial to optimize chances for a successful extubation. Sedatives must be discontinued or weaned if administered over a prolonged course. Nutrition must be optimized to assure sufficient caloric reserves for the patient to breathe on his own. Enteral feedings should be held for at least 4 hours prior to extubation in the event that emergent control of the airway is required following extubation. If neuromuscular blocking agents have been used, sufficient time on a support mode of ventilation must be anticipated to allow the patient to regain muscle strength and endurance. If an air leak at less than 20 cm water is not present around the endotracheal tube,[69] downsizing to a smaller tube may be helpful prior to extubation. Alternatively, if an air leak is not present within reasonable levels, the patient may not be a reasonable candidate for extubation.

The use of a short-term course of intravenous steroids, such as dexamethasone, given every 6 to 8 hours, to decrease subglottic edema prior to extubation is often considered helpful although evidence is conflicting.[70,71] The decision to use steroids should be discussed with the pediatric intensivist or anesthesiologist and otolaryngologist. If long-term systemic steroids are administered, side effects such as glucose intolerance, gastritis and bleeding, adrenal suppression, infection, mental status alterations, hypertension, and hypokalemia should be anticipated and the child should be monitored closely. H2 antagonists or other agents for gastrointestinal prophylaxis should be considered.

Weaning with a Tracheostomy Tube

The tracheostomy tube facilitates weaning by reducing airway resistance and functional dead space ventilation by bypassing the upper airway. In general, weaning a patient with a tracheostomy tube from mechanical ventilation is approached in a similar fashion to weaning a child with an endotracheal tube. With the tracheotomy tube in place and simultaneous decannulation not planned, the critical clinical issues for weaning from mechanical ventilation are identical to those detailed earlier for intubated children.

CARE OF THE CHILD FOLLOWING EXTUBATION

General Considerations

Long-term management issues of extubation sequelae are discussed in Chapter 22 (extubation problems). Short-term extubation complications or failures will manifest within minutes to hours after the tube has been removed from the child. Following extubation, the child must be closely observed for signs of respiratory distress or failure. Distress may result from airway obstruction secondary to edema or excessive secretions, anatomic obstruction such as the tongue or upper airway structures, tracheal collapse due to malacia, or excessive sedation impairing normal ventilatory drive. The cumulative effect of initially mild to moderate airway restriction may not be appreciated until manifested by gradual breathing fatigue.

Excessive secretions can be managed by suctioning and pulmonary toilet. Nasopharyngeal airways may help to alleviate upper airway obstruction and also facilitate suctioning of secretions from the hypopharynx. Diuretics may be beneficial by eliminating retained fluid once positive pressure ventilation has been terminated. Partial reversal of narcotics with naloxone (Narcan®) will help alleviate depressed respiratory effort secondary to prolonged effects of narcotics.

Adjunctive Intervention

Oxygen and Heliox

Oxygen supplementation after extubation is rarely regretted; it may be deferred for children who become agitated with the application of the oxygen delivery device if they are not hypoxemic while breathing room air. Cool humidification may also be useful. Heliox, a mixture of helium and oxygen, improves airflow through constricted airways by decreasing gas density.[72-75] The beneficial effects of helium are obtained with concentrations of 60 to 70% helium (i.e., 40 to 30% oxygen), limiting its use if the patient is hypoxic. Heliox combined with aerosolized racemic epinephrine or steroids (see below) may be beneficial to the child with severe airway obstruction. The high thermal conductivity of Heliox can result in hypothermia;[74] therefore, close observation for thermal instability in the infant or small child is important when this agent is used.

Steroids and Epinephrine

Systemic steroids may be beneficial by relieving airway soft tissue edema. Aerosolized racemic epinephrine (2.25% solution) is effective in relieving postextubation stridor. A dose of 0.25 mL in infants and 0.5 to 1.0 mL in older children, mixed with 2.5 to 3 mL of normal saline, is nebulized at a frequency not greater than every hour. Aerosolized steroids such as budesonide or dexamethasone have been shown to relieve stridor associated with croup.[76-79] They can be added to racemic epinephrine; however, their efficacy for postextubation stridor remains unclear. Use of bronchodilators such as albuterol may promote beta adrenergic stimulation, thus resulting in vasodilation with resultant tissue edema and potentiating upper airway obstruction. Therefore, the use of beta adrenergic agonists should be minimized[80] and children should be monitored for potential return of airway symptoms.

Additional Interventions

Using continuous positive airway pressure (CPAP) — particularly in infants — placement of a nasopharyngeal airway, and placing the patient in a high Fowler's position or the patient's position of comfort may be helpful. Antibiotics may be useful and should be guided by recent culture and sensitivity information when feasible.[81]

TRANSPORT OF THE PEDIATRIC PATIENT WITH A CRITICAL AIRWAY

BACKGROUND

Evolution of pediatric critical care medicine has dictated the need for specialized transport teams to evaluate and safely transport critically ill and injured children to a regional pediatric center. These specialized teams are designed to meet the special needs of pediatric patients. The pediatric transport team is an integral component of any pediatric facility providing care for children ranging in age from newborns to adolescents. Many acutely ill children will have respiratory-related problems; therefore, the need for expertise in airway management is crucial. A dedicated transport team can significantly reduce major adverse events, thus improving patient care.[82–85] Although team composition and skill levels may vary, care provided for the child with a critical airway should be managed by the most experienced person who is adept at managing a pediatric airway.

PLANNING AND PREPARATION

Appropriate planning and anticipation of adverse events is crucial to ensure the safe, efficient transport of any child. Following stabilization of the child with a critical airway problem in the referring facility, transfer to a pediatric center with a pediatric intensive care unit for ongoing monitoring and support should be arranged. The goal of the pediatric transport team is to provide rapid assessment, stabilization, and safe transport of the critically ill child to a center where ongoing care can be provided. The team must anticipate problems during transport and maintain stability and ongoing monitoring of major organ system functions, thus preventing morbidity and mortality.

Transport begins with communication of the child's condition, which allows the receiving center to prepare for the admission. The referring center needs to document events and laboratory studies, make copies of appropriate records and radiographic studies, and keep the referring center informed while the transport team is en route.

Prior to transport, the team should secure the airway; document the endotracheal tube position, including recording the position of the artificial airway relative to the lip or teeth; and establish appropriate monitoring for transport. Stabilization of the child with a critical airway should occur in a setting such as the emergency department or operating suite as discussed earlier. Team composition may vary, but it is preferable that the most skilled person experienced with the pediatric airway escort the patient, along with a respiratory therapist, transport nurse, or paramedic. In children with a critical airway, a physician skilled in pediatric airway management can enhance care and reduce morbidity.[84–85] Emergency care providers who do not routinely deal with pediatric airway emergencies have intubation success rates of 60% or less in children less than 1 year of age, and higher complication rates in children with normal airways.[86–89] Therefore, it is unlikely that successful intubation would occur in the child with a critical airway when performed by an inexperienced provider.

Provisions for securing the airway include ready availability of an appropriately sized endotracheal tube in case the tube becomes dislodged during transport and having an alternative plan in the event that the child cannot be reintubated. As the patient is packaged for transport, confirmation of the ETT should have occurred as well as ensuring proper placement of the ETT. The child should be suctioned and the security of the ETT should be rechecked. Appropriate monitoring, including cardiac and respiratory monitoring and pulse oximetry, in addition to $ETCO_2$ monitoring, should be established.

The decision to ventilate the child manually or mechanically during transfer will be determined by the equipment available to each team. Smaller transport ventilators providing various modes of ventilation are available and can be used on a variety of patients ranging from infants to adolescents. Manual ventilation results in greater fluctuation of ventilation parameters (as noted by Dockery and colleagues) in addition to limiting the role of the respiratory therapist during transport.[90]

Additionally, adverse effects from hypo- or hyperventilation can be more easily controlled with mechanical ventilation. When used, ventilator management should be done in collaboration with an intensivist (or anesthesiologist) and a respiratory therapist skilled in caring for children requiring assisted ventilation.

Secure IV access for administration of IV fluids, sedatives, and neuromuscular blocking agents should be obtained prior to transport. IV sedation with a benzodiazepine or pain control with IV opioids should be administered, and the use of neuromuscular blocking agents combined with a benzodiazepine should be considered for the active, agitated, or uncooperative child. Appropriate use of these agents may help reduce the risk of complications or patient deterioration.[83] All medical records, consent for transport, and radiographs should be copied and transported with the patient. Communication with the accepting physician and ICU team is crucial to ensure a safe and successful transport.

The decision to transport by air or ground is an institutional one. Factors to take into consideration include availability of a transport vehicle, equipment compatibility, weather and traffic conditions, geography, distance, the urgency of the transport to a pediatric center, and appropriate landing area at the referring center to support air transport. In some instances, air transport may not have an impact on the time difference if patient transport by ground must also occur to reach the receiving center.

TRANSPORT COMPLICATIONS

Complications from transport of the pediatric patient primarily occur secondary to inadequate stabilization of the airway and lack of appropriate monitoring. Additionally, severity of illness and duration of transport are associated with adverse events.[91] Combative or unrestrained patients may extubate themselves or dislodge IVs. Lack of appropriate monitoring may result in hypoxemia secondary to tube dislodgment, which may go unrecognized for a prolonged period, especially in the chemically paralyzed patient.

If the endotracheal tube becomes dislodged during transport, airway support must be provided immediately. Attempting to secure the airway again in the back of a moving transport vehicle or helicopter can be difficult and may result in further complications such as airway trauma secondary to repeated or failed attempts at intubation. Diversion to the closest emergency department is a reasonable alternative and should be considered. Lack of appropriate monitoring also may lead to inadequate ventilation and oxygenation, resulting in hypoxia and acidosis. Airway obstruction secondary to secretions or mucus plugging can result in hypoxemia and hypercarbia. Lack of or inadequate sedation can be psychologically traumatic to the pediatric patient. Sedation and pain control should be routinely administered in any child who is intubated and mechanically ventilated.

CONCLUSIONS

A rapid and thorough evaluation should identify children with severe respiratory distress and impending respiratory failure who require immediate stabilization of their airway. Adequate preparation, appropriate monitoring, and the use of pharmacologic adjuncts can assist the physician in stabilizing the difficult airway in this child. Following intubation, attention to sedation, pain control, and prevention of secondary injury are crucial to the successful treatment of any child who has an artificial airway.

Care of the child with an artificial airway requires a dedicated team of specialists caring for all aspects of the child. In addition to securing the difficult airway, provisions for emergent reintubation should be established and appropriate equipment and personnel readily available if this event occurs. Complications from mechanical ventilation can be minimized when treated in a tertiary care facility with trained individuals competent in mechanically ventilating infants and children. Continuous bedside monitoring of respiratory parameters to alert caregivers of potential complications associated with mechanical ventilation is imperative.

Ongoing nutritional support, pain and sedation control, and management of fluids and electrolytes require close observation and intervention by trained personnel to prevent alteration of the cardiovascular and respiratory systems and nutritional deprivation. Neuromuscular blocking agents should be used as needed and should always be combined with sedatives. Attention to eye and skin care is essential to prevent secondary injury.

A coordinated effort between referring and accepting physicians to transport the child with a critical airway safely and efficiently to a tertiary care facility with trained pediatric subspecialists is imperative. Collaboration between medical and surgical disciplines will enhance overall quality of care and can minimize potential morbidity and mortality in this specialized patient population.

REFERENCES

1. Helfaer, M.A., Nichols, D.G., and Rogers, M.C. Developmental physiology of the respiratory system. In *Textbook of Pediatric Intensive Care,* 3rd ed. Rogers, M.C., Ed., Baltimore, MD: Williams and Wilkins. 1996, 97.
2. Davidson, D., Stalcup, S.A., and Mellins, R.B. Systemic hemodynamics affecting cardiac output during hypocapnic and hypercapnic hypoxia. *J. Appl. Physiol.,* 1986, 60, 1230–1236.
3. Wohl, D. Traumatic vocal fold avulsion injury in a newborn. *J. Voice,* 1996, 10, 106–108.
4. Saracino, D.P., Jones, G.P., and Lee, Y.M. Esophageal perforation: case reports and review of the principles in diagnosis and management. *Resident Staff Phys.,* 1992, 38, 89–96.
5. Reyes, G., Galvis, A.G., and Thompson, J.W. Esophagotracheal perforation during an emergency intubation. *Am. J. Emerg. Med.,* 1992, 10, 223–225.
6. Gerardi, M.J., Sacchetti, A.D., Cantor, R.M. et al. Rapid-sequence intubation of the pediatric patient. *Ann. Emerg. Med.,* July 1996, 28, 55–74.
7. Bhende, M.S. and Thompson, A.E. Evaluation of an end-tidal CO_2 detector during pediatric cardiopulmonary resuscitation. *Pediatrics,* 1995, 95, 395–399.
8. Bhende, M.S., Thompson, A.E., Cook, S.R. et al. Validity of a disposable end-tidal CO_2 detector in verifying endotracheal tube placement in infants and children. *Ann. Emerg. Med.,* 1992, 21, 142–145.
9. Wee, M.Y.K. and Walker, A.K.Y. The oesophageal detector device: an assessment with uncuffed tubes in children. *Anaesthesia,* 1991, 46, 869–871.
10. Haynes, S.R. and Morton, N.S. Use of the esophageal detector device in children under one year of age. *Anesthesia,* 1990, 45, 1067–1069.
11. American Heart Assoc. Pediatric advanced life support. *Circulation,* 2000, 102 Suppl(8), I291–I342.
12. McGowan, P. and Skinner, A. Preoxygenation: the importance of a good face mask seal. *Br. J. Anaesth.,* 1995, 75, 777–778.
13. Levy, F., Bratton, S.L., and Jardine, D.S. Routine chest radiographs following repositioning of endotracheal tubes are necessary to assess correct position in pediatric patients. *Chest,* 1994, 106, 1508–1510.
14. Volker, D., Harmut, O., Volker, W., and Schmucker, P. The laryngeal tube: a new simple airway device. *Anesth. Analg.,* 2000, 90, 1220–1222.
15. Peak, D. and Roy, S. Needle cricothyroidotomy revisited. *Pediatr. Emerg. Care,* 1999, 15, 224–226.
16. Doobinin, K. and Nakagawa, T.A. Rapid sequence intubation. American Heart Association, *Pediatric Advanced Life Support Manual.* 2002.
17. Morell, R.C., Berman, J.M., Royster, R.I. et al. Revised label regarding use of succinylcholine in children and adolescents. *Anesthesiology,* 1994, 80, 242–245.
18. Hopkins, P.M.L. Use of suxamethonium in children. *Br. J. Anaesth.,* 1995, 75, 675–677.
19. Lerman, J., Berdock, S.E., Bissonnette, B. et al. Succinylcholine warning [letter]. *Can. J. Anaesth.,* 1994, 41, 165.
20. Badgwell, J.M., Hall, S.C., and Lockhart, C. Revised label regarding use of succinylcholine in children and adolescents. *Anesthesiology,* 1994, 80, 243–245.
21. Bevan, D.R. Succinylcholine. *Can. J. Anaesth.,* 1994, 41, 465–468
22. Doobinin, K.A. and Nakagawa, T.A. Emergency department use of neuromuscular blocking agent in children. *Pediatr. Emerg. Care,* 2000, 16, 441–447.

23. Marini, J.J. New options for the ventilatory management of acute lung injury. *New Horizons*, 1993, 1, 489.
24. Chao, D.C. and Steinhorn, D.J. Weaning from mechanical ventilation. *Crit. Care Clin.*, 1998, 14, 799.
25. Page, N.E., Giehl, M., and Luke, S. Intubation complications in the critically ill child. *AACN Clin. Issues*, 1998, 9(1), 25–35.
26. Spence, K. and Barr, P. Nasal versus oral intubation for mechanical ventilation of newborn infants (Cochrane Review). Cochrane Lib., Issue 4, 2000. Oxford, Update Software.
27. Angelos, G.M., Smith, D.R., Jorgenson, R., and Sweeney, E.A. Oral complications associated with neonatal oral tracheal intubation: a critical review. *Pediatr. Dentistry*, 1989, 11(2), 133–140.
28. Heffner, J.E. Airway management in the critically ill patient. *Crit. Care Clin.*, 1990, 6, 533.
29. Derkay, C.S., Bluestone, C.D., Thompson, A.E., and Kardatske, D. Otitis media in the pediatric intensive care unit: a prospective study. *Otolaryngol. Head Neck Surg.*, 1989, 100, 292–299.
30. McCulloch, T.M. and Bishop, M.J. Complications of translaryngeal intubation. *Clin. Chest Med.*, 1991, 12(3), 507–521.
31. Balestrieri, F. and Watson, C.B. Intubation granuloma. *Otolaryngol. Clin. North Am.*, 1982, 15(3), 567–579.
32. Macey-Dare, L.V., Morales, D.R., Evans, R.D., and Nixon, F. Long-term effect of neonatal endotracheal intubation on palatal form and symmetry in 8- to 11-year-old children. *Eur. J. Orthodontics*, 1999, 21, 703–710.
33. Rivera, R. and Tibballs, J. Complications of endotracheal intubation and mechanical ventilation in infants and children. *Crit. Care Med.*, 1992, 20, 193–199.
34. Dreyfuss, D., Solar, P., and Saumon, G. Spontaneous resolution of pulmonary edema caused by short periods of cyclic overinflation. *J. Appl. Physiol.*, 1992, 72, 2081.
35. Muscedere, J.G., Mullen, J.B.M., and Slutsky, A.S. Tidal ventilation at low airway pressures can augment lung injury. *Am. J. Respir. Crit. Care* Med., 1994, 149, 1327.
36. Pierson, D.J. Aveolar rupture during mechanical ventilation: role of PEEP, peak airway pressure, and distending volume. *Respir. Care*, 1988, 33, 472.
37. Cournand, A., Motley, H.L., Werko, L., and Richards, D.W. Physiological studies of the effects of intermittent positive pressure breathing on cardiac output in man. *Am. J. Physiol.*, 1948, 152, 162.
38. Scharff, F.M., Caldini, P., and Ingram, R.H., Jr. Cardiovascular effects of increasing airway pressure in the dog. *Am. J. Physiol.*, 1977, 232, H35.
39. Laver, M.B. Dr. Starling and the "ventilator" kidney. *Anesthesiology*, 1979, 50, 383.
40. Baratz, R.A., Philbin, D.M., and Patterson, R.W. Plasma antidiuretic hormone and urinary output during continuous positive-pressure breathing in dogs. *Anesthesiology*, 1971, 34, 510.
41. Hall, S.V., Johnson, E.E., and Hedley–Whyte, J. Renal hemodynamics and function with continuous positive-pressure breathing in dogs. *Anesthesiology*, 1974, 41, 452.
42. Davis, A. Atrial natriuretic factor in the pediatric intensive care unit. *Crit. Care Clin.*, 1988, 4, 803–813.
43. Stein, F. and Trevino, R. Nosocomial Infections in the pediatric intensive care unit. *Pediatr. Clin. North Am.*, 1994, 6, 1245–1257.
44. Craven, D.E., Make, B., McCabe, W.R. et al. Risk factors for pneumonia in patients receiving continuous mechanical ventilation. *Am. Rev. Respir. Dis.*, 1986, 133, 792.
45. Craven, D.E. and Steger, K.A. Pathogenesis and prevention of nosocomial pneumonia in the mechanically ventilated patient. *Respir. Care*, 1989, 34, 85.
46. Durbin, C.G. Sedation in the critically ill. *New Horizons*, 1994, 2, 64.
47. Loper, K.A., Butler, S., Nessly, M. et al. Paralyzed with pain: the need for education. *Pain*, 1989, 37, 315.
48. Prielipp, R.C., Coursin, D.B., Wood, K.E. et al. Complications associated with sedative and neuromuscular blocking drugs in critically ill patients. *Crit. Care Clin.*, 1995, 11, 983–1003.
49. McArdle, P. Intravenous analgesia. *Crit. Care Clin.*, 1999, 15, 89.
50. Armstrong, P.J. and Bersen, A. Normeperidine toxicity. *Anesth. Analg.*, 1986, 65, 536–538.
51. Romsing, J. and Walther–Larson, S. Peri-operative use of nonsteroidal anti-inflammatory drugs in children: analgesic efficacy and bleeding. *Anaesthesia*, 1997, 52, 673.
52. Tung, A. and Rosenthal, M. Patients requiring sedation. *Crit. Care Clin.*, 1995, 11, 791–802.
53. Tobias, J.D. Tolerance, withdrawal, and physical dependency after long term sedation and analgesia of children in the pediatric intensive care unit. *Crit. Care Med.*, 2000, 28, 2122–2132.

54. Anand, K.J.S. and Arnold, J.H. Opioid tolerance and dependence in infants and children. *Crit. Care Med.*, 1994, 22, 334–342.
55. Tobias, J.D. Outpatient therapy of iatrogenic opioid dependency following prolonged sedation in the pediatric intensive care unit. *J. Intensive Care Med.*, 1996, 11, 284–287.
56. Hirsch, I.A. and Zaauder, H.L. Chloral hydrate: a potential cause of arrhythmias. *Anesth. Analg.*, 1986, 65, 691–692.
57. Pershad, J., Palmisano, P., and Nichols, M. Chloral hydrate: the good and the bad. *Pediatr. Emerg. Care*, 1999, 15, 432–435.
58. Parke, T.J., Steven, J.E., Rice, A.S.C., Greenaway, C.L., Bray, R.J., Smith, P.J., Waldmann, C.S., and Verghese, C. Metabolic acidosis and fatal myocardial failure after propofol infusion in children: five case reports. *Br. Med. J.*, 1992, 305, 613–616.
59. Bray, R.J. Propofol infusion syndrome in children. *Paediatr. Anaesth.*, 1998, 8, 491–499.
60. Lavandosky, G., Gomez, R., and Montes, J. Potentially lethal misplacement of femoral central venous catheters. *Crit. Care Med.*, 1996, 24, 893–896.
61. Galvis, A. and Nakagawa, T.A. Hydrothorax as a late complication of central venous catheterization in children. Diagnosis and management. *Anaesth. Intens. Care*, 1992, 20, 75–77.
62. Bar-Joseph, G. and Galvis, A.G. Perforation of the heart by central venous catheter in infants; guidelines to diagnosis and management. *J. Pediatr. Surg.*, 1983, 18, 284–287.
63. Kudsk, K.A. Clinical applications of enteral nutrition. *Nutr. Clin. Pract.*, 1994, 9, 165.
64. Schears, G.J. and Deutchsman, C.S. Common nutritional issues in pediatric and adult critical care medicine. *Crit. Care Clin.*, 1997, 13, 669.
65. Chao, D.C. and Steinhorn, D.J. Weaning from mechanical ventilation. *Crit. Care Clin.*, 1998, 14, 799.
66. Khan, H., Brown, A., and Venkataraman, S.T. Predictor of extubation success and failure in mechanically ventilated infants and children. *Crit. Care Med.*, 1996, 24, 1568–1579.
67. Manczur, T., Greenough, A., Pryor, D., and Rafferty, G. Comparison of predictors of extubation from mechanical ventilation in children. *Pediatr. Crit. Care Med.*, 2000, 1, 28–32.
68. Deakers, T.W., Reynolds, G., Stretton, M., and Newth, C.J.L. Cuffed endotracheal tubes in pediatric intensive care. *J. Pediatr.*, 1994, 125, 57–62.
69. Seid, A.B., Godin, M.S., Pransky, S.M., Kearns, D.B., and Peterson, B.M. The prognostic value of endotracheal tube-air leak following tracheal surgery in children. *Arch. Otolaryngol. Head Neck Surg.*, 1992, 118(4), 448–449.
70. Tellez, D.W., Galvis, A.G., Storgion, S.A., Amer, H.N., Hoseyni, M., and Deakers, T.W. Dexamethasone in the prevention of postextubation stridor in children. *J. Pediatr.*, 1991, 118, 289–294.
71. Anene, O., Meert, K.L., Uy, H., Sompson, P., and Sarnaik, A.P. Dexamethasone for the preventions of postextubation airway obstruction: a prospective, randomized, double-blind, placebo-controlled trial. *Crit. Care Med.*, 1996, 24, 1666–1669.
72. Tobias, J.D. and Nichols, D.G. *Pediatric Critical Care. The Essentials. Croup, Upper Airway Obstruction, and Status Asthmaticus.* Armonk, NY: Futura Publishing Company. 1999. 37–56.
73. Tobias, J.D. Heliox in children with airway obstruction. *Pediatr. Emer. Care*, 1997, 13, 29–32.
74. Fleming, M.D., Weigelt, J.A., Brewer, V., and McIntire, D. Effect of helium and oxygen on airflow in a narrowed airway. *Arch. Surg.*, 1992, 127, 956–960.
75. Eileau, C., Galperine, R.I., Guenard, H., and Demarquez, J.L. Helium–oxygen mixture in respiratory distress syndrome. A double-blind study. *J. Pediatr.*, 1993, 122, 132–136.
76. Johnson, D.W., Schuh, S., Koren, G., and Jaffe, D.M. Outpatient treatment of croup with nebulized dexamethasone. *Arch. Pediatr. Adolesc. Med.*, 1996, 150, 349–355.
77. Klassen, T.P., Feldman, M.E., Watters, L.K., Sutcliffe, T., and Rowe, P.C. Nebulized budesonide for children with mild to moderate croup. *N. Engl. J. Med.*, 1994, 331, 285–289.
78. Husby, S., Agertoft, L., Mortensen, S., and Pedersen, S. Treatment of croup with nebulised steroid (budesonide): a double blind, placebo controlled study. *Arch. Dis. Child*, 1993, 68, 352–355.
79. Fitzgerald, D., Mellis, C., Johnson, M., Allen, H., Cooper, P., and Van Asperen, P. Nebulized budesonide is as effective as nebulized adrenaline in moderately severe croup. *Pediatrics*, 1996, 97, 722–725.
80. Barr, F.E., Patel, N.T., and Newth, C.J.L. The pharmacologic mechanism by which inhaled epinephrine reduces airway obstruction in respiratory syncytial virus-associated bronchiolitis. *J. Pediatr.*, 2000, 136, 699–700.

81. Weymuller, E.A., Jr. Prevention and management of intubation injury of the larynx and trachea. *Am. J. Otolaryngol.*, 1992, 13(3), 139–144.
82. Link, J., Krause, H., Wagner, W. et al. Intrahospital transport of critically ill patients. *Crit. Care Med.*, 1990, 18, 1427–1429.
83. Beyer, A.J., Land, G., and Zaritsky, A. Non physician transport of intubated pediatric patients: a system evaluation. *Crit. Care Med.*, 1992, 20, 961–966.
84. Macnab, A.J. Optimal escort for interhospital transport of pediatric emergencies. *J. Trauma*, 1991, 31, 205–209.
85. Edge, W.E., Kanter, R.K., Weigle, D.G.M., and Walsh, R. Reduction of morbidity in interhospital transport by specialized pediatric staff. *Crit. Care Med.*, 1994, 22, 1186–1191.
86. Gausche, M., Lewis, R.J., Stratton, S.J., Haynes, B.E., Gunter, C.S. Goodrich, S.M. et al. Effect of out-of-hospital pediatric endotracheal intubation on survival and neurological outcome. *JAMA*, 2000, 283, 783–790.
87. Aijian, P., Tsia, A., Knopp, R., and Kallsen, G.W. Endotracheal intubation of pediatric patients by paramedics. *Ann. Emerg. Med.*, 1989, 18, 489–494.
88. Losek, J.D., Bonadio, W.A., Walsh, K.C., Hennes, H., Smith, D.S., and Glaeser, P.W. Prehospital pediatric endotracheal intubation performance review. *Pediatr. Emerg. Care*, 1989, 5, 1–4.
89. Brownstein, D., Shugerman, R., Cummings, P., Rivara, R., and Copass, M. Prehospital endotracheal intubation of children by paramedics. *Ann. Emerg. Med.*, 1996, 28, 34–39.
90. Dockery, W.K., Futterman, C., Keller, S.R., Sheridan, M.J., and Akl, B.F. A comparison of manual and mechanical ventilation during pediatric transport. *Crit. Care Med.*, 1999, 27, 802–806.
91. Wallen, E., Venkataraman, S.T., Grosso, M.J., Kiene, K., and Orr, R.A. Intrahospital transport of critically ill pediatric patients. *Crit. Care Med.*, 1995, 23, 1588–1595.

7 Pediatric Otolaryngology Imaging

Michelle S. Whiteman and Bernadette Koch

There are some people who see a great deal and some who see very little in the same things.

T.H. Huxley

CONTENTS

AVAILABLE IMAGING TOOLS

Diagnostic imaging is an integral part of the preoperative evaluation of pediatric patients with disorders of the head and neck region. When performed properly and interpreted correctly, radiology can provide critical information regarding normal anatomy as well as details and boundaries of disease. The otolaryngologist armed with such information can reduce the number of potential complications associated with the disease and his surgical procedures.

In order to select the study that will offer the best information to diagnose and treat the child accurately, it is essential that the pediatric otolaryngologist and the radiologist work as a team. Plain films, computed tomography (CT), ultrasound, magnetic resonance imaging (MRI), and nuclear evaluation medicine examinations comprise the basic exams used (see Table 7.1).

Plain films are commonly used in the evaluation of the pediatric chest and abdomen, but the soft tissue resolution of plain films is often inadequate for the assessment of the head and neck region. Facial films obtained following trauma are very good for detection of facial fractures, but subtle fractures may require further examination using CT. Plain films of the paranasal sinuses are of limited utility. If the clinical concern for chronic sinusitis or a complication of acute sinusitis is strong, CT is recommended. The typical skin dose for a child undergoing a CT scan of the neck is approximately 20 to 25 mGy (2000 to 2500 mrad).[1] This dose is compared with the 1 to 2 mGy (100 to 200 mrad) for screen film radiography of the same anatomic region. Plain films of the

TABLE 7.1

Suggested Initial and Subsequent Imaging Studies for Some More Common Clinical Disorders of the Ear, Nose, Throat, and Head and Neck

Imaging of Pediatric Otolaryngology		
Clinical disorder	Start with ...	May need to add
Facial trauma	Plain films of the face	CT, axial and coronal (plain)
Chronic sinusitis/preop FESS	CT (coronal if possible)	Contrast CT or MRI if suspect orbital or intracranial complications
Mastoiditis and cholesteatoma	High-resolution (noncontrast) CT of the temporal bones	MRI if suspect intracranial extension
Neck mass (other than suspected thyroglossal duct cyst or fibromatosis colli)	CT with contrast	Ultrasound or MRI for selected cases
Parapharyngeal/retropharyngeal abscess	CT with contrast	
Epiglotittis	Lateral plain film neck, soft tissue technique	
Congenital loss of hearing	High-resolution CT temporal bones (noncontrast)	
Vascular malformation and hemangioma	MRI with contrast preferably, or contrast	MRA or MRV, conventional angiography for therapeutic embolization
Thyroglossal duct cyst	Ultrasound	Contrast CT or MRI if atypical
Fibromatosis colli	Ultrasound	Contrast CT or MRI if atypical

Note: MRI = magnetic resonance imaging; MRA = magnetic resonance angiogram; MRV = magnetic resonance venogram.

mastoids do not aid significantly in the evaluation of a child with suspected mastoiditis. High-resolution CT of the temporal bones provides much greater detail, especially regarding bone destruction and complications such as labyrinthine fistula. Plain films are indicated, however, in the radiologic evaluation of a child with suspected epiglotittis. A single lateral view of the neck can be obtained in the radiology department, as long as the appropriate personnel and equipment are available. The referring otolaryngologist needs to be in close proximity in the event that the child decompensates, and a pediatric crash cart needs to be immediately available.

CT imaging is often used in the evaluation of neck masses and can provide rapid (especially with spiral scanners) images with excellent resolution. It is preferable that these studies be obtained with contrast because (1) lymph nodes can be easily distinguished from vessels and (2) the enhancement characteristics are often very helpful in establishing a differential diagnosis. In general, if neoplasm or infection is under consideration, a contrast study is preferred. Sinusitis that does not respond to conservative treatment may be imaged with a noncontrast exam, but if complications such as orbital or intracranial involvement are suspected, a contrast-enhanced CT or MR will be needed. Ultrasound can add significant information, especially regarding the evaluation of neck masses, and can also be used to provide an ultrasound guided biopsy. Color doppler is also helpful in evaluation of vascular abnormalities.

CT is invaluable in the evaluation of suspected mastoiditis and cholesteatoma, and in the child with congenital loss of hearing. CT of the temporal bone is also essential to the evaluation of pulsatile tinnitus as well as for patients with a vascular mass seen behind the tympanic membrane. High-resolution CT of the temporal bones must be obtained in axial and coronal projections with slice thickness of no greater than 1.0 to 1.5 mm. CT of the temporal bone is most often obtained as a noncontrast exam because the bony detail, rather than the soft tissues, is the primary focus of this study. However, if intracranial extension is suspected, contrast is helpful in delineating the spread of tumor or infection.

CT is also an excellent exam for evaluation of the upper airway and tracheobronchial tree. Extrinsic airway compression is well demonstrated, although endoluminal lesions are better evaluated with clinical endoscopy. Helical CT can provide three-dimensional reconstructions and can also be used to navigate the lumen of the airway, thus providing a "virtual endoscopy" of the upper airway. This technique, however, requires specific software and a workstation and may not be available on all scanners. When available, this study is particularly useful in the evaluation of patients with subglottic stenosis.

The soft tissue resolution of MRI is excellent; however, this study takes considerably longer than a CT and requires the patient to be completely still for a longer period of time. This increases the total dose and duration of sedation. MRI is, therefore, most helpful in answer to a specific question such as, "Is the cavernous sinus involved?" "Is retrobulbar extension present?" or "Is there associated meningitis?"

These studies are usually obtained without and with contrast. A contrast-enhanced (gadolinium) MR study can be obtained in the child who has an iodine allergy and cannot have a contrast CT. MR studies can be obtained in coronal, axial, and sagittal planes and can provide a better depiction of normal anatomy and the extent of a disease process. Vascular abnormalities can be investigated with MR angiography (MRA) or MR venography (MRV). MR spectroscopy can be used to differentiate intracranial abscess from tumor, providing a local biochemical profile within a voxel positioned over the area of interest.

Nuclear medicine studies are also exams that can be used to answer a particular clinical question. One can use 99^m Tc pertechnetate, ^{123}I, or ^{131}I to determine if functional thyroid tissue is present and, if so, its location. Thallium (201Tl) is a potassium analogue often used to distinguish intracranial tumor from infection. Metabolically active tissue, such as a neoplasm, will show increased uptake of 201Tl relative to adjacent brain parenchyma, whereas an abscess does not. FDG-PET (fluorodeoxyglucose positron emission tomography) can be used to localize a neoplastic process in the head and neck or to differentiate tumor from infection (increased activity is seen with neoplasm). This study is also of great utility in postoperative patients when conventional imaging such as CT or MR is unable to distinguish scar from recurrent disease.

A bone scan can identify osseous metastases, but is nonspecific in that fracture and infection, as well as metastasis, will show increased uptake. A bone scan/gallium scan can be obtained to confirm a suspected osteomyelitis. Gallium is a weak bone agent and thus will accumulate at the site of any acute bony pathology. However, when read in conjunction with a bone scan, a very positive gallium scan is more indicative of osteomyelitis. Indium[III]–white blood cell study can also be used to localize infection, but is preferred for soft tissue infection.

An additional nuclear scintigraphic exam is the octreotide study. Octreotide is a somatostatin analogue; neuroendocrine tumors are known to possess somatostatin receptors. Thus, octreotide (which is bound to [III]In) can be used to localize neuroendocrine tumors such as paragangliomas. Because paragangliomata can be multicentric, this exam can also be used to screen for additional paragangliomas that may not be clinically evident.

MIBG (metaiodobenzylguanidine) is a nuclear agent that can be tagged to Iodine-131 or Iodine-123. It is a useful agent in the detection of pediatric neuroblastoma. Less than 5% of neuroblastoma occurs in the neck. Cervical neuroblastoma can be a primary lesion or metastatic disease and MIBG can be used to locate other sites of involvement.

Conventional angiography is usually reserved for vascular malformations, aneurysms, and treatment of vascular tumors. In many cases, MRI and MRA may be most helpful as initial studies with conventional angiography reserved for definitive diagnosis and possibly therapeutic embolization. Angiography is an invasive procedure that requires careful sedation of the patient and should only be performed at institutions that have significant experience with these studies. Similarly, endovascular embolization needs to be planned by a treatment team with sufficient training and expertise in these specialized procedures.

The information provided by a radiographic study is dependent upon the technical quality of the exam as well as the radiologic interpretation. The radiologist reading the study may be less familiar with pediatric disorders, as well as with the normal variation of anatomy seen in the developing child, than with those affecting adults. Thus, if the interpretation of a study seems to be at odds with the physician's clinical impression, it is certainly worth reviewing the study with the radiologist; in more complex cases, a second or third opinion may be sought.

SEDATION VS. GENERAL ANESTHESIA

With the distraction of video equipment during sonography, nearly all children undergo ultrasound (US) examination without sedation. In newer generation CT technology, the majority of children can also be imaged without sedation. However, most children under 6 years of age and some older children are unable to cooperate for optimal MR imaging and therefore require sedation to obtain high-quality images. A complete sedation program should be in place prior to sedating children in the radiology department. Collaboration among the physician responsible for sedation, nursing staff, anesthesiology, and referring physician is required. A safe, effective formulary of medications should be used. The sedated child must be monitored continuously during imaging and recovery. Extensive documentation of the complete process is necessary, and a quality assessment program should be in place

Prior to the child's arrival at the imaging department, a pre-sedation mailing to the parents containing the time of the exam, the NPO (nothing by mouth) instructions, and a brief description of what to expect during the sedation process is suggested. The mailing should include a sedation education sheet describing why children need sedation, the sedation process, and the risks. In addition, a short description of the recovery and what to expect when returning home is helpful. A confirmation phone call 24 hours prior to the exam is useful for reiterating the NPO instructions and answering parental questions.

According to the American Academy of Pediatrics guidelines,[2] dietary restrictions call for no milk or solids:

- 4 hours prior to sedation for children 0 to 5 months of age
- 6 hours prior to sedation for children 6 to 36 months of age
- 8 hours prior to sedation for children older than 36 months

All children may have clear liquids until 2 hours prior to sedation.

A brief pre-sedation physical exam should include vital signs, assessment of airway, and auscultation of lungs and heart as well as assessment of neurologic baseline. Pre-sedation history should include review of systems, recent illness, medications, allergies, and gestational age at birth. Note of whether the patient snores should be made because adenoidal and tonsillar hypertrophy may increase the risk of potential airway obstruction during sedation.

Using the American Society of Anesthesiology (ASA) physical status classification, children in Class I and Class II are, in general, considered appropriate candidates for deep sedation. Patients in ASA Class III to Class V require individual consideration, including general anesthesia as an option. Additional patients who may be better suited for general anesthesia include patients with documented sleep apnea or airway obstruction, and patients with a prior history of severe paradoxical reaction to sedatives. Preterm infants less than 60 weeks postconception may have an increased incidence of postanesthesia apnea; therefore, continuous monitoring for at least 12 hours after general anesthesia or sedation is recommended to prevent apnea-related complications.

The decision to sedate should always be based on urgency and/or necessity of the exam relative to the overall health of the child. If sedation is felt to be safe, a limited formulary with maximal dose limits within the margin of safety is recommended. The most popular medications currently used in pediatric radiology departments include oral chloral hydrate, intravenous and oral pentobarbital sodium (Nembutal), midazolam (Versed), fentanyl citrate (Sublimaze), and diazepam (Valium). Appropriate resuscitation equipment, including an oxygen delivery system, positive pressure ventilation bag and mask, resuscitation cart, appropriate medications, suction catheters, laryngoscope blades, electrocardiogram machine, and defibrillator, should always be readily accessible.

Prior to discharge, patients should meet appropriate discharge criteria.[2] Written and verbal instructions, including postsedation care, a phone number to call with questions, and what to do in case of an emergency, should be provided to a responsible caregiver. A follow-up phone call the day after sedation is helpful to answer parental questions and gather quality assessment information.

The physician administering medication should have a clear understanding of its pharmacokinetics and pharmacodynamics, as well as an appreciation of drug interactions. Preprinted patient management forms allow easy documentation of the history, physical exam, and vital signs during sedation and recovery. Heart rate, respiratory rate, and oxygen saturation should be recorded by the nurse at appropriate intervals during the imaging study (every 5 minutes) and during recovery (every 10 minutes). Blood pressure should be routinely taken before sedation and while in the recovery room. Routine blood pressure measurements during the examination, in an otherwise stable patient, may awaken the patient and require additional sedative. If the patient cannot be safely sedated with appropriate monitoring, if emergency equipment is not available, or if the physicians and nurses are not appropriately trained, sedation or general anesthesia by an anesthesiologist should be considered.[2,4–6]

SINONASAL IMAGING

The majority of children with sinonasal disease are treated on the basis of clinical assessment and do not require imaging at all. When indicated, CT is the preferred method of imaging the sinonasal cavity in children with chronic sinusitis, orbital complications of sinusitis, and mass lesions involving the osseous structures. MR imaging is superior to CT in the evaluation of intracranial complications of sinusitis and intracranial extension of neoplasm, as well as in distinguishing inflammatory sinus disease from sinonasal neoplasm. In the evaluation of congenital nasal masses, CT and MRI may be necessary and complementary; CT demonstrates the osseous defects better and MRI shows intracranial involvement.

SINUSITIS

Acute, uncomplicated sinusitis is a common childhood illness, usually requiring no imaging. Conventional sinus radiographs lack sensitivity and specificity,[7–9] and the correlation between findings on routine radiographs and CT examinations in children with chronic sinusitis is poor.[10,11] CT frequently demonstrates abnormalities that are clinically insignificant or not related to acute bacterial sinusitis. There is a high incidence of abnormalities of the sinuses on cranial CT of infants, with (87%) and without (59%) recent upper respiratory infections, in the absence of clinical evidence of sinusitis.[12] On MR imaging, up to 3 mm of mucosal thickening has been noted in asymptomatic adults.[13,14] Because MRI changes may last up to 8 weeks, the use of imaging is discouraged in the evaluation of children with uncomplicated acute sinusitis.

In children with chronic sinusitis or suspected orbital or intracranial complications, imaging is recommended. In the preoperative evaluation for functional endoscopic sinus surgery, thin section (3 mm or less) coronal CT imaging is recommended[15] because it offers the most detailed anatomic evaluation of the paranasal sinuses. Incidence of anatomic variants is lower in children than in adults because pneumatization of the paranasal sinuses increases with age. Additional abnormalities that can be ideally assessed with CT imaging include Haller cells, concha bullosa, paradoxical middle turbinate, Onodi cells, congenital or post-traumatic deformities of the lamina papyracea, and low position of the roof of the ethmoidal labyrinth. In addition to viewing the images in bone windows, standard soft tissue windows should also be reviewed to rule out unexpected hydrocephalus or intracranial mass, which may be the cause of the patient presenting symptoms such as headache (Figure 7.1).

Conventional radiographs and CT expose the face, including the lens of the eye, to ionizing radiation. Estimated entrance dose exposure in roentgens in a 15-year-old patient is 0.210 to 0.250 R for a single Water's view, 0.44 to 0.52 R for a three-view sinus series, and 0.9 to 1.3 R for a complete coronal CT of the paranasal sinuses.

A
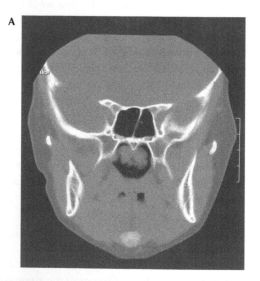

B
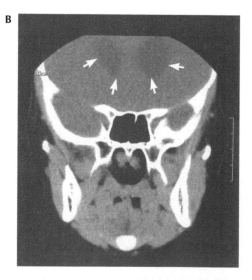

FIGURE 7.1 Hydrocephalus on sinus CT obtained for evaluation of headaches. A. Coronal bone window image through the sphenoid sinus inadequately visualizes the intracranial contents. B. Coronal soft tissue window clearly shows enlargement of the frontal horns of the lateral ventricles (arrows). In this patient, hydrocephalus secondary to a craniopahryngioma was the cause of headaches.

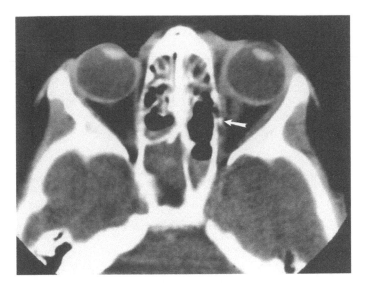

FIGURE 7.2 Lamina papyrecea defect status post FESS. Axial CT shows osseous defect in the medial aspect of the left orbital wall with displacement of a small fragment (arrow) and deviation of the medial rectus muscle.

Complications of functional endoscopic sinus surgery (FESS) include cerebrospinal fluid (CSF) leak, cephalocele, orbital hematoma, damage to extraocular muscles or optic nerve, and perforation of the cribriform plate.[16,17] Defects in the lamina papyracea may also be a complication of FESS (Figure 7.2). These complications can be imaged with CT as the initial modality. MR imaging may provide additional information in certain cases.

The most common complications of acute sinusitis include periorbital/orbital cellulitis and subperiosteal/orbital abscess. In cases of the latter, axial and coronal postcontrast CT images show low attenuation collections, which may or may not have enhancing walls (Figure 7.3). Although

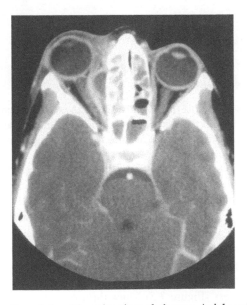

FIGURE 7.3 Orbital complication of sinusitis: subperiosteal abscess. Axial postcontrast CT shows extensive ethmoid and sphenoid sinus opacification. There is preseptal and postseptal soft tissue edema as well as an elliptically shaped low-attenuation, rim-enhancing, extraconal fluid collection in the medial right orbit. Mild proptosis results.

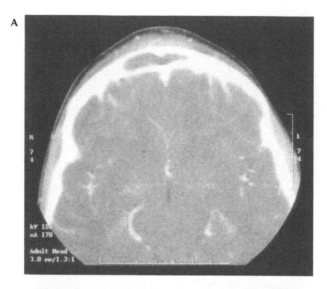

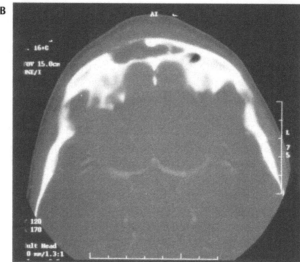

FIGURE 7.4 Frontal sinus osteomyelitis (Pott's puffy tumor). A. Axial postcontrast CT demonstrates opacification of the frontal sinus with soft tissue swelling and edema of the forehead. B. Axial postcontrast bone window images reveal osseous disruption of the anterior wall of the right frontal sinus.

suspicious for drainable abscess, a phlegmonous inflammatory mass prior to liquefaction may have a similar appearance.[18,19] Since the advent of antibiotics, osteomyelitis of the frontal bone (Pott's puffy tumor) is a rare complication of frontal sinusitis (Figure 7.4).

Intracranial complications of acute sinusitis are less frequent than orbital complications in children and can be imaged with CT or MR. In the acute setting, while imaging the orbits, a postcontrast CT of the brain is often helpful to evaluate the intracranial contents in patients with suspected intracranial complications of sinusitis. MR imaging is superior to CT for evaluation of meningeal enhancement, extra-axial collections (subdural/epidural effusions or empyemas), foci of cerebritis, parenchymal abscess (Figure 7.5), sinus thrombus, and early infarction.

Patients with fungal sinusitis often present with sinus disease unresponsive to usual medical therapy, and many are immunocompromised. Imaging findings are frequently nonspecific and may be similar to those of nonfungal disease. Mucosal thickening, complete opacification, reactive sclerosis, or frank osseous erosion may take place. CT shows hyperdense intrasinus contents

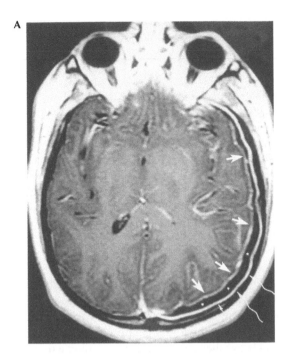 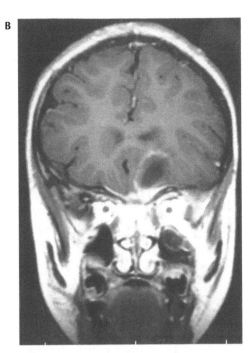

FIGURE 7.5 Intracranial complication of sinusitis. A. Axial postcontrast T1-weighted image shows diffuse left hemisphere leptomeningeal contrast enhancement (arrows), low signal intensity subdural fluid collection (asterisks), and thickening and contrast enhancement of the dura (wavy arrows). B. Coronal postcontrast T1-weighted image shows a focal area of low signal intensity with mild rim enhancement in the left frontal lobe consistent with abscess and enhancement of the adjacent meninges as well as posterior ethmoid sinus disease.

(differential diagnosis includes hemorrhage, polyposis, and dessicated secretions). MR may reveal hypointensity or hyperintensity on T2-weighted images, but the presence of hypointense signal is strongly suggestive of fungal rather than bacterial sinus disease.[20–25] Aggressive fungal disease such as aspergillus or mucoromycosis should be suggested if there is bony erosion or cavernous sinus involvement.

SINONASAL POLYPS

Nasal polyps are uncommon in children less than 5 years of age. The pathogenesis is unknown, but these polyps may be more common in children with atopic hypersensitivity. When polyps protrude through a sinus ostia and extend into the choana, they are termed choanal polyps. Choanal polyps may arise from the sphenoid ostia (spenochoanal polyp), the ethomoid ostia (ethmoidochoanal polyp), or the maxillary ostia (antrochoanal polyp). Antrochoanal polyps are the most common. Imaging shows the polyp with enlargement of the ostia, often with associated postobstructive sinus disease.

The term "sinonasal polyposis" is applied when polyps are present throughout the nasal cavity and paranasal sinuses. There may be high attenuation central material surrounded by a lower attenuation material at the periphery of the air cells. Differential diagnosis of this appearance includes sinonasal polyposis, desiccated secretions, and much less commonly, fungal sinusitis.[26] In addition, patients with sinonasal polyposis often have bulging of the nasal walls, demineralization of the ethmoid septations, and enlargement of the infundibulum.[27]

Children with cystic fibrosis (CF) have an increased incidence of sinusitis and polyposis. CT imaging of the paranasal sinuses is frequently requested to evaluate the extent of disease. In these children, one may see the typical appearance of sinusitis, or more advanced disease may be present, such as mucocele or sinonasal polyposis. If sinonasal polyposis or a sinus mucocele is identified in a child without a known diagnosis of CF, it is prudent to test the child for that condition.

SINONASAL NEOPLASMS

In the evaluation of sinonasal neoplasm, masses that involve bone are best evaluated with CT; however, if intracranial extension is suspected, MR imaging is quite useful, for example, in patients with rhabdomyosarcoma or juvenile nasopharyngeal angiofibroma. The multiplanar capability of MRI provides complete evaluation of intraorbital or intracranial extension. Patients with sinonasal tumors should be evaluated with MRI because it is helpful in distinguishing between changes related to postobstructive inflammation and those related to the intrinsic neoplasm.[28] Cavernous sinus disease and perineural extension are also best evaluated with contrast MRI, and fat saturation technique is essential when imaging the skull base. As described later in this chapter, angiography is performed for therapeutic intervention in children with juvenile nasopharyngeal angiofibroma.

CONGENITAL NASAL MASSES

The differential diagnosis of congenital nasal masses includes dermoid, nasal glioma, and cephalocele. Although imaging cannot always definitively determine the nature of these masses, CT is ideal to evaluate for osseous defects while MR imaging better shows intracranial connection. Therefore, both imaging modalities may be necessary for optimal preoperative evaluation. Occasionally, CT cisternography is useful (although not always diagnostic) in distinguishing a dermoid cyst from a meningocele. In patients with meningocele, free communication may be seen between the intracranial subarachnoid space and the meningocele.

IMAGING OF THE NECK AND PHARYNX

The most common reasons to image the pediatric neck and pharynx are for evaluation of the airway in children with suspected tracheal stenosis or tracheomalacia and in the evaluation of neck masses. The majority of neck masses in the pediatric population are related to congenital malformations or inflammation, with malignancy much less common than in the adult population. The most common congenital masses in children include thyroglossal duct cyst, branchial apparatus anomalies, hemangiomas of infancy and vascular malformations, and fibromatosis colli. The most common neoplasms are lymphoma and rhabdomyosarcoma.

CROUP VS. EPIGLOTTITIS

Croup (laryngotracheobronchitis) is the most common cause of stridor in children, usually caused by viral disease. Most children can be treated based on history and physical exam, without imaging. Radiographs are obtained primarily to exclude other causes of stridor, such as epiglottitis, foreign body, subglottic hemangioma, or subglottic stenosis, or to confirm presumed diagnosis of croup. Radiographically, the most significant narrowing usually occurs just below the vocal cords. AP radiographs typically show loss of normal "shouldering" appearance of the subglottic trachea and resultant "steeple" appearance of the lumen. Inspiratory lateral radiographs show distension of the hypopharynx and narrowing of the subglottic trachea.[29]

Membranous croup is usually caused by bacterial infection and typically occurs in older children. Historically, these patients present with more severe respiratory and systemic symptoms than do children with viral croup. In addition to the typical radiographic findings of croup, identification of intraluminal soft tissue densities or irregular tracheal walls should raise the question of membranous croup in any child. If this is identified on airway films, emergent referral to an otolaryngologist is advised to prevent aspiration of membranes and potential hypoxic/ischemic injury.[30]

Epiglottitis is uncommon, fortunately. These children are acutely ill and in grave danger of sudden airway obstruction. If imaging is desired, a single lateral view should be obtained while the patient is in the upright position, with care not to agitate the patient. A physician should remain with the patient at all times and equipment necessary for emergency ventilation or tracheostomy must be immediately available. Lateral radiograph will show enlargement of the epiglottis and thickening of the aryepiglottic folds.

COMPLETE TRACHEAL RINGS

Tracheal stenosis secondary to complete tracheal rings is an uncommon cause of respiratory symptoms in children. Associated vascular anomalies such as pulmonary artery sling may be present in up to 40% of these patients.[31-38] Therefore, imaging should be tailored to evaluate the tracheal stenosis and the vascular anatomy.

Conventional radiographs may show narrowing of the tracheal lumen; however, they are insufficient for evaluating the vascular anatomy. Preoperative CT with contrast is recommended in these children. Thin section helical CT using CT angiography technique (with sagittal and coronal reformation) ideally images the airway and the vascular anomalies rapidly, often without the need for sedation. The airway and vascular anatomy may also be imaged with MRI; however, nearly all of these children would require sedation for MR imaging. Conventional radiographs and coronal CT or MR images will show short- or long-segment circumferential tracheal narrowing. If the stenosis is distal, the distal trachea and proximal right and left main bronchi will have an inverted-T shape on frontal radiographs or coronal images. On cross-sectional axial images, the involved segment of trachea has a characteristic "O" shape rather than the usual inverted "U" shape.

INFLAMMATORY MASSES

Children with suspected retropharyngeal cellulitis or abscess are often initially imaged with airway radiographs to assess prevertebral soft tissue swelling. These should be obtained in inspiration with the child's neck extended. Because children have redundant prevertebral/retropharyngeal tissues, lateral film in neutral or flexed position will cause nonpathologic thickening of the soft tissues. When good inspiratory films with the neck extended cannot be obtained, lateral fluoroscopy is very helpful. The radiologist can dynamically view the airway and prevertebral soft tissue as the child breathes, cries, and arches his or her neck in order to move away from the examiner. When prevertebral soft tissue swelling is present, the differential diagnosis includes cellulitis, adenopathy, and abscess. Conventional radiographs can only confirm the presence of an abscess if gas is identified within the soft tissue.

Ultrasound (US) is the most reliable modality to differentiate between cystic and solid masses.[39-42] Therefore, this type of imaging is often used in the initial evaluation of inflammatory neck masses in children to identify the preoperative location of focal suppurative abscess and to differentiate this from nonsuppurative adenopathy. When a more detailed evaluation of the extent of inflammation and evaluation of deep neck infection is desired (such as retropharyngeal abscess), CT imaging with contrast is recommended. A focal low-attenuation mass with peripheral rim of enhancement is highly suggestive, but not diagnostic, of a drainable abscess. CT findings are reported to be accurate in differentiating phlegmon from abscess (Figure 7.6) in approximately 75% of patients, with a false negative rate of 14% and a false positive rate of 11%.[43,44] It should be noted that an infected congenital cyst or lymphatic malformation may have similar imaging characteristics.

When evaluating any abnormality of the neck, in addition to evaluating the palpable mass, one must carefully and judiciously search for all normal anatomic structures, particularly the vessels of the carotid sheath. Narrowing of the internal carotid artery, compression or thrombosis of the jugular vein, and aberrant position of the internal carotid artery must be identified and related to the surgeon preoperatively. Internal carotid artery narrowing in children with retropharyngeal

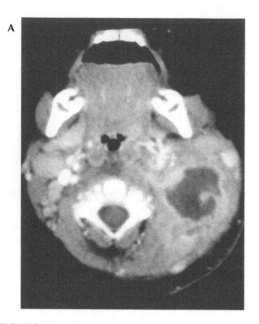 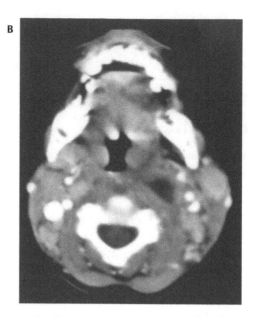

FIGURE 7.6 Inflammatory collections-drainable abscess vs. phlegmon. A. Axial postcontrast CT of the neck shows an irregularly shaped fluid collection with an irregular rim of contrast enhancement in the left posterior triangle. Drainable purulent material was found at surgery. B. Axial poscontrast CT at the level of the tonsils shows a low attenuation collection deep to the carotid sheath in the left lateral retropharyngeal space suggesting suppurative adenitis or abscess. However, a well-defined rim of contrast enhancement is not present; therefore, phlegmonous material is most likely. Only phlegmonous material was found at surgery.

lymphadenitis and abscess may be quite marked.[45] However, this usually does not result in a neurologic deficit and, therefore, does not require specific treatment other than treatment of the primary infection (Figure 7.7).

Lemierre syndrome consists of septic thrombophlebitis of the internal jugular vein secondary to oropharyngeal infection.[46] In these patients, the radiologist and the surgeon must be sure to differentiate abscess from inflammatory venous thrombosis (thrombophlebitis). On all imaging studies, the two may be confused if the lesion is not recognized as an enlarged thrombus-filled, noncompressible jugular vein (Figure 7.8). The key to this diagnosis is to identify the absence of a normal jugular vein and to recognize that the inflammatory lesion is tubular in nature and becomes contiguous with the normal vein above or below the level of disease.

ABERRANT INTERNAL CAROTID ARTERY

In the general population, 1 to 16% have a surgically vulnerable cervical internal carotid artery detectable as pulsations in the lateral wall of the pharynx. Aberrant positioning of the cervical portion of the internal carotid artery is bilateral in up to 31% of cases; it is present in up to 44% of children with velocardiofacial syndrome and may also be seen in otherwise healthy children (Figure 7.9). This is an important anomaly to recognize because it poses a risk of hemorrhage during oropharyngeal surgery such as adenoidectomy and tonsillectomy. In fact, death, secondary to surgical injury,[47–50] has been reported several times in the literature.

THYROGLOSSAL DUCT CYST

Approximately 70% of congenital abnormalities in the pediatric neck are thyroglosal duct (TGD) cysts.[51] Complications include infection, rupture, fistula, and coexisting carcinoma.[52,53] Historically,

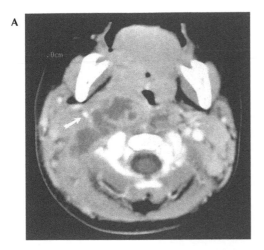 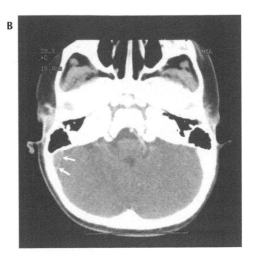

FIGURE 7.7 Internal carotid artery narrowing, jugular vein/sigmoid sinus thrombosis. Axial postcontrast CT shows an irregularly shaped low-attenuation collection with partial rim enhancement in the right retropharyngeal/peritonsillar region deviating the internal carotid artery anteriorly (arrow). Notice that the right internal carotid artery is smaller in caliber than the left. The right jugular vein is not identified. B. Axial postcontrast CT through the posterior fossa in the same child shows intermediate attenuation clot with minimal surrounding enhancement in the sigmoid sinus (arrows).

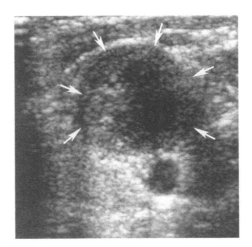

FIGURE 7.8 Jugular vein thrombosis simulating abscess. Axial ultrasound image shows a well-defined hypoechoic mass (arrows) with increase through transmission anterior to the right internal carotid artery. If not recognized as an enlarged thrombus filled jugular vein by its location and an absence of flow in the jugular vein, this might be mistaken for an abscess or suppurative adenitis.

nuclear scintigraphy has been used to document the presence of normal thyroid tissue. However, US has recently been advocated as the imaging modality of choice to evaluate the mobile cystic midline neck mass and confirm the presence of thyroid gland that appears to be normal.[54] Ultrasound shows a well-defined midline or paramidline mass with variable echogenicity, usually hypoechoic. The presence of internal echoes does not correlate with prior hemorrhage or infection.[55] CT and MRI show a mass in the appropriate location that appears to be cystic. The imaging characteristics will be altered by the presence of intralesional hemorrhage or infection.

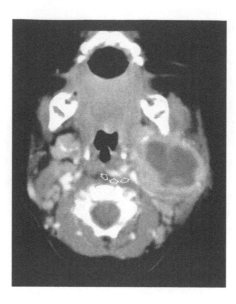

FIGURE 7.9 Aberrant internal carotid artery in a child with neck abscess. Axial postcontrast CT of the neck shows a thick-walled, rim-enhancing fluid collection in the anterior triangle of the left neck. Notice the curvilinear enhancing structure in the left paramidline retropharyngeal space (arrowheads), which represents an aberrant internal carotid artery.

BRANCHIAL APPARATUS ANOMALIES

Branchial apparatus anomalies may result in a cyst, sinus tract, or fistula and may be anomalies of one of the six pairs of branchial arches, the five pairs of endodermal pharyngeal pouches, or the five pairs of ectodermal branchial clefts. Cysts may be imaged with US, CT, or MRI. US is best at differentiating cystic from solid masses. However, CT and MRI better delineate the extent, location, and relationship to normal structures such as carotid sheath, parotid gland, and sterno-cleidomastoid (SCM) muscle.

First branchial anomalies are usually located near the ear — anterior or posterior to the pinnae, superficial or deep to the parotid gland.[56,57] MRI is particularly helpful in delineating the course of Type I anomalies relative to the external auditory canal (EAC) and parotid gland. Second branchial cleft cysts are the most common anomalies of the branchial apparatus. According to Bailey's classification, they can be located superficial or deep to the SCM, between the internal and external carotid arteries, or adjacent to the pharyngeal wall.[56,58] Lesions located anterior to the SCM are the most common, displacing the SCM posteriorly, the submandibular gland anteriorly, and the carotid sheath posteromedially. All imaging modalities show a cystic mass in the appropriate location. When infection is present, they may show a peripheral rim of contrast enhancement simulating suppurative adenopathy/abscess and edema of adjacent subcutaneous fat (cellulitis) or muscle (myositis). Third branchial anomalies are rare. Remnants of the thyropharyngeal duct result in thymic cysts, which may occur anywhere from the skull base to the upper mediastinum,[59,60] usually closely associated with the carotid sheath. When large, they may compromise the airway.

Pyriform sinus fistula is a rare cause of recurrent thyroiditis in children and is thought to be secondary to a remnant of the third or fourth pharnygeal pouch. Barium swallow shows barium filling the fistula extending from the inferior aspect of the pyriform sinus.[61,62] CT of the neck obtained after the patient swallows barium optimally shows the tract and the relationship to the pyriform sinus and thyroid gland.

FIBROMATOSIS COLLI

Fibromatosis colli (sternocleidomastoid tumor of infancy) is a well-recognized cause of neck mass associated with a torticollis in infants. The etiology is uncertain but the incidence is increased in children with history of a breech presentation and forceps delivery. Children typically present at 2 to 4 weeks of age with torticollis and a palpable neck mass. US examination is quick and inexpensive and allows a confident diagnosis in patients with the appropriate history. US shows a hypoechoic or mixed echogenicity mass, which conforms to the enlarged SCM muscle.[63,64] CT and MRI show variable attenuation and signal characteristics of the enlarged SCM muscle; however, this should not be required to make the diagnosis.

HEMANGIOMAS AND VASCULAR MALFORMATIONS

Soft tissue vascular anomalies can be divided into hemangiomas and vascular malformations based on the endolthelial characteristics and clinical behavior of these lesions.[65] Hemangioma of infancy is a benign neoplasm of proliferating endothelial cells that gradually increases in size during the first year of life and usually spontaneously involutes over the next several years. Vascular malformations are lesions that grow commensurate with the patient, lack proliferating endothelium, and do not involute. Although CT or MRI can define the extent of these lesions, MR characteristics are better able to predict the type of vascular lesion.[66,67] Hemangiomas of infancy are well-defined masses, intermediate signal on T1-weighted and hyperintense signal on T2-weighted images with intense diffuse postcontrast enhancement. During the proliferative phase, these lesions frequently contain intralesional flow voids indicative of the high-flow nature of this vascular lesion. Later, in the involutional phase, there may be intralesional foci of high T1 signal secondary to fatty replacement.

Vascular malformations may be arteriovenous malformations, venous malformations, lymphatic malformations, or mixed lesions. Arteriovenous malformations typically contain flow voids with multiple serpiginous channels secondary to arteriovenous shunting. They usually have less mass effect than hemangiomas because they lack intervening parenchyma. Venous malfomations (cavernous hemangiomas) lack intralesional flow voids, may be well-defined or infiltrative, and typically contain hyperintense areas on T2-weighted images in regions of venous lakes, which enhance after contrast. Phleboliths are typically seen with venous malformations. Lymphatic malformations are composed of lymphatic sacs of varying sizes, hypointense on T1-weighted images and hyperintense on T2-weighted images, without significant contrast enhancement. There may be mild enhancement of intervening septations. They may also contain fluid levels secondary to intralesional hemorrhage.

Of all of the vascular malformations, the most common to hemorrhage is the lymphatic malformation. Treatment of these vascular malformations depends on the primary cell type within the lesion and requires an experienced medical team. On rare occasion, children with extracranial hemangiomas have a constellation of coexisting abnormalities that has recently been termed PHACE syndrome, including Posterior fossa malformations; large cervicofacial Hemangioma; Arterial anomalies; Coarctation of the aorta and cardiac defects; and Eye abnormalities.[68]

NEOPLASMS

The most common primary malignant neoplasms of the head and neck in children are lymphoma and rhabdomyosarcoma. Malignant lymphoma may be Hodgkin's or non-Hodgkin's lymphoma, unilateral or bilateral, or primarily nodal or extra-nodal (Waldeyer ring, paranasal sinuses, and nasal cavity). Imaging should include CT of the neck, chest, abdomen, and pelvis as well as gallium-67 nuclear scintigraphy.

Rhabdomyosarcoma is the most common childhood soft tissue sarcoma, occurring in the head and neck in 40% of patients.[69–71] Initial imaging can be accomplished with CT because osseous erosion is frequent. MR imaging is helpful to exclude intracranial extension in children with parameningeal disease (middle ear, paranasal sinus, nasopharynx). Imaging should include the primary mass and the entire neck to exclude metastatic lymphadenopathy.

Neuroblastoma is the most common malignant tumor in children less than 1 year of age and usually arises within the adrenal gland, although it may be extra-adrenal. Primary cervical neuroblastoma is uncommon. The mass is usually posterior to the vascular sheath in the neck, rarely extends intraspinal, and may or may not be partially calcified. These lesions can be imaged with MRI or CT. Whole-body meta-iodobenzylguanidine (MIBG) imaging should also be performed to assess the primary lesion and to rule out metastatic disease. In addition, skeletal scintigraphy should be performed to rule out bony metastasis.

IMAGING THE PEDIATRIC TEMPORAL BONE

A wide variety of pathology may affect the pediatric temporal bone. Inflammatory disease is the most frequent disorder affecting this area and the associated complications are well demonstrated on CT and MR. Congenital, traumatic, vascular, and neoplastic disorders are also well visualized on imaging studies. The radiologic appearance of this varied pathology is described in this section, with an emphasis on the information that can be derived from each imaging modality.

The primary imaging modalities used for the pediatric temporal bone are high-resolution computed tomography (HRCT) and magnetic resonance imaging (MRI). Occasionally, magnetic resonance angiography (MRA), conventional angiography, and/or nuclear medicine studies may be used to answer a particular question. CT studies are obtained with a high-resolution bone algorithm using 120 kV and 140 mA. The plane for axial scanning is parallel to the hard palate, which delivers less radiation to the lens compared with the plane along the orbitomeatal line.[72] Images are obtained with a thickness of 1.0 to 1.5 mm at 1.0 mm intervals. The images are targeted to each side and viewed with bone windows (a window of approximately 3000 Houndsfield units (HU) and a level of approximately 350 HU) as well as soft tissue windows. Contrast is added for cases of complicated acute otomastoiditis or suspected neoplasm, with soft tissue windows as well.

MR imaging usually includes a T2-weighted spin echo or fast spin echo axial image of the brain and a FLAIR (fluid-attenuated inversion recovery) axial image through the brain. Thin section T1-weighted axial and coronal images are then obtained through the temporal bones pre- and postcontrast. Finally, axial three-dimensional Fourier transformation (3DFT) gradient echo (T2-weighted) images are obtained in a volume acquisition, permitting very thin sections of 1 mm thickness or less. These gradient echo images are extremely useful in evaluating the membranous labyrinth. In selected cases, MRA or MRV may be used, usually accomplished without the use of contrast (gradient echo sequences that produce flow-related enhancement are used).

As a general approach, CT is used for evaluation of a conductive hearing loss (CHL) as well as congenital sensorineural hearing loss (SNHL) in children, with MR for evaluation of acquired SNHL in adults and older children. In many cases, CT and MR provide complementary information. CT is best for visualization of the ossicles and other bony structures, whereas MR is preferred for detection of soft tissue masses, especially in the internal auditory canal (IAC) and cerebellopontine (CP) angle. Because of its depiction of bony detail, CT is used for identification of fractures as well as in cases of suspected middle ear disease (inflammation, cholesteatoma, etc.). For evaluation of congenital anomalies, CT is usually the initial study, although MR may be added as needed. Acquired disease of the inner ear (fibrosis resulting from meningitis/labyrinthitis) is best detected on the thin section T2-weighted MR images. Petrous apex lesions are also best characterized with MR, although CT may provide some useful information (calcification, hyperostosis, etc.). CT is an informative initial study for patients with pulsatile tinnitus, but if the CT study is negative, an MRI and/or MRA may be required to complete the evaluation.

CONGENITAL/DEVELOPMENTAL ABNORMALITIES

The External Ear

Congenital aural dysplasia includes malformations of the pinna (microtia) and external auditory canal (EAC). Occurrence is most often sporadic, unilateral, and nonsyndromic, although up to one third of EAC atresia may be bilateral.[73] The external and middle ear derive from the branchial apparatus, whereas the inner ear arises from neuroectoderm.[74,75] Thus, EAC dysplasia is commonly associated with anomalies of the middle ear and mastoid, while associated labyrinthine malformations are seen in only 11 to 13%.[76]

The EAC dysplasia ranges in severity from an EAC stenosis to complete atresia and may be bony, membranous, or mixed. Schuknecht's classification[77] stratifies the bony atresias into Type A (meatal, with stenosis involving the fibrocartilage of the EAC), type B (partial, with bony and fibrocartilage stenosis), type C (total), and type D (hypopneumatic total).[77] Membranous atresia consists of a soft tissue plug in the location of the tympanic membrane (TM).

Associated middle ear anomalies include hypoplasia of the middle ear, as well as absence, deformity, and/or fusion of the ossicular chain. The most common finding is fusion of the malleus and incus with fusion as well to the bony atresia plate, which is in the expected location of the TM.[78] The course of the facial nerve is often anomalous with anterior displacement of the mastoid segment. Thus, coronal CT images may reveal the mastoid segment of the nerve at the level of the vestibule, which normally demonstrates the tympanic segment of the nerve running just below the lateral semicircular canal. EAC dysplasia may also be associated with cholesteatoma within a stenotic EAC (congenital or acquired) or in the middle ear (congenital cholesteatoma).

In a child with aural atresia, CT is used to help plan the surgical reconstruction. Critical information must be determined from the CT regarding the severity of the ossicular deformity; the patency of the oval and round windows; the size of the middle ear cavity; the degree of mastoid pneumatization; and the course of the facial nerve. Other important findings include the presence of cholesteatoma, position of the sigmoid sinus, location of the mandibular condyle, and presence of any inner ear abnormalities.[78–80] Surgery may be deferred in some patients with bilateral atresia to allow for development of the mastoid air cells. Therefore, CT is best obtained close to the date of planned surgery, unless cholesteatoma or inner ear anomalies are suspected.[73]

The Middle Ear

Congenital ossicular anomalies may occur in association with EAC dysplasia, as described earlier, or may occur in isolation. Bilateral anomalies may be associated with autosomal dominant inheritance.[81,82] The most common isolated congenital ossicular deformity is an incudostapedial disconnection, wherein the long process of the incus is absent or elongated and oriented more posteriorly than normal with respect to the oval window.[73] The stapes superstructure may also be abnormal or absent.

In cases of congenital stapes fixation associated with dysplasia of the inner ear, a perilymph "gusher" can occur at surgery upon removal of the stapes footplate. Congenital stapes fixation may not be apparent on CT,[82] but can be associated with other radiologic findings that suggest a greater risk of perilymph gusher. These imaging findings include enlargement of the lateral portion of the IAC, dysplasia of the cochlea, and a dilated vestibular aqueduct.[83]

A cholesteatoma may be considered congenital in origin if the tympanic membrane (TM) is intact and there is no prior history of ear drainage or TM perforation and no previous trauma or surgery.[84] These lesions arise from displaced epithelial rests present at birth and are identical to epidermoid cysts.[85] Congenital cholesteatoma is most commonly seen in the middle ear, but can also arise in the petrous apex, the mastoid bone, or the EAC. Congenital cholesteatoma occurs three times more often in males than in females[84] and is often present with a conductive hearing loss.[86] About 28% of middle ear cholesteatoma in children under 13 years old is congenital in origin.[87] A white retrotympanic mass may be visible on otoscopy,[88] and CT reveals a soft tissue mass, which may be associated with bone erosion. Ossicular erosion is often seen at surgery.[87,89]

The Inner Ear

About 20% of children with congenital SNHL have radiographic abnormalities of the inner ear identified on imaging studies.[90] The normal cochlea contains a 3-cm-long spiral canal that wraps around a central bony axis, the modiolus, with 2 1/2 turns. Labyrinthine aplasia (Michel deformity) denotes absence of the cochlea, vestibule, and semicircular canals (SCC). This results from developmental arrest in the third gestational week. Failure of development in the fourth to fifth weeks results in formation of a common cavity, which replaces the cochlea, vestibule, and semicircular canals. This anomaly accounts for 26% of cochlear malformations.[91]

The classic Mondini malformation makes up 55% of all inner ear deformities and results from developmental arrest in the seventh gestational week.[73] The cochlea has fewer than 2.5 turns and the apical and middle turns appear confluent (known as incomplete partition).[73] On HRCT, the basal turn is seen connected to a single ovoid cavity. In 20% of cases, there may be coexistent deformity of the vestibule, SCC, and/or endolymphatic duct/sac.[73] Risk of perilymph fistula is also increased, which may result in recurrent meningitis or CSF otorrhea.[92] The Mondini malformation is seen in conjunction with a number of syndromes, including Klippel–Feil, Wildervanck, Alagille, Waardenburg, Pendred, DiGeorge, and Pierre–Robin syndromes.[93] There is also an association with the CHARGE (coloboma, heart defects, atresia of the choanae, retardation of growth, genital/urinary abnormalities, ear abnormalities/hearing loss) syndrome, congenital CMV infection, and trisomy 21.[94]

An enlarged vestibular aqueduct (VA) is the most common abnormal imaging finding in children with congenital SNHL.[93] It is bilateral in 72% of cases.[95] A VA is considered to be dilated if it measures >1.5 mm in width at its midpoint. Approximately 16 to 26% of ears with large VA also have an abnormality of the cochlea.[95,96] In patients with a dilated VA, the endolymphatic duct and sac are usually enlarged, which can be seen on the T2-weighted 3DFT axial MR images. These MRI findings can also be present in the absence of a dilated VA on CT.[97] Hearing loss in these patients is often fluctuating or progressive. The high-resolution T2-weighted images are also helpful in identifying hypoplasia or aplasia of the vestibulocochlear nerve.

Perilymphatic Fistula

Congenital perilymphatic fistula (PLF) results from an abnormal connection between the inner and middle ear, allowing perilymph to leak into the middle ear or mastoid air cells. This can also provide a route for the spread of infection from the middle ear to the meninges and can be the cause of recurrent meningitis.[98] Symptoms include episodic vertigo; sudden, progressive, or fluctuating hearing loss; otorrhea; rhinorrhea; or mimicking of an otitis media (OM).[94] These PLF can be bilateral. The most frequent site of the fistula is at the oval window, with the next most frequent location being the round window.[99]

Middle ear abnormalities are often identified in these patients, and the most common of these is a malformed stapes superstructure.[99] Inner ear abnormalities may be seen in about one third of patients with PLF; this most commonly includes a large VA followed in frequency by a Mondini malformation.[99] CT demonstration of a middle or inner ear anomaly increases the likelihood that a leak will be seen at surgery.[100] Surgery is indicated to stabilize or improve hearing, to decrease vertigo, or to prevent recurrent meningitis.[101]

IMAGING OF COCHLEAR IMPLANT CANDIDATES

Preoperative CT is essential for surgical planning in cochlear implant candidates. CT is used to identify congenital malformations, cochlear ossification, patency of the round window, and any unusual anatomy that may complicate the surgical procedure. A narrowed IAC of <2.5 mm diameter suggests absence of the vestibulocochlear nerve,[102] which can be confirmed with MRI. MRI is also useful in identification of cochlear fibrosis (following meningitis/labyrinthitis). Cochlear aplasia and absence of the cochlear nerve preclude implantation.[102,103] Severe dysplasia of the cochlea has a greater risk of overinsertion of the electrode and of perilymphatic gusher.[103,104]

VASCULAR ANOMALIES

One or both of the internal carotid arteries (ICA) may be aplastic.[105] CT reveals absence of the carotid canal. Much more commonly, an aberrant ICA is identified. This occurs due to a lack of development or regression of the cervical segment of the ICA during embryogenesis. The inferior tympanic artery enlarges and anastamoses with an enlarged caroticotympanic artery to reestablish flow in the horizontal petrous ICA.[106] Patients may present with pulsatile tinnitus and/or conductive hearing loss. The aberrant vessel passes through the middle ear posterolateral to the expected location of the vertical ICA. The aberrant carotid then courses anteriorly to join the horizontal carotid canal through a bony defect in the carotid plate. CT reveals absence of the normal bony plate which covers the lateral aspect of the ICA. This is seen well on axial and coronal images. The horizontal carotid canal appears elongated, extending laterally into the hypotympanum. The aberrant ICA is usually smaller in caliber than the normal contralateral ICA.

A persistent stapedial artery is a rare anomaly that may occur with or without an aberrant ICA.[107,108] This may occur bilaterally. The persistent stapedial artery emerges from the ICA in the vertical petrous canal and travels to the middle ear where it enters the tympanic segment of the facial nerve canal, which appears enlarged on CT. The vessel then courses to the middle cranial fossa, posterolateral to the absent foramen spinosum. The artery then divides into the middle meningeal artery and a sphenoidal branch.[109]

A high-riding jugular bulb may be defined as rising above the inferior rim of the tympanic ring or rising to the inferior margin of the round window.[110] A bony dehiscence may be present in the overlying bony plate with protrusion of the jugular vein into the hypotympanum. This is best visualized on axial or coronal CT images. The dehiscent jugular bulb may present as a bluish middle ear mass, which may be pulsatile or nonpulsatile, and/or with pulsatile tinnitus, or with bleeding after myringotomy[94] (Figure 7.10).

INFLAMMATORY DISEASE

Uncomplicated acute OM does not require imaging of the temporal bone; however, CT and MR are useful in depicting the complications of acute and chronic OM. OM with effusion results in opacification of the middle ear (ME) and mastoid air cells on CT. Persistent infection may be complicated by mastoiditis, with opacification of mastoid air cells. Coalescent mastoiditis refers to bony resorption and erosion in conjunction with a pus-filled mastoid. The bone erosion is well seen on HRCT. Complications that may occur with continued infection include subperiosteal abscess, epidural or subdural abscess, meningitis, cerebritis, and/or brain abscess as well as venous sinus thrombosis (Figure 7.11). Subperiosteal abscess is most often retroauricular in location and the adjacent mastoid bone is eroded. A contiguous ring-enhancing mass is seen at the site of bone erosion.

If intracranial extension is suspected, MR is the study of choice. Meningeal enhancement and epidural and/or subdural collections are best imaged using gadolinium-enhanced MR. Thrombosis

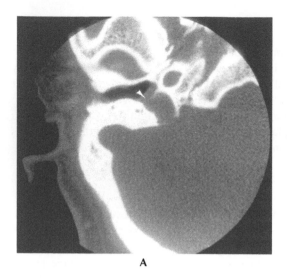
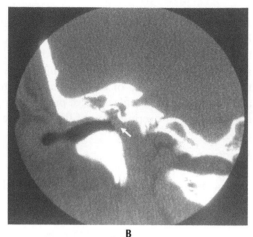

A   B

FIGURE 7.10 Dehiscent jugular bulb. A. Axial CT image at the level of the hypotympanum demonstrates a prominent jugular bulb with a dehiscence in the overlying bony plate (arrowhead). Some inflammatory debris is also present in the hypotympanum. B. Coronal image of the same patient reveals opacification of the epitympanum, mesotympanum, and hypotympanum by inflammatory disease. There are chronic sclerotic changes in the bone and blunting and thickening of the scutum. Again, note absence of the bony plate overlying a prominent jugular bulb (arrow). The inflammatory disease had been described in the preoperative CT report, but the dehiscence of the jugular bulb had not been mentioned. This anatomic variant was recognized intraoperatively, however, by the surgeon who was operating to clear the inflammatory disease.

or thrombophlebitis of the sigmoid sinus and/or jugular vein will appear as a filling defect on contrast-enhanced CT. On MR, T2-weighted images will lack the normal flow void seen in the dural venous sinuses, and MR venography (MRV) reveals a loss of flow-related enhancement on the affected side. Extra-axial empyemas appear as subdural or epidural fluid collections with intense enhancement of the adjacent dura. There may be significant mass effect on the subjacent brain. Increased signal on FLAIR and T2-weighted images in the brain parenchyma may indicate an early cerebritis. Brain abscess as a complication of otomastoiditis is most commonly found in the temporal lobe and demonstrates the typical pattern of ring enhancement with surrounding edema and mass effect.

Bone destruction related to otomastoiditis indicates osteomyelitis. Spread to the petrous apex results in petrous apicitis and may be accompanied by focal abscess formation within the petrous apex (Figure 7.12). This may be suggested clinically by Gradenigo's syndrome, with a triad of sixth nerve palsy, pain along the distribution of the fifth nerve, and purulent otorrhea. In such cases, CT and MR provide complementary information, with the CT providing greater bony detail and the MR providing better soft tissue resolution.

Otomastoiditis or meningitis may result in a labyrinthitis that is best seen on MR imaging. Contrast-enhanced T1-weighted images may demonstrate enhancement of the affected membranous labyrinth. A delayed sequela of labyrinthitis/meningitis is fibrous obliteration of the membranous labyrinth. On the thin section T2-weighted MR sequence, the bright signal of the fluid within the membranous labyrinth is replaced by low-signal fibrous tissue. This fibrous obliteration is more common than the bony changes seen with labyrinthitis ossificans,[90] which can also be a delayed sequela of labyrinthitis/meningitis. In the latter, CT reveals bony density filling the membranous labyrinth, which appears effaced.

Chronic otitis media (COM) commonly produces some granulation tissue, which is nonspecific in appearance on CT studies but usually enhances on contrast MR studies.[111] This tissue is quite friable and may cause some hemorrhage. In the absence of cholesteatoma, conductive hearing loss (CHL) may occur in the setting of COM as a result of ossicular erosion or fixation or from

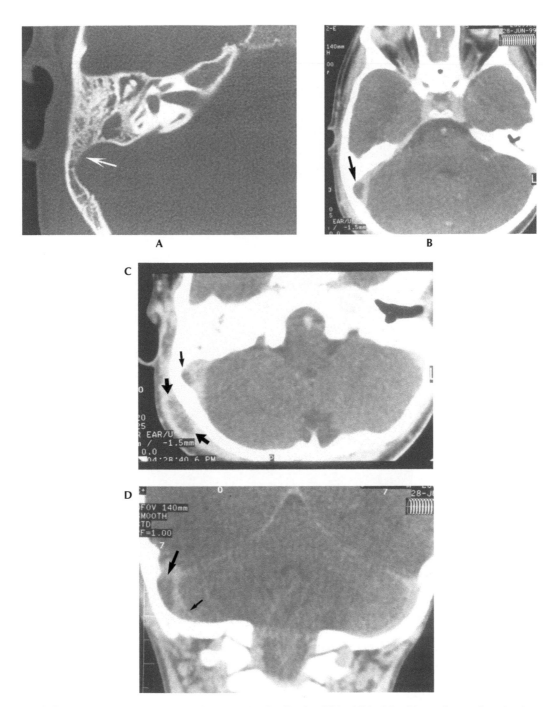

FIGURE 7.11 Acute mastoiditis with focal epidural collection. This child with otitis media was found to have severe pain over the right mastoid. A. Axial CT reveals complete opacification of the middle ear and mastoid. Note bony demineralization of the mastoid adjacent to the sigmoid sinus (arrow) indicating early erosion and coalescent mastoiditis. The ossicles appear intact. B. Contrast-enhanced axial CT reveals an epidural collection just lateral to the sigmoid sinus (arrow). The sigmoid sinus is displaced medially. C. Contrast-enhanced CT again reveals the epidural collection (small arrow). In addition, this extracranial soft tissue density (large arrows) was found to be an abscessed lymph node at surgery. D. Coronal contrast-enhanced CT again demonstrates the epidural collection (large arrow) that displaces the sigmoid sinus medially. There is a filling defect in the right sigmoid sinus (small arrow) suggesting clot and partial sigmoid sinus thrombosis.

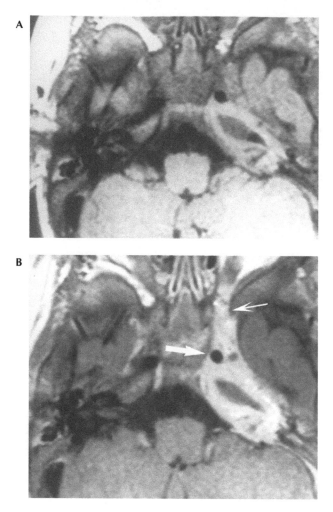

FIGURE 7.12 Petrous apicitis. A. Noncontrast T1-weighted axial MR image reveals abnormal soft tissue replacing the left petrous apex. The hypointense signal seen centrally represents pus within an abscess cavity. This 10-month-old child had draining ears, bilaterally. CT (not shown) showed opacification of the right middle ear/mastoid and complete destruction of the left temporal bone. B. Postcontrast image reveals intense enhancement of the thick walls of this petrous abscess. The circular flow void (thick arrow) seen along the anterior margin of the mass is the cavernous internal carotid artery. Note the abnormal enhancement extending forward along the cavernous sinus (thin arrow) toward the left orbital apex.

tympanosclerosis. The ossicular erosion most commonly involves the long and lenticular processes of the incus and can be seen on HRCT.[112]

CHOLESTEATOMA

Cholesteatoma may be congenital (2%) or acquired (98%) in origin and consists of a mass of stratified squamous epithelium containing exfoliated keratin.[113] Primary acquired cholesteatoma is the most common type of ME cholesteatoma.[73] It is thought to arise from retraction of the pars flaccida of the TM, resulting in an epithelial pocket that becomes trapped and enlarges.[112] Secondary acquired cholesteatoma arises in association with COM, with perforation of the pars tensa of the TM. Pars flaccida cholesteatoma begins in Prussak's space, between the scutum and the ossicular chain. Pars tensa cholesteatoma commonly involves the posterior recesses of the middle ear. Involvement of the posterior recesses is well visualized on CT, but may not be as evident intraoperatively. In such cases, the preoperative CT is very helpful in surgical planning and reduces the possibility that residual disease will be left in the posterior recesses.

Expansion of the pars flaccida cholesteatoma results in bone erosion, especially of the scutum and ossicles. Conductive hearing loss may result from ossicular erosion. Other complications may include erosion of the mastoid and the tegmen, and erosion of the facial nerve canal. Erosion into the lateral semicircular canal can be seen on axial and coronal CT images indicating a labyrinthine fistula. Intracranial extension can occur via a defect in the tegmen with resulting intracranial abscess, meningitis, and venous sinus thrombosis. Characteristic findings of a typical pars flaccida cholesteatoma on CT imaging include a soft tissue mass in the epitympanum with displacement of the ossicles medially, blunting of the scutum, and ossicular erosion.

BELL'S PALSY

Bell's palsy is thought to result from viral inflammation and is sudden in onset. Most cases are not imaged and show gradual resolution of the facial nerve paralysis. Imaging is urged, however, when the paralysis has an atypical course — if it is gradual in onset, prolonged or without improvement, or recurrent. In these cases, other pathology must be excluded. Abnormal enhancement of the facial nerve can be seen on T1-weighted contrast-enhanced MR studies in patients with Bell's palsy. This may involve the intracanalicular portion of the nerve as well as the labyrinthine, tympanic, and mastoid segments. Enhancement is usually linear and involves multiple continuous segments, in contrast to that seen with a neuroma, which is more focal and bulbous. The normal facial nerve does show mild enhancement in the labyrinthine, tympanic, and mastoid segments; however, it is normally discontinuous and does not involve the IAC.

POSTOPERATIVE IMAGING

CT is preferred in the evaluation of the postoperative temporal bone. The imaging assessment should include recognition of the type of surgery performed (canal-wall-up vs. canal-wall-down mastoidectomy), appearance of the surgical defect, integrity of the remaining ossicular chain, and presence or absence of persistent soft tissue debris. The tegmen should be carefully examined and the semicircular canals should be evaluated for the possibility of labyrinthine fistula.

TRAUMA

CT is the procedure of choice in evaluation of temporal bone trauma. CT delineates well the orientation of temporal bone fractures, as well as the presence of ossicular fracture or subluxation, and detects involvement of the facial nerve canal and bony labyrinth.

Longitudinal fractions are most common, accounting for 70 to 90% of temporal bone fractures.[114] These fractures are parallel to the long axis of the petrous bone and commonly cause CSF otorrhea.[115] Facial nerve paralysis may be seen in 10 to 20%, usually from injury to the tympanic segment just distal to the geniculate ganglion.[116,117] This paralysis is often delayed and incomplete. The bony labyrinth is usually spared but the ossicles are commonly involved, resulting in a conductive hearing loss.[114]

Transverse fractures are less common but often involve the IAC and bony labyrinth (Figure 7.13). The facial nerve may be injured, usually in the labyrinthine segment. Facial paralysis occurs in 40 to 50% of patients with transverse fractures of the temporal bone, and it is often immediate and complete.[114] The ossicles are often unaffected in the transverse type of fracture. Opacification of the middle ear or mastoid air cells may be due to hemorrhage. In reality, many or most temporal bone fractures are mixed, with longitudinal and transverse components.

Additional complications that may arise after trauma include CSF otorrhea or rhinorrhea, meningitis, and perilymph fistula. In addition to ossicular fracture, ossicular subluxation/dislocation may be evident on CT. Subluxation of the incudostapedial joint is the most common post-traumatic

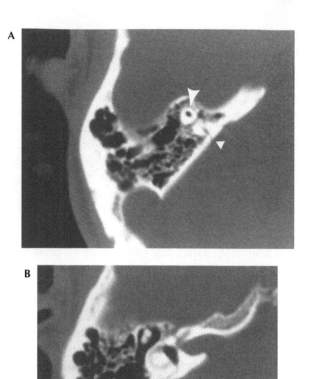

FIGURE 7.13 Fracture of the superior semicircular canal, pneumolabyrinth. A. Axial CT reveals a transverse fracture through one limb of the superior semicircular canal (small arrowhead). Air is seen within the other limb of the superior semicircular canal (large arrowhead). B. Axial CT reveals air within the vestibule as a result of the transverse fracture in (A).

ossicular derangement.[118] Although CT can demonstrate compression of the facial nerve by a bony fragment, contrast-enhanced MR can show enhancement in an edematous nerve.[90] Noncontrast MR is also able to demonstrate intralabyrinthine hemorrhage, which is of increased signal intensity on T1- and T2-weighted images.

Post-traumatic vertigo and/or fluctuating SNHL can be due to a perilymph fistula (PLF). This is most often due to a tear in the round window or in the ligamentous attachment of the stapes footplate at the oval window. CT is usually negative. Enhancement of the cochlea or vestibule on gadolinium-enhanced MRI is supportive evidence for a PLF.[119] MRI is also helpful in detection of any post-traumatic encephalocele in which brain or CSF is seen extending through a bony defect (Figure 7.14).

Mass Lesions of the Temporal Bone

A variety of mass lesions may affect the petrous apex and skull base, the IAC, and cerebellopontine angle (CPA). Lesions of the petrous apex include cholesterol cyst (cholesterol granuloma), epidermoid, mucocele, cartilaginous tumors, metastases, meningioma, and trigeminal schwannoma. Lesions affecting the skull base in children also include lymphoma, eosinophilic granuloma, and

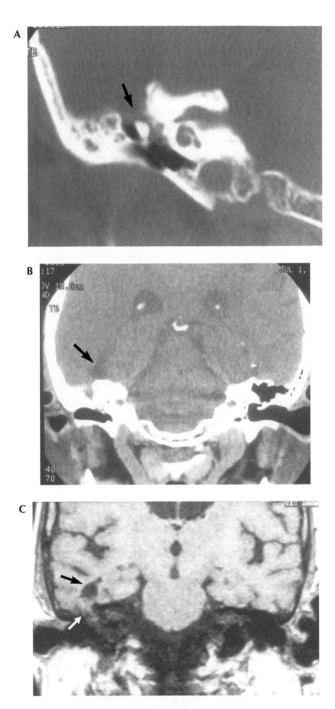

FIGURE 7.14 Post-traumatic encephalocele with CSF leak. A. Coronal CT image reveals a large defect in the tegman tympani (arrow). Some opacity is also seen in the epitympanum, medial to the ossicular chain. The history of trauma was not originally elicited. The defect in the tegmen was thought to be the result of infection and/or cholesteatoma. B. Coronal CT again reveals the defect of the tegmen on the right. A hypodensity is seen within the right temporal lobe (arrow). C. Coronal T1-weighted MR image reveals cystic encephalomalacia in the right temporal lobe (black arrow). Brain parenchyma is also seen extending down into the tympanic cavity (white arrow). The patient was questioned and did reveal a remote history of trauma. A diagnosis of post-traumatic encephalocele was made. The patient had been suffering for several years from recurrent meningitis and a CSF leak, although the site of the leak had never been documented.

rhabdomyosarcoma. Most of these are best delineated with a combination of CT and MR imaging. CT provides a roadmap for planning the route of access to a lesion.

A cholesterol cyst (cholesterol granuloma) can occur anywhere from the ME cavity to the petrous apex. Otoscopy may reveal a bluish TM, which needs to be differentiated from a vascular variant or vascular tumor. Cholesterol granuloma are lined by fibrous connective tissue, which is quite friable with a propensity to hemorrhage. Brownish fluid containing cholesterol crystals, multinucleated giant cells, red blood cells, and hemosiderin fills the lesion. On CT, this appears as a nonspecific expansile soft tissue mass, while the MR appearance is quite characteristic. Because of the hemorrhagic nature of these cysts, methemoglobin is present, thus resulting in hyperintense signal on the T1- and T2-weighted images. Because the imaging appearance is fairly specific, a cholesterol cyst can be strongly suspected from the preoperative imaging studies.

Epidermoid and mucocele are most often hypointense on T1-weighted images and hyperintense on T2-weighted images. However, due to variability in protein content and other internal debris, these lesions may appear somewhat hyperintense to CSF on the T1-weighted sequence. The central portion does not enhance. Some minimal peripheral enhancement may be due to adjacent fibrosis and inflammation. Diffusion MR imaging can be used to differentiate an epidermoid from other cystic lesions. Because of its complex internal contents, an epidermoid will show restricted fluid motion, whereas a cyst does not. The normal petrous apex may contain marrow and is therefore bright on T1-weighted images. Alternatively, the petrous apex may be aerated and is thus hypointense on all sequences. In any particular patient, the petrous apices may be asymmetric and thus one side may have a signal that is very different from the other petrous apex on MR imaging. This should not be mistaken for a lesion.

The primary lesions affecting the skull base in children include rhabdomyosarcoma, lymphoma, and eosinophilic granuloma (Langerhan cell histiocytosis). Rhabdomyosarcoma is the most common primary malignancy of the temporal bone. It is a locally aggressive lesion with a propensity for meningeal invasion as well as metastatic disease. CT reveals an extensive lesion with bone destruction. MR imaging demonstrates the full extent of disease, with identification of any intracranial involvement or extension to the cavernous sinus. Meningeal disease is readily identified on postgadolinium studies. These skull base masses may have a similar appearance on imaging studies, with specific identification only possible by biopsy.

IAC and CPA Masses

Lesions of the IAC/CPA are suspected when unilateral or asymmetric hearing loss (retrocochlear pathology) occurs. MR imaging is the study of choice for imaging this region. In many cases, MR characteristics are sufficiently specific to permit differentiation among the common lesions in this area, including vestibular nerve schwannoma, meningioma, arachnoid cyst, epidermoid, and trigeminal schwannoma. Vestibular schwannomas are rare in childhood,[120] and thus the presence of even a unilateral vestibular schwannoma in a child should suggest the possibility of neurofibromatosis type 2.[73] Vestibular schwannoma are iso- to hypointense on T1-weighted noncontrast images and are hyperintense on T2-weighted images. Some lesions may have a cystic component.

Postcontrast images reveal intense enhancement. Smaller lesions may reveal purely intralabyrinthine or intracanalicular enhancement. The T2-weighted thin section gradient echo images permit visualization of the individual nerves and a small nodule can be easily seen arising from the vestibulocochlear nerve surrounded by high-signal CSF. Labyrinthitis can also show intralabyrinthine enhancement on contrast images but will not demonstrate a focal nodule on the gradient echo images[90] (as is seen with schwannomas).

Noncontrast T1-weighted images may reveal a focal bright signal in the IAC, consistent with a lipoma or hemangioma. Meningioma is rare in childhood but has the typical appearance of a dural-based mass with intense enhancement, centered on the CPA rather than the IAC. An arachnoid cyst appears hypointense on T1-weighted images and hyperintense on T2-weighted images without enhancement. An epidermoid may have similar imaging characteristics or may appear somewhat brighter on the T1-weighted images due to the complex contents. Again, diffusion imaging can be used to identify the epidermoid lesion that has restricted fluid motion on diffusion imaging. Trigeminal schwannomas show intense enhancement and are often identified by their location.

Glomus Tumors

Glomus tumors are rare in children.[121] Lesions can be multicentric, especially if familial.[85] A glomus tympanicum can be seen on CT as a soft tissue density adjacent to the cochlear promontory. A vascular retrotympanic mass may be seen at otoscopy. The CT must be carefully evaluated to differentiate this lesion from a vascular variant such as an aberrant ICA or a dehiscent jugular bulb. A glomus jugulare will show bony erosion in the region of the jugular foramen on CT, and MR imaging will reveal the typical appearance of "salt and pepper" on T2-weighted images.[122] Multiple flow voids are seen within these lesions due to prominent tumor vascularity, resulting in the "salt and pepper" appearance on these weighted images. The vascular nature of glomus tumors also produces prominent enhancement on contrast studies.

Fibrous Dysplasia

Approximately one fifth of patients with fibrous dysplasia of the skull have involvement of the temporal bone.[123] The disease is usually monostotic.[91] Clinical presentation includes painless mass, progressive hearing loss, and possibly, narrowing of the EAC. The latter can result in canal cholesteatoma from partial obstruction.[124] The CT appearance is characteristic with often marked bony expansion and the classic "ground glass" appearance of the bone.

CONCLUSION

This section has provided an overview of imaging issues in the pediatric temporal bone with an emphasis on what each imaging modality has to offer. In many cases, HRCT and MR provide different but complementary information. These studies are used most effectively when the clinical question to be answered is clearly defined and when there is open communication between the referring clinician and the radiologist.

REFERENCES

1. Vade, A., Demos, T.C., Olson, M.C. et al. Evaluation of image quality using 1:1 pitch and 1.5:1 pitch helical CT in children: a comparative study. *Pediatr. Radiol.*, 1996, 26, 891–893.
2. Kaufmann, R., Banner, W., and Berlin, C. American Academy of Pediatrics Committee on Drugs: guidelines for monitoring and management of pediatric patients during and after sedation for diagnostic and therapeutic procedures. *Pediatrics*, 1992, 89, 1110–1115.
3. Kurth, C.D., Spitzer, A.R., Broennle, A.M., and Downes, J.J. Postoperative apnea in preterm infants. *Anesthesiology*, 1987, 66, 483–488.
4. Cote, C.J. Sedation for the pediatric patient. A review. *Pediatr. Clin. North Am.*, 1994, 41, 31–58.
5. Egelhoff, J.C., Ball, W.S., Jr., Koch, B.L., and Parks, T.D. Safety and efficacy of sedation in children using a structured sedation program. *Am. J. Roentgenol.*, 1997, 168, 1259–1262.
6. Pruitt, A., Striker, T., Anyan, W.R. et al. Guidelines for the elective use of conscious sedation, deep sedation, and general anesthesia in pediatric patients. Committee on Drugs. Section on anesthesiology. *Pediatrics*, 1985, 76, 317–321.
7. Maresh, M.M. and Washbum, A.H. Paranasal sinuses from birth to late adolescence. *Am. J. Dis. Child*, 1940, 60, 841.

8. Shopfner, C.E. and Rossi, J.O. Roentgen evaluation of the paranasal sinuses in children. *Am. J. Roentgenol.,* 1973, 118, 176.

9. Glasier, C.M., Ascher, D.P., and Williams, K. Incidental parasinal sinus abnormalites on CT of children: clinical correlation. *Am. J. Neuroradiol.,* 1986, 7, 861.

10. McAlister, W.H., Lusk, R., and Muntz, H.R. Comparison of plain radiographs and coronal CT scans in infants and children with recurrent sinusitis. *Am. J. Roentgenol.,* 1989, 153, 1259.

11. Gwaltney, J.M., Phillips, C.D., Miller, R.D., and Riker, D.K. Computer tomographic study of the common cold. *New Engl. J. Med.,* 1994, 330, 25.

12. Glasier, C.M., Mallory, G.B.J., and Steele, R.W. Significance of opacification of the maxillary and ethmoid sinuses in infants. *J. Pediatr.,* 1989, 114, 45.

13. Rak, K.M., Newell, J.D.I., and Yakes, W.F. Paranasal sinuses on MR images of the brain: significance of mucosal thickening. *Am. J. Neuroradiol.,* 1990, 11, 1211.

14. Leopold, D.A., Stafford, C.T., Sod, W.W. et al. Clinical course of acute maxillary sinusitis documented by sequential MRI scanning. *Am. J. Rhinol.,* 1994, 8, 19–28.

15. Clement, P.A.R., Bluestone, C.D., Gordts, F. et al. Management of rhinosinusitis in children. *Arch. Otolaryngol. Head Neck Surg.,* 1998, 124, 31–34.

16. Hudgins, P.A., Browning, D.G., Gallups, J. et al. Endoscopic paranasal sinus surgery: radiographic evaluation of severe complications. *Am. J. Neuroradiol.,* 1992, 13, 1161–1167.

17. Stankiewicz, J.A. Complications of endoscopic sinus surgery. *Otolaryngol. Clin. North Am.,* 1989, 22, 749.

18. Towbin, R., Han, B.K., Kaufman, R.A., and Burke, M. Postseptal cellulitis: CT in diagnosis and management. *Radiology,* 1986, 158, 735–737.

19. Andrews, T.M. and Myer, C.M.I. The role of computed tomography in the diagnosis of subperiosteal abscess of the orbit. *Clin. Pediatri.,* 1992, 31, 37.

20. Som, P.M., Dillon, W.P., and Fullerton, G.D. Chronically obstructed sinonasal secretions: observations on T1 and T2 shortening. *Radiology,* 1989, 172, 515.

21. Som, P.M., Dillon, W.P., and Curtin, H.D. Hypointense paranasal sinus foci: differential diagnosis with MR imaging and relation to CT findings. *Radiology,* 1990, 176, 777.

22. Dillon, W.P., Som, P.M., and Fullerton, G.D. Hypointense MR signal in chronically inspissated sinonasal secretion. *Radiology,* 1990, 174, 73.

23. Zinreich, S.J., Kennedy, D.W., and Malat, J. Fungal sinusitis: diagnosis with CT and MR imaging. *Radiology,* 1988, 169, 439.

24. Som, P.M. and Curtain, H.D. Chronic inflammatory sinonasal disease including fungal infections: the role of imaging. *Radiologic Clin. North Am.,* 1993, 31, 33.

25. Kopp, W., Fotter, R., and Steiner, H. Aspergillosis of the paranasal sinuses. *Radiology,* 1985, 156, 715.

26. Chang, T., Teng, M.M.H., and Wang, S.F. Aspergillosis of the paranasal sinuses. *Neuroradiology,* 1992, 34, 520.

27. Babbel, R.W., Harnsberger, H.R., Sonkens, J., and Hunt, S. Recurring patterns of inflammatory sinonasal disease demonstrated on screening sinus CT. *Am. J. Neuroradiol.,* 1992, 13, 903–912.

28. Som, P.M., Shapiro, M.D., Biller, H.F., Sasaki, C., and Lawson, W. Sinonasal tumors and inflammatory tissues: differentiation with MR imaging. *Radiology,* 1988, 167, 803–808.

29. Currarino, G. and Williams, B. Lateral inspiration and expiration radiographs of the neck in children with laryngotracheitis (croup). *Radiology,* 1982, 145, 365–366.

30. Han, B.K., Dunbar, J.S., and Striker, T.W. Membranous laryngotracheobronchitis (membranous croup). *Am. J. Roentgenol.,* 1979, 133, 53–58.

31. Cotter, C.S., Jones, D.T., Nuss, R.C., and Jonas, R. Management of distal tracheal stenosis. *Arch. Otolaryngol. Head Neck Surg.,* 1999, 125, 325–328.

32. Oshima, Y., Yamaguchi, M., Ohashi, H. et al. [Pulmonary artery sling with tracheal stenosis—primary repair in infancy]. *Jpn. J. Thorac. Cardiovasc. Surg.,* 1998, 46, 347–353.

33. Rimell, F.L. and Stool, S.E. Diagnosis and management of pediatric tracheal stenosis. *Otolaryngol. Clin. North Am.,* 1995, 28, 809–827.

34. Dunham, M.E., Holinger, L.D., Backer, C.L., and Mavroudis, C. Management of severe congenital tracheal stenosis. *Ann. Otol. Rhinol. Laryngol.,* 1994, 103, 351–356.

35. Pawade, A., de Leval, M.R., Elliott, M.J., and Stark, J. Pulmonary artery sling. *Ann. Thorac. Surg.,* 1992, 54, 967–970.

36. Sailer, R., Zimmermann, T., Bowing, B., Scharf, J., Zeilinger, G., and Stehr, K. Pulmonary artery sling associated with tracheobronchial malformations. *Arch. Otolaryngol. Head Neck Surg.*, 1992, 118, 864–867.

37. Lowe, G.M., Donaldson, J.S., and Backer, C.L. Vascular rings: 10-year review of imaging. *Radiographics*, 1991, 11, 637–646.

38. Berdon, W.E., Baker, D.H., Wung, J.T. et al. Complete cartilage-ring tracheal stenosis associated with anomalous left pulmonary artery: the ring-sling complex. *Radiology*, 1984, 152, 57–64.

39. Friedman, A.P., Haller, J.O., Goodman, J.D., and Nagar, H. Sonographic evaluation of noninflammatory neck masses in children. *Radiology*, 1983, 147, 693.

40. Kraus, R., Han, B.K., Babcock, D.S., and Oestreich, A.E. Sonography of neck masses in children. *Am. J. Roentgenol.*, 1986, 146, 609.

41. Kreutzer, E.W., Jafek, B.W., Johnson, M.L., and Zunkel, D.E. Ultrasonography in the preoperative evaluation of neck abscesses. *Head Neck Surg.*, 1982, 4, 290.

42. Yamaguchi, M., Takeuchi, S., and Matsuo, S.I. Ultrasonic evaluation of pediatric superficial masses. *J. Clin. Ultrasound*, 1987, 15, 107.

43. Nyberg, D.A., Jeffrey, R.B., and Brant–Zawadzki, M. Computed tomography of cervical infections. *J. Comput. Assist. Tomogr.*, 1985, 9, 288.

44. Stone, M.E., Walner, D.L., Koch, B.L., Egelhoff, J.C., and Myer, C.M. Correlation between computed tomography and surgical findings in retropharyngeal inflammatory processes in children. *Int. J. Pediatr. Otorhinolaryngol.*, 1999, 49, 121–125.

45. Hudgins, P.A., Dorey, J.H., and Jacobs, I.N. Internal carotid artery narrowing in children with retropharyngeal lymphadenitis and abscess. *Am. J. Neuroradiol.*, 1998, 19, 1841–1843.

46. Weesner, C.L. and Cisek, J.E. Lemierre syndrome: the forgotten disease. *Ann. Emerg. Med.*, 1993, 22, 256–258.

47. Davis, H.J. Case of abnormal artery wall of pharynx. *Proc. R. Soc. Med.*, 1914, 7, 104.

48. Foreign Letters. Paris letter. *JAMA*, 1921, 76, 532.

49. Schaeffer, J.P. Aberrant vessels in the surgery of the palatine and pharyngeal tonsils. *JAMA*, 1921, 77, 14–19.

50. Carmack, J.W. Aberrant internal carotids and their relation to surgery of the pharynx. *Laryngoscope*, 1929, 39, 707–720.

51. Thomas, J.R. Thyroglossal-duct cysts. *Ear Nose Throat J.*, 1979, 58, 21.

52. Allard, R.H. The thyroglossal duct. *Head Neck Surg.*, 1982, 5, 134.

53. Choy, F.J. and Ward, R. Carcinoma of the thyroglossal duct. *Am. J. Surg.*, 1964, 108, 361.

54. Lim–Dunham, J.E., Feinstein, K.A., Yousefzadeh, D.K., and Ben–Ami, T. Sonographic demonstration of a normal thyroid gland excludes ectopic thyroid in patients with thyroglossal duct cyst. *Am. J. Roentgenol.*, 1995, 164, 1489.

55. Wadsworth, D.T. and Seigel, M.J. Thyroglossal duct cysts: variability of sonographic findings. *Am. J. Roentgenol.*, 1994, 163, 1475.

56. Benson, M.T., Dalen, K., and Mancuso, A.A. Congenital anomalies of the branchial apparatus: embryology and pathologic anatomy. *Radiographics*, 1992, 12, 943.

57. Mukherji, S.M., Tart, R.P., and Slattery, W.H. Evaluation of first branchial anomalies by CT and MR. *J. Comput. Assist. Tomogr.*, 1993, 17, 576.

58. Bailey, H. *Branchial Cysts and Other Essays on Surgical Subjects in the Faciocervical Region.* London: Lewis, 1929.

59. Cressman, W.R. and Myer, C.M.I. Cervical thymic cyst. *Arch. Otolaryngol. Head Neck Surg.*, 1992, 118, 774.

60. Guba, A.M., Adam, A.E., Jaques, D.A., and Chambers, R.G. Cervical presentation of thymic cysts. *Am. J. Surg.*, 1978, 136, 430.

61. Lucaya, J., Berdon, W.E., Enriquez, G., Regas, J., and Carreno, J.C. Congenital pyriform sinus fistula: a cause of acute left-sided suppurative thyroiditis and neck abscess in children [see comments]. *Pediatr. Radiol.*, 1990, 21, 27–29.

62. Taylor, W.E., Jr., Myer, C.M.D., Hays, L.L., and Cotton, R.T. Acute suppurative thyroiditis in children. *Laryngoscope*, 1982, 92, 1269–1273.

63. Youkilis, R.A., Koch, B.L., and Myer, C.M.I. Ultrasonographic imaging of sternocleidomastoid tumor of infancy. *Ann. Otol. Rhinol. Laryngol.*, 1995, 104, 323.

64. Chan, Y.L., Cheng, J.C., and Metreweli, C. Ultrasonography of congenital muscular torticollis. *Pediatr. Radiol.*, 1992, 22, 356.

65. Mulliken, J.B. and Glowacki, J. Hemangiomas and vascular malformations in infants and children: a classification based on endothelial characteristics. *Plastic Reconstr. Surg.*, 1982, 69, 412.

66. Baker, L.L., Dillon, W.P., Hieshima, G.B., Dowd, C.F., and Frieden, I.J. Hemangiomas and vascular malformations of the head and neck: MR characterization. *Am. J. Neuroradiol.*, 1993, 4, 307.

67. Meyer, J.S., Hoffer, F.A., Barnes, P.D., and Mulliken, J.B. Biological classification of soft-tissue vascular anomalies: MR correlation. *Am. J. Roentgenol.*, 1991, 157, 559.

68. Frieden, I.J., Reese, V., and Cohen, D. PHACE syndrome. The association of posterior fossa brain malformations, hemangiomas, arterial anomalies, coarctation of the aorta and cardiac defects, and eye abnormalities. *Arch. Dermatol.*, 1996, 132, 307–311.

69. Castillo, M. and Pillsbury, H.C.I. Rhabdomyosarcoma of the middle ear: imaging features in two children. *Am. J. Neuroradiol.*, 1993, 14, 730.

70. Latack, J.T., Hutchinson, R.J., and Heyn, R.M. Imaging of rhabdomyosarcomas of the head and neck. *Am. J. Neuroradiol.*, 1987, 8, 353.

71. Schwartz, R.H., Movassaghi, N., and Marion, E.D. Rhabdomyosarcoma of the middle ear: a wolf in sheep's clothing. *Pediatrics*, 1980, 65, 1131.

72. Torizuka, T., Hayakawa, K., Satoh, Y. et al. High-resolution CT of the temporal bone: a modified baseline. *Radiology*, 1992, 184, 109–111.

73. Robson, C.D., Robertson, R.L., and Barnes, P.D. Imaging of pediatric temporal bone abnormalities. *Neuroimaging Clin. N. Am.*, 1999, 9, 133–155.

74. Kenna, M.A. Embryology and developmental anatomy of the ear. In Bluestone, C.H., Stool, S.E., and Kenna, M.A., Eds. *Pediatric Otolaryngology*. Philadelphia: W.B. Saunders, 1996, 113.

75. Moore, K. The eye and ear. In Moore K., Ed. *The Developing Human: Clinically Oriented Embryology*. Philadelphia: W.B. Saunders, 1988, 402.

76. Jafek, B.W., Nager, G.T., Strife, J., and Gayler, R.W. Congenital aural atresia: an analysis of 311 cases. *Trans. Am. Acad. Ophthalmol. Otolaryngol.*, 1975, 80, 588–595.

77. Schuknecht, H.F. Congenital aural atresia. *Laryngoscope*, 1989, 99, 908–917.

78. Remley, K.B., Swartz, J.D., and Harnsberger, H.R. The external auditory canal. In Swartz, M.D. and Harnsberger, H.R., Eds. *Imaging of the Temporal Bone*. New York: Thieme Medical Publishers, 1998, 16.

79. Jahrsdoerfer, R.A., Yeakley, J.W., Aguilar, E.A., Cole, R.R., and Gray, L.C. Grading system for the selection of patients with congenital aural atresia. *Am. J. Otol.*, 1992, 13, 6–12.

80. Yeakley, J.W. and Jahrsdoerfer, R.A. CT evaluation of congenital aural atresia: what the radiologist and surgeon need to know. *J. Comput. Assist. Tomogr.*, 1996, 20, 724–731.

81. Bluestone, C.D. and Klein, J.O. Otitis media, atelectasis, and eustachian tube dysfunction. In Bluestone, C.D., Stool, S.E., and Kenna, M.A., Eds. *Pediatric Otolaryngology*. Philadelphia: W.B. Saunders, 1996, 388.

82. Swartz, J.D. and Harnsberger, H.R. The middle ear and mastoid. In Swartz, J.D. and Harnsberger, H.R., Eds. *Imaging of the Temporal Bone*. New York: Thieme Medical Publishers, 1998.

83. Talbot, J.M. and Wilson, D.F. Computed tomographic diagnosis of X-linked congenital mixed deafness, fixation of the stapedial footplate, and perilymphatic gusher. *Am. J. Otol.*, 1994, 15, 177–182.

84. Levenson, M.J., Michaels, L., and Parisier, S.C. Congenital cholesteatomas of the middle ear in children: origin and management. *Otolaryngol. Clin. North Am.*, 1989, 22, 941–954.

85. Schuknecht, H.F. *Pathology of the Ear*. 2nd ed. Philadelphia: Lea & Febiger, 1993.

86. McGill, T.J., Merchant, S., Healy, G.B., and Friedman, E.M. Congenital cholesteatoma of the middle ear in children: a clinical and histopathological report. *Laryngoscope*, 1991, 101, 606–613.

87. Sade, J. and Shatz, A. Cholesteatoma in children. *J. Laryngol. Otol.*, 1988, 102, 1003–1006.

88. Bellet, P.S., Benton, C., Jr., Matt, B.H., and Myer, C.M.D. The evaluation of ear canal, middle ear, temporal bone, and cerebellopontine angle masses in infants, children, and adolescents. *Adv. Pediatr.* 1992, 39, 167–205.

89. Karmarkar, S., Bhatia, S., Khashaba, A., Saleh, E., Russo, A., and Sanna, M. Congenital cholesteatomas of the middle ear: a different experience. *Am. J. Otol.*, 1996, 17, 288–292.

90. Casselman, J.W. Temporal bone imaging. *Neuroimaging Clin. N. Am.*, 1996, 6, 265–289.

91. Swartz, J.D. and Harnsberger, H.R. The otic capsule and otodystrophies. In Swartz, M.D. and Harnsberger, H.R., Eds. *Imaging of the Temporal Bone*. New York: Thieme Medical Publishers, 1998, 240.

92. Wolfowitz, B. Spontaneous CSF otorrhea simulating serous otitis. *Arch. Otolaryngol.*, 1979, 105, 496–499.

93. Mafee, M.F., Charletta, D., Kumar, A., and Belmont, H. Large vestibular aqueduct and congenital sensorineural hearing loss. *Am. J. Neuroradiol.*, 1992, 13, 805–819.

94. Benton, C. and Bellet, P.S. Imaging of congenital anomalies of the temporal bone. *Neuroimaging Clin. N. Am.*, 2000, 10, 35–53, vii–viii.

95. Valvassori, G.E. and Clemis, J.D. The large vestibular aqueduct syndrome. *Laryngoscope*, 1978, 88, 723–728.

96. Okumura, T., Takahashi, H., Honjo, I., Takagi, A., and Mitamura, K. Sensorineural hearing loss in patients with large vestibular aqueduct. *Laryngoscope*, 1995, 105, 289–293; discussion 293–284.

97. Dahlen, R.T., Harnsberger, H.R., Gray, S.D. et al. Overlapping thin-section fast spin-echo MR of the large vestibular aqueduct syndrome. *Am. J. Neuroradiol.*, 1997, 18, 67–75.

98. Wetmore, S.J., Herrmann, P., and Fisch, U. Spontaneous cerebrospinal fluid otorrhea. *Am. J. Otol.*, 1987, 8, 96–102.

99. Weber, P.C., Perez, B.A., and Bluestone, C.D. Congenital perilymphatic fistula and associated middle ear abnormalities. *Laryngoscope*, 1993, 103, 160–164.

100. Weissman, J.L., Weber, P.C., and Bluestone, C.D. Congenital perilymphatic fistula: computed tomography appearance of middle ear and inner ear anomalies. *Otolaryngol. Head Neck Surg.*, 1994, 111, 243–249.

101. Reilly, J.S., Weber, P.C., and Bluestone, C.D. Perilymphatic fistulas in infants and children. In Bluestone, C.D., Stook, S.E., and Kenna, M.A., Eds. *Pediatric Otolaryngology*. Philadelphia: W.B. Saunders, 1996, 371.

102. Shelton, C., Luxford, W.M., Tonokawa, L.L., Lo, W.W., and House, W.F. The narrow internal auditory canal in children: a contraindication to cochlear implants. *Otolaryngol. Head Neck Surg.* 1989, 100, 227–231.

103. Slattery, W.H., III and Luxford, W.M. Cochlear implantation in the congenital malformed cochlea. *Laryngoscope*, 1995, 105, 1184–1187.

104. Lo, W.W. Imaging of cochlear and auditory brain stem implantation. *Am. J. Neuroradiol.*, 1998, 19, 1147–1154.

105. Okuchi. K., Kamada, K.S.I. et al. Bilateral absence of the internal carotid artery. *Neurol. Med. Clin.*, 1988, 28, 685–689.

106. Lo, W.W., Solti-Bohman, L.G., and McElveen, J.T., Jr. Aberrant carotid artery: radiologic diagnosis with emphasis on high-resolution computed tomography. *Radiographics*, 1985, 5, 985–993.

107. Guinto, F.C., Jr., Garrabrant, E.C., and Radcliffe, W.B. Radiology of the persistent stapedial artery. *Radiology*, 1972, 105, 365–369.

108. Pirodda, A., Sorrenti, G., Marliani, A.F., and Cappello, I. Arterial anomalies of the middle ear associated with stapes ankylosis. *J. Laryngol. Otol.*, 1994, 108, 237–239.

109. Govaerts, P.J., Marquet, T.F., Cremers, W.R., and Offeciers, F.E. Persistent stapedial artery: does it prevent successful surgery? *Ann. Otol. Rhinol. Laryngol.*, 1993, 102, 724–728.

110. Wadin, K. and Wilbrand, H. The jugular bulb diverticulum. A radioanatomic investigation. *Acta Radiol.* [Diagn] (Stockh), 1986, 27, 395–401.

111. Martin, N., Sterkers, O., and Nahum, H. Chronic inflammatory disease of the middle ear cavities: Gd-DTPA-enhanced MR imaging. *Radiology*, 1990, 176, 399–405.

112. Swartz, J.D. Temporal bone inflammatory disease. In Som, P.M. and Curtin, H.D., Eds. *Head and Neck Imaging*. St. Louis: C.V. Mosby Year Book, 1996, 1391.

113. Swartz, J.D. Cholesteatomas of the middle ear. Diagnosis, etiology, and complications. *Radiol. Clin. North Am.*, 1984, 22, 15–35.

114. Swartz, J.D. and Harnsberger, H.R. Trauma. In Swartz, J.D. and Harnsberger, H.R., Eds. *Imaging of the Temporal Bone*. New York: Thieme Medical Publishers, 1992, 247.

115. Parisier, S.C. and McGuirt, W.F. Injuries of the ear and temporal bone. In Bluestone, C.H., Stool, S.E., and Kenna, M.A., Eds. *Pediatric Otolaryngology*. Philadelphia: W.B. Saunders, 1996, 687.

116. Holland, B.A. and Brant-Zawadzki, M. High-resolution CT of temporal bone trauma. *Am. J. Roentgenol.*, 1984, 143, 391–395.

117. Lindeman, R.C. Temporal bone trauma and facial paralysis. *Otolaryngol. Clin. North Am.*, 1979, 12, 403–413.

118. Hough, J.V. Surgical aspects of temporal bone fractures. *Proc. R. Soc. Med.*, 1970, 63, 245–252.

119. Mark, A.S. and Fitzgerald, D. Segmental enhancement of the cochlea on contrast-enhanced MR: correlation with the frequency of hearing loss and possible sign of perilymphatic fistula and autoimmune labyrinthitis. *Am. J. Neuroradiol.*, 1993, 14, 991–996.

120. Stram, J.R. Tumors of the ear and temporal bone. In Bluestone, C.H. and Stool. S.E., Eds., *Pediatric Otolaryngology*. Philadelphia: W.B. Saunders, 1990, 77.

121. Bartels, L.J. and Gurucharri, M. Pediatric glomus tumors. *Otolaryngol. Head Neck Surg.*, 1988, 99, 392–395.

122. Olsen, W.L., Dillon, W.P., Kelly, W.M., Norman, D., Brant-Zawadzki, M., and Newton, T.H. MR imaging of paragangliomas. *Am. J. Roentgenol.*, 1987, 148, 201–204.

123. Nager, G.T., Kennedy, D.W., and Kopstein, E. Fibrous dysplasia: a review of the disease and its manifestations in the temporal bone. *Ann. Otol. Rhinol. Laryngol.*, 1982, 92, Suppl., 1–52.

124. Brown, E.W., Megerian, C.A., McKenna, M.J., and Weber, A. Fibrous dysplasia of the temporal bone: imaging findings. *Am. J. Roentgenol.*, 1995, 164, 679–682.

Section III

Cognitive Impairment

8 Hearing Loss

Kenneth M. Grundfast, Mary Jo Schuh, and Nancy Sculerati

I am just as deaf as I am blind...the problems of deafness are deeper and more complex, if not more important than those of blindness...Deafness is a much worse misfortune, for it means the loss of that most vital stimulus, the sound of the human voice, which brings language, sets thoughts astir, and keeps us in the intellectual company of man.

Helen Keller

CONTENTS

INTRODUCTION

Complications do not occur often in the management of children with hearing loss. Instead, the problems inherent in the evaluation and management of children with hearing loss primarily involve: (1) failure to identify an underlying cause, (2) failure to communicate effectively with parents about alternatives for management, and (3) recommending inappropriate medical or surgical intervention. Of course, with otologic surgery, complications such as worse hearing postoperatively, injury to the facial nerve, damage to the dura with cerebrospinal fluid (CSF) leak, and even meningitis from postoperative infection can occur. This chapter provides information about pearls and pitfalls in the management of a child with hearing impairment as well as the audiologic evaluation. Useful approaches in hearing measurement, medical diagnosis, and the habilitation of hearing-impaired children are described.

CONDUCTIVE HEARING LOSS

FAILURE TO IDENTIFY A SYNDROME ASSOCIATED WITH CONDUCTIVE HEARING LOSS

When a child has conductive hearing loss without middle ear effusion and without otoscopic or radiographic evidence of chronic middle ear disease, a reasonable possibility is that the child has a congenital ossicular abnormality. If a child has bilateral conductive hearing loss or bilateral mixed conductive and sensorineural hearing loss, then the child's face should be carefully examined for constricted midface and antimongolid slant of the palpebral fissures that might help to make a diagnosis of mandibulo-facial dysostosis (Treacher–Collins syndrome). A severely retracted eardrum and a CT of the temporal bones with almost nonexistent mastoid antrum are findings that should raise suspicion about Treacher–Collins syndrome.

If a child has a unilateral conductive hearing loss not easily attributed to ossicular erosion from choesteatoma or chronic ear disease, then a diagnosis of facio-auriculo-vertebral dysplasia (Goldenhar syndrome) should be considered. To make a diagnosis of Goldenhar syndrome, it is necessary to look carefully for assymetry of the face — especially the mandible. If the mandible ipsilateral to the conductive hearing loss appears to be smaller than the contralateral mandible or if the ipsilateral ear canal appears smaller or more tortuous than the ear canal on the side with normal hearing, then the examiner should look carefully for other findings that might support the diagnosis of Goldenhar syndrome. Other findings helpful in making this diagnosis are flattened malar eminence, epibulbar dermoid, and vertebral abnormalities. Also, a child with conductive hearing loss and congenital ossicular abnormalities could have a syndrome such as ectodermal dysplasia, so the hair and skin should be examined for abnormalities such as thick, scaly skin or extremely coarse hair.

FAILURE TO CLOSE AIR/BONE GAP WITH OSSICULOPLASTY

Good closure of an air/bone gap with ossiculoplasty in young children is more difficult to achieve than with ossiculoplasty or stapes surgery in adults. The child less than 5 years of age with congenital conductive hearing loss and no history of chronic otitis media is likely to have a congenital abnormality in the area of the oval window or fixation of the head of the malleus. In some children — especially children with Treacher–Collins syndrome — there may be no well-defined stapes footplate and only an indentation cephalad to the promontory and caudad to the facial nerve. In addition, the incus may be malformed, thus making fenestration into the vestibule and insertion of a prosthesis extremely difficult.

A common pitfall in operating on a child with congenital ossicular abnormality is failure to discuss with the parents and then obtain operative permit for mastoidectomy so that access to the epitympanum can be achieved during surgery. That is, exploration of the middle ear may reveal that the stapes is mobile, the incus is questionably normally mobile, and the malleus apparently fixed. In such a case, release of the malleus fixation is likely to require opening of the epitympanum and bimanual manipulation of the malleus with possible removal of the incus followed by incus interposition. Therefore, when operating on a child less than 5 years of age with congenital conductive hearing loss and presumed congenital ossicular abnormality, the surgeon should always obtain an operative permit for mastoidectomy in addition to securing permission for the middle ear approach.

In children older than 5 years of age who have had problems with chronic otitis media or who have had cholesteatoma, erosion of the lenticular process of the incus is the most likely cause of conductive hearing loss. If erosion of the incus is confirmed at surgery, ossiuloplasty should be considered. Depending upon the extent of erosion, presence or absence of cholesteatoma, and structural integrity of the stapes superstructure, an incus interposition or insertion of an incudostapedial joint prosthesis or a partial ossicular replacement prosthesis (PORP) should suffice to improve hearing.

OSSICULOPLASTY RESULTING IN AN ANACUSTIC EAR

Perhaps no surgical outcome in otology is more devastating for a child and disheartening for the surgeon than the complete loss of hearing after surgery in the operated ear in a child with bilateral conductive or mixed hearing loss. Therefore, it is imperative that parents know and understand that there is always a risk that a child could completely lose hearing in an operated ear following surgery that attempted to improve hearing. Whenever this surgery involves opening into the vestibule, there is risk of total sensorineural hearing loss following the surgery. After all, the child who has absence of a stapes footplate or congenital fixation of the stapes may have other microanatomic abnormalities.

A child with bilateral conductive hearing impairment who might be reluctant to use hearing aids may be hopeful that surgery will obviate the need for a hearing aid in one ear. However, parents of that child must realize that surgery could result in total loss of hearing in the operated ear after surgery and that the result of surgery could be an anacustic (operated) ear and conductive hearing loss in the only remaining (unoperated) hearing ear. A general guideline in this regard is that the ear with maximum conductive hearing loss and computerized tomography (CT) scan demonstrating some slight abnormality of inner ear anatomy without evidence of ossicular abnormality is most likely to be at risk for severe sensorineural hearing loss following surgery to close an air/bone gap. Accordingly, children with Treacher–Collins syndrome are not usually good candidates for stapes or other ossiculoplasty surgery.

MIXED HEARING LOSS

NOT REALIZING THAT A SENSORINEURAL COMPONENT EXISTS

The younger a child is, the more difficult can be the task of identifying that a hearing loss is conductive as well as sensorineural. Not infrequently, a child with middle ear effusions and elevated hearing thresholds has undergone an insertion of tympanostomy tubes. Then, at some point after the insertion, a subsequent audiogram reveals elevated bone conduction scores and evidence of sensorineural hearing loss. When this occurs, parents often have difficulty understanding why the underlying sensorineural hearing loss had not been known or suspected prior to inserting the tubes. Sometimes, parents will even wonder if "something happened" during insertion that might have caused the sensorineural hearing loss.

To avoid this situation, it is worthwhile to know when to suspect that a child with persistent otitis media and elevated hearing thresholds may have conductive hearing loss from middle ear effusion and also a congenital mild sensorineural hearing impairment. The surgeon should suspect concomitant sensorineural hearing impairment in the child with conductive hearing loss from middle ear effusion when

- The child has significant delay in developing speech
- The pure tone average or speech reception threshold is higher than 30 dB
- Family members previously have been diagnosed with childhood sensorineural hearing loss

If the child is too young to cooperate for behavioral hearing testing, then an auditory brainstem response test may provide clues to the presence of a sensorineural component to a mixed hearing loss. In general, the more elevated a child's hearing thresholds presumably caused by middle ear effusions are, the more important is the need after tube placement to obtain a postoperative hearing test to be sure that hearing has returned to normal after the middle ear fluid is no longer present.

CAUSING PERILYMPH GUSHER WHEN OPERATING ON A CHILD WITH A CONGENITAL HEREDITARY DISORDER

Males with a hereditary disorder known as "X-linked mixed hearing loss (MHL) with stapes gusher" present with mixed conductive and sensorineural hearing loss. Not infrequently, a surgeon will recommend exploration of the middle ear in an attempt to diminish the air–bone gap; at the time of surgery, a poorly mobile stapes will be detected. Prior to recommending surgery in a child with mixed hearing loss, a CT scan should always be obtained and the size and shape of the internal auditory canals should be assessed carefully. Males with MHL with stapes gusher syndrome often have a bulbous internal auditory canal that may raise suspicion that perilymph gusher will occur if the stapes is removed or the footplate of the stapes is fenestrated to insert a prosthesis. In other words, males with MHL, especially those who have other family members with similar hearing loss, should be evaluated carefully. The medical professional should look for evidence in the family or on the CT scan of the temporal bones that might indicate potential for developing perilymph gusher during stapes surgery.

OSSICULOPLASTY RESULTING IN AN ANACUSTIC EAR

As discussed earlier, ossiculoplasty in a child can result in complete loss of hearing in the operated ear. For reasons not entirely clear, children with congenital mixed hearing loss seem to have a higher risk of severe hearing loss following stapes surgery compared with children who have purely conductive hearing loss.

PROFOUND CONGENITAL SENSORINEURAL HEARING LOSS

FAILURE TO DETECT AT AN EARLY AGE

Many states require universal newborn hearing screening (UNHS); thus, the chances that congenital profound hearing impairment in babies will go undetected are diminishing. Nonetheless, otolaryngologists must remain vigilant so that all deaf children will be identified as early as possible. By 1998, 10 states had enacted laws requiring the creation of UNHS screening programs. One year later, the United States Congress passed the Newborn Hearing Screening Act of 1999. Despite this federal mandate, in 2002, one quarter of the states had not yet implemented screening programs or had done so variably. Particular hospitals may only perform chart reviews and not actually test babies. Testing technology varies, using different forms of otoacoustic evoked response (OAE) and auditory brainstem-evoked response (ABR) screening tools and interpretation. Rhode Island is the only state to have achieved screening of 95% or more of the infant population; however, some neonates have left the hospital without having been screened, and some of the babies who failed a screen have not undergone required follow-up testing.

Even though high-risk factors and screening programs can help in early identification of deaf infants, otolaryngologists should keep in mind this dictum:

Whenever a parent or caregiver expresses concern that a baby or young child is hearing impaired, proceed immediately to assess hearing using any objective method of assessment deemed appropriate. However, do not ever attempt to reassure a parent or other caregiver or attempt to allay concerns about hearing impairment without some assessment of the baby's auditory thresholds.

An infant who had normal hearing at birth can suffer the onset of a noncongenital deafness; therefore, children require clinical suspicion of hearing loss and auditory validation later in life if indicated by a change in behavior, poor speech, or parental suspicion of hearing loss. When hearing loss is not detected early, children can suffer impairment in the acquisition of language and cognitive skills. Failures in these areas have a dramatic impact on the quality of life and not only during the childhood years. Intervention is required before the age of 6 months to prevent language delay in children with congenital hearing impairment.[1] After that age, the later the intervention actually occurs, the worse the correlating language outcome will be as measured in the 5-year-old.[2]

FAILURE TO IDENTIFY SYNDROME ASSOCIATED WITH HEARING LOSS

About 200 syndromes include hearing impairment. In some of the syndromes, the impairment is congenital and profound, while in others it may be delayed in onset and slowly progressive. Every child with hearing loss that cannot be attributed to an identifiable cause such as otitis media or cholesteatoma should be viewed as possibly having hearing loss as part of a syndrome. Although there is always a tendency to focus on auditory threshold levels whenever hearing loss is discovered in a child, there is also a need to consider that the hearing loss could be the first manifestation of a constellation of findings that might lead to diagnosis of a syndrome.

Identifying a syndrome is of more than academic interest. If a child has hearing loss as part of Alport syndrome, then assessment of renal function and follow-up with a urologist might be indicated. Similarly, if a child has hearing loss as part of Usher syndrome, an ophthalmologist should be involved with the child's medical management. In most cases, if one suspects that a child might have a syndrome, referral to a clinical geneticist is worthwhile. In addition, because approximately 40 oculo-auditory syndromes are known, referral to a pediatric ophthalmologist for evaluation can be helpful in determining whether a child has a syndrome.

INSENSITIVITY IN PRESENTING OPTIONS FOR CHILD'S METHODS FOR COMMUNICATING AND EDUCATIONAL SETTING

A mistake commonly made in providing advice to the parent of a child newly diagnosed with severe or profound sensorineural hearing loss is to be judgmental in advising the parents that the child *should* enter an oral–aural program because "this is what's best." Such a simplistic and biased approach can be insensitive. When parents first are informed that their child has severe hearing impairment or is deaf, they can quickly become depressed, fearful, and easily confused.

The parents often are bombarded with a lot of information and conflicting advice. Some will say that the child is deaf but must learn how to talk "like a normal person." Others will say that life in the world of the hearing is too difficult for a deaf child — that the deaf daughter will have no friends and a terrible social life if the parents try to push her toward learning to speak with her voice rather than using sign language and that she should go to a school for the deaf to learn sign language. Still others may say that the way to go is for the deaf child to learn "total communication" or to have a cochlear implant immediately. In some cases, the parents may even receive well-meaning phone calls from representatives of the Alexander Graham Bell Association for the Deaf, who will advocate for and provide information about oral–aural communication (listening and talking). Other calls from the National Association for the Deaf extol the advantages of learning sign language and bonding with the deaf community.

The otolaryngologist who is interacting with and providing advice to parents confronted with so much conflicting information must keep in mind that they are likely feeling considerable stress and angst. They want to make the right choices for their young child, but they need time to think and talk to others. They need nonjudgmental advice from their child's otolaryngologist. The otolaryngologist providing advice to parents should be knowledgeable about all the options for the hearing-impaired or deaf child. Furthermore, he or she should be able to facilitate the information-gathering and decision-making processes for the parents without trying to influence their decisions based on personal bias.

DELAY IN BEGINNING APPROPRIATE HELPFUL INTERVENTION

Without doubt, the earlier a child's hearing loss is identified and the earlier the child gets one or two hearing aids or a cochlear implant, the better will be the child's ability to acquire communicative skills. Failure to give credence to a parent or caregiver's concern about a child's seemingly difficult hearing and subsequent delay in obtaining testing that can confirm or negate the presence of a hearing loss can needlessly delay the beginning of intervention for the child. Therefore, whenever a parent or caregiver expresses concern about a child's hearing, there should be some sense of urgency about testing hearing and beginning to consider the options for further management.

PROGRESSIVE SENSORINEURAL HEARING LOSS

FAILURE TO FIND A TREATABLE UNDERLYING CAUSE

Although adults with progressive sensorineural hearing loss are likely to have presbycusis or an autoimmune disorder, the cause of a child's sensorineural hearing loss can be difficult to determine precisely. Even though no specific cause can be identified in about half of children who have progressive sensorineural hearing loss, many disorders can be identified. For example, a child with progressive sensorineural hearing loss could have a disorder such as congenital syphilis or cytomeglaovirus, Alport syndrome, Usher syndrome Type-2, nonsyndromic hereditary delayed-onset progressive sensorineural hearing loss, or an enlarged vestibular aqueduct.

When a child manifests progressively worsening sensorineural hearing loss, the medical history and physical exam findings must be carefully analyzed in order to find out if the hearing loss might be associated with other findings that could help make a unifying diagnosis. Diagnostic studies likely to be most helpful are

- A CT scan looking for enlarged vestibular aqueduct or cochlea dyplasis
- Urinalysis to check for blood or protein in the urine
- Exam by an ophthalmologist looking for evidence of retinitis pigmentosa
- Exam by a clinical geneticist to discover any dysmorphic features on exam that may have gone unrecognized and to conduct genetic tests looking for abnormalities in the connexin-26 gene or in mitochondrial DNA

MISLEADING PARENTS BY OFFERING TO PERFORM A SURGICAL PROCEDURE WITH LITTLE LIKELIHOOD OF PREVENTING FURTHER HEARING LOSS

In general, the parent of a child who is severely hearing impaired or who is losing hearing will accept almost any recommendation made by a physician that offers the possibility of preventing further hearing loss or improving hearing. Thus, physicians — and especially otologic surgeons — have the ethical responsibility of using caution in giving advice about surgical procedures that might help prevent a child's further hearing loss or improve hearing. Several years ago, otolaryngologists were recommending that children's ears be explored for a perilymph fistula that might need to be patched or repaired in order to avert further hearing loss or improve hearing; however, little evidence supported the concept that surgery was of benefit in most cases. Accordingly, otolaryngologists should be reticent to mention surgical exploration of the middle ear for children with progressive sensorineural hearing loss unless there is specific, compelling evidence to suggest that a perilymph fistula is the cause of the hearing loss.

ESSENTIAL CONSIDERATIONS OF PEDIATRIC DIAGNOSTIC AUDIOLOGY

DELAY IN DIAGNOSIS OR MISSING A HEARING LOSS

No clinician wants to delay identification of a hearing-impaired child or miss the diagnosis of deafness, yet this complication does occur. In the U.S., the average age of a congenitally deaf child at identification was nearly 3 years as recently as 1997. The great majority of these late-identified deaf children had received regular health care from competent physicians.

What accounted for such a delay in diagnosis? Hearing tests in infants and young children were often inconsistent and inaccurate in the past. Referring pediatricians commonly received results stating "not able to test" and request for follow-up "after the age of 6 months." Primary care providers strove to avoid unnecessary tests that fit those descriptions; parental concerns over possible hearing loss were handled by reassurance instead of referral. Minimal, unilateral, and progressive hearing losses often were unsuspected and no referral was warranted until communication and learning were affected during school-age years. Hearing screening programs for at-risk newborns still missed over 50% of congenital deafness and were expensive and time consuming.[3] However, rapid and accurate hearing evaluation tools are now reliably reproducible for virtually all children. In addition, more highly trained professionals are available to assess children at any age accurately.

Elliot and Elliot[4] have confirmed physiologically that the human cochlea has normal adult function after the 20th week of gestation; thus, the newborn infant has been hearing sounds for at least 4 months. Eisenberg[5] has demonstrated that most newborns, including those with known central nervous system abnormalities, can discriminate sound on the basis of frequency and intensity. The development of auditory behavior follows a hierarchy of auditory function, and when a disruption occurs anywhere in the system, sound is not heard.

Various measurable auditory subskills are present in the very young; thus, two approaches are available to assess hearing accurately and reliably: behavioral and physiological. For newborns and young infants, a physiological measure is the initial approach of choice. Older infants and children can be tested efficiently and effectively with behavioral as well as physiological measures. Because ear-specific type, degree, and configuration of hearing loss are obtainable with greater precision with today's improved technology, appropriate intervention can be initiated in a timely fashion. However, the astute clinician will be aware that pitfalls can still occur.

BEHAVIORAL AUDIOMETRIC TESTING

AUDIOGRAM IS THE ONLY "TRUE" HEARING TEST

Behavioral assessment of auditory function is based on the observation of overt responses to controlled auditory signals and is the only true test of hearing.[6] The state of the infant or child, type of the auditory stimulus, and subsequently defined response pattern influence the likelihood of obtaining reliable responses. This strategy has been criticized for examiner bias influences.

The behavioral observation audiometry (BOA) technique introduces a high-intensity, wide-band burst of noise with monitoring or observation of various startle responses (Moro reflex) with no reinforcement. This method is used for infants from birth through 6 months of age for gross auditory l response levels. A restriction with BOA is that thresholds (minimal response levels) show a wide range that qualifies as normal with high intersubject variability in ages 3 months to 4 years.[7] BOA can have a high incidence of false-positive and false-negative results and should not be used as an isolated tool. In conjunction with electrophysiologic measures within a battery of tests, BOA can be highly informational in assessment beyond the brainstem auditory functioning. It is useful as an alternative for older children who are severely developmentally delayed and for younger children who cannot be conditioned using reinforcement.

The modified auditory behavior index for infants, by Northern and Downs,[8] is a highly regarded study of norms for infant auditory behavior commonly used in pediatric audiology settings. Other variations include the use of air and bone conduction stimuli to check neurological response patterns associated with strength of stimuli.

At 6 months of age, normally developing children can consistently demonstrate a specifically defined motor response; thus, reinforcement coupled with behavioral observation is highly success-ful. Visual reinforcement audiometry (VRA) is a successful assessment procedure for children 6 months through 2 years of age. In VRA, an animated lighted toy reinforces conditioned turns of the head toward a sound source. This method is generally performed in a sound field environment using loudspeakers; results do not indicate a specific ear. Responses are described as representing "hearing in at least one ear." If the child is cooperative for insert earphone or standard earphone placement, ear-specific test results can be obtained and should be attempted. Speech, music, and warbled pure tone stimuli are most effective. Once again, air- and bone-conducted stimuli should be used to gain information on the influences of the middle ear system.

Conditioned play audiometry (CPA) yields the most information because the child engages in some play activity each time he hears something. This technique is the most widely accepted procedure for children between the ages of 2 and 6 years. Diefendorf indicated thresholds obtained at levels of 10 dB or better for preschoolers aged 30 to 48 months, who overwhelmingly cooperated with this method.[9] Although insert earphone usage is preferable, sound field testing may be needed for the earphone-resistant child. Speech detection and recognition thresholds and word recognition ability assessment should be obtained easily with the aid of CPA. Standard techniques used for adults are typically employed for children 6 years and older with normal developmental skills. Motivation to keep the child's attention, social approval, and good rapport will enhance the reliability of responses.

No Child Is Too Young or Difficult to Test

Behavioral testing requires skills of highly trained and talented audiologists to reliably test the very young, the difficult to test, and those who do not speak or co-operate. Many pediatricians and other physicians, including otolaryngologists, once were trained to defer formal measurements of hearing in patients under the age of 2 years and instead reassure concerned parents of slow development of speech in their children until 3 years of age. At this time, "hearing screens" involving clapping and key jiggling behind the back or similar informal methods are not only performed in the offices of many well respected clinicians, but also still taught in some pediatric residency training programs. Consequently, the quality and availability of pediatric speech and hearing services vary. Facilities may accept referrals for infants and children despite limited experience or possession of appropriate equipment. The referring medical professional is responsible for seeking the most appropriate services for the child. Serial audiograms are essential for valid testing of the peripheral and central auditory function; the utilization of a pediatric test battery cannot be overemphasized inclusive of objective measures.

OBJECTIVE HEARING MEASURES

Hearing Tools, Not Hearing Tests

The autistic-like child, the child with ENS impairment, infants, and the obstinate "normal" child make up the "difficult-to-test" patient label. In addition to the behavioral approach, these patients require an objective hearing measure that measures a patient's hearing ability without the patient's active participation — usually related to an autonomic physiologic response. The presence of some physiologic response, seemingly related to the presence of an auditory signal, does not ensure that the child does indeed hear. Physiologic measures are not tests of hearing, but only indicators of auditory function. The use of physiologic measures in estimating hearing levels makes some presumptions regarding the concept of hearing. Objective hearing procedures used in children include immitance audiometry, OAEs, and ABRs.

Acoustic immitance measures introduced in the early 1970s are an acceptable and widely used component of hearing assessment; within medical offices, they have recently been used to validate middle ear status. This is an objective method of evaluating the integrity and function of the peripheral auditory system, although not beyond the middle ear. Tympanometers can quickly determine middle ear pressure, tympanic membrane mobility, eustachian tube function, continuity and mobility of the middle ear ossicles, and aural acoustic reflex thresholds. This electroacoustic technique uses a probe placed in the external auditory canal that measures the acoustic energy reflected back after mechanically varied air pressures are placed in the canal. Jerger's convenient classification system of tympanometry curves and relationships to conditions of the middle ear[10] is used routinely.

Tympanometry, physical volume test, and eustachian tube function tests have clinical applications for physician management of middle ear disease and determination of the presence and amount of conductive components in audiometry. An acoustic stapedial reflex threshold test can assist the audiologist in determining loudness recruitment in cochlear losses, hearing threshold estimates, functional hearing losses, and confirmation of conductive components.

TECHNICALLY POOR MEASURES LEAD TO MISINTERPRETATION AND INACCURATE DIAGNOSES

Caution should be used by those who perform the test. The canal and tympanic membrane should be visually inspected before testing, and repeat testing should be performed if needed or if results are in question. Paradise et al.[11] and Howie et al.[12] concluded that the use of tympanometry was valid and offered much in the diagnosis of middle ear effusion. However, this test is not advocated in infants less than 7-months-old due to the highly compliant influences of the external auditory canal in this age group. The recent development of a high-frequency 600-Hz probe tone instead of the standard 220-Hz tone and proper probe placement are essential in the pediatric population to minimize this effect.

A classic misinterpretation of mobility of the tympanic membrane measures occurs routinely in primary care offices. A flat tympanogram tracing, usually indicative of a nonmobile intact tympanic membrane, can be confused with the presence of a functioning pressure equalizing tube or tympanic membrane perforation. Also, an abnormally small physical volume may be related to cerumen occluding the external canal or probe tip or, perhaps, to a probe tip pressed against the canal wall. It is imperative that the physical volume measurements be read to determine status.

An abnormal tympanogram will not necessarily produce an air/bone gap on the audiogram or produce reduced hearing sensitivity levels. Medical treatment may not be needed with all abnormal readings. Chronic middle ear disease, postoperative conditions, intersubject differences, and trauma may affect standard tympanometric classification. Caution must be used when intrepreting immitance testing without correlating with the history and examination of the patient. Repeat immitance measures are recommended when indicated due to the changing nature of the middle ear system.

OTOACOUSTIC EMISSIONS MEASURE OUTER HAIR CELL FUNCTION, NOT HEARING

Otoacoustic emissions are sounds generated in the inner ear that can be recorded by sensitive microphones in the external ear canal.[13] These sounds are thought to be generated by the outer hair cells in the cochlea and are indirect measure of the function of these hair cells; they are not necessary for hearing.[14] Transient OAEs use a broadband click, and distortion product OAEs use two frequencies presented by a probe in the external auditory canal. The response is recorded by a sensitive microphone. Emissions can be measured quickly, without active participation of the patient.

Clinical applications are significant in determining the presence of hearing with some frequency-specific information, but not the degree of loss. In neonatal hearing screening programs, particularly in the late 1990s with the advent of universal screening programs in hospital nursery, OAE has been the tool of choice. Probe placement is critical and the main reason for high false positive results. Practice with probe location and use of highly skilled technicians in assessing outer ear status for obstructions are recommended. Automated pass/fail criteria are reducing false readings.

Diagnostic use of OAEs is growing; all pediatric centers use this method as part of the pediatric battery of testing for all children. Combined transient otoacoustic emissions (TEAOEs) and distortion product otoacoustic emissions (DPOAES) are used. The limitation of OAE testing to sensory rather then neural cause of hearing loss has led some authors to question its value for mass screening of infants or school-age populations. OAE research has also produced a new disorder named "auditory neuropathy."[15] In a subset of affected infants and children, there is normal cochlear function (i.e., OAE is present) but dysfunction of the auditory nerve and or brainstem (i.e., ABR is absent). The incidence of this disorder is unknown and probably low, but it is important because management of nonconductive hearing loss is traditionally amplification. Amplification destroys outer hair cell function and is not effective. Also, newborn hearing screening programs based on OAE technology alone will fail to identify such children as hearing impaired.

ABR Is Not the Definitive Answer

More then 60 years ago, Davis reported recording changes in electroencephalic activity when subjects heard sound.[16] The application of signal-averaging computer technology during the 1960s has led to the use of auditory brainstem response recordings as a means to predict hearing sensitivity. Endorsed by the Joint Committee on Infant Hearing (JCIH) since 1989, the ABR has been used as a method to screen for hearing loss in the neonate population, as well as to assess auditory function in pediatrics. ABR does not provide a direct measure of hearing. The recorded waveforms or their absence does not document that the child perceives the acoustic signal. Rather, ABR data are used to estimate hearing sensitivity based on norms, instrumentation, age of the patient, general health, and neurological status.

ABR is the method of choice for predicting hearing sensitivity in most infants between birth and 2 years of age. The accuracy and reliability of measurements and clinically acceptable level of predictive accuracy for hearing sensitivity have been well defined. The major disadvantage is cost and the relatively long amount of time necessary to complete an assessment.

Early ABR potentials obtained from neonates differ from those of adults. In neonatal infant populations, morphology of the ABR waveforms varies systematically as a function of maturation and health status. Whereas the normal adult ABR can be conceptualized as a rather static response, the ABR in infants is a dynamic process. For example, the inverse relationship between stimulus intensity and absolute wave latency is well known; however, there is a confounding interaction between wave latency and age. Thus, without normative data that specify wavy latency as a function of gestational age, appropriate interpretation of ABR can be misleading.

ABR results are an objective measure, but the clinical interpretation based on these results is subjective. One must have theoretical knowledge as well as practical experience in "peak picking," i.e., identifying waveforms. Mislabeling can lead to over- or underestimation of hearing loss. Outer and middle ear disease interferes technically and can mask true sensory components; when possible, the ABR study should be postponed until active disease is resolved. Errors of interpretation have resulted from poorly conducted technical studies; when a baby is subjected to sedation, a technically flawless outcome is expected.

CROSS-CHECK PRINCIPLE

The cross-check principle is a requisite for pediatric audiological assessment. This principle for pediatric auditory assessment stipulates that the results of a single test are never accepted as conclusive proof of the nature or site of auditory disorder without support from at least one additional independent test. It is not limited in application to the age group from birth to 6 months, but applies equally to older infants and young children. Application of the cross-check principle requires not only appreciation for various measurement strategies, but also recognition of the importance of selecting strategies based on the patient's age and physical and developmental levels. In summary, accurate diagnosis for a significant fraction of children requires a battery of audiological and medical tests over a series of follow-up visits (Table 8.1). The clinician should test any age and not delay.

TABLE 8.1
Pearls and Pitfalls of Pediatric Audiology Testing Techniques

Assessment Tools	Problems	Specifics	Solutions
Behavioral Testing			
Pure tone	Age adjustment	Elevated AC levels mimic hearing loss	Assess developmental and neurological
Air conduction (AC)	Performing AC levels only with elevated response	Misdiagnosing SNHL component	Always attempt BC at one or two frequencies
Bone conduction (BC)	Collapsing canals	Testing induced hearing loss	Use insert earphones instead of cup earphones
	Uncooperative child	Resisting earphones, nonresponsive behavior	Move to objective testing
Speech tests	Functional/malingerers	Elevated speech recognition compared with pure tones; question neurological status	Perform Stenger test
Speech detection (SD)	Failure to perform SD gives inaccurate reliability (checks and balances)	Elevated pure tones compared with speech; question malingering	Perform objective tests
Speech recognition			Neurological consultation
Objective Testing			
Immittance testing	Flat tympanogram interpretation confusion	Effusion vs. cerumen impaction vs. TM perforation	Visual inspection and pneumatic otoscopy
Tympanometry	Misinterpretation of hearing loss	Absent reflexes due to middle ear disease, probe placement, blocked probe, or neurological status	Do not perform during active middle ear disease
Stapedial acoustic reflexes			Caution interpretation with chronic middle ear disease
			Perform AC and BC audiogram
Physiologic Testing			
ABR (BAER, BERA, BSER)	Name confusion	Can be screen or diagnostic tool	Use as estimation of hearing and in conjunction with behavioral testing
	ABR is not hearing test	Early latency ABR (standard) does not test auditory cortical activity	(1) Serial testing
	This objective test has subjective component	Misinterpretation can lead to diagnosis of hearing loss	(2) Second opinion of interpretation/training
	Outer/middle ear disease influences	Delayed latency can cause misinterpretation of sensory component	(3) Check technical issues
			Postpone ABR until middle ear disease resolves
			Correct underlying middle ear disease
OAE (DPOAEs/TEOAEs)	OAEs do not determine level of hearing — outer hair cell function only	Present OAE and absent ABR do not mean hearing is present	Consider auditory dysynchrony
	Middle ear disease influences	Absent OAE with middle disease	Consider BC testing with middle ear disease
	High technical errors	Probe placement — false positives	More training needed
		Probe blocked — false positives	Defer until middle ear disease corrected

REFERENCES

1. Yoshinaga–Itano, C., Sedey, A.L., Coulter, B.A., and Mehl, A.L. Language of early and later identified children with hearing loss. *Pediatrics*, 1998, 102, 1168–1171.
2. Moeller, M.P. Early intervention and language development in children who are deaf and hard of hearing. *Pediatrics*, 2000, 106(3), 4E3.
3. Mauk, G.W., White, K.R., Mortensen, L.B., and Behrens, T.R. The effectiveness of screening programs based on high-risk characteristics in early identification of hearing loss. *Ear Hearing*, 1991, 12, 312–319.
4. Elliot, G.B. and Elliot, K.A. Some pathological, radiological and clinical implications of the precocious development of the human ear. *Laryngoscope*, 1964, 74, 1160–1171.
5. Eisenberg, R.B. The development of hearing in man: an assessment of current status. *American Speech and Hearing Association,* 1970, 12, 119–123.
6. Diefendorf, A.O. *Hearing Impairment in Children: Behavioral Evaluation of Hearing-Impaired Children*, Austin, TX: York Press, 1988, 133–159.
7. Thompson, G. and Weber, B. Responses of infants and young children as a function of auditory stimuli and test method. *J. Speech Hearing Disorders*, 1974, 39, 140–147.
8. Northern, J.L. and Downs, M.P. *Clinical Audiologic Testing: Hearing in Children*, Baltimore: Williams & Wilkins, 1974, 113–122.
9. Diefendorf, A.O. The effect of a pre-play period on play audiometry. Paper presented at the Tennessee Speech–Language–Hearing Association Annual Convention, Memphis, 1981.
10. Jerger, J.J. Clinical experience with impedance audiometry. *Arch. Otolaryngol.*, 1970, 92, 311–324.
11. Paradise, J.L., Smith, C., and Bluestone, C.D. Tympanometric detection of middle ear effusion in infants and young children. *Pediatrics*, 1976, 58, 198–206.
12. Howie, V.M., Ploussard, J.H., and Sloyer, J.L. Natural history of otitis media. *Ann. Otol. Rhinol. Larynogol.*, Suppl. 25, 1976, 85, 18.
13. Kemp, D.T. Stimulated acoustic emissions from within the human auditory system. *J. Acoust. Soc. Am.*, 1978, 64, 1386–1391.
14. Norton, S.J. and Widen, J.E. Evoked otoacoustic emissions in normal-hearing infants and children: emerging data and issues. *Ear Hearing*, 1990, 11, 121–127.
15. Berlin, C.I., Hood, L.J., Hurley, A., and Wen, H. Hearing aids: only for hearing-impaired patients with abnormal otoacoustic emissions. In Berlin, C.I. (Ed.), *Hair Cells and Hearing Aids*. San Diego: Singular Publishing Group, Inc., 1996.
16. Davis, P.A. Effects of acoustics stimuli on the waking human brain. *J. Neurophysiol.*, 1939, 2, 494–499.

9 Language Development

Suzanne Hasenstab, Ralph F. Wetmore, and Tara Eggleston

To be conscious that you are ignorant of the facts is a great step towards knowledge.

Benjamin Disraeli

CONTENTS

INTRODUCTION

Communication development begins in earliest infancy and extends through adolescence and adulthood. Deficits or disorders can result from interruptions or inhibitions at any time during the communication learning process. Current measures in developmental pediatrics may assess only general communication growth in infants. An in-depth awareness and understanding of early communication stages, therefore, can result in a more precise evaluation and an early diagnosis. We must strive to identify early children born "at risk" for language learning deficits and monitor them closely, as well as any child not developing according to expectations, so that interventions that can offset long-term effects can be initiated.

COMMUNICATION DEVELOPMENT AND LANGUAGE CODE ACQUISITION

Communication is informational exchange between or among persons. Language is the code or medium of exchange that allows communication. If there is no exchange of meaning, there is no communication. Communication emerges from the social demand for interaction and the necessity of a code to exchange information. Existing "at the intersection of cognition and social behavior,"[1] communication allows one to share and develop information (knowledge, ideas, values, etc.) with others through culturally agreed upon social protocols. *Communication learning* requires acquisition of a language code — a system of established and agreed upon spoken or written symbols organized according to rules to convey meaning. *Meaning* is knowledge shared by people with similar experiences and is central to communication.

LANGUAGE CODE FORMS

The two primary language code forms are s*poken language* and *written language.* Spoken language develops first and uses the auditory–vocal–speech system for communication comprehension and production. Once a child enters school, the demand increases for mastery of written language that uses the visual–motor–graphic system. The two language code forms are independent but share social protocols and a generic knowledge base. Both code forms use input (reception), understanding (comprehension), and output (expression) processes. However, the different sensory modalities necessitate separate systematic rules for structure and use. For example, in written language, punctuation signals the end of a phrase or sentence, while in spoken language, pauses and emphasis are used.

LANGUAGE CODE DEVELOPMENT

Interruptions or inhibitions at any point in development can cause fragmented, deficient, or inaccurate operation of the processes necessary for language code acquisition.

Metalinguistic Competency

A child in school is expected to function independently in receptive (listening, reading) and expressive (speaking, writing) communication by the fourth grade in order to support learning in academic subjects (i.e., the language of math or history books). In order to reach that stage, knowledge about rules of spoken and written language — "metalinguistic competency" — needs to be developed. A child with rule mastery of pragmatics, semantics, syntax, morphology, and phonology/graphology can play with, develop, discuss, and increasingly express communication in accepted language code forms.

Metalinguistic competency is present at every stage of language development. Vocal play is the earliest manifestation as infants and toddlers rehearse phoneme prototypes and babbling strings. By kindergarten, children play with rhymes and invent words. By first grade, recognition of beginning sounds, phonics, and word blending are major metalinguistic tasks imposed by school and reflect a child's ability to disassemble words, match spoken and written symbols, and reconstruct phoneme patterns.

EDUCATIONAL OBSTACLES

School curricula often neglect differences in children's knowledge of language code rules and assume all children have the same experiences and communication ability. However, children do not enter school with identical backgrounds and their experiences are not the same throughout the academic years. For example, a student may appear to have competent language code systems, but be unable to use them effectively in the communication demands of school.

STAGES OF COMMUNICATION DEVELOPMENT AND SPOKEN LANGUAGE ACQUISITION

Human interactive communication evolves from eye contact and physical closeness between parent and child into independent conversational dialogue within just 2.5 to 3 years. It is beyond the scope of this chapter to elaborate in detail the intricacies of each stage of communication development. Nonetheless, it is incumbent upon the clinician to be able to recognize the gradations and progressive developmental stages in order to identify variations from expected norms. A cognitive summary and a broader generalization are presented below. For more specific information sources, refer to the Selected Reading section at the end of this chapter.

TERMINOLOGY

- *Pragmatics*: the correct use of language in social context.
- *Phonology*: the vowels and consonants *(phonemes)* that make up the sound system of the language code form *(speech)*.
- *Semantics*: the communication of meaning and intent.
- *Syntax*: the underlying structure of phrases and sentences.
- *Morphology*: words or word markers that cue nuances of meaning.
- *Prenatal development*: the child's auditory system begins functioning by the 20th prenatal week. It requires vast listening experiences before reaching full sophistication, but physiological structures and neurological pathways are operating and the fetus hears by midterm pregnancy.
- *Newborn development*: young babies demonstrate auditory awareness, turn their heads toward the source of speech-like sounds, and present anticipatory behaviors such as eye fixation, pupil dilation, visual searching, and breath holding. The fact that a newborn prefers his or her mother's voice over others indicates that processing and auditory learning have already begun.
- *Infant development*: the infant begins to develop an intact neuromotor system to produce speech sounds or to form patterns of letters in written language. Furthermore, he or she develops the axial muscle coordination, mobility, and fine motor dexterity needed to investigate the environment and create a sensory knowledge base.
- *Early childhood development*: the child's genetic nature will drive his or her ability to analyze, organize, classify, comprehend, restructure, and use information gathered by input channels to make sense of the world (cognition).

PREVERBAL COMMUNICATION: THE FIRST YEAR

Birth through 4 Months

Pragmatics and phonology are the first language systems to debut and are evident at 3 to 4 months of age, with nonverbal behaviors that allow the infant to interact with caretakers, such as the alerting cry, eye contact and gazing, posturing, facial expression, and vocalization. The earliest infant vocalizations (birth to 6 weeks) are made in association with parenting and nurturing and are called *reflexive vocalizations* (crying or fussing sounds) and *vegetative vocalizations* (gurgles, grunts). Subsequently, *nonreflexive vocalizations* (phonation) are observed between 6 weeks and 4 months. These purposeful and controlled vocalizations are best observed when interacting with a baby at close range with constant eye contact.

5 Months through 1 Year

Pragmatic development. Sound differences between phonemes continue to be increasingly recognized and result from contrasts or changes in movement of the tongue, lips, and pharynx (vocal tract). With increasing motor freedom, the infant becomes action oriented in communication, using upper extremity movement and finger dexterity to point, gesture, and wave "bye-bye." Vocalizations show more variation as the baby makes specific discomfort, calling, and request sounds. The preverbal child uses personal intents including imperatives (requests), declaratives (statements), and negatives (protest and rejection).

Phonological development. All babies experiment with all possible production contrasts (closure, resonance, pitch, intensity, and timing) to produce a broad orchestration of playful sounds. Vocal play is the basis for consonant features and pitch, intensity, and timing aspects of phonology. In the babbling stages, babies organize spontaneous vocal play into syllable patterns that characterize the adult language code. The sequential substages of babbling include marginal babbling, canonical or reduplicated babbling, variegated babbling or jargon, and babbling strings that sounds like elaborated sentences.

VERBAL COMMUNICATION: THE SECOND AND THIRD YEAR

Single-Word Utterances

In the second year of life, semantics is the communication priority. The baby is able to represent persons, objects, actions, and events cognitively and to symbolize these realities in words. The central characteristic of first words is the baby's ability to use an arbitrary symbol, a word, to communicate meaning and intent.

Pragmatic development. Children understand that by producing a consistent pattern of sounds they get results. Interactions can be initiated with a single word: "Mommy" or "Daddy." Responses can be made to questions: "No." Topic contracting emerges as children expand joint attention and use a word to introduce their own topic.

Phonological development. Children apply the phonemes produced during babbling stages to early first words. Additional consonants also occur but many will be used only in a specific word context (e.g., /s/ as in soup). By age 12 months, a child in the English language culture is able to produce all English vowels, but there is a pervasive use of "front consonants" (/m/, /b/, /p/, /d/, /t/, etc.) that characterize late babbling. No child's repertoire of initial consonants is totally identical with that of any other child; however, all children will produce certain sounds, attempt others, and actually avoid some consonants.

Two-Word Utterances

In response to new demands, children begin to sequence words into short, concise, telegraphic sentence patterns called *protosentences*. Syntax, the focal component of the protosentence, emerges and governs phrase and sentence structure. Words are arranged in specific, predictable, rule-governed formats (semantic–syntactic relationships). Children intentionally place words in a specific order and know that such word order is appropriate. Meaning is direct and children use content words (nouns, verbs, adjectives) and omit functors (articles, prepositions, auxiliary verbs, forms of "be"). Children also delete morphological inflections that mark tense, plurality, and passive forms. Examples of two-word sentence patterns include, "mommy pretty," "more cookie," and "no outside."

Pragmatic development. Children become informative and are able to convey information about an object or event that is not present in the immediate context. True dialogue is observed, but topic closures are still indicated by nonverbal performatives (breaking eye contact, walking away). Ending a topic or conversation using spoken cues requires more social awareness and cognitive sophistication than these young children possess.

Phonological development. As children gain greater control of their vocal structures and neuromusculature system, finer articulatory movements and production of more complex phonemes and phoneme patterns are possible. Children still avoid or replace some consonants, such as /w/ for /r/ or /f/ for /th/. Phonological production at the two-word level reflects children's attempts to cope with adult phonology, resulting in temporary overgeneralizations of phonological rules. It is not unusual, for example, for a 2-year-old to master phonemes in a word such as "doggie"; several months later the word becomes "goggie," but the phoneme /d/ remains intact in other words such as "daddy" or other positions like "bad." Complete mastery of English consonants is not accomplished until 5 or 6 years of age.

Semantic development. At the two-word level, children's comprehension of words, phrases, and different communication demands surges; however, meaning still depends on context and interpretation must always be viewed from the perspective of the child. Through protosentences, children begin to understand and express relational meanings of and between persons, objects, actions, and events not possible with single words. As context changes, meaning changes. Children always understand more than they are able to express, and word understanding is twice that of expression.

LANGUAGE EXPRESSION AND REFINEMENT: PRESCHOOL AND ELEMENTARY SCHOOL YEARS

Multiword Utterances

Pragmatic development. Children between ages 3 and 5 refine their ability to communicate needs, ideas, feelings, and experiences. They become better communicators and listeners and have less difficulty determining intent and meaning. They comprehend more and begin to combine words into complex phrase and sentence patterns.

Turn-taking and turn-maintaining. The late preschooler engages in more reciprocity in social situations and willingly shares toys, attention, time, and space, but is equally righteous if his or her turn is not respected. Children with problems in turn roles do not cue turns nor do they appropriately interpret the cues of others. Primary nonverbal cues (eye contact and gazing) and suprasegmental features (intonation variations and pauses) may be misused or absent.

Intent and discourse. By age 3, children request information and expand declarative intents. They also can elaborate, describe, comment, affirm, and appropriately label. By age 4, children should understand that discourse rules apply to speaker and listener and must be respected for successful dialogue. Children unable to do so will have difficulty in communication. Many of these children, however, have developed a broad vocabulary, adequate syntax, and accurate articulation, so they are frequently seen as behavior problems or rude children rather than being appropriately identified as language deficient.

Conversational clarification. Clarification requests from the listener and clarification provisions by the speaker establish a mutual meaning base and allow conversation to proceed. Five-year-old children adapt to clarification needs of children and adults and make meaning understandable through paraphrase or revisions rather than simply repeating. Failure to request and/or attempt to provide clarification is a strong indicator of a communication problem.

Syntax and morphological development. From ages 3 to 12 years, children understand and produce ever more elaborate and complex sentences. Phrasing and clausal structure provide nuances of meaning to words. Morphological markers, such as past tense forms (*-ed* or *run/ran*), possessive markers (*'s*), and plural markers (*-s/es*), permit more explicit coding of subtle word meanings as well as structural extensions within sentences.

Phonological development. During the preschool years, children's pronunciation forms may still differ from adult models but intelligibility improves. In the case of children with obvious phonological language disorders, in-depth evaluation is necessary to determine the nature and extent of the overall language deficit and the role of phonology in the disorder. Acquisition lists are helpful in charting progress of phonological development, but should be treated as guidelines and not rigid rules of production. Application of suprasegmental features to sentences, phrases, and words occurs as phonological development refines to adult pronunciation between ages 3 and 8. For example, in connected speech, precise articulation of each phoneme is neither necessary nor always possible. The child's words may merge into phrasal chunks to respect time requirements.

Semantic development. Semanticity continues to refine, alter, and restructure throughout life; it is highly idiosyncratic because meaning emerges from experiential learning and new meanings are always affected by existing knowledge. Word meaning is much more than dictionary (denotative) meaning. However, developmental tests, intelligence or cognitive measures, and reading and content evaluation instruments often rely heavily on vocabulary subtests to determine verbal ability. Vocabulary size alone is often an inappropriate factor in determining language progression once a child enters school. It must be recognized that development in semantics is a function of depth and breadth of word use and not merely the number of words. By the time a child enters school, a functional vocabulary of 2000 to 3000 words is common. Semantic development includes how the child can comprehend and code modifications of meaning, which, in large part, depends on context and previous experiences.

COMMUNICATION DISORDERS

EARLY DEVELOPMENTAL

Cognitive impairments and medical conditions that affect general development can have a significant impact on language development. Examples include children with Down syndrome or fragile X syndrome and some children born prematurely. In these children, the onset of phonological expansion, babbling stages, and first words can be significantly behind that seen with unimpaired children. Comprehensive intervention programs should offer a team approach with services of speech–language pathologists, audiologists, educators, social workers, occupational therapists, physical therapists, and developmental specialists.

Children with structural airway or orofacial abnormalities are at risk for communication delays. One example is the infant or toddler with a long-term tracheotomy who is aphonic and does not engage in vocal play or exploration of the vocal tract. The child's communication is inhibited because he or she lacks reinforcement for purposeful sound production and is thus at risk for general linguistic and specific phonological delays. This condition can be at least partially remedied by early placement of a "speaking valve" (if tolerated) over the tracheotomy tube. The valve allows air intake through the tracheotomy tube and channels the exhaled air through the larynx and pharyngeal area, thus permitting vocalization.

LATE DEVELOPMENTAL

Most pediatric language problems become evident between the ages 2 and 5 years. Once problems are identified, prompt therapeutic intervention by a qualified speech–language pathologist and, possibly, other subspecialists is critical. It is important, therefore, to understand the major categories of disorders.

Communication/language delay is a lag in acquisition. The child progresses in the correct manner but at a slower rate than expected. Communication delays are evident in receptive and expressive language. Receptive delay affects language comprehension and may include depressed vocabulary, difficulty understanding language syntax and different parts of speech (pronouns, adjectives, etc.), and limited conceptual development based on age expectations. The child frequently has difficulty following verbal directions without visual cues and understanding even simple word meanings. Expressive delay is manifest in a child's inability to express himself or herself to meet age-appropriate demands. Restricted word use and difficulty constructing sentences to form complete thoughts are typical characteristics.

ASSOCIATED MEDICAL CONDITIONS

Pervasive developmental disorders (PDD) and *autism* affect pragmatics and general language performance. PDD describes conditions that differ from general autism and include Asperger's syndrome, Rett's syndrome, sensory integration disorder, and atypical autism. Children with these conditions present with varying degrees of atypical social and play interaction and language deficits.

Children with autism and some forms of PDD may show language development milestones at expected times but apply communication and language rules inappropriately or perseverate beyond the expected age. For example, echolalia is part of normal linguistic development; however, autistic or PDD children notably extend use for several years and apply it in irrelevant situations. Autistic children also have extensive pragmatic deficits and lack social reciprocity. As a result, they have severely impaired peer relationships. They demonstrate fleeting eye contact, have difficulty learning and applying greetings and social "small talk," and do not respect conversational turn-taking. Difficulty with turn-taking is seen in communication as well as in play, thus restricting ability to play with other children and develop normal peer interactions.

Acquired brain injuries, including focal lesions, seizure disorders, brain damage after tumors, radiation, infection, and traumatic brain injury, affect communication. Acquired language deficits and disorders differ from those that are developmental. In general, acquired deficits and disorders present later and are usually evidenced by direct neurological impairment. Prevailing problems in short-term memory, new information acquisition, communication consistency, and overall linguistic function may be seen. Direct intervention in a multidisciplinary team setting is the suggested treatment delivery for these patients.

ARTICULATION DISORDERS

Phonology development disorders present as speech error patterns and misarticulations that adversely affect intelligibility. Similar to children with normal systematic acquisition of speech sounds within a language system (phonology), children with disordered phonological development exhibit distinct and predictable patterns in speech production and their evaluation is incomplete and incorrect if only based on age-appropriate expectations. These children require structured speech therapy emphasizing phonological rule development using auditory and kinesthetic modes.

Articulation delays, disorders, or *deficits* may become evident at any time during the procurement of speech. Phonemes and syllable structures must be compared with developmental expectations to determine the nature and extent of the problem. Effective intervention considers problem severity, the child's age, current developmental abilities, and attention and focus. Speech sound errors are generally categorized by sound omissions (/ba/ for bat), sound substitutions (/tat/ for bat), sound additions (/galu/ for glue), and sound distortions (a frontal lisp).

Speech apraxia or *dyspraxia* is a neurologically based speech–motor disorder. However, MRIs show no evidence of focal or global abnormalities, so the actual existence of apraxia is considered controversial. Children with speech apraxia have difficulty coordinating necessary oral movements, exhibit limited ability in correct sound imitation, and may show "groping" movements of the tongue or lips during imitative attempts. Because speech production can be inconsistent, sounds and words may be vocalized differently with subsequent attempts. Children with apraxia may have normal receptive language abilities, but expressive speech ability is severely impaired or absent. Reasonable expectations of the potential benefits of therapy need to be firmly established at the outset.

Dysarthria is weakness, paresis, or malfunction in muscle tone of the oral cavity articulators secondary to intracranial pathology. Reduced movement and weakness of the articulators and slurred speech are common. Respiration, phonation, resonation, and prosody may also be affected. Dysarthria is categorized by the affected anatomic area: spastic (bilateral upper motor neuron lesion), flaccid (lower motor neuron lesion), ataxic (cerebellar lesion), hypokinetic (basal ganglia lesion), and unilateral upper motor neuron dysarthria. Each subtype results in characteristic speech symptoms. Dysarthrias are uncommon in children, and it may be difficult to distinguish the various subtypes with limited experience.

VOICE DISORDERS

Voice disorders can arise from multiple anatomical or physiological conditions. Sound production is a direct result of vocal fold variation. The acoustic output of the larynx is produced by interruptions of airflow by the anterior membranous edges of the vocal folds, resulting in a mucosal sound wave. Changes in airflow pressure (a function of the diaphragm as well as the larynx), thickness of the vocal folds, approximation of the vocal folds, and elasticity of the vocal fold tissue can affect the quality of the sound produced.[2] Once generated, the sound wave is altered by changes in the resonance chamber of the pharynx (nasopharynx and velopharyngeal sphincter), nose, and oral cavity (tongue, lips, and teeth). Given the complexity of the multiple coordinated systems required for voice production, it can be difficult, at times, to identify the pathology appropriately.

The incidence of pediatric vocal disorders is estimated to range from a conservative 6–9% to 18–33%.[2-6] Hoarseness and other vocal disorders appear to be more common in children living in urban environments and those who attend summer camp.[7-9] Reasons for the higher incidence in these populations are unknown but may stem from the intensity of social interactions in these settings. Surprisingly, hoarseness is not more common in children who sing,[10] perhaps due to good breathing and vocal techniques. The assumption that most children "outgrow" hoarseness is not necessarily true and problems with hoarseness may continue into adulthood. Many children with chronic hoarseness remain undiagnosed in part because of less concern that the etiology is a neoplastic process. Benign vocal nodules are the usual cause of hoarseness in children; however, other treatable conditions, such as laryngeal papillomas or allergic vocal fold edema, may be present. Children with persistent or progressive hoarseness should receive, at the very least, a baseline laryngeal evaluation.

AGE-RELATED VOICE CHANGES

As children grow, the larynx descends from a cervical spine level of C2–3 in an infant to C6–7 by age 15. In infancy, the angle of the thyroid ala approximates 130°. By puberty, this angle decreases to 120° in girls and 110° in boys.[7] Increased length of the vocal folds and anterior growth of the thyroid cartilage produce a noticeable decrease in fundamental frequency in pubescent males and females.[2] Increased thyroarytenoid muscle mass increases the vertical thickness of the vocal fold, thus creating bulging of the medial contour of the fold, and also contributes to this deepening voice pitch.[8]

Although the pediatric larynx and respiratory tract are smaller, most children are able to match the vocal intensity of adults. Lung volumes in children are less than those in adults, and children must work harder to achieve the same airflow pressure. By the age of 10 years the need for extra respiratory effort to achieve adult vocal intensity has diminished.

ETIOLOGY

Prompt identification of vocal disorders in children minimizes the negative impact on communication development. The following overview is presented to maintain the reader's familiarity with some of the diverse developmental and physiologic etiologies that can affect a child's voice.

Congenital Disorders

- *Vocal fold paresis* or *paralysis* may be truly idiopathic or result from hydrocephalus, Arnold–Chiari malformation, intraventricular hemorrhage, or congenial anomalies that involve the left recurrent laryngeal nerve in the chest or the vagal nuclei or nerves. Neurophysiologic testing is of limited clinical benefit.[9] Symptoms depend on whether one or both sides are involved and whether complete paralysis or paresis is present. Children with *unilateral paresis/paralysis* usually have a soft, breathy, weak, or absent voice, and aspiration may be an associated problem. Children with *bilateral paresis/paralysis* usually have near normal vocal quality and minimal or no problems with aspiration.
- *Anterior glottic webs* result in vocal symptoms ranging from mild hoarseness to complete aphonia. Respiratory symptoms depend on web size.[11]
- *Laryngeal cysts,* depending on size and location, may affect voice. *Subglottic cysts* can partially block the airway, decrease airflow, and cause turbulence resulting in diminished vocal intensity. Large *saccular* or *supraglottic cysts* may distort the larynx, causing a muffled cry.
- *Hemangiomas* and *vascular malformations* may affect airflow and laryngeal closure, causing weak voice, hoarseness, or stridor.
- *Craniofacial anomalies*, including *cleft palate with velopharyngeal insufficiency*, may affect vocal quality as well as vocal production.
- *Laryngomalacia* is the most common cause of congenital *stridor*. Because the cry is usually normal, an abnormal cry suggests the possibility of a secondary disorder.

Acquired Disorders

- *Vocal nodules* are common in children and account for 39 to 78% of pediatric hoarseness.[2] They are usually the result of vocal strain or abuse, although allergy or gastroesophageal reflux may be contributory causes.
- *Benign laryngeal neoplasms* are uncommon. The most common is recurrent respiratory papillomatosis. They have a propensity to recur even after repeated treatment and secondary voice changes due to laryngeal scar tissue may result.[12]
- *Malignant laryngeal neoplasms* in children also are infrequent. In young children, rhabdomyosarcoma seldom affects the larynx. Occasionally, laryngeal squamous cell carcinoma is found in older children or adolescents.[13]
- *Vocal fold hemorrhage*, or *varix*, is rare vocal fold lesions in children; they can result from trauma, such as severe vocal abuse.
- *Blunt larngeal trauma* to the neck can produce injury to the larynx from a vocal fold hematoma to a thyroid cartilage fracture.
- *Penetrating neck injuries* may cause severe injury to the vocal folds. Traumatic endotracheal intubation or instrumentation may affect the voice by arytenoid dislocation, avulsion of a vocal ligament, vocal fold paresis, or vocal fold granuloma.[14,15]

- *Smoke exposure or thermal injury* may also affect laryngeal function.
- *Gastroesophageal reflux* to the level of the larynx may cause posterior laryngeal edema and erythema, mucosal hyperplasia, and true vocal fold edema.
- *Infectious disorders* range from acute viral laryngitis, which is the most common cause of transient hoarseness, to uncommon bacterial infections and granulomatous fungal infections of the larynx that may be seen in immunocompromised or chronically ill children.
- *Systemic illnesses* such as juvenile rheumatoid arthritis or relapsing polychondritis may affect the larynx and cause hoarseness, local discomfort, and dysphagia.
- *Aerosolized and inhalant medications* may adversely affect the larynx. Asthma inhalers may cause atrophy of the vocal muscle and/or the superficial lamina propria.[16] Aerosolized recombinant DNAase I may cause vocal fold edema.
- *Acquired unilateral* or *bilateral vocal fold paresis* may result from hydrocephalus secondary to shunt dysfunction, surgical trauma, or viral neuropathy.
- *Metabolic disorders*, such as hypocalcemia and other electrolyte abnormalities, may affect vocal production physiology. Myxedema resulting from hypothyroidism and lipid storage disorders with infiltration of the vocal folds can alter sound quality produced by the larynx.
- *Laryngeal foreign bodies* rarely cause hoarseness but should be considered in acute onset of hoarseness or voice change.
- *Psychogenic vocal disorders* may be a form of a conversion hysteria ranging from mild hoarseness to complete aphonia and is most often seen in older children and adolescents. Examination of the larynx may reveal false vocal fold approximation, bowed vocal folds, or hypoadducted vocal folds. Normal voice can often be elicited by having the patient cough or laugh.

EVALUATION

The evaluation of voice disorders in very young children often requires the ability to ferret out clues in the history as to the onset of vocal changes and accompanying symptoms of stridor or respiratory compromise. The evaluation of voice disorders in children age 2 and older should include a speech–language pathology assessment of vocal characteristics such as hoarseness, coarseness, harshness, pitch, range, loudness, breathiness, nasality, and intelligibility. A voice recording can be helpful in analyzing pitch, loudness, range, jitter (frequency pertubation), and shimmer (intensity pertubation).

Flexible fiberoptic laryngeal examination of the larynx can be successfully performed using topical anesthesia with children at any age including infants.[17] The examination should be confined to evaluation of the supraglottic larynx and true vocal folds and the endoscope need not enter the trachea. If airway compromise is detected or suspected, this examination should be performed under more controlled conditions. The nose and nasopharynx should be evaluated for patency and evidence of velopharyngeal insufficiency or adenoidal hypertrophy. Large palatine tonsils may protrude into the pharynx and produce a muffled voice quality. Erythema of the posterior larynx and hypopharynx may suggest gastroesophageal reflux. Inspection of laryngeal mobility during speech and breathing is essential to exclude the presence of vocal fold paresis or paralysis. The vocal folds should be closely inspected for the presence of lesions affecting laryngeal closure.

Electroglottography (EGG) enables indirect assessment of vocal fold contact using surface electrodes to measure changes in electrical impedance in the neck. It is possible to calculate pitch, jitter, and incomplete glottic closure. Cooperation is needed and testing is more appropriate with older children and adolescents.

Aerodynamic assessment permits indirect measurement of glottal airflow rate, subglottic air pressure, and glottal resistance to airflow and is helpful in patients with breathy vocal quality or suspected vocal fold paresis or paralysis. Cooperation is necessary, so this technique is best used with older children and adolescents.

Stroboscopic videolaryngoscopy has gained increasing versatility in the pediatric age group. This examination requires cooperation and a skillful endoscopist. A good study will allow analysis of supraglottic compression, arytenoid movement, vocal fold edge irregularity, glottic closure, the mucosal wave and phrase symmetry of vocal fold vibration, and the presence of swelling of the larynx or secretions.[17]

Operative assessment of the larynx by an experienced endoscopist is indicated when the larynx cannot be safely examined by a fiberoptic endoscope in the office and when it is necessary to assess the condition of the vocal folds accurately under the microscope with possible microsurgical intervention.

MANAGEMENT

Voice therapy is the mainstay of treatment. The speech–language pathologist must be comfortable with identifying poor vocal habits and vocal misuse in children and with educating parents in supportive home therapy. He or she must recognize when psychotherapy is indicated for functional disorders. For best results, pediatric voice therapists must be competent with the basics as well as with listening training, posture modifications, breathing exercises, and relaxation techniques in children. Unfortunately, it is sometimes difficult to obtain medical insurance coverage for therapy if public services are available — even if therapists in the public sector, although appropriately motivated, are not the most qualified.

Medical therapy often involves management of allergies and gastroesophageal reflux. Awareness of physiologic and emotional side effects from antihistamines, nasal steroid inhalers, allergen avoidance, and immunotherapy is important (see Chapter 11). Treatment of reflux may include elevation of the head of the bed, a change in eating habits, avoidance of citrus and products containing caffeine, and/or use of antacids, H^2 antagonists, or proton pump inhibitors, each of which may present its unique compliance and complications issues (see Chapter 19).

Surgical therapy has a limited but vital role in the management of pediatric vocal disorders. Any surgical procedure on the vocal folds carries the risk of progressive injury to the delicate mucosal surfaces and should be approached cautiously. In and of itself, surgery alone is rarely curative and continued voice therapy is often warranted.

As children mature and the true vocal fold lengthens, vocal nodules may decrease in size. Newer microsurgical techniques are available to the trained laryngologist but should be limited to children refractory to intensive vocal therapy. A unilateral vocal fold lesion suggests pathology other than nodules and warrants more serious attention. Modifying adult surgical techniques to pediatric vocal pathology may be indicated in selected cases of confirmed, permanent vocal fold paralysis.[18] Microlaryngeal resection remains the mainstay of treatment for recurrent respiratory papillomatosis, with less emphasis on lasers and increased use of various antiviral medications, interferon, and other immune boosting agents as adjuvant therapy.

It is critical to establish reasonable expectations with any proposed surgical intervention because many of these procedures improve voice at the expense of airway caliber or vice versa. Although maintenance of the airway should always be the first consideration in any laryngeal procedure, knowledgeable care should be taken to preserve the voice.

CONCLUSION

A FINAL WORD

Communication problems can underlie difficulties in learning, reading and writing, social acceptance, and self-image. Early and appropriate intervention is critical for the development of cognitive, social, and communicative growth of all children. Children with identified communication difficulties should be referred for evaluation, diagnosis, and recommendations for intervention to a speech–language pathologist trained in pediatric cases. In many cases, speech therapy can accelerate communication skills to meet age-appropriate norms. In more severe situations, speech therapy can assist a child and his or her family in finding an appropriate alternative to expected verbal communication.

SELECTED READING

1. Wallach, G.P. and Butler, K.G., Eds. *Language Learning Disabilities in School Age Children*. Baltimore, MD: Williams & Wilkins, 1984.
2. Hasenstab, M.S. and Laughton, J. *The Language Learning Process*. Rockville, MD: Aspen, 1986.
3. Hasenstab, M.S. *Language Learning and Otitis Media*. Boston, MA: College Hill Press, 1987.
4. Murdock, B.E., Ed. *Acquired Speech/Language Disorders in Childhood*. New York: Taylor & Francis, 1990.
5. Crary, M.A. *Developmental Motor Speech Disorders*. San Diego, CA: Singular Publishing Group, 1993.
6. Alpiner, J.G. and McCarthy, P.A., Eds. *Rehabilitative Audiology*, 3rd ed. Philadelphia, PA: Lippincott, Williams & Wilkins, 2000.
7. Paul, R. *Language Disorders from Infancy through Adolescence*. St. Louis, MO: Mosby, 1995.

REFERENCES

1. Whitehurst, G. Commentary by Grover S. Whitehurst, *Monogr. Soc. Res. Ch. Dev.*, 1981, 46, 5.
2. Gray, S.D., Smith, M.E., and Schneider, H. Voice disorders in children. *Pediatr. Clin. North Am.*, 1996, 43, 1357–1384.
3. Choi, S.S. and Zalzal, G.H. Voice Disorders. In Cummings, C.W., Fredrickson, J.M., Harker, L.A. et al., Eds. *Otolaryngology Head and Neck Surgery*. St. Louis: Mosby, 1988, 335–346.
4. Baynes, R.A. An incidence study of cronic hoarseness among children. *J. Speech Hearing Disorders*, 1966, 31, 172–176.
5. Silverman, E.M. and Zimmer, C.H. Incidence of chronic hoarseness among school-age children. *J. Speech Hearing Disorders*, 1975, 40, 211–215.
6. Casper, M., Abramson, A.L., and Forman-Franco, B. Hoarseness in children: summer camp study. *Int. J. Pediatr. Otorhinolaryngol.*, 1981, 3, 85–89.
7. Kahane, J.C. A morpholoical study of the human prepubertal and pubertal larynx. *Am. J. Anat.*, 1978, 151, 11–20.
8. Sell, D. and Maccurtain, F. Speech and language development in children with acquired subglottic stenosis. *J. Laryngol.*, 1988, 17 (Suppl): 35–38.
9. Wohl, D.L., Kilpatrick, J.T., Leshner, R.T., and Shaia, W.T. Intraoperative pediatric laryngeal electromyography: experience with monopolar electrodes. *Ann. Otol. Laryngol. Rhinol.*, 2001, 110(6), 524–531.
10. Mulutinovic, Z. Social environment and incidence of voice disturbances in children. *Folia Phoniatr. Logop*, 1994, 46, 135–138.
11. Cohen, S.R. Congential glottic webs in children: a retrospective review of 51 patients. *Ann. Otol. Rhinol. Laryngol.*, 1985, 94 (Supp. 121), 1–16.
12. Ossoff, R.H., Werkhaven, J.A., and Dere, H. Soft-tissue complications of laser surgery for recurrent respiratory papillomatosis. *Laryngoscope*, 1991, 101, 1162–1166.
13. McGuirt, W.F., Jr. and Little, J.P. Laryngeal cancer in children and adolescents. *Otolaryngol. Clin. North Am.*, 1997, 30(2), 207–214.
14. Wohl, D.L. Traumatic vocal fold avulsion injury in a newborn. *J. Voice*, 1996, 10(1), 106–108.
15. Heller, A.J. and Wohl, D.L. Vocal fold granuloma induced by rigid bronchoscopy. *Ears, Nose Throat J.*, 1999, 78(3), 176–180.

16. Hanania, N.A., Chapman, K.R., and Kesten, S. Adverse effects of inhaled corticosteroids. *Am. J. Med.*, 1995, 98, 196–208.
17. Nuss, R.C. Disorders of the voice. In Wetmore, R.F., Muntz, H.R., and McGill, T.J., Eds. *Pediatric Otolaryngology: Principles and Practice Pathways*. New York: Thieme, 2000, 753–762.
18. Smith, M. and Gray, S. Laryngeal framework surgery in children. *Adv. Oto Head Neck Surg.*, 1994, 8, 91–106.

10 Coagulopathy

Joanna A. Davis and Jeanne Lusher

A physician is obligated to consider more than a diseased organ, more even than the whole man — he must view the man in his world.

Harvey Cushing

CONTENTS

INTRODUCTION

In dealing with infants, children, and adolescents, the otolaryngologist may be called to see a patient with unexplained epistaxis, profuse bleeding from a tonsil, or excessive bleeding following an ENT surgical procedure. The child's medical history, family history, and physical examination will often be quite helpful in sorting out possible reasons for excessive bleeding. This should precede the ordering of a large number of laboratory tests.[1] When the cause for bleeding is not readily apparent, it will also be helpful to obtain a pediatric hematology consult. If the child is known to have an underlying coagulation disorder, such as von Willebrand's disease, and surgery is being planned, close cooperation (with frequent communication) among surgical, medical, nursing, and laboratory personnel is essential. An awareness of the more common pediatric coagulation disorders plus the ability to identify patient risk factors and appropriately interpret available screening tests can help to minimize patient risk significantly.[2]

HEMOSTASIS

The process of hemostasis occurs in three phases. Primary hemostasis begins with the injury. The blood vessel constricts in an attempt to slow the bleeding. The break in the endothelial lining exposes proteins, which attract platelets to the area and facilitate platelet adhesion. Von Willebrand's protein (or von Willebrand factor antigen) is released from the endothelial cells. This protein serves as a "bridge" between the blood vessel wall and a platelet surface receptor, glycoprotein Ib/IX. The bound platelets attract others and a loose platelet plug is formed, which also helps to slow the bleeding. The platelet plug is relatively weak and easily dislodged. A deficiency in platelet number, impaired platelet function, or a deficiency of von Willebrand's protein will result in a prolonged bleeding time and/or characteristic mucocutaneous bleeding.[3]

Secondary hemostasis results in the formation of cross-linked fibrin strands that stabilize and solidify the platelet plug. Fibrin formation represents the end of the clotting cascade. This is an orderly, sequential activation of the clotting factors — soluble proteins that are inactive in plasma. Two possible activation pathways lead to the common pathway of fibrin formation: the intrinsic pathway, measured by the partial thromboplastin time or PTT, and the extrinsic pathway, measured by the prothrombin time or PT. Qualitative or quantitative deficiencies in any one of the clotting factors may prolong either or both the PT and PTT. The deficiencies may be congenital or acquired. Bleeding manifestations vary from mucocutaneous bleeding, as in von Willebrand's disease, to joint and soft tissue bleeds as in classical hemophilia A or hemophilia B.[4]

PREOPERATIVE EVALUATION

A basic preoperative screening panel should include a complete blood count (CBC), PT, and activated PTT. A review of the peripheral blood smear is done to identify abnormalities in any of the three blood cell lines (red cells, white cells, and platelets). Patients at risk for potentially serious bleeding may be missed, however, by routine screening. Although surgeons do not need a comprehensive knowledge of hematology, an awareness of the interpretations and limitations of the screening panel and familiarity with the patient's personal and family medical histories may well avoid catastrophe.[5]

Table 10.1 lists a battery of preoperative screening tests, normal values, and parameters measured.[6] In addition to physiologic explanations for abnormal results, the physician should be aware that mechanical or technical factors may interfere with the testing processes.

PLATELET DISORDERS

PLATELETS

A numerical platelet count, if requested, is part of the CBC. A normal count does not predict adequate platelet function. Review of the peripheral smear may help the physician recognize platelet dysmorphology (such as microthrombocytes in patients with Wiskott–Aldrich syndrome) or suggest a possible reason for a low platelet count (e.g., circulating leukemia cells in a patient with thrombocytopenia.) In many cases, however, a review of the peripheral smear is of limited usefulness in identifying the etiology of thrombocytopenia. Qualitative platelet function is in no way manifest in light microscopic examination of the platelets.

Thrombocytopenia is defined as a platelet count greater than two standard deviations below the mean of the general population, i.e., less than 150,000/mm³. Clinically significant spontaneous bleed-

---

TABLE 10.1
Coagulation Screening Tests

Test	Normal range[a]	Measures
PT	11.0–12.0 sec	Factors II, V, VII, X; fibrinogen
APTT	20.0–35.0 sec	Factors VIII, IX, XI, XII, II,V, X
Bleeding time (BT)[b]	3–9 min	Platelet numbers; platelet function; von Willebrand factor; vascular integrity
Platelet count	150,000–400,000/μL	Platelet numbers

[a] Normal control ranges will vary somewhat from laboratory to laboratory. In particular, APTT normal range will vary depending on reagents and instruments used.

[b] Bleeding time is difficult to standardize and is least reliable of these screening tests.

Source: Lusher, J.M. *Am. J. Obstetr. Gynecol.*, 1996, 175(3pt2), 778–783. Reprinted with permission.

---

ing in the absence of injury is unusual if the platelet count is over 50,000/mm^3. Spontaneous bleeding is not uncommon with a platelet count less than 30,000/mm^3, and a count of less than 20,000/mm^3 may be associated with potentially life-threatening spontaneous or post-traumatic bleeding.[7]

Table 10.2 lists a differential diagnosis of thrombocytopenia in the pediatric population. Thrombocytopenia in neonates, however, may additionally be attributed to congenital hematopoietic disorders, maternal alloantibodies and autoantibodies, and sepsis. Careful attention to the newborn's medical history, maternal medical history, and circumstances surrounding the pregnancy, labor, and delivery is of utmost importance.

PLATELET FUNCTION ASSAYS

Platelet function may be assessed by two conventional methods: bleeding time and platelet aggregation studies. The template bleeding time is often inaccurate, especially if the patient has a platelet count of less than 75,000 mm^3.[8] A blood pressure cuff is inflated on the upper arm of the patient to 40 mm of mercury. A calibrated incision is made within 30 to 60 seconds of inflating the cuff. The incision is made with a device equipped with a blade and a spring mechanism. The incision is made on the volar surface of the forearm, in an area free of superficial blood vessels, scars, or bruises. As blood wells up from the laceration, it is absorbed by a filter paper. The droplets are siphoned off every 30 seconds. The time that elapses until no more blood stains the filter paper is the bleeding time, which can range from 3 to 9 minutes. Standardization is difficult.[9]

A prolonged bleeding time may reflect a platelet count of less than 75,000 or platelet dysfunction that may be constitutional or drug induced. In young children, lack of cooperation during the test (such as arm movements, resistance, and crying) may falsely prolong the bleeding time. Other variables that influence the accuracy of the test include the skill of the technician, skin temperature, type of device used for the incision, consistency of the application of the venous pressure, and the orientation of the incisional cut (vertical incisions stop bleeding sooner than do horizontal ones). Although the results of the bleeding time are known immediately at the bedside, the difficulty in performing an accurate test limits its usefulness, and it is not routinely recommended for use in children.[8] Additionally, clinical bleeding during surgery does not accurately correlate with the length of the bleeding time.

Platelet aggregation studies provide more accurate results than do bleeding times. These studies also help to differentiate between drug-induced acquired thrombocytopathies and congenital disorders. Platelet-rich plasma is exposed to a variety of agents that stimulate platelet aggregation. The assays measure the formation of platelet clumps, and a series of clotting tracings is generated.[4]

TABLE 10.2
Differential Diagnosis of Thrombocytopenia in Children

Acutely ill child

Sepsis	Thrombotic; thrombocytopenic purpura
Disseminated intravascular coagulation	Massive transfusion or hemorrhage
Liver disease	Hypothermia
Hemolytic-uremic syndrome	Hyperthermia (e.g., heat stroke)
Malignant infiltrative marrow disease	Cardiopulmonary bypass
Purpura fulminans	

Chronically ill child

Human immunodeficiency virus	Hypersplenism
Systemic lupus erythematosus or other connective tissue disease	Prosthetic heart valve
Liver disease	Cyanotic heart disease
Chemotherapy/radiotherapy	Nutritional deficiencies (e.g., iron, folate, B_{12})

Child who appears to be well

Destructive thrombocytopenia

Immune

Immune thrombocytopenic purpura (ITP)
Drug-induced thrombocytopenia
Systemic lupus erythematosus or other mixed connective tissue disease
Posttransfusion purpura
Allergy and anaphylaxis

Nonimmune

Hypersplenism
Kasabach–Merritt syndrome
Catheters, vascular prostheses, artificial heart valves
Congenital or acquired heart disease

Decreased or impaired production

Aplastic anemia	Fanconi anemia
May–Hegglin anomaly	Mediterranean thrombocytopenia
Bernard–Soulier syndrome	Wiskott–Aldrich syndrome
Congenital megakaryocytic thrombocytopenia	Other rare familial syndromes

Source: Murphy, S., Nepo, A., and Sills, R. *Pediatr. Rev.*, 1999, 20(2), 64. Reprinted with permission.

Care must be taken during the sampling and handling process to avoid activating the platelets prematurely. Studies should always be done on fresh specimens. A delay may result in loss of platelet function and abnormal results. These tests usually require several days for completion and are best done in an elective setting and not as part of a preoperative screening process.[9]

Congenital disorders of platelet function are relatively uncommon. These are characterized by the mucocutaneous bleeding or bruising typical of thrombocytopenia or platelet dysfunction. These disorders are best defined by platelet aggregation studies. Some of these disorders include the Bernard–Soulier syndrome, Glanzman's thrombasthenia, and Wiskott–Aldrich syndrome.[4]

Medications may also interfere with platelet function. These include aspirin and other nonsteroidal anti-inflammatory drugs, penicillin derivatives, and some cephalosporins. Because the life span of normal platelets is about 10 days in the peripheral circulation, a preoperative history must include questions about any medications taken by the patient within the several weeks prior to the operative date.[4]

COAGULOPATHIES

PROTIME AND PARTIAL THROMBOPLASTIN TIME

The protime (PT) and activated partial thromboplastin times (PTT) are run on plasma derived from whole blood samples collected in sodium citrate (light blue topped tubes). Both tests measure the time to formation of a fibrin clot by the activation of one of the two pathways of the clotting cascade. Spectrophotometry is used. Each lab has its own range of reference values. At the University of Miami Special Coagulation Lab, the PT values range from 12.0 to 15.0 seconds and the activated PTT ranges from 25.4 to 37.4 seconds.[8]

A prolonged protime may be explained by

- A deficiency in extrinsic pathway factors (V, VII, X, II, I)
- The use of Coumadin as an oral anticoagulant
- The presence of liver disease
- Disseminated intravascular coagulation (DIC)
- The presence of an acquired or congenital inhibitor to one or more of the clotting factors

The activated partial thromboplastin time may be prolonged because of

- A qualitative or quantitative deficiency in the intrinsic pathway factors (VIII, IX, XI, XII) or fibrinogen (I), and the common pathway factors (II, V)
- A lupus-like inhibitor or specific factor inhibitor
- The presence of heparin, e.g., sample drawn through an indwelling line
- DIC
- Deficiencies or abnormalities of high molecular weight Kininogen or pre-Kallikrein factor

Technical mishandling during collection may lead to falsely prolonged results. The specimen must be nonhemolyzed because hemolysis interferes with spectrophotometric analysis. The specimen must be brought on ice immediately to the laboratory. A clean venipuncture with free-flowing blood ("an easy stick") is necessary because even a small clot in the sample may falsely prolong the results. The ratio of plasma to anticoagulant is critical. An insufficient sample will give inaccurate results. Patients with unusually high or low hematocrits will need to have adjustments made.[8]

MEDICAL HISTORY

Careful attention to personal and family bleeding histories will help the surgeon decide which screening tests are most appropriate. Underlying blood coagulation disorders may be hereditary or acquired. By far the most common of the hereditary disorders of coagulation is von Willebrand's disease (affecting 1 to 2% of the population);[10-14] thus, one should have a high index of suspicion of von Willebrand's disease in a child with excessive mucous membrane bleeding and/or postoperative bleeding. This disorder affects all racial and ethnic groups worldwide; unfortunately, the majority of affected individuals are not diagnosed. This is true in the United States as well as elsewhere. This is unfortunate because user-friendly treatment is available once the diagnosis is made.[10] Factor XI deficiency occurs most often in Ashkenazi Jews and can cause a prolonged PTT and clinical bleeding. Therefore, as part of the personal history, the family ethnic background also needs to be identified.[8]

Acquired disorders of blood coagulation may be secondary to hepatocellular disease, malabsorption syndromes, renal failure, cyanotic congenital heart disease, disseminated intravascular coagulation (DIC), bone marrow failure syndromes, or certain drugs.[1] Symptoms that may be related to a collagen vascular disease indicate a need to screen for acquired inhibitors. Children with frequent head and neck infections, multiple antibiotic exposures, and those on chronic anticonvulsant therapy may develop inhibitors to clotting proteins. Although these are not usually associated with clinical bleeding, the PTT may be prolonged. This knowledge will help the surgeon, and eventually the hematologist, interpret an abnormal panel of results and will also help with decisions regarding further work-up and evaluation[6] prior to a rescheduled surgical date.

Although it is beyond the scope of this chapter to review each of these in detail, a few of the more common entities that the otolaryngologist may encounter (sometimes quite unexpectedly), are discussed next.

VON WILLEBRAND'S DISEASE (vWD)

vWD is the most common of the hereditary disorders of blood coagulation, affecting an estimated 1 to 2% of the population worldwide. It is inherited as an autosomal dominant trait; boys as well as girls are affected. The disorder was first described in 1926 by Dr. Eric von Willebrand of Helsinki, Finland. He studied a large kindred living on the Åland Islands (between Sweden and Finland), many of whom had major bleeding problems. The index case, Hjordis, bled to death during her fourth menstrual period at age 12; four of Hjordis' siblings had already died of hemorrhage between the ages of 2 and 4 years. Dr. von Willebrand noted that affected members of the kindred had prolonged bleeding times, normal appearing platelets, and mucous membrane-type bleeding.[15] It was not until much later that the underlying abnormality causing the bleeding tendency was identified.

Although there is quite a wide spectrum of clinical severity, vWD is characterized by mucous membrane bleeding, excessive bruising, and bleeding following surgical procedures and invasive dentistry. Because of the frequency of vWD and its variation in clinical severity, excessive bleeding during or immediately following surgery may well be the first indication that a child has an underlying bleeding disorder. Although a preoperative medical history and family history will often be "positive" for mucous membrane bleeding in a child and/or one of his or her parents, it may not be. This is particularly true in the case of mild type I vWD, especially if the individual has had no prior surgical procedures.

The underlying abnormality in vWD is in a large, multimeric plasma glycoprotein called von Willebrand factor (vWf), which has two major functions: (1) it serves as a "bridge" between platelets and injury sites in the vessel wall; and (2) it circulates as a complex with factor (F) VIII, protecting F VIII from rapid proteolytic degradation. If vWf is lacking (or quite low), platelets will not adhere to the injury site. Bleeding will continue, and if one orders a template bleeding time (BT), it will be prolonged. The patient's F VIII level will also be low because it will not be protected by vWf.

Laboratory tests for suspected vWD are listed in Figure 10.1 Of the usual coagulation "screening tests" (PT, APTT, and BT), the BT may be abnormally prolonged, but may be normal in mild vWD. The APTT may be prolonged (above the normal range for the particular laboratory); however, with

---

- APTT*

- Bleeding Time†

- Ristocetin Cofactor Assay (R:Cof)

- F VIII

- VWf:Ag

FIGURE 10.1 *The APTT may or may not be abnormally prolonged, depending on the patient's F VIII assay. With most APTT reagents, the APTT will not be prolonged unless the F VIII value is <35%. † The BT may be normal in mild vWd.

most APTT reagents, the APTT will be normal if F VIII is ≥ 35%. Thus, in an individual with mild type I vWD who has 40% vWf, 40% vWf antigen (vWf:Ag), and 40% F VIII, the APTT will be normal.

A more definitive battery of tests of suspected vWD consists of assays for vWf (usually measured by the ristocetin cofactor assay, R Cof), vWf:Ag, and F VIII, and multimeric analysis of the individual's vWf:Ag (using SDS gels and a radiolabelled antibody to vWf:Ag). The highest molecular weight bands are the most important hemostatically.[16,17] It should be noted that vWf levels can be influenced by many things. vWf levels rise in stressful situations, in hyperthyroidism, in DIC, and with hormonal changes (as seen during the menstrual cycle, in late pregnancy, or in women on oral contraceptive agents). Persons with blood group O have roughly 30% less vWf than do persons of blood type AB.[18]

Although over 20 types and subtypes of vWD have been described, most affected individuals (~80%) have type I vWD. Persons with type I vWD do not produce enough vWf, but what they do produce is structurally and functionally normal. Their vWf functional activity (as measured by the R Cof assay), vWf:Ag, and F VIII will be proportionately low, and the BT will generally be prolonged (>9 min.). All multimeric bands will be present on SDS gels.

In the type 2 variants (which account for ~20% of persons with vWD), the vWf produced is structurally and functionally abnormal.[19,20] On SDS gels the higher molecular weight multimers are absent in types 2A and 2B. In the so-called "Normandy variant" (type 2N), vWf lacks a binding site for F VIII; thus, F VIII levels may be very low (often 3%), and the child may be erroneously diagnosed as having hemophilia A (the two conditions can be separated by a kinetic binding assay). In vWD type 2M, the vWf platelet binding site is abnormal.

In the rare vWD type 3, the individual has inherited a gene for vWD from each parent and will have a more severe bleeding tendency. In addition to mucous membrane bleeding, he or she may have recurrent joint and intramuscular bleeding due to extremely low levels of F VIII (as well as vWf). Such individuals will usually come to medical attention early in life (and probably will have been diagnosed properly).

Treatment of von Willebrand's Disease

The treatment of choice for bleeding (or for preventing excessive bleeding as with surgery) in children and adolescents (as well as adults) with vWF type I is the synthetic agent, 1-deamino-8D-arginine vasopressin (DDAVP).[1,21,22] An analog of the naturally occurring antidiuretic hormone, vasopressin, DDAVP acts by releasing preformed vWf from storage sites in endothelial cells. It is available in several formulations, for parenteral or intranasal (IN) use. For in-hospital use, most use the drug intravenously (IV). The recommended dose is 0.3 μg/kg/dose; if necessary, repeat doses can be given every 12 to 24 hours. DDAVP has relatively few side effects; however, it is a potent antidiuretic agent. Thus, in operative or postoperative situations, one should avoid the concurrent use of hypotonic IV fluids and monitor fluids and electrolytes. DDAVP is not recommended for use in infants because fluid balance problems are more likely to occur in this age group. A highly concentrated IN spray formulation[23] (Stimate nasal spray) is also available and is ideal for home or out-patient use in children ≥6 years of age (i.e., children who are old enough to use the metered spray pump properly, under supervision).

For infants, children, and adolescents with the type 2 variants or with type 3 vWD, DDAVP will generally be ineffective (and may be harmful). In type 2, DDAVP will effect a release of vWf from the endothelial stores, but it will be structurally and functionally abnormal and thus not hemostatically effective. In the severe type 3, storage sites have nothing to be released. The treatment of choice in these situations is a plasma-derived F VIII concentrate rich in the hemostatically most important high molecular weight multimers of vWf (such as ZLB–Behring's Humate P or Alpha Therapeutics' Alphanate).

Adjunctive Treatment

For bleeding in the oral cavity (such as tongue or mouth lacerations, post-tonsillectomy bleeding, invasive dentistry), one should also use an antifibrinolytic agent (epsilon aminocaproic acid [EACA; Amicar®] or tranexamic acid [Cyclokapron®]) for a period of 7 to 10 days in order to prevent rapid clot lysis. Recommended dosage for EACA is 75 mg/kg/dose, given every 6 hours; for tranexamic acid, dosage is 25 mg/kg, given every 8 hours.

One should avoid the use of acetylsalicylic acid (aspirin and all aspirin-containing compounds) in children with an underlying bleeding disorder because this results in a platelet function abnormality that lasts the lifetime of "aspirinated" platelets. In the case of vWD, the child's BT will be prolonged even further. Certain antihistamines and nonsteroidal anti-inflammatory agents (e.g., ibuprofen and indomethacin) can also interfere with platelet function, but by different mechanisms than those of aspirin. Additionally, their inhibition of platelet function is short lived compared with aspirin.[24]

F XI DEFICIENCY

F XI deficiency occurs most commonly (but not exclusively) in persons of Ashkenazi Jewish descent. It may or may not be associated with a bleeding tendency.[25] In families with certain F XI genotypes, excessive bleeding may occur with surgery, as well as mucous membrane bleeding. Whether or not members of a particular family bleed excessively seems to have little or no relationship to the individuals' F XI levels. In F XI deficiency, the APTT will be prolonged as a result of subnormal F XI. If surgery is planned in a child and it is not known whether affected family members bleed excessively (for example, none have had surgery), one should be prepared to give solvent-detergent-treated fresh frozen plasma (SD FFP) or "FFP, donor retested" if excessive bleeding is encountered. F XI has a long half-life in the circulation (2.5 to 3 days). FFP, when necessary, should be given as follows: 15 to 20 mL/kg initially, followed by half that amount (7.5 to 10 mL/kg) every 12 to 24 hours. If surgery involves mucosal surfaces, an antifibrinolytic agent should be given as well.

F VIII AND F IX DEFICIENCIES

Hemophilia A (F VIII deficiency) and hemophilia B (F IX deficiency) are inherited as sex-linked recessive traits and thus affect males almost exclusively. It is noteworthy that among newly diagnosed infants, roughly one third have no family history of hemophilia. There are different degrees of severity, with most having severe hemophilia (<1% F VIII or F IX activity), while other families have moderate (1 to 5% F VIII or F IX activity), or mild hemophilia (>5 to 35% F VIII or F IX). Those with severe hemophilia can have spontaneous bleeding into joints, as well as soft tissue hemorrhages and internal bleeding (usually secondary to trauma). Boys with mild or moderate hemophilia generally bleed only secondary to trauma or surgery. Most boys with severe or moderate hemophilia will have been diagnosed before they are seen by an otolaryngologist; however, it is possible that a boy with mild hemophilia may not have been diagnosed.

If ENT surgery is being considered, there should be communication and close cooperation with a pediatric hematologist. Plasma-derived and recombinant (r) F VIII and F IX concentrates are available; most pediatric age patients in the U.S. are on rF VIII or rF IX concentrates. Approximately 25 to 30% of boys with severe hemophilia A develop inhibitors (inhibitory antibodies) to F VIII. These will destroy infused F VIII; thus, other therapeutic measures are often used for patients with significant inhibitors to F VIII. These include activated prothrombin complex concentrates (APCCs), rF VIIa, and highly purified porcine F VIII concentrate. For surgery involving mucosal surfaces, an antifibrinolytic agent should also be used.

LOW-LEVEL "CARRIERS" OF HEMOPHILIA

Due to random inactivation of the X chromosome in somatic cells, girls who have inherited one gene for hemophilia A or B may have very low levels of F VIII or F IX. If such a "carrier" female has < 20% F VIII or F IX activity, she may bleed excessively during and following surgery. Thus, if a girl who is a known or possible carrier is being scheduled for an ENT surgical procedure, one should check her F VIII (or F IX) level prior to the procedure. Low-level carriers of F VIII deficiency can be treated with IV DDAVP (0.3 µg/kg/dose) or with rF VIII concentrates. Very low-level carriers of F IX deficiency can be treated with rF IX concentrates.

ACQUIRED DISORDERS OF HEMOSTASIS

Although there are a number of acquired disorders of hemostasis, including acute and chronic forms of ITP, DIC, etc., the following subsections give a few examples of those which the pediatric otolaryngologist may encounter, particularly in a hospital setting.

Bleeding Associated with Vitamin K Deficiency

In the absence of vitamin K, the N-terminal domains of certain coagulation factors (Fs II, VII, IX, and X, as well as protein C and protein S) are not adequately gamma-carboxylated. This results in circulation of noncarboxylated proteins (PIVKA: protein induced by vitamin K absence or antagonism). Decarboxy-prothrombin is referred to as PIVKA II. These decarboxylated vitamin K proteins have abnormal calcium bindings, which interfere with their ability to bind to surfaces and participate in hemostasis. The lack of functional activity of Fs II, VII, IX, and X can lead to bleeding, particularly mucous membrane bleeding, bruising, and oozing from puncture sites.

Vitamin K deficiency is usually seen in chronically ill infants and children who have inadequate intake of vitamin K, or in disorders that interfere with absorption of vitamin K (e.g., cystic fibrosis, chronic diarrhea, celiac disease, biliary atresia). It can also be seen in children with poor nutrition who are on broad spectrum antibiotics (which alter the child's normal intestinal flora).

Laboratory testing will reveal a prolonged PT and APTT due to low levels of Fs II, VII, IX, and X. In a positive PIVKA II test (factor VII and Protein C have the shortest half-lives of the vitamin K-dependent proteins), F VII is the first of the procoagulants to decrease, resulting in an isolated prolongation of the PT. Levels of F II, IX, and X then fall, prolonging the APTT as well. The bleeding tendency can be corrected by giving parenteral (or oral) vitamin K. Subcutaneous vitamin K will correct the PT in 2 to 6 hours; if absorption is not impaired, vitamin K can be given orally, although correction of hemostasis will be somewhat slower (6 to 8 hours).

Hepatocellular Disease

Liver disease can also result in a bleeding tendency. Almost all of the coagulation factors are synthesized by hepatocytes. Thus, in acute hepatitis or in cirrhosis, there will be impaired hepatic synthesis of most clotting proteins and activation of the coagulation and fibrinolytic systems. Poor hepatic clearance of activated clotting factors (resulting in a consumptive coagulopathy) and loss of coagulation proteins into ascitic fluid can also occur. There may be concurrent vitamin K deficiency, thrombocytopenia, and abnormal platelet function. The PT and APTT are usually prolonged; platelets may be decreased and the bleeding time prolonged. Because F VIII is produced elsewhere, it will be normal (as will von Willebrand factor). Although spontaneous bleeding is relatively uncommon, bruising and hemorrhage secondary to invasive procedures can occur. In cirrhotic patients, bleeding from esophageal and gastric varices can be life threatening.[26]

If an ENT surgical procedure is being considered, one should consult a pediatric hematologist regarding management of this often complex coagulopathy.

End Stage Renal Disease

In children (and adults) with end stage renal disease, the risk of bleeding is related to the degree of uremia. In uremic children (with blood urea nitrogen values of ≥100 mg/dL), one may see quantitative as well as qualitative platelet defects, with impaired platelet aggregation and a prolonged bleeding time. The most common causes of bleeding in uremic children are impaired platelet function and heparin therapy for dialysis. Bleeding is usually mucosal (for example, epistaxis, gastrointestinal), but may occur with invasive procedures. Treatment options to improve hemostasis include cryoprecipitates, DDAVP (0.3 µg/kg/dose, IV) and effective dialysis. Cryoprecipitates and DDAVP transiently increase vWf and shorten the bleeding time.[26]

Nephrotic Syndrome

Thrombotic problems (particularly renal vein thrombosis and pulmonary embolism) can occur in children with nephrotic syndrome. Levels of procoagulant factors are increased and the major inhibitor of coagulation, AT III, is reduced. Anticoagulants and/or thrombolytic therapy have been used for such complications.

CONCLUSION

The otolaryngologist may encounter a child with a coagulopathy for referral for recurrent epistaxis, an intraoperative or postoperative hemorrhage after a surgical procedure, or in consultation to perform a surgical procedure on an already diagnosed child with a hematologic disorder. A thorough history, as well as good communication with a pediatric hematologist, will enable the otolaryngologist to manage these patients appropriately while avoiding complications.

A list of hemophilia treatment centers is available through the National Hemophilia Foundation (www.hemophilia.org) or the World Federation of Hemophilia (wfhewfh.org).

ACKNOWLEDGMENTS

The author would like to acknowledge Celeste Bowen especially for her invaluable help in preparing the manuscript.

REFERENCES

1. Lusher, J.M. Approach to the bleeding patient. In Nathan, D.G. and Oski, S.H., Eds. *Hematology of Infancy and Childhood*, 5th ed., Vol. 2, Philadelphia, PA: W.B. Saunders Company, 1998, 1574–1584.
2. Nierman, E. and Zakrzewski, K. Recognition and management of preoperative risk. *Rheumatic Dis. Clin. North Am.*, 1999, 25(3), 585–622.
3. Ewenstein, B.M. The pathophysiology of bleeding disorders presenting as abnormal uterine bleeding. *Am. J. Obstetr. Gynecol.*, 1996, 175(3 pt2), 770–777.
4. Nathan, D.G. and Oski, F.A. *Hematology of Infancy and Childhood*. 4th ed. Philadelphia, PA: W.B. Saunders Company, 1993, 1040.
5. Fuller, A.M. Evaluation and management of coagulation disorders in elective surgical patients. *Laryngoscope*, 1981, 91(9 pt1), 1484–1500.
6. Lusher, J.M. Screening and diagnosis of coagulation disorders. *Am. J. Obstetr. Gynecol.*, 1996, 175(3 pt2), 778–783.
7. Murphy, S., Nepo, A., and Sills, R. *Thrombocytopenia. Pediatr. Rev.*, 1999, 20(2).
8. *Procedure Manual, Special Coagulation Laboratory,* University of Miami Hospital and Clinics/Jackson Memorial Medical Center, Miami, FL, 1999.
9. Berkowitz, S.D., Frelinger, A.L., III, and Hillman, R.S. Progress in point-of-care laboratory testing for assessing platelet function. *Am. Heart J.*, 1998, 136 (Suppl), 51–65.
10. Lusher, J.M. and Sarnaik, S. Hematology (Contempo issue). *JAMA*, 1996, 275, 1814–1815.
11. Rodeghiero, F., Castaman, G., and Dini, E. Epidemiological investigations of the prevalence of von Willebrand's disease. *Blood*, 1987, 69, 454–459.

12. Werner, E.J., Broxson, E.H., Tucker, E.L. et al. Prevalence of von Willebrand's disease in children: a multiethnic study. *J. Pediatr.*, 1993, 123, 893–898.

13. Ewenstein, B.M. von Willebrand's disease. *Ann. Rev. Med.*, 1993, 48, 525–542.

14. Montgomery, R.R., Gill, J.C., and Scott, J.P. Hemophilia and von Willebrand's disease. In Nathan, D.G. and Oski, S.H., Eds. *Hematology of Infancy and Childhood*, 5th ed., Vol. 2, Philadelphia, PA: W.B. Saunders, 1998, 1631–1659.

15. von Willebrand, E. Hereditary pseudo-hemofili. *Finska Lak Handi*, 1926, 68, 87.

16. Meyer, D. and Girma, J.P. von Willebrand's factor: structure and function. *Thromb. Haemost.*, 1993, 70, 99.

17. Montgomery, R.R. and Coller, B.S. von Willebrand's disease. In Colman, R.W., Hirsh, J., Marder, V.J. et al., Eds., *Hemostasis and Thrombosis: Basic Principles and Clinical Practice*. Philadelphia, PA: J.B. Lippincott, 1994, 134–168.

18. Gill, J.C., Endres–Brooks, J., Bauer, P.J. et al. The effect of ABO blood group on the diagnosis of von Willebrand's disease. *Blood*, 1987, 69, 1691–1695.

19. Sadler, J.E. A revised classification of von Willebrand's disease. *Thromb. Haemost.*, 1994, 71, 520–525.

20. Federici, A.B. Diagnosis of von Willebrand's disease. *Haemophilia*, 1998, 4, 654–660.

21. Mannucci, P.M. Treatment of von Willebrand's disease. *Haemophilia*, 1998, 4, 661–664.

22. Mannucci, P.M., Bettega, D., and Cattaneo, M. Consistency of responses to repeated DDAVP infusions in patients with von Willebrand disease and haemophilia A. *Br. J. Haematol.*, 1992, 82, 87–93.

23. Lethagen, S. and Ragnarson, T.G. Self-treatment with desmopression intranasal spray in patients with bleeding disorders: effect on bleeding symptoms and socioeconomic factors. *Ann. Hematol.*, 1993, 66, 257–260.

24. Shattil, S.J. and Bennett, J.S. Acquired qualitative platelet disorders due to diseases, drugs, and foods. In Beutler, E., Lichtmann, M.A., Coller, B.S., and Kipps, T.J., Eds. *William's Hematology*, 5th ed. New York: McGraw–Hill, Inc., 1995, 1386–1400.

25. Smith, J.K. Factor XI deficiency and its management. *Haemophilia*, 1996, 2, 128–136.

26. Andrew, M. and Montgomery, R.R. Acquired disorders of hemostasis. In Nathan, D.G. and Oski, S.H., Eds. *Hematology of Infancy and Childhood*, 5th ed. Vol. 2, Philadelphia, PA: W.B. Saunders 1998, 1677–1718.

11 Allergy and Immunology

Dale Schrum and Louis M. Mendelson

What is called understanding is often no more than a state where one has become familiar with what one does not understand.

Edward Teller

CONTENTS

INTRODUCTION

Many issues overlap the subspecialties of otolaryngology and allergy/immunology. Even though the domain of allergy/immunology is systemic in nature and not anatomical, the target organs most often affected by allergic disease are part of the upper respiratory tract, especially the nasal mucosa and sinus cavities. Furthermore, the use of pharmacotherapy for otolaryngologic disease can lead to adverse drug reactions — another allergy domain. A working knowledge of the immune system, its deficiencies (immunocompromise), and the potential for over-reaction (allergy) is essential to any physician taking care of children. This chapter offers the clinician an understanding of disease entities that may complicate otolaryngologic care and its therapy.

IMMUNODEFICIENCY

The immune system is a highly integrated cellular and biochemical network designed to protect us from infectious pathogens such as viruses, bacteria, and parasites. Much of the immune response is specific, in that it is targeted to unique molecular structures on different microbes or to chemicals that they secrete. These foreign structural molecules and chemicals are called antigens; they are almost always proteins or glycoproteins.

An example of this specific immune response is the production of antibodies by specialized lymphocytes called B-cells against bacterial toxins. The antibody is specific to the toxin in an almost lock-and-key fit. Other specialized lymphocytes called T-cells have antigenically specific receptors. Once T-cells are stimulated by microbial antigens they orchestrate a complex immune attack called cell-mediated immunity. Certain aspects of the immune system, such as enzymes within mucosal barriers that are destructive to bacteria, are nonspecific. Many components of the immune system have specific and nonspecific attributes, such as phagocytic cells (e.g., neutrophils and macrophages). The immune system has much redundancy, but dysfunction in any one of the "parts" leads to increased risk of infection called immunocompromise or immunodeficiency.

The term "primary immunodeficiency" refers to inborn errors leading to a malfunction in one or more of the many aspects of immune function. The unifying clinical presentation in these patients is an increased rate of infection. Because these immune abnormalities are genetic, the presentation almost always occurs in childhood. Depending on which aspect of the immune system is affected, one sees infections with different types of organisms and, to some degree, in different areas of the body.

An increase in sinopulmonary bacterial infections is most commonly seen with deficiencies of the humoral immune system, which is the aspect of the immune system involved with production of antibodies. Antibody deficiencies are the most common type of primary immune deficiency, accounting for around 50% of known immunodeficiencies.[1] The bacteria most commonly cultured from the middle ear and sinus cavities of children with humoral immunodeficiencies are *Moraxella catarrhalis*, *Streptococcus pneumonia*, and *Haemophilus influenza*.

IgA with IgG Subclass Deficiency

The most common antibody deficiency is selective IgA deficiency. IgA is the major immunoglobulin isotype found in secretions of the sinopulmonary tract. As such it serves as the first line of antibody defense against infection. Many individuals have been found through blood donor screening to have very low or undetectable levels of IgA, but have no obvious clinical immune abnormality.[2] The reason for this phenotypic variance is not completely understood.

Patients with IgA deficiency have a higher incidence of autoimmune disease, especially connective tissue disorders.[3] This historical clue may heighten the clinician's suspicion of an IgA deficiency in the child with recurrent sinusitis. Deficiencies of the IgG subclasses 2 and 4 have been associated with IgA deficiency patients.[4] These individuals tend to have more severe and frequent infections[5] because most of the antibodies against polysaccharide antigens (found on the external surfaces of common pyogenic bacteria) are of the IgG 2 subclass. Further lab analysis of IgG subclass levels should be undertaken in patients with clinical IgA deficiency. Circulating anti-IgA antibodies are found in 30 to 40% of patients with IgA deficiency. These individuals are at risk of anaphylaxis if they receive blood products containing IgA. Blood transfusions in IgA-deficient patients should always be with washed RBCs or blood from another IgA-deficient patient.

Bruton's Disease (X-Linked Agammaglobulinemia)

A less common but more severe humoral immunodeficiency is Bruton's or x-linked agammaglob-ulinemia. In this condition, levels of all immunoglobulin isotypes (IgG, IgA, IgM, IgE) are extremely low or absent, secondary to the absence of B-cells (the sole producer of immunoglobulins). Recurrent or chronic sinusitis and otitis is inevitable, along with more severe infections such as pneumonia and sepsis. Chronic disseminated echo virus infection with encephalitis has an unusually high prevalence rate in these patients.[6]

Another complicating feature of this particular immunodeficiency syndrome is arthritis with sterile effusions. Children with x-linked agammaglobulinemia are always male because it is an x-linked recessive syndrome. There may be a family history on the maternal side of males with severe childhood infections, early childhood deaths, or diagnoses of immunodeficiency. Recurrent infections usually start after 6 months to 1 year of age because transplacentally acquired maternal antibodies are protective the first few months of life and therefore offer humoral immunity to these patients.

A common abnormal physical finding in these patients is absence of or very underdeveloped tonsilar and adenoidal tissue. This is due to an inability of lymphoid tissue to form germinal centers because no B-cells are present in the body. Lymph nodes throughout the body are small or absent. Any of the preceding historical or physical findings may make the diagnosis of x-linked agammaglobulinemia evident before laboratory confirmation.

COMMON VARIABLE IMMUNODEFICIENCY

Another primary immunodeficiency of antibody production associated with sinusitis and otitis media is common variable immunodeficiency. This is a heterogeneous condition that comprises numerous immunological defects. All patients have very low levels of the major immunoglobulin isotypes — especially IgG, IgA, and usually, IgM. Patients have increased incidence of infections, especially with encapsulated bacteria. The exact type and degree of immunoglobulin or antibody abnormality as well as the age of onset is variable, as the name implies. Infections usually start in early childhood, around ages 1 to 5, or in late adolescence, around ages 16 to 20.[7]

Common variable immunodeficiency differs from x-linked agammaglobulinemia in several ways. Immunoglobulins are not completely absent and B-cells are present in most patients with common variable immunodeficiency. Tonsils, adenoids, and lymph nodes are usually present and often enlarged. There is often splenomegally. These patients have a high incidence of chronic diarrhea secondary to gastroenteritis from Camphylobacter and *Giardia lamblia* infestation. They also have a very high incidence of hemolytic abnormalities such as anemia, thrombocytopenia, and leucopenia, often from autoimmune responses.

OTHER IMMUNE DEFICIENCY CATEGORIES

A few other immunodeficiency diseases are even less common in occurrence, but often lead to recurrent or chronic rhinosinusitis and otitis media. The hyper-IgM syndrome is a disease in which patients have very low levels of IgG, IgA, and even IgE, but normal to high levels of IgM. They have sinuopulmonary bacterial infections similar to those of patients with agammaglobulinemia, but also have a high rate of opportunistic infections such as PCP pneumonia. These patients have a tendency toward neutropenia and chronic diarrhea; lymphoid hyperplasia is usually present. The mode of inheritance is usually x-link recessive.

Wiskott–Alderich syndrome is another x-link recessive immunodeficiency disease with cell-mediated as well as humoral immunological defects. It presents clinically as a triad of conditions including thrombocytopenia with associated bleeding, eczema, and recurrent bacterial infections, as well as severe viral and opportunistic infections. An increased incidence of autoimmune disease and lymphoid malignancies is found in Wiskott–Alderich patients. Ataxia-telangiectasia is yet another syndrome with cell-mediated and humoral deficiencies as part of a triad of multisystem disorders including cerebellar ataxia and occulocutaneous teleangiectasia. Patients usually present in early childhood with ataxia and related neuromotor conditions. There is a high association with endocrine abnormalities including glucose intolerance and ovarian failure. The inheritance for ataxia-telangiectasia is autosomal recessive.

Clinical Evaluation

Even though most recurrent sinuopulmonary infections are related to mechanical, anatomical, or environmental etiologies, a high index of suspicion for immunodeficiency should be maintained by the otolaryngologist. A basic knowledge of immunodeficiency disease will prompt appropriate patient and family history and directed physical exam, which may lead to earlier diagnosis of these children.

Frequency and severity of infections is the first clue to possible immunodeficiency. These children usually have a history of numerous antibiotic courses and often inadequate response to antibiotics. There may be a history of other organ systems infected besides the upper respiratory tract. Pneumonia, bronchiectasis, chronic gastroenteritis, skin abscesses, meningitis, and sepsis are often diagnosed in different immunodeficiency diseases. A chronic or recurrent cough may be secondary to bronchiectasis or to sinusitis. The age of onset of infections and the organisms involved may give a clue to the type of immunodeficiency present.

A family history is very important because most immunodeficiency diseases are inherited. A history should include early childhood or infant deaths from infections, especially in male relatives on the maternal side. This fact reflects the preponderance of x-link recessive inheritance for many immunodeficiency diseases. Over 80% of children with an immunodeficiency are male.

On physical exam, the clinician should look for acute or chronic infection of the upper respiratory tract. Auscultation of the lungs may demonstrate localized or scattered course crackles suggestive of bronchiectasis. The presence of enlarged lymph nodes and tonsillar tissue or their absence may suggest an immunodeficient state. The skin is examined to identify acute or healed abscesses, eczema, or telangiectasia.

An initial laboratory screening should be performed to include a cell blood count (CBC) with differential, platelet count, and quantitative immunoglobin levels for IgG, IgA, and IgM. Isohemagglutinin titers and antibody titers to tetanus and pneumococcus serotypes may also be included. The CBC with differential and platelet count can detect leukopenia, lymphopenia, anemia, or thrombocytopenia — all found in varying combinations with many different immunodeficiency diseases. A quantitative immunoglobulin assay is the most important screening lab test for detecting deficiencies of antibody production and can be diagnostic for the most common immunodeficiency disease, IgA deficiency. Isohemagglutinins detect a functioning IgM response to antigen. Even more important is the detection of antibody function through the measurement of specific antibody titers to antigens. Tetanus titers measure the IgG antibody response to protein-based antigens and pneumococcal titers measure the antibody response to polysaccharide-encapsulated antigen. These are separate responses and either can be impaired.

ASTHMA

Pediatricians, allergists, and pediatric pulmonologists commonly treat asthma. This bronchospastic/inflammatory disease of the lower airway is the most common chronic pediatric illness with around 7% of the pediatric population affected. Clinically, asthma presents as episodes of cough, wheezing, or shortness of breath due to reversible airway obstruction. These episodes are recurrent and can vary from intermittent symptoms occurring a few times a year with upper respiratory infections to persistent symptoms occurring on a daily basis. At its least, asthma leads to diminished quality of life; at its worst, it can be fatal.

A major controversy exists among physicians who specialize in asthma management as to whether a relationship exists among allergic rhinitis, sinusitis, and asthma. Recent review articles have been published regarding this issue.[8,9] There is little doubt that a significantly higher incidence of allergic rhinitis occurs in asthmatics, with up to 80% of all asthma sufferers having concomitant allergic rhinitis.[10] Studies also suggest a significant increase in the incidence of sinusitis in pediatric asthmatics,[11] although other studies show no such relationship.[12]

Much of the problem lies with the difficulty in defining and diagnosing sinusitis. Plain radiographs have poor sensitivity and specificity, while CT scans have fair sensitivity with poor specificity. Diagnosis from clinical symptoms is variable and subjective. Epidemiological studies looking at the incidence of sinusitis in asthmatics have potential flaws secondary to the possible over or under diagnosis of sinusitis.

An equally controversial issue is whether asthma is triggered or worsened by sinusitis or chronic rhinitis. Indirect evidence indicates cause and effect because treating sinusitis often improves asthma, but these were not controlled studies.[13] Better evidence through controlled studies confirms that allergic rhinitis treatment improves asthma symptoms.[14]

One proposed mechanism of linkage between upper and lower respiratory pathology is a rhinosinobronchial reflex through parasympathetic neurologic inervation; however, this has never been consistently proven. It is also possible that aspiration of inflammatory or infectious material from the upper airway leads to lower airway symptoms due to the deposition of inflammatory mediators. This hypothesis has also not been proven. It is generally agreed that aggressive management of allergic rhinitis or sinusitis should be pursued in asthmatics on the principle of coexisting disease causing comorbidity.[15]

A specific consideration with regard to asthma in the otolaryngologic patient is perioperative management. The airways of asthmatic children are always hyper-responsive to some degree. Hyper-responsitivity of airways means that they will go into bronchospasm with certain types of stimulation. Intubation and manipulation of the upper airway is one such stimulation that will lead to bronchospasm and airway obstruction of the lower airways of asthmatics. Furthermore, airway hyper-responsiveness is directly related to the degree of airway inflammation and the severity or frequency of asthma symptoms at any given time. A thorough history of baseline asthma symptoms and recent asthma exacerbation is important for deciding the timing of an elective surgery and perioperative prophylactic management.

The perioperative management of pediatric asthma usually comes under the domain of the anesthesiologist. In more severe asthmatics, consultation with an allergist or pediatric pulmonologist may be warranted. Only a few studies in the medical literature concern perioperative asthma management in children.[16] Most anesthesiologists use inhaled bronchodilators, such as albuterol, the evening before and the day of surgery. Albuterol is a short-acting medication lasting about 4 hours after use and thus may need to be used intraoperatively as well. In children with an asthma exacerbation within 1 month prior to surgery or persistent symptoms occurring two or more times a week, ongoing inflammation in the airways should be assumed. If there is a history of a recent exacerbation or persistent symptoms, oral corticosteroids such as prednisone should be given 2 to 3 days before surgery, the day of surgery, and the day after surgery. Oral corticosteroids are the most effective treatment for the rapid reduction of asthmatic inflammation.

The most severe asthmatics may be on daily or every-other-day oral corticosteroids for long-term management of chronic asthma. Stress-dose steroids for adrenal suppression are crucial in perioperative management of these children. As well, stress-dose steroids should be considered in children on high doses of inhaled corticosteroids for daily asthma management because high-dose daily inhaled steroids can cause adrenal suppression in some cases. Elective surgery should usually be delayed until optimal asthma management is achieved.

In some cases, such as the pediatric patient requiring sinus surgery for chronic infectious sinusitis, the surgical management is a crucial part of optimal asthma management. Therefore, these patients should proceed with surgery even though baseline symptoms may be present. However, aggressive perioperative asthma management must be performed. This may require preoperative hospital admission so that these patients can be aggressively, medically managed by the pulmonologist and/or allergist.

ALLERGIC RHINITIS

Approximately 50 million Americans have allergic rhinitis (AR), which affects 10 to 30% of adults and up to 40% of children.[17] The prevalence of AR has increased dramatically in the past 30 years and may still be rising.[18,19] The direct and indirect costs of AR are considerable. U.S. health care expenditures were estimated to be $5.93 billion in 1996, and this does not include the indirect costs of the 3.5 million work days and 2 million school days lost each year because of AR.[20]

Allergic rhinitis involves IgE-mediated reactions of the nasal mucosa to one or more allergens. It may be seasonal, perennial, or both. Risk factors for allergic rhinitis include family history of atopy, serum IgE greater than 100 IU/ml before age 6 years, exposure to indoor allergens (e.g., animals, dust mites), eczema, and small family size.[21] Although allergic rhinitis may have its onset at any age, it generally begins before 20 years of age, with the greatest rate of onset between 12 and 15 years of age.[22] It is unusual in children under 3 years of age, but occasionally symptoms may appear in infants. It usually takes two to three seasons of exposure to a new antigen for the symptoms to appear.

The long-term outlook for patients with allergic rhinitis varies. Usually, once symptoms develop, they gradually worsen. Although some symptoms will improve with time, most will not and they tend to persist indefinitely after clinical symptoms appear. In 15 to 25% of patients, spontaneous remission of seasonal allergic rhinitis symptoms occurs in early to mid-life. Perennial allergic rhinitis is much less likely to undergo spontaneous remission. The severity of symptoms may vary from year to year, depending on the quality of pollen released and patient exposure during the specific pollinating season.

PRESENTATION AND SYMPTOMS

Seasonal Allergic Rhinitis

In seasonal allergic rhinitis, patients experience an IgE-mediated reaction in the nasal mucosa to one or more seasonal allergens. The symptoms are periodic, correlating with seasonal variation in aeroallergens. They occur during the pollinating season of the plants to which the patient is sensitive. Tree, grass, and weed pollens and mold spores are the allergens responsible for seasonal allergic rhinitis. The pollens important in causing allergic rhinitis are from plants that depend on the wind for cross-pollination. Plants that depend upon insect pollination, such as goldenrod, dandelions, and most flowers, rarely cause seasonal allergic rhinitis symptoms.

The pollinating season of the various plants depends on the individual plants and on the various geographic locations in the United States. Generally, trees pollinate early to mid-spring. Grasses pollinate late spring and early summer. Weeds pollinate late summer to early fall. Pollination may occur year round in the southern U.S. For any particular plant in a given locale, however, the pollinating season is constant from year to year. Weather conditions such as temperature and rainfall influence the amount of pollen produced but not the actual onset or termination of a specific season.[23,24]

Characteristic symptoms of seasonal allergic rhinitis include paroxysms of sneezing, clear rhinorrhea, nasal pruritus, nasal congestion, and palatal itching. Sneezing is the most characteristic symptom, and it is not uncommon to have attacks of 10 or more sneezes at a time. These episodes are especially common in the morning, but may arise without warning or may be preceded by itching or irritated feeling in the nose. During the pollen season, nonspecific factors such as dust exposure, air pollutants, or noxious irritants also may trigger sneezing episodes.[25]

Rhinorrhea is typically a thin discharge, which may be profuse and continuous. Nasal congestion resulting from swollen turbinates is a frequent complaint and may be the only presenting symptoms, particularly in children.[26] It may be intermittent at the onset of the pollen season and become more symptomatic as the pollen season progresses. Itching of the nose also may be a prominent feature, inducing frequent rubbing of the nose, particularly in children. Because of irritating sensations in the throat and the postnasal drainage, a hacking, nonproductive cough may be present.

For patients who also complain of constricted feeling of the chest and shortness of breath, the diagnosis of coexisting asthma should be considered.[27] In severe cases, mucous membranes of the eyes, eustachian tube, middle ear, and paranasal sinus may be involved. This produces symptoms of conjunctival irritation, redness and tearing, ear fullness and popping, and pressure over the cheeks and forehead. Malaise, weakness, irritability, fatigue, and anorexia may also be present.[28]

Perennial Allergic Rhinitis

Perennial allergic rhinitis is characterized by intermittent or continuous nasal symptoms resulting from an IgE-mediated reaction to allergens that show little or no seasonal variation. The symptoms are generally persistent throughout the year. The patient often complains of a persistent cold or chronic sinusitis.

The major perennial allergens are house dust mites, mold spores, cockroaches, and animal proteins. Exposure to airborne allergens at work may produce symptoms during the week with a symptom-free period at weekends. Occupational allergic rhinitis has been seen in persons who work with laboratory animals, detergent, and wood, among others.[29] Ingested food allergens rarely produce IgE-mediated rhinitis in adults without the involvement of other organs.[30] Symptoms that promptly follow eating a food may suggest a causal etiology, but this may not be IgE mediated. This is the case with beer, wine, and other alcoholic drinks with which symptoms are produced by local vasodilation. Food allergy is an uncommon cause of allergic rhinitis in infants and children.

Characteristic symptoms of perennial allergic rhinitis are prominent nasal congestion and postnasal drainage. Rhinorrhea and sneezing are less prominent than in seasonal allergic rhinitis. Nasal obstruction is the major complaint, particularly in children, in whom the passageways are relatively small. This may cause mouth breathing, snoring, and a nasal twang to the speech. Because of constant mouth breathing, patients complain of dry, irritated, or sore throat. Loss of the sense of smell may occur in patients with marked chronic nasal obstruction. In children, episodes of serous otitis media may recur.[31] Constant postnasal drainage may be associated with a chronic cough or a continual clearing of the throat.

The symptoms of allergic rhinitis often extend beyond the nose. Patients frequently experience headaches, fatigue, impaired concentration, reduced productivity, loss of sleep, a decrease in emotional well-being and social function, and increased occupational risks. In patients with perennial symptoms, the degree of impairment of health-related quality of life is similar to that seen in patients with asthma.[32] When allergic rhinitis is untreated or inadequately treated, symptoms may become chronic and contribute to associated conditions such as sinusitis, asthma, and/or otitis media. Treatments have been shown to improve health-related quality of life in allergic rhinitis and to prevent worsening of associated conditions.

DIFFERENTIAL DIAGNOSIS

Rhinitis is an inflammation of the mucous membranes of the nose and the characteristic symptoms are sneezing, itching, nasal discharge, and congestion.[33] Infectious rhinitis is characterized predominantly by cloudy (white, yellow, or green) nasal secretions with many neutrophils and, less commonly, bacteria. Noninfectious rhinitis is characterized by clear (watery or mucoid) discharge that often contains eosinophils. The noninfectious rhinitis can be allergic, nonallergic, or both (Table 11.1).

Symptoms of nonallergic rhinitis are similar to those of allergic rhinitis, but there is usually no pruritus and no evidence of allergic disease as determined by skin testing or serum levels of IgE to specific allergens. Nonallergic rhinitis can be due to anatomic obstruction, including choanal atresia, cleft palate, deviated septum, pharyngeal stenosis, tumors, adenoid hypertrophy, and foreign

---

TABLE 11.1
Classification of Rhinitis

Allergic rhinitis
Seasonal allergic rhinitis
Perennial allergic rhinitis

Nonallergic rhinitis
Infectious rhinitis
Idiopathic nonallergic, or vasomotor rhinitis
Nonallergic rhinitis with eosinophils
Rhinitis medicamentosa
Hormonal rhinitis
Anatomical causes of rhinitis

---

body obstruction. Nonanatomic causes include nonallergic eosinophilic rhinitis, infectious rhinitis, idiopathic nonallergic or vasomotor rhinitis, rhinitis medicamentosa, and hormonal rhinitis. Systemic immunologic diseases may also affect the nose. These include Wegener's granulomatosis, sarcoidosis, relapsing polychondritis, and midline granuloma.[34] Infections, such as tuberculosis, syphilis, leprosy, sporotrichosis, blastomycosis, histoplasmosis, and coccidiodomycosis, also may cause granuomatous nasal lesions.

Nonallergic eosinophilic rhinitis (NARES) is characterized by marked nasal eosinophilia, perennial symptoms of sneezing, nasal obstruction, profuse watery rhinorrhea, nasal itching, and occasionally, loss of smell.[35] There may be coexistent eosinophilic inflammation of the paranasal sinuses and nasal polyps. Patients with nonallergic asthma can also have NARES and some patients develop aspirin sensitivity.

Patients with idiopathic nonallergic or vasomotor rhinitis display nasal hyper-responsiveness to a variety of nonspecific factors, including chemical irritants, strong smells, and environmental changes in humidity, temperature, or barometric pressure. Symptoms are variable, consisting mainly of nasal obstruction and hypersecretion. Sneezing and pruritis are less common. No evidence exists of abnormal cellularity of nasal secretions and the mechanism has not been identified. The syndrome of copious watery rhinorrhea occurring immediately after ingestion of hot, spicy foods has been termed gustatory rhinitis and is vagally mediated.[36]

Overuse of topical decongestant is the most common cause of rhinitis medicamentosa. Other drugs producing rhinitis medicamentosa include antihypertensives, antipsychotics, oral contraceptives, and cocaine. Aspirin and nonsteroidal anti-inflammatory drugs may also cause rhinorrhea.

In hormonal rhinitis, patients experience rhinitis related to changes in hormonal status. Pregnancy can produce nasal obstruction and/or hypersecretion. Symptoms may also be associated with puberty, menses, and hypothyroidism.

PHYSICAL EXAMINATION AND LABORATORY EVALUATION

The physical examination should concentrate on the upper respiratory tract, but also include the eyes, ears, mouth, chest, and skin.[37] The patient may have mouth breathing and repeated nose wiggling, wiping, and pushing (allergic salute). A transverse nasal crease may be across the lower third of the nose where the soft cartilaginous portion meets the rigid bony ridge. Allergic shiners, a darkening of the infraorital skin resulting from venous dilation, are indicative of chronic nasal congestion — particularly in children — but are not diagnostic for allergic disease. The eyes may exhibit excessive lacrimation, the sclera and conjunctiva may be reddened, and chemosis may be present.

Examination of the nose with high illumination using a nasal speculum discloses pale blue and boggy nasal turbinates with a clear watery discharge or inflamed erythematous mucosa. Swollen turbinates may completely occlude the nasal airway. Nasal polyps may be present in cases of chronic perennial allergic rhinitis of long duration. Occasionally, fluid is in the middle ear. In children affected with perennial allergic rhinitis early in life, narrowing of the arch of the palate may occur. In addition, these children may develop facial deformities, such as dental malocclusion or gingival hypertrophy.[38] The throat is usually normal on examination, although cobblestone appearance of posterior pharyngeal wall may be seen.

The diagnosis of seasonal allergic rhinitis usually presents no difficulty by the time the patient has had symptoms severe enough to seek medical attention. The seasonal nature of the condition, the characteristic symptom complex, and the physical finding should establish a diagnosis in almost all cases. Skin testing is the diagnostic method of choice to demonstrate IgE antibodies.[39] Positive skin tests to aeroallergens are important confirmatory findings in patients whose history and physical examinations suggest chronic allergic rhinitis. The radioallergosorbent test may be a useful diagnostic aid when skin testing cannot be performed.

Nasal smears usually contain eosinophils in an allergic patient and are useful in determining if chronic rhinitis has an infectious origin where polymorphonuclear neutrophils present. They do not differentiate allergic from nonallergic eosinophilic rhinitis. Absence of eosinophils does not exclude an allergic cause.

Many research studies have used nasal provocation challenge to simulate rhinitis syndromes. Currently, no standardized technique can be applied to clinical practice. Standardized nasal provocation challenge has the potential to become a more frequently used additional clinical test in the diagnosis of allergic rhinitis.[40] Similarly, rhinomanometry and acoustic rhinometry provide the best methods for objective assessment of nasal obstruction; however, further studies are needed to validate their use for long-term comparisons of nasal obstruction in clinical practice.[41]

MANAGEMENT

Avoidance Measures

In treating patients with allergic rhinitis, the most important first step in achieving symptomatic improvement is avoidance of the offending allergen. Whenever practical, the patient should minimize exposure to allergens known to exacerbate symptoms, and the patient's family should be educated on how to eliminate or reduce exposure to allergens and other irritants in the patient's surroundings. Airborne pollens should be kept out of the immediate environment by keeping windows and doors closed and using air conditioning in the house and in automobiles.[42] Window or attic fans that draw in outside air should be avoided. Peak pollination occurs at different times of the day for different pollens (e.g., ragweed in the late morning and grasses in the afternoon), and outdoor activities should be minimized during times of high pollen counts. Following outdoor activity, the patient should shower or bathe, and change clothes.

To decrease the mold exposure, in addition to following pollen avoidance recommendations, patients should refrain from walking through uncut fields, working with compost or dry soil, and raking leaves. Mold growth in the home can be controlled by keeping the indoor humidity less than 50%, cleaning any moldy surface, and fixing all water leaks or seepage.

For pet allergy, removal of the pet from the home is obviously important and can control the allergic rhinitis symptoms completely; however, this recommendation is rarely followed. If removal of the animal is not possible, then the pet should be kept out the patient's bedroom and the bedroom door should be kept closed. Use of a HEPA-type air cleaner in the bedroom will help reduce animal allergen.[43]

For dust mite allergy, allergen-proof covers for mattress, pillow, and box springs; frequent washing of linens in hot water ($\geq130°F$); and reducing indoor humidity to <50% are the first steps to minimize exposure. Removing carpets from the bedroom and carpets laid on concrete from any room and minimizing upholstered furniture can be done for more complete control. These simple measures often enable the patient to have fewer and milder symptoms.

Pharmacotherapy

Avoidance measures are the mainstay of treatment. However, if such measures fail or are unrealistic, several pharmacologic therapies can successfully control the symptoms of allergic rhinitis.

Antihistamines

Antihistamines are the mainstay of pharmacotherapy for allergic rhinitis and first-line therapy for mild disease. They may be given alone or in combination with intranasal corticosteroids. H_1-receptor antagonist activity blocks histamine-induced symptoms, including rhinorrhea, pruritus, and sneezing. They have a onset of action of 1 to 2 hours and may reduce related symptoms in eyes and throat. However, they are generally considered ineffective for treating nasal congestion.[44] Although first-generation antihistamines are readily available in over-the-counter preparation, it is prudent to avoid their use because of their side effect profile. They have sedating side effects and may affect cognitive and motor functions even without obvious sedation.[45] Other adverse effects include blurry vision, dry eyes, constipation, urinary retention, bradycardia, restlessness, and insomnia.

Second- and third-generation antihistamines are potent H_1-receptor blockers and, except for cetirizine and azelastine, are no more sedating than placebo. They are generally free of anticholinergic effects and adverse GI effects. They have rapid onset and long duration of action, often up to 24 hours. Cetirizine, loaratadine, desloratadine, and fexofenadine all have been shown to be more effective than placebo for treatment of allergic rhinitis. Intranasal azelastine is an effective and well-tolerated alternative for symptomatic relief of allergic rhinitis; however, significant systemic absorption may occur, resulting in drowsiness, and it may have bitter taste.[46]

Decongestants

Sympathomimetic drugs are used as vasoconstrictors for the nasal mucous membrane to relieve symptoms of nasal congestion. Decongestants may have mild effects in treating rhinorrhea but are not helpful in treating nasal itching, sneezing, or ocular symptoms. Consequently, these medications are often given in combination with antihistamines. In large doses, these drugs induce elevated blood pressure, nervousness, and insomnia; they should be used with caution in patients with heart disease, hypertension, diabetes, or prostate hypertrophy. Intranasal decongestants act more rapidly and effectively than oral decongestants to relieve nasal congestion and have fewer systemic side effects. Patients should be warned that overuse of these medications may cause rebound congestion, nasal hyper-reactivity, tolerance, and rhinitis medicamentosa.

Intranasal Corticosteroids

Intranasal corticosteroids are the first-line medication in treating patients with moderate or severe allergic rhinitis.[47] Corticosteroids can

- Reduce inflammatory cell infiltration in the superficial nasal mucosa
- Reduce endothelial and epithelial permeability
- Increase sympathetic vascular tone
- Decrease response of mucous glands to cholinergic stimulation
- Reduce nasal hyper-reactivity[48]

Intranasal corticosteroids provide effective relief for the complex of nasal symptoms associated with allergic rhinitis, as well as relief from congestion and even ocular symptoms, to a certain extent. Time to onset and to maximum benefit is longer than with antihistamines. Initial relief may be 4 to 12 hours after the first dose, and maximum therapeutic benefit usually occurs within 2 weeks.[49] Patients need to be instructed that to maintain effectiveness, intranasal steroids must be administered regularly, even in the absence of symptoms.

Local side effects are relatively uncommon, with about 10% of patients reporting nasal irritation, nasal burning, or sneezing after use. Approximately 2% report bloody nasal discharge, and there are a few case reports regarding septal perforations and delayed hypersensitivity reactions. Systemic side effects are not considered a serious risk with intranasal corticosteroids. Studies have failed to show significant effects on serum markers of bone metabolism or cortisol concentrations after stimulation with adrenocorticotropic hormone. Some intranasal corticosteroids have been shown to cause a reduction in growth velocity when administered to children, but this effect may be transient and there is no significant effect on final adult height.[50] Oral or intramuscular steroids are not routinely indicated for treatment of allergic rhinitis. A short course of oral corticosteroids may be appropriate for some patients with severe symptoms or to gain control of symptom exacerbation.

Mast Cell Stabilizers

Cromolyn sodium is considered a mast cell stabilizing agent that prevents mediator release in experimental models; however, the mechanism of action of cromolyn sodium remains uncertain and may not be related to mast cell stabilization. It blocks the early- and late-phase nasal allergic responses and relieves sneezing, rhinorrhea, nasal congestion, and nasal pruritus. It has an excellent safety profile with few side effects, but is not as effective as nonsedating oral antihistamines or topical nasal corticosteroids. For treating seasonal symptoms, it is advisable to being therapy 2 weeks before expected allergen exposure. Cromolyn sodium may be used immediately before an anticipated exposure to prevent rhinitis symptoms, but it is most effective when used prophylactically four to six times a day. Unfortunately, this frequent dosing schedule makes compliance a challenge.

Anticholinergics

Ipratropium bromide reduces fluid secreted by the nose regardless of cause. It significantly and rapidly reduces secretions associated with allergic rhinitis, without excessive dryness or potential cholinergic side effects. Because it does not relieve nasal congestion, pruritus, or sneezing, it is indicated for use in patients with rhinorrhea as their main complaint.[51] Excessive use may lead to irritations, crusting, and epistaxis. Long-term use of topical ipratropium bromide appears safe.

Leukotriene Modifiers

Leukotriene modifiers are selective and competitive receptor antagonists of leukotriene D_4 and E_4. They have been shown to relieve nasal congestion more than sneezing or rhinorrhea in patients with seasonal allergic rhinitis.[52] They may also help manage nasal allergy in patients being treated for concomitant asthma.[53]

Monoclonal Anti-IgE Antibody

The monoclonal anti-IgE antibody omalizumab is a recombinant humanized antibody that binds to the Fc portion of human IgE, inhibiting the binding of IgE to its receptor. Recent studies indicate that omalizumab decreases serum IgE level, provides symptomatic relief in patients with allergic rhinitis, and improves patients' quality of life in a dose-dependent manner.[54] It may help treat patients with moderate to severe seasonal allergic rhinitis who have not achieved symptomatic relief from or cannot tolerate other therapies. The FDA has not yet approved this therapy.

Immunotherapy

Immunotherapy is the subcutaneous introduction of increasing doses of the allergen vaccines to which the patient is sensitive. Clinical studies have demonstrated the effectiveness of immunotherapy in treating symptoms of allergic rhinitis.[55] Potent and standardized vaccines are available for common allergens such pollen, dander, and dust mites. Immunotherapy is antigen specific; thus, the skin test sensitivity of the patient must be known before formulating vaccines for therapy. About 80 to 85% of patients will derive significant long-lasting symptomatic relief.[56]

TABLE 11.2
Classification of Adverse Reactions to Drugs

Predictable reactions	Example
Overdosage	Acetaminophen — hepatic necrosis
Side effect	Antihistamines — lethargy
Secondary effect	Clindamycin — Clostridium difficile pseudomembraneous colitis
Drug–drug interaction	Terfenadine/erythromycin — torsade de pointes arrhythmia

Unpredictable reactions	Example
Intolerance	Aspirin — tinnitus (at usual dosage)
Idiosyncratic	Chloroquinie — hemolytic anemia in G6PD-deficient patient
Allergic	Penicillin — anaphylaxis
Pseudoallergic	Radiocontrast material — anaphylactoid reaction

Immunotherapy is considered for long allergen season, perennial symptoms, and poor response to, poor tolerance of, or unwillingness to use symptomatic medication. It may prevent the worsening or development of asthma,[57] chronic or recurrent rhinosinusitis, and chronic or recurrent middle ear disease. Immunotherapy is not without risk and, although the annual fatality rate from immunotherapy is low at about one fatality per 2 million doses, prospective patients should be informed of this potential.[58]

DRUG ALLERGY

The ENT physician is frequently confronted with children with a history of various medication allergies. In the pediatric population, antibiotics are by far the most commonly implicated medication in allergic drug reactions. Although most adverse reactions to medications are labeled "allergic," this label should be applied only to reactions that are known (or presumed) to be mediated by immunologic mechanisms. Adverse reactions are divided into predictable and unpredictable reactions. Predictable reactions occur in otherwise healthy individuals, are generally dose dependent, and are related to the known pharmacology of the drug. Approximately 80% of drug reactions are predictable. Unpredictable reactions occur only in susceptible individuals, are dose dependent, and are not related to pharmacologic actions of the drugs. Examples of both of these types of reactions can be found in Table 11.2.[59]

Allergic reactions, which are considered unpredictable, account for less than 10% of all adverse reactions. The overall incidence of allergic drug reactions is difficult to estimate in pediatrics due to the wide spectrum of disorders they encompass and lack of good diagnostic tests. The frequency of anaphylactic reactions to antibiotics is rare in the pediatric population. In a study of 1740 children and young adults who received intramuscular injections of penicillin G, for an average of 3.4 years, the incidence of anaphylaxis was 1.23 per 10,000 injections. The incidence of allergic reactions was 3.2%.[60]

Allergic reactions to drugs are classified according to the Gell and Coombs classifications. Although this classification system is helpful in classifying allergic reactions to drugs, no single classification scheme is able to account for all allergic drug reactions. The reason for this is that the mechanisms responsible for most drug reactions are not known. As can be seen in Table 11.3, reactions are divided into four types.[59]

Because of their small size, most medications are unable to elicit an immune response independently. They must first covalently bind with a larger carrier molecule, such as serum proteins or normal tissue, to form a large molecule capable of eliciting an immune response. This process

TABLE 11.3
Gell and Coombs Classification Scheme Allergic Reactions

Type	Mechanism	Example
I	IgE reaction	Penicillin — anaphylaxis
II	Cytotoxic reaction (IgG/IgM mediated)	Quinidine — hemolytic anemia
III	Immune complex reaction	Cephalexin — serum sickness
IV	Delayed T-cell-mediated reaction	Neomycin — contact dermatitis

is called haptenization and the small metabolite of the drug is referred to as a hapten. The responses may be humoral with elicitation of specific antibodies, cellular with elicitation of a T-cell response, or both. Most medications in their native state are not chemically reactive, but rather must be first converted into reactive metabolites enzymatically, usually in the liver, before they can combine with a larger molecule and be immunologically reactive. One of the reasons that adequate testing materials for antibiotic allergies have not been developed is that the reactive metabolites formed by most drugs are unknown.[59,61]

The important exception to this is penicillin, which, under physiologic conditions, undergoes spontaneous degradation to form reactive metabolites. Of the metabolites formed, 90% are in the form of penicillolyl and this is referred to as a major antigenic determinate. The remainder stays as penicillin or degrades to pinilloate or penicilloate, both of which are referred to as the minor determinants and are associative with the most severe allergic reactions to penicillin.[61–63] Unfortunately, even though researchers have known about the breakdown products of penicillin since the late 1960s, the minor determinants for skin testing are not available for commercial use. Therefore, many allergists associated with medical centers must synthesize these reagents for local use.

The majority of children labeled as allergic to penicillin can take this antibiotic without fear of a life-threatening reaction for several reasons:

- Children can lose their sensitivity to penicillin with time.
- A virus or bacteria cause reaction and not the penicillin.
- The interaction of penicillin and/or amino penicillins with certain viral infections can cause reaction.
- Of children who take amino penicillins, 7 to 10% develop a maculopapular rash 8 to 10 days into the course, which usually does not lead to an allergic reaction upon subsequent use.[64,65]

Patients with an uncertain allergic history to penicillin, or those for whom penicillin-type drugs may be most appropriate for treatment, can have skin testing to determine whether penicillin-type drugs can be tolerated. When the major and minor determinants are used for penicillin skin testing, the procedure is safe and highly accurate in predicting a life-threatening reaction to penicillin. No one has ever reported a severe life-threatening reaction in a child who had negative skin tests to the major and minor determinants and subsequently received penicillin.

Skin testing for penicillin allergy is useful in predicting only IgE reactions to penicillin. It does not predict non-IgE reactions such as hemolytic anemia, nephritis, Steven Johnson syndrome, or contact dermatitis. Evaluation for penicillin allergy by RAST or ELISA is not reliable in ruling out penicillin allergy. The reasons for this are that no minor determinant is available using these tests, and the tests are not as sensitive as skin testing. In addition, results are not immediate.[62,64,65]

Because the majority of children labeled as allergic to penicillin can safely take this antibiotic without fear of a life-threatening reaction, children should be skin tested. These children can be tested in an outpatient setting. The ideal time to test them is when they are well and not in immediate need of penicillin. It has been shown that elective skin testing and provocative challenge testing done by allergists in the outpatient setting are safe and highly reliable and seldom cause resensitization.[64]

In children who are penicillin skin test positive and require treatment with a penicillin antibiotic because no acceptable alternative antibiotic is available, rapid desensitization should be considered. Despite various theories, the immunologic mechanisms behind acute desensitization remain unknown. Desensitization does not prevent non-IgE reactions such as serum sickness, hemolytic anemia, and interstitial nephritis. Once a child is desensitized to the penicillins, in order to maintain the desensitization, the patient must receive penicillin daily. If penicillins are discontinued for 48 hours or more, the patient is again at risk for anaphylactic reaction, and desensitization should be repeated if need for penicillin arises again. Penicillin desensitization should be performed in a hospital setting with intravenous access and resuscitative medications and equipment available.[65]

Amoxicillin has replaced penicillin as the most common antibiotic used in the outpatient setting for children. Approximately 7 to 10% of children treated with amoxicillin will develop a nonpruritic maculopapular rash 7 to 10 days into the treatment course. This increase is up to 72 to 100% if the patient has a concurrent infection with infectious mononucleosis or a cytomegallic virus. Children with a history of having had the classic, nonpruritic maculopapular rash to amoxicillin or who developed this rash with one of the underlying diseases previously mentioned usually can tolerate penicillin or amoxicillin in the future without a severe life-threatening reaction. In such children, skin testing with the penicillin determinants and amoxicillin for late reaction can be helpful in determining whether a child will have the same reaction again. In children with a history of an IgE reaction to these antibiotics, in addition to the major and modern determinants, ampicillin is added to the skin testing reagents. In children suspected of a late reaction to amoxicillin, the skin tests are observed for 72 hours for late reactions.[65]

The administration of cephalosporins to patients who have a history of penicillin allergy deserves additional comments. Because cephalosporins and penicillin share a common beta-lactam ring, one might expect moderate allergic cross-reactions between these two classes of antibiotics. However, in clinical practice, cross-reactivity occurs much less frequently. A life-threatening reaction rarely occurs in children taking oral second- and third-generation cephalosporins. The incidence of reactions to these cephalosporins in individuals with a history of penicillin allergy and positive penicillin skin tests is 2% in the first 24 hours.

Approximately 1 to 3% of children will develop a cutaneous reaction to the cephalosporins. Because the metabolites of the cephalosporins are not known, no skin testing reagents for the cephalosporins are available. At least 80% of children with a history of penicillin allergy are skin-test negative, and only 2% of skin-test positive patients will react to cephalosporins, so the chance of a child with a history of penicillin allergy reacting to a cephalosporin is probably less than 1%. Because some of these reactions are life-threatening, a cautious graded challenge using a third-generation cephalosporin is suggested in penicillin skin-test positive patients if a cephalosporin is required. In patients requiring a cephalosporin who have a history of penicillin allergy testing with the cephalosporins, the result is only helpful to the clinician if the skin test is positive. This is because no reagents for cephalosporin skin testing are available. The meaning of a negative skin test is not helpful.[65]

Penicillin skin testing can help guide physicians in their approach to patients with a history of penicillin allergy requiring treatment with a cephalosporin. Children with a history of penicillin allergy who are found to have negative penicillin skin tests are at no greater risk for having an allergic reaction and can safely receive a cephalosporin. Because the vast majority of children labeled as allergic to penicillin can safely take this antibiotic, this is a further indication for elective skin testing in children.

For antibiotics other than the penicillins, the immunochemistry is poorly understood and no reliable diagnostic tests for drug-specific IgE antibodies are currently available. Despite this fact, some less reputable commercial diagnostic laboratories offer serologic testing for allergies to a

TABLE 11.4

False Assumptions in the Management of Anaphylaxis

Severe anaphylaxis is always preceded by hives.

Epinephrine is always effective.

Antihistamines and corticosteroids are effective for acute anaphylaxis.

Mild symptoms will not progress to severe anaphylaxis.

wide spectrum of antibiotics. These tests purport to measure drug-specific IgE or IgG antibodies, but the measurements are meaningless because no recorded standards are available. Therefore, the only way to prove or disapprove unequivocally whether an antibiotic allergy to these antibiotics exists is to challenge the patient with the suspected antibiotic. These provocative challenges are more risky and should be undertaken only if no acceptable alternative antibiotic can be substituted. No child should be challenged with an antibiotic that previously caused a Steven Johnson or exfolliative dermatitis reaction.

ANAPHYLAXIS

Anaphylaxis is a generalized, potentially life-threatening, immediate allergic reaction resulting from IgE-mediated release of mediators from mast cells and basophils (see Table 11.4).[66–69] The term "anaphylactoid reaction" refers to a clinically indistinguishable event that is not mediated by IgE antibodies. In children, the most common causes are foods (e.g., peanuts, tree nuts, crustaceans), medicines, venoms, immunotherapy vaccines, and latex.[69–71] Signs and symptoms of anaphylaxis usually occur within 5 to 30 minutes after introduction of the antigen; however, the reactions may not develop for several hours, occurring usually after oral ingestion of the antigen.[68] Late-phase or biphasic reactions, which occur 4 to 12 hours after the initial attack, can also occur. Usually, the more rapid the onset of symptoms is, the more severe are the reactions.[66,67,69] In addition, asthmatics are more likely to suffer severe reactions than those who are not asthmatic.

Anaphylaxis can involve the cutaneous, respiratory, gastrointestinal, and/or cardiovascular systems.[72] Generalized urticaria and angioedema are the most common manifestations of cutaneous involvement, but pruritus and flush can occur without hives. However, cutaneous manifestations might be delayed or absent in some cases of fatal anaphylaxis.[73,74] The second most common set of symptoms, consisting of stridor with upper airway edema, shortness of breath, and/or wheezing, involves the respiratory tract. Hypotension is the third most common feature with symptoms consisting of dizziness, disorientation, syncope, and a feeling of impending doom. Gastrointestinal symptoms with nausea, vomiting, diarrhea, and cramping abdominal pain follow in frequency. On rare occasions, rhinitis, substernal pain, and itch without rash can occur.

In children, the differential diagnosis is most commonly a vasodepressor reaction. An important marker in the differential diagnosis of vasodepressor reaction and anaphylaxis is that the heart rate is slow (usually less than 60 beats per minute) with the former.[69] The use of serum tryptase levels, a mast cell marker, can be useful in differentiating an anaphylactic from nonanaphylactic reaction. This peaks 1 to 1.5 hours after onset and can remain elevated up to 15 hours.[75]

All ENT specialists involved with allergy management of children should be prepared to prevent and treat an anaphylactic reaction. The most important principle in treatment of anaphylaxis is early recognition and prompt treatment with appropriate medications. There are no clues to predict how an anaphylactic reaction is going to progress; therefore, treatment with intramuscular epinephrine is essential in all but the mildest cases (Table 11.5).[66,67,73] An antihistamine or corticosteroids have no place as a first line treatment of anaphylaxis because neither has an effect on acute anaphylaxis.

The elements of optimal treatment of anaphylaxis are early and aggressive administration of intramuscular epinephrine,[74,76] delivery of 100% oxygen, early and aggressive administration of

TABLE 11.5
Key Features in Treatment of Anaphylaxis

Rapid and aggressive IM administration of epinephrine

Delivery of 100% oxygen

Maintenance of adequate intravascular volume with early and aggressive administration of saline or Ringers lactate if BP
< 80 in child after epinephrine

Prompt and safe transport to the hospital

Be prepared:

Detailed emergency plan and practice regularly

Attach check list and flow sheet with proper dosages to crash cart

Sources: Kemp, S.F. and Lockey, R.F. *J. Allergy Clin. Immunol.*, 2002, 110, 341–348; Kemp, S.F. *Immunol. Allergy Clin. North Am.*, 2001, 21, 611–634; and Joint Task Force on Practice Parameters. *J. Allergy Clin. Immunol.*, 1998, 101, S465–528.

TABLE 11.6
Physician-Supervised Management of Anaphylaxis

Immediate intervention

Assessment of airway, breathing, circulation, and adequacy of mentation

Epinephrine IM. Dose: 1:1000 aqueous, 0.01 ml/kg up to 0.3 ml intramuscularly into arm (deltoid) every 5 min as necessary to control symptoms and blood pressure. Administer in the anterolateral thigh to children with moderate, severe, or progressive anaphylaxis.

Epinephrine IV if not responding to IM epinephrine and volume replacement. Dose: 1:10,000 (1 ml of 1:1000 in 9 ml of saline) at 0.01 ml/kg aqueous 10–20 min

General measures

Place child in supine position and elevate lower extremities

Administer 100% oxygen and monitor using pulse oximeter

Get IV access

Administer normal saline intravenously for fluid replacement and venous access if blood pressure is not responding to epinephrine (systolic <80 to 100 after epinephrine) and pulse remains weak, at rate of 20 cc/kg

If any problem is anticipated, call 911 to transfer child to hospital

fluids, and prompt and safe transport to hospital (Table 11.5 and Table 11.6). It is essential that any ENT specialist who performs procedures in his or her office that could cause an anaphylactic reaction be prepared. A designated crash cart should be available with attached checklist for equipment needed to treat anaphylaxis, and proper dosages of medications should be available. This cart should be checked monthly by a designated person. Mock drills should be planned in timely fashion so that everyone knows his or her responsibilities.

REFERENCES

1. Stiehm, E.R. Immunology disorders: general considerations In Stiehm, E.R., Ed. *Immunologic Disorders in Infants and Children.* 3rd ed. Philadelphia PA: W.B. Saunders Company, 1989, 157–195.
2. Ropars, C., Muller, A., Paint, N., Beige, D., and Avenard, G.V. Large-scale deletion of IgA-deficient blood donors. *J. Immunol. Methods*, 1982, 54, 183–189.
3. Cassidy, J.T., Burt, A., Petty, R., and Sullivan, D.V. Large IgA deficiency in connective tissue disease. *New Engl. J. Med.*, 1969, 280, 275.
4. Oxelius, V.A. et al. IgG subclasses in selective IgA deficiency: importance of IgG2–IgA deficiency. *New Engl. J. Med.*, 1981, 304, 1476–1477.

5. Ugazio, H.G. et al. Recurrent infections in children with "selective" IgA deficiency: association with IgG2 and IgG4 deficiency. *Birth Defects*, 1983, 19, 169–171.
6. Wilfert, C.M. et al. Persistent and fatal central nervous system echovirus infections in patients with agammaglobulinemia. *New Engl. J. Med.*, 1977, 296, 1485–1489.
7. Hermaszewski, R.A. and Webster, A.D.B. Primary hypogammaglobulinemia: survey of clinical manifestations and complications. *Q. J. Med.*, 1993, 86, 31–42.
8. Campanella, S.G. and Asher, M.I. Current controversies: sinus disease and the lower airway. *Pediatr. Pulmonol.*, 2001, 31, 165–172.
9. Benedictis, F.M. and Bush, A. Rhinosinusitis and asthma: epiphenomenon or casual association. *Chest*, 1999, 115, 550–556.
10. Smith, J.M. Epidemiology and natural history of asthma, allergic rhinitis, and atopicdermatitis (eczema) In Middleton, E., Jr., Reed, C.E., Ellis, E.F., Adkinson, N.F., Jr., and Yunginger, J.W., Eds. *Allergy Principles and Practice*, 3rd ed. St. Louis MO: Mosby Company, 1988, 891–929.
11. Slavin, R.G. Asthma and sinusitis. *J. Allergy Clin. Immunol.*, 1992, 90, 534–537.
12. Lombard, E., Stein, R.T., Wright, A.L., Morgan, W.J., and Martinez, F.D. The relationship between physician-diagnosed sinusitis, asthma, and skin test reactivity to allergens in 8-year-old children. *Pediatr. Pulmonol.*, 1996, 22, 141–146.
13. Rachelefsky, G.S., Katz, R.M., and Siegel, S.C. Chronic sinus disease with associated reactive airways disease in children. *Pediatrics*, 1984, 73, 526–529.
14. Friedman, R., Ackerman, M., Wald, E. et al. Asthma and bacterial sinusitis in children. *J. Allergy Clin. Immunol.*, 1984, 74, 185–189.
15. Wetson, W.T., Becker, A.B., and Simons, F.E. Treatment of allergic rhinitis with intranasal corticosteroids in patients with mild asthma: effect on lower airway responsiveness. *J. Allergy Clin. Immunol.*, 1993, 91, 97–101.
16. Scalfaro, P., Sly, P.D., Sims, C., and Hbre, W. Salbutamol prevents the increase of respiratory resistance caused by tracheal intubation during sevoflurane anesthesia in asthmatic children. *Anesth. Analg.*, 2001, 93, 898–902.
17. Nathan, R.A., Meltzer, E.O., Selner, J.G., and Storms, W. The prevalence of allergic rhinitis in the United States. *J. Allergy Clin. Immunol.*, 1997, 99, S808–S814.
18. Linna, O., Kokkonen. J., and Lukin, M. A 10-year prognosis of childhood allergic rhinitis. *Acta Pediatr.*, 1992, 81, 100–102.
19. Sibbald, B., Rink, E., and O'Souza, M. Is the prevalence of atopy increasing? *Br. J. Gen. Pract.*, 1990, 40, 338–340.
20. Malone, D.C., Lawson, K.A., Smith, D.H. et al. A cost of illness study of allergy rhinitis in the United States. *J. Allergy Clin. Immunol.*, 1997, 99, 22–27.
21. Wright, A.L., Holberg, C.J., Martinez, F.D. et al. Epidemiology of physician-diagnosed allergic rhinitis in childhood. *Pediatrics*, 1994, 94(6), 895–901.
22. Fleming, D.M. and Crombie, D.A. Prevalence of asthma and hay fever in England and Wales. *Br. Med. J.*, 1987, 294, 279–283.
23. Jelks, M. *Allergy Plants That Cause Sneezing and Wheezing*. Tampa: Worldwide Publications, 1986.
24. Lewis, W.H., Vinay, P., and Zenger, V.E. *Airborne and Allergic Pollen of North America*, Baltimore: Johns Hopkins University Press, 1983.
25. Druce, H.M. Allergic and nonallergic rhinitis. In Middleton, E., Reed, C.E., Ellis, E.F. et al., Eds. *Allergy: Principles and Practice*, 5th ed. St. Louis: C.V. Mosby, 1998, 770–782.
26. Sknoer, D.P., Doyle, W.J., Boehm, S., and Fireman, P. Late phase eustachian tube and nasal allergic responses associated with inflammatory mediator elaboration. *Am. J. Rhinol.*, 1988, 2, 155–161.
27. Settipane, R.A. Complications of allergic rhinitis. *Allergy Asthma Proc.*, 1999, 20, 209–213.
28. Meltzer, E.O. Quality of life in adults and children with allergic rhinitis. *J. Allergy Clin. Immunl.*, 2001, 108, S45–S53.
29. Murphy, E.E. and Slavin, R.S. Occupational rhinitis: when to suspect, what to do. *J. Respir. Dis.*, 1995, 16, 135–142.
30. Atkins, F.M., Steinber, S.S., and Metcalfe, D.D. Evaluation of immediate adverse reactions to foods in adult patients. I. Correlation of demographic, laboratory, and prick skin test data with response to controlled oral food challenge. *J. Allergy Clin. Immunol.*, 1985, 75, 348.

31. Bernstein, J.M. The role of IgE-mediated hypersensitivity in the development of otitismedia with effusion. *Otolaryngol. Clin. North Am.*, 1992, 25, 197–211.
32. Meltzer, E.O. Quality of life in adults and children with allergic rhinitis. *J. Allergy Clin. Immunl.*, 2001, 108, S45–S53.
33. Dykewicz, M.S. and Fineman, S. Diagnosis and management of allergic rhinitis: parameter documents of the Joint Task Force on Practice Parameters in Allergy, Asthma, and Immunology. *Ann. Allergy Asthma Immunol.*, 1998, 81, 463–518.
34. Falkoff, R.J. *Nasal Manifestations of Systemic Disease*. Providence: Oceanside, 1991.
35. Jacobs, R.L., Freedman, P.M., and Boswell, R.N. Nonallergic rhinitis with nasal eosinophilia (NARES syndrome). *J. Allergy Clin. Immunol.*, 1981, 67, 253–262.
36. James, J.M., Bernhisel-Broadbent, J., and Sampson, H.A. Respiratory reactions provoked by double-blind food challenges in children. *Am. J. Respir. Crit. Care Med.*, 1994, 149, 59–64.
37. Kaliner, M.A. and Lemanske, R. Rhinitis and asthma. *JAMA*, 1992, 268, 2807–2829.
38. Shapiro, G. The role of nasal airway obstruction in sinus disease and facial development. *J. Allergy Clin. Immunol.*, 1988, 82, 935–940.
39. Bernstein, I.L. and Storms, W.W. Practice parameters for allergy diagnostic testing. Joint Task Force on Practice Parameters for the Diagnosis and Treatment of Asthma. The American Academy of Allergy, Asthma and Immunology and the American College of Allergy, Asthma, and Immunology. *Ann. Allergy Asthma Immunol.*, 1995, 75, 543.
40. Malm, L., Gerth van Wijk, R., and Bachert, C. Guidelines for nasal provocations withaspects on nasal patency, airflow, and airflow resistance. International Committee on Objective Assessment of the Nasal Airways, International Rhinologic Society. *Rhinology*, 2000, 38, 1–6.
41. Clarke, R.W. and Jones, A.S. The limitation of peak nasal flow measurement. *Clin. Otolaryngol.*, 1994, 19, 502–504.
42. Solomon, W.R., Burge, H.A., and Boise, J.R. Exclusion of particulate allergens by window air conditioners. *J. Allergy Clin. Immunolol.*, 1980, 65, 305–308.
43. Wood, R.A., Johnson, E.F., Van Natta, M.L., Chen, P.H., and Eggleston, P.A. A placebo-controlled trial of a HEPA air cleaner in the treatment of cat allergy. *Am. J. Respir. Crit. Care Med.*, 1998, 158(1), 115–120.
44. Simons, K.S. and Simons, F.E.R. H1-Receptor antagonists: pharmacokoinetics and clinical pharmacology. In Simons, F.E.R., Ed. *Histamine and H1-Receptor Antagonists in Allergy Disease*. New York: Marcel Dekker. 1996, 175–214.
45. Gengo, F.M. and Manning, C. A review of the effects of antihistamines on mentalprocesses related to automobile driving. *Allergy Clin. Immunolol.*, 1990, 186, 1034–1039.
46. Anonymous. Astelin (azelastine hydrochloride) nasal spray product insert (Rev.10/96).
47. Van Cauwenberge, P., Bachert, C., Passalacqua, G. et al. Consensus statement on the treatment of allergy rhinitis. *Allergy*, 2000, 55, 116–134.
48. Pauwels, R. Mode of action of corticosteroids in asthma and rhinitis. *Clin. Allergy.*, 1986, 16, 251–258.
49. Corren, J. Allergic rhinitis: treating the adult. *J. Allergy Clin. Immunol.*, 2000, 105, S611–S615.
50. LaForce, C. Use of nasal steroids in managing allergic rhinitis. *J. Allergy Clin. Immunol.*, 1999, 103, S388–S394.
51. Kaiser, H.B., Findlay, S.R., Georgitis, J.W. et al. The anticholinergic agent, ipratropiumbromide, is useful in treatment of rhinorrhea associated with perennial allergicrhinitis. *Allergy Asthma Proc.*, 1998, 19, 23–29.
52. Donnely, A.L., Glass, M., Minkwitz, M.C., and Casale, T.B. The leukotriene D4-receptorantagonist, ICI 204, 219, relieves symptoms of acute seasonal allergic rhinitis. *Am. J. Respir. Crit. Care Med.*, 1995, 151, 1734–1739.
53. Meltzer, E.O., Malmstrom, K., Lu, S. et al. Concomitant montelukast and loaratadine as treatment for seasonal allergic rhinitis: a randomized, placebo-controlled clinical trial. *J. Allergy Clin. Immunolol.*, 2000, 105, 917–922.
54. Casale, T., Condemi, J., LaForce, C. et al. Effect of omalizumab on symptoms of seasonal allergic rhinitis: a randomized controlled trial. *JAMA*, 2001, 286, 2956–2967.
55. Bernstein, R.A., Nicklas, R., Greenberger, P. et al. Practice parameter for allergen immunotherapy. *J. Allergy Clin. Immunol.*, 1996, 341, 468–475.
56. Weber, R.W. Immunotherapy with allergens. *JAMA*, 1997, 278, 1881–1887.

57. Jacobsen, L. Preventative allergy treatment. *Clin. Exp. Allergy*, 1996, 26, 80–85.
58. Norman, P.S. and Van Metre, T.E., Jr. The safety of allergenic immunotherapy. *J. Allergy. Clin. Immunol.*, 1990, 85, 522–525.
59. Adkinson, N.F. Drug allergy. In Middleton, E. et al., Eds. *Allergy Principles and Practice*, 5th ed. St. Louis: Mosby, 1998, 1679–1694.
60. International Rheumatic Fever Study Group. Allergic reactions to long-term benzathine penicillin prophylaxis for rheumatic fever. *Lancet*, 1991, 337, 1308–1310.
61. Parker, C.W., deWeck, A.L., Kern, M. et al. The preparation and some properties of penicillenic acid derivatives relevant to penicillin hypersensitivity. *J. Exp. Med.*, 1962, 115, 803–819.
62. Levine, B.B. and Ovary, Z. Studies on the mechanism of the formulation of the penicillin antigen. *J. Exp. Med.*, 1961, 114, 875–904.
63. Levine, B.B. and Redmond, A.P. Minor haptenic determinant-specific regions of penicillin hypersensitivity in man. *Int. Arch. Allergy Appl. Immunol.*, 1969, 35, 445–455.
64. Mendelson, L.M. Adverse reactions to B-lactam antibiotics. *Immunol. Allergy Clin. North Am.*, 1998, 18, 745–757.
65. Solensky, R. and Mendelson, L.M. Systemic reactions to antibiotics. *Immunol. Allergy Clin. North Am.*, 2001, 21, 679–697.
66. Kemp, S.F. and Lockey, R.F. Anaphylaxis: a review of causes and mechanisms. *J. Allergy Clin. Immunol.*, 2002, 110, 341–348.
67. Kemp, S.F. Anaphylaxis: current concepts in pathophysiology, diagnosis, and management. *Immunol Allergy Clin. North Am.*, 2001, 21, 611–634.
68. Joint Task Force on Practice Parameters. The diagnosis and management of anaphylaxis. *J. Allergy Clin. Immunol.*, 1998, 101, S465–S528.
69. Sampson, H.A., Mendelson, L., and Rosen, J.P. Fatal and near fatal anaphylactic reactions to foods in children and adolescents. *New Engl. J. Med.*, 1992, 327, 380–384.
70. Lieberman, P. Distinguishing anaphylaxis from other serious disorders. *J. Resp. Dis.*, 1995, 16, 411–420.
71. Yocum, M.W., Buttterfield, J.H., Klein, J.S. et al. Epidemiology of anaphylaxis in Olmsted County. A patient population based study. *J. Allergy Clin. Immunol.*, 1999, 104, 452–456.
72. Brown, A.F.T., McKinnon, D., and Chu, K. Emergency department anaphylaxis. A review of 142 patients in a single year. *J. Allergy Clin. Immunol.*, 2001, 108(5), 861–866.
73. Kemp, S.F., Lockey, R.F., Wolf, B.L., and Lieberman, P. Anaphylaxis: a review of 266 cases. *Arch. Intern. Med.*, 1995, 155, 1749–1754.
74. Lieberman, P. Anaphylaxis: guidelines for prevention and management. *J. Resp. Dis.*, 1995, 16, 456–462.
75. Simons, F.E.R., Roberts, J.R., Gu, X., and Simons, K.J. Epinephrine absorption in children with a history of anaphylaxis. *J. Allergy Clin. Immunol.*, 1998, 101, 33–37.
76. Lin, R.Y., Schwartz, L.B., Curry, A. et al. Histamine and tryptase levels in patients with acute allergic reactions: an emergency department based study. *J. Allergy Clin. Immunol.*, 2000, 106, 65–71.
77. Simons, F.E.R., Gu, X., and Simons, K.J. Epinephrine absorption in adults: intramuscular versus subcutaneous injection. *J. Allergy Clin. Immunol.*, 2001, 108, 871–873.

12 Caring for Children with Syndromic Features

Joann N. Bodurtha, Walter E. Nance, and David N. Madgy

The most basic principle of lateral thinking is that any particular way of looking at things is only one from among many other possible ways.

Edward de Bono, in *Lateral Thinking: Creativity Step by Step*

CONTENTS

INTRODUCTION

We see what we know. An important component of the genetic approach to otolaryngology is an enhanced sensitivity to distinctive clinical features that may define a specific syndrome. The ever expanding array of new syndromes being identified and understanding of the molecular bases of birth defects and genetic diseases require every specialist to stay up to date. All otolaryngologists are encouraged to develop a collegial referral network for genetic evaluation and syndrome identification.

Children with complex syndromes are often best managed by interdisciplinary teams. This chapter's goal is to bridge the gap for the majority of otolaryngologists who do not see a consistent variety of children with syndromic features. We emphasize a set of key points to improve recognition and care of children with syndromic features, review variations in the physical exam of the head and neck, describe significant new developments in syndrome identification and genetics, provide a brief list of major complications, suggest some measures to improve family-centered care, and provide a list of resources for additional information.

BACKGROUND

Syndromes and birth defects are individually rare and collectively common. A syndrome is a particular set of anomalies that repeatedly occurs in a consistent pattern. More than 150,000 children are born with recognizable birth defects and syndromes annually in the United States. Congenital anomalies are the leading cause of infant mortality in the postneonatal period.[1] Genetically influenced conditions have been estimated to account for over one third of pediatric admissions[2] and approximately one fifth of pediatric deaths in intensive care units.[3] Discoveries derived from mapping of the human genome are likely to increase diagnostic and treatment capabilities for a wide array of genetic conditions.

KEY POINTS TO IMPROVE RECOGNITION AND CARE

- Take a family history in every patient. Ask about consanguinity, early deaths, and occurrence of similar and related conditions in first-degree relatives individually (e.g., syncope, sudden death, or drowning in a deaf child with prolonged QT interval).
- Avoid reassuring a family about "little" chance of a recurrence unless you know the underlying genetic or other etiologic mechanism.
- Consider referral to a geneticist, especially if multiple consultants have seen the child for a variety of problems.
- Remember that external anomalies may be correlated with internal malformations (e.g., single central incisor and holoprosencephaly, severe micrognathia and glossoptosis, or congenital heart defects in Down syndrome).
- Train your instincts so that you can trust your assessment that a child looks distinctive.
- Use person-first, family-centered language. Avoid using terms such as "FLK," "dwarf case," or "mongolism." The Golden Rule of personal respect is a useful guide in working with families.
- Diagnosis is not complete until the etiology has been established.

VARIATIONS IN PHYSICAL EXAMINATION OF THE HEAD AND NECK

Accurate physical assessment, especially of infants, is essential for identifying those who will need more thorough examination, medical or support services, and family counseling. A dysmorphic feature is an abnormally developed body component that can be measured and/or characterized. The ability to appreciate the broad range of human variation while distinguishing the truly unusual requires ongoing attention to the physical examination.

FAMILY HISTORY

Family history questions should include: any relatives with features of any syndrome being considered in the child's ethnic background, complications of pregnancy, and potential presence of consanguinity. Ask directly about the following genetic conditions:

- Blindness or nightblindness
- Brain malformations

- Cleft lip and palate
- Congenital heart disease
- Deafness
- Epilepsy
- Kidney disease
- Mental retardation
- Recurrent sycope or sudden death
- Sickle cell disease
- Cutaneous or pigmentary abnormalties

Also ask the more general question, "Do any illnesses or conditions run in the family?" Then ask about the health status of all first-degree relatives individually.

MINOR OR SUBTLE ANOMALIES

Minor or subtle anomalies (e.g., preauricular skin tag, a couple of café au lait spots, and flat occiput) are minor physical defects that occur in fewer than 4% of children. The presence of three or more of these dysmorphic features in the absence of an explanatory diagnosis (e.g., flattened features secondary to oligohydramnios with amniotic fluid leak) warrants consideration of chromosome analysis. The presence of three or more minor anomalies, nearly 50% of which involve the head and face, has been associated with a 20% risk for the presence of a major birth defect.[4]

A child may appear striking because of disproportion or because a feature or features are particularly distinctive. The presence of certain clear-cut facial birth defects, such as cleft lip or a missing external ear, should stimulate the examiner to scrutinize the face more closely because additional abnormalities are more likely. Knowledgeable pattern recognition is a skill developed by paying attention to the details of every child's exam and by review of resource materials that characterize distinctive syndromes.[5–8] Conscious comparison of one side of the face and body to the other side can reveal significant asymmetries of growth associated with underlying structural problems or intrauterine influences. Symmetrical anomalies tend to be of genetic etiology, whether benign familial traits or significant syndromes.

MEASUREMENT TABLES

Measurement tables for physical features (e.g., canthal index, ear length, mouth size) are available.[5,9] Measurements are useful in supporting the "gestalt" observation that a particular feature is disproportionate. They are also useful in assessing possibly familial traits, such as large head and small ears. Documentation of measurements in infancy is imperative for assessing growth or its deficiency in later childhood.

Measurement of the head circumference, palpation of the sutures and fontanels, and description of the overall facial shape and proportion should be documented in every infant. Examination of the scalp for defects, which may be seen in infants with trisomy 13, and the neck for webbing, which may be seen in children with Turner syndrome or Noonan syndrome, is important. Because the infant's forehead is generally fairly straight, sloping back or protruding (usually called bossing) should be noted.

SPECIFIC EXAMINATION FEATURES

Paired organs should be systematically compared side to side. With the head positioned straight on the neck, each ear should be examined for setting, configuration, and the presence of tags, pits, bronchial clefts and creases. Ears are considered low set if the top part of the helix does not touch an imaginary line drawn across the canthi of the eyes. The ears are measured in their longest axis and compared with data in standard tables. Small ears (2.5 cm or smaller) are often seen in children with Down syndrome.

The eye exam deserves attention, with initial focus on complete development of the structures. Specifically, are the brows, lids, lashes, irises, pupils, and sclera present and symmetric? The slant of the eyes is described by the location of the outer canthus relative to the inner canthus, so children with Down syndrome often have upslanted eyes with epicanthus, a fold of skin over the inner canthus. Missing pieces are among the most important physical findings to note about the eye of the newborn. The presence of brows and lashes with intact lid margins should first be assessed. Whenever possible, usually in a darkened room, spontaneous eye opening and movements should be observed for the presence of any paralysis. Any alteration in bilaterally intact irises and red reflexes should be noted. A canthal index ≥ 1.95 is consistent with a diagnosis of Waardenburg syndrome.

Most newborns have low nasal bridges and relative midface hypoplasia compared with older children. Distinctive nasal findings to be noted include asymmetric nares and a notched or broad nasal tip. Clefting should be carefully examined for its boundaries. The presence of only a nasal tip and no nasal bridge may indicate underdeveloped choanae, possible warfarin exposure, or a genetic skeletal condition.

The mouth region is distinctive in a variety of syndromes. The philtrum may be flattened and elongated with a thin vermilion border in children with fetal alcohol syndrome. The posterior palate, especially the uvula, and the movement and any disproportion of the tongue should be noted. A relatively large tongue may be seen in children with Down syndrome, hypothyroidism, and the macrosomia condition Beckwith–Wiedemann syndrome in which hypoglycemia, umbilical hernia, and Wilms tumor may occur. Micrognathia may be associated with the posteriorly displaced tongue and U-shaped cleft palate of Pierre Robin sequence.

NEW DEVELOPMENTS IN SYNDROME IDENTIFICATION

22q11.2

The broad range of findings encompassed by 22q11.2 deletion syndrome, including diGeorge, velocardiofacial, conotruncal anomaly face syndromes, and some patients with autosomal dominant Opitz G/BBB syndrome, has been described over the past 10 years.[10] Features vary from patient to patient, but include some combination of the following:

- Conotruncal cardiac anomalies
- Palatal defects including overt and submucosal cleft palate and/or velopharyngeal incompetence
- Thymic hypoplasia or aplasia
- T-cell abnormalities
- Learning disabilities
- Some mild distinctive facial features

Feeding difficulties and short stature are also common. Specific testing by fluorescent *in situ* hybridization (FISH) of a chromosome sample is currently the optimal diagnostic technique. The autosomal dominant nature of this condition in many families, as well as the clinical importance of diagnosing immune and cardiac problems early, supports clarifying family history, doing a complete physical exam, and asking for a medical genetics evaluation in any child with two or more of the preceding findings.

CRANIOSYNOSTOSIS

Although the current recommendation that children sleep on their backs to avoid SIDS may have resulted in a recent increase in cranial deformations, asymmetry of the head is frequently associated with craniosynostosis on a genetic basis. Mutations of fibroblast growth factors have been found in classic syndromes with craniosynostosis, often with additional involvement of the limbs and palate, such as Apert, Crouzon, Jackson–Weiss, and Pfeiffer syndromes. In addition, isolated craniosynostosis — if not due to other conditions, such as hyperthyroidism, a severe anemia like thalassemia, or a metabolic condition such as a mucopolysaccharidosis — may also be associated with gene changes in fibroblast growth factors.[11]

Children with significantly asymmetric heads need assessment for torticollis and consideration of skull radiographs and CT or other scanning, a complete physical exam, and a careful family history in order to define syndromes and address family questions about recurrence risk. Complications of craniosynostosis can include

- Increased intracranial pressure
- Visual disturbances
- Stridor
- Apnea
- Malocclusion
- Airway problems
- Increased ear infections
- Hearing problems
- Psychosocial concerns

CONNEXIN

After years of recognizing that an autosomal recessive pattern of inheritance was likely in many children with congenital sensorineural hearing loss, mutations involving the gene encoding the gap junction protein, connexin 26, have been found to be the most important single cause of genetic hearing loss in European and American populations. Rapid advances in molecular biology have revealed that the family of gap junction proteins is indispensable for various cellular functions and involved in a variety of conditions, including x-linked Charcot–Marie–Tooth syndrome and some cataract and heart malformations, as well as connexin 26 hearing loss.

The carrier rate for mutations in connexin 26 is about 3%, similar to that for cystic fibrosis. In the Ashkenazi Jewish population, the carrier rate is about 4%. Clinical studies have shown that the recessive hearing loss can vary from mild to profound, even within the same sibship. Other mutations in the same gene have also been found to be associated with dominant nonsyndromic hearing loss, and many of these individuals exhibit dermatologic abnormalities. With earlier identification of hearing loss by newborn screening and the availability of genetic testing, families have the opportunity to consider proper audiologic, medical, educational, and genetic counseling.[12]

WAARDENBURG

Waardenburg syndrome is a group of autosomal pigmentary auditory syndromes caused by physical absence of melanocytes from the skin, hair, eyes, or the stria vascularis of the cochlea. Individuals with this condition may have patchy, abnormal pigmentation of the eyes, hair, and skin and varying degrees of sensorineural hearing loss. At least four types of Waardenburg syndrome have now been described resulting from mutations on at least eight different loci on the basis of the patients' clinical patterns and underlying gene changes:

- Waardenburg syndrome, type 1, is caused by loss function mutations in the PAX3 gene at chromosomal location 2q35. Dystopia canthorum (lateral displacement of the inner canthi) is the hallmark of this type.
- Type 2 is heterogeneous with a minority of persons heterozygous for mutations in the human microphthalmia gene on chromosome 3p. Heterochromia iridum is an important marker in type 2.
- Type 3 may involve gene changes in PAX3 on chromosome 2q and have abnormalities of the arms and myelomeningocele.
- Type 4, also known as Shah–Waardenburg syndrome with Hirschsprung disease, is autosomal recessive and can be caused by mutations in the genes for endothelin-3 or one of its receptors, EDNRB. Gastrointestinal abnormalities including gastrointestinal dysmobility and chronic constipation also can be seen in Types 1 and 2 Waardenburg syndrome.

The first three types appear to be dominant. All types show marked variability, even within families. Even when a mutation is found, the severity of findings cannot be reliably predicted.[13]

Cleft Lip and Palate

Hundreds of syndromes have been described in which cleft lip and palate are frequently found.[6] However, the majority of children with cleft lip and palate have nonsyndromic forms without obvious other birth defects. Genetic factors are likely to be involved in syndromic and nonsyndromic cleft lip and palate. Inheritance is generally considered to involve multiple genes with internal variations determining fractions of genetic risk. Some pedigrees are clearly due to single gene changes consistent with autosomal dominant or recessive inheritance.

Much recent research has focused on genetic susceptibility changes — for example, polymorphisms in transforming growth factor-alpha found in higher frequency in some children with cleft lip with or without cleft palate. Other gene changes, not yet known, and environmental exposures, most also yet unknown, also need to be present in order for the embryo to have a cleft. Certain drugs are clearly teratogens, including ethanol, retinoids, and folate antagonists. Thus, the cumulative risk for clefting is a combination of environmental and genetic factors, including their interaction. The fusion of palatal shelves and labial buds is a multistep process. The newborn with clefting needs a full physical examination with a detailed family and pregnancy history to address the syndromic or nonsyndromic basis and recurrence risk.[14]

Superficial Siderosis

There is growing recognition of the importance of chronic subarachnoid hemorrhage as a cause for progressive high-frequency hearing loss. Hemoglobin breakdown products specifically damage the 1st and 6th cranial nerves. The tonotopic localization of high-frequency sound fibers within the auditory nerve accounts for the high frequency loss. The condition can be diagnosed using a T2-weighted MRI. Several genetic forms of syndromic and nonsyndromic deafness are known or suspected to share this pathogenic mechanism.[15]

MEASURES TO IMPROVE FAMILY-CENTERED CARE

Recognition that the daily and ultimate responsibility for a child's health resides with the family should guide the practice. The reality of short hospital stays and least restrictive environments means that children with complex health concerns live in bedrooms and schoolrooms more than hospital environments. This requires effective and supportive communication and focus on the optimal education of families about their child's health condition and care. The health care professional needs to be guided first by effective listening to the parents and child's concerns. The incorporation of child life specialists and the interdisciplinary teams of occupational, speech, physical, and other therapists in the child's in-hospital care support the continuity of effort to optimize a child's well-being.

Knowledge of community resources is vital for sustaining continuity of care. Supporting a family's desire to network with other helpful parents can enhance care. Information can help families make the best choices.

RESOURCES

The Internet has enhanced families' abilities to access information. Not all families access information well, and the reliability of resource materials is quite variable. The following resources have a history of concern about presenting balanced information, distinguishing opinions from established medical evidence, and working collaboratively with families and health care providers. We have found it helpful to encourage families to share with us information they are reading and to work together to find reliable information to guide a child's health care. We remind families to use reliable sites and to be wary of advertising and unproven therapies.

- The Alliance (formerly Alliance of Genetic Support Groups) http://www.geneticalliance. org
- *Exceptional Parent Magazine* http://www.familyeducation.com
- Family Voices http://www.familyvoices.org
- Genetics Education Center, University of Kansas Medical Center http://www.kumc.edu/gec/
- March of Dimes http://www.modimes.org
- The National Genome Research Institute http://www.nhgri.nih.gov/
- National Organization for Rare Disorders http://www.rarediseases.org
- Office of Genetics and Disease Prevention http://www.cdc.gov/genetics/
- Woodbine House Book Publishers, Publishers of the Special Needs Collection http://www.woodbinehouse.com

REFERENCES

1. Guyer, B. et al. Annual summary of vital statistics–1998. *Pediatrics*, 104, 1999, 1229–1246.
2. McCandless, S.E. et al. The burden of genetic disease on inpatient care in a children's hospital. *Am. J. Hum. Genet.* 74, 2004, 121–127.
3. Cunniff, C. et al. Contribution of heritable disorders to mortality in the pediatric intensive care unit. *Pediatrics*, 95(5), 1995, 678–681.
4. Leppig, K.A. et al. Predictive value of minor anomalies. Part 1: association with major malformations. *J. Pediatrics*, 110(4), 1987, 531–537.
5. Jones, K.L. *Smith's Recognizable Patterns of Human Malformation*. Philadelphia: W.B. Saunders, 1997.
6. Gorlin, R.J., Cohen, M.M., and Levin, L.S. *Syndromes of the Head and Neck*, 4th ed. New York: Oxford University Press, 2001.
7. Winter, R.M. and Baraitser, M. *London Dysmorphology Database and Photo Library*. 3rd ed. Oxford: Oxford Electronic Publishing, 1995.
8. Bankier, A. et al. *POSSUM: Pictures of Standard Syndromes and Undiagnosed Malformations*, 4th ed. Melbourne: Computer Power Pty Ltd. and the Murdoch Institute for Research into Birth Defects, 1995.
9. Hall, J.G., Forster–Iskenius, U.G., and Allanson, J.E. *Handbook of Normal Physical Measurements*. Oxford: Oxford Medical Publications, 1989.
10. McDonald-McGinn, D. et al. The 22q11.2 deletion: screening, diagnostic work-up, and outcome of results; report on 181 patients. *Genet. Testing*, 1, 1997, 99–108.

11. Renier, D. et al. Fibroblast growth factor receptor 3 mutation in nonsyndromic coronal synostosis: clinical spectrum, prevalence and surgical outcome. *J. Neurosurg.*, 92, 2000, 631.

12. Cohn, E.S. and Kelley, P.M. Clinical phenotype and mutations in connexin 26 (DFNB/GJB2), the most common cause of childhood hearing loss. *Am. J. Med. Genet.*, 89, 1999, 130–136.

13. Read, A.P. and Newton, V.E. Waardenburg syndrome. *J. Med. Genet.*, 34, 1997, 656–665.

14. Houdayer, C.l. and Bahuau, M. Orofacial cleft defects: inference from nature and nurture. *Ann. Genet.*, 41, 1998, 89–117.

15. Dodson, K.M. et al. Superficial siderosis: a potentially important cause of genetic as well as non-genetic deafness. *Amer. J. Med. Genet.* 130A, 2004, 22–25.

13 Caring for Children with Cancer

Paul A. Pitel and Cynthia A. Gauger

Much wisdom I have learned from my teachers, more from my colleagues, from my pupils most of all.

Maimonides

CONTENTS

INTRODUCTION

Although childhood cancers are uncommon, the otolaryngologist will be confronted relatively commonly with children for whom cancer is in the differential diagnosis. Childhood cancer has an incidence of approximately 17.6 per 100,000 children per year below the age of 15.[1] Although 5% of the malignant neoplasms arise in the head and neck region, 25% of pediatric malignancies will ultimately involve the head and neck.[2–4] Despite tremendous advances in the diagnosis, treatment, and cure of these disorders, cancer remains the second leading cause of childhood mortality, following only trauma.[1] Clearly, recognition of these diseases, timely diagnosis, and collaboration with pediatric oncologists is necessary to provide these children with optimal therapy with minimal long-term sequelae.

OVERVIEW OF PEDIATRIC ONCOLOGY

In 1998, only 12,400 children and adolescents younger than age 20 were diagnosed with cancer in the United States.[1] This relative rarity of pediatric cancer, combined with its devastating effects on the child and family, led to interinstitutional cooperation in the early 1960s. The development of national protocols for the evaluation and treatment of these children and the application of transitional research to their problems resulted in extraordinary progress over the ensuing decades. Today, approximately 70% of children in the U.S. are enrolled in clinical trials, and it is estimated that greater than 70% of all children diagnosed with cancer will enjoy long-term, disease-free survival.[1] It is therefore incumbent upon all health care providers to make these advances available to their patients.

The Children's Oncology Group (COG) has been the single, unified vehicle for pediatric cancer trial in the U.S. since 2000 (http://www.childrensoncologygroup.org). Arising from four preceding organizations, it has permitted the focus of expertise in research, diagnosis, and therapeutic intervention. Many diseases now require multimodality therapy — surgery, chemotherapy, and radiation — to optimize treatment results. Laboratory studies once available in only a few sites are now nationally accessible. Central pathology review can help assure appropriate diagnosis and staging, and national safety monitoring helps assure the safety and efficacy of newer treatment approaches.

HEAD AND NECK MALIGNANCIES

Primary malignant head and neck tumors in pediatrics make up approximately 5% of childhood cancer. The spectrum of malignancies of the head and neck in children and adolescents is different from that seen in adults and the elderly.[5–8] Squamous cell carcinoma is essentially unknown in children; nasopharyngeal carcinoma is rare. The more common primary malignant tumors include lymphomas, thyroid carcinoma, rhabdomyosarcoma, and retinoblastoma. Other malignant head and neck tumors that may present include salivary gland neoplasms, malignant teratomas, and other sarcomas (Table 13.1). It is important to remember that the age of the child is an important consideration in the initial evaluation because some malignancies are far more common in very young infants and children and others are more common in adolescents and young adults (Table 13.2).

CLINICAL PRESENTATION

LYMPHADENOPATHY

Lymphadenopathy is a common complaint and physical finding in children and may be the cause of an initial referral to an otolaryngologist. Although potential presentation varies widely, a lymph node is considered enlarged if it is more than 10 mm in any dimension. The two major exceptions to this guideline are epitrochlear nodes, which should not exceed 5 mm, and inguinal nodes, which may be normal up to 15 mm.[9]

The diagnostic work-up for lymphadenopathy may involve antibiotic therapy, a complete blood count (CBC) with differential, and a chest radiograph to exclude mediastinal adenopathy. In general, if a lymph node is unresponsive to antibiotics and continues to grow over a 2-week period, it should be biopsied. Within 2 to 3 weeks, most noncancerous nodes should begin to regress. Not all such nodes are malignant; diseases such as TB, viral and fungal infections, and atypical mycobacteria should be considered (see Chapter 16).

TABLE 13.1
**Types of Malignancies Identified in the Head and Neck
in the Pediatric Population**

Lymphomas
Hodgkin's lymphoma
Non-Hodgkin's lymphoma
Rhabdomyosarcoma
Thyroid carcinoma
Nasopharyngeal carcinoma
Salivary gland neoplasms
Neuroblastoma
Malignant teratomas
Other sarcomas
Osteosarcomas
Chondrosarcomas
Fibrosarcoma
Malignant fibrous histiocytoma
Synovial sarcoma
Angiosarcoma
Liposarcoma
Malignant schwannoma
Leiomyosarcoma
Unclassified sarcomas

TABLE 13.2
Predominant Pediatric Head and Neck Tumors by Age

Newborn (<1 year)	Infancy (1–3 years)	Childhood (3–11 years)	Adolescent and young adult (12–21 years)
Retinoblastoma	Retinoblastoma	Rhabdomyosarcoma	Lymphoma
Neuroblastoma	Neuroblastoma	Lymphoma	Soft tissue sarcoma
Rhabdomyosarcoma	Rhabdomyosarcoma		

The need for lymph node biopsy is particularly suggested by the following:

• A persistently enlarging node after 2 to 3 weeks of appropriate coverage
• Nodes that do not regress after 5 to 6 weeks, particularly if associated with fever, weight loss, night sweats, or hepatosplenomegaly
• Enlarging nodes associated with an abnormal chest radiograph

OTHER MASSES

Awareness of the major malignancies of the head and neck in children is necessary when discriminating among the potential differential diagnosis of a tumor. Asymmetric physical findings should always be viewed cautiously, even in a child. An enlarging mass — essentially, regardless of site of origin — demands a careful and complete evaluation. Unless the mass or node is clearly of typical infectious origin, appropriate imaging studies and, probably, a biopsy will be needed. Although many head and neck masses are of noninfectious embryologic origin (Chapter 17), it is incumbent upon assessing physicians to arrive at an accurate diagnosis in a timely manner. Malig-

TABLE 13.3
Symptoms and Signs of Childhood Cancer Mimicking
Normal Childhood Illnesses: Initial Evaluation for Cancer,
Usually Not Warranted

Symptom (sign)	Possible malignancy
Headache, nausea, vomiting	Brain tumor
Febrile, seizure	Brain tumor
Earache	STS
Rhinitis	STS
Epistaxis	Leukemia, STS
Pharyngitis	STS
Adenopathy	Neuroblastoma, thyroid, lymphoma, leukemia

Note: STS = soft tissue sarcoma.

TABLE 13.4
Unusual Symptoms or Signs of Cancer Warranting Immediate Evaluation

Symptoms/signs	Evaluation	Possible malignancy
	Brain	
Headache, vomiting early in A.M., dilated pupil, papilledema, afibrile, seizures, paralysis	CT scan, MR	Brain tumor
	Eyes	
White reflex, proptosis, intraorbital hemorrhage	Ophthalmology evaluation	Retinoblastoms, LCH, RMS, neuroblastoma
	Ears	
Bulging mass ear canal, mastoid tenderness, swelling, puffy face, and neck	Imagery, ENT evaluation	LCH, RMS
	Pharyngeal mass	
Bulging, painful pharyngeal mass	ENT, dental evaluation	LCH, NHL, NBL, osteosarcoma

Note: LCH = Langerhan's cell histiocytosis; RMS = rhabdomyosarcoma; ENT = ear, nose, and throat; NHL = non-Hodgkin's lymphoma; NBL = neuroblastoma.

nancies, unfortunately, do arise most commonly from muscle (rhabdomyosarcoma); nasopharynx (nasopharyngeal carcinoma); retina (retinoblastoma); connective tissue (soft tissue sarcomas); bone (osteosarcoma and Ewing's sarcoma); salivary gland (microepidermoeal carcinoma); and thyroid (thyroid carcinoma) (Table 13.3 and Table 13.4).

TISSUE SAMPLING

Optimal treatment for the child with cancer can begin only after the tumor has been accurately diagnosed and the extent of disease precisely defined. Before any tissue is obtained for pathologic study it has become increasingly important that the surgeon work in a collaborative fashion with the pediatric oncologist and pathologist to discuss the site to biopsy, appropriate lymph node sampling, the amount of tissue needed, and the specimens to be obtained. Excisional and incisional biopsies are standard techniques for obtaining diagnostic material with minimal risk of residual scarring. The use of ultrasound-guided cutting needle core biopsy of neck masses is established in the pediatric population.[10] This procedure offers the advantage of a tissue core rather than cytology alone from fine needle aspiration (FNA) and may be performed under local anesthesia. In contrast, an excisional or incisional biopsy yields a greater amount of tissue with fewer artifactual distortions; although anesthesia is generally required, this is often the selected diagnostic technique.[11]

Assurance of an adequate tumor specimen for analysis must be verified with the pathology team. Limited sampling of surrounding inflammatory tissue or biopsies of central necrosis, for example, may yield false negative results. Frozen section analysis can help reduce this potential for false negative sampling or inadequate specimen, with the understanding that the definitive diagnosis will be based on permanent sections. Regardless of the particular biopsy technique, routine handling of childhood cancer tissue for optimal pathologic and biologic studies, as prescribed by the COG, has contributed to significant improvements in diagnostic accuracy. Although many local institutions lack the laboratory facilities to perform many of the specialized molecular diagnostics, proper handling of tissue by prescribed protocols (e.g., fresh, viable tumor tissue, short-term culture, or fresh frozen tissue) and shipment to central reference laboratories provide access to necessary diagnostic and prognostic studies.

In order to further limit the potential for false negative or inconclusive biopsy results, tissue must be collected fresh. The single most important principle in the collection of cancer tissue in the operating room is that tissue must *not* be immediately placed into fixative. Fixed tissue has limited utility for most molecular genetic diagnostic procedures and cell cultures, and precludes reliable fluorescence-activated cell sorter (FACS) analysis. Furthermore, tissue should be placed in 0.9% saline and immediately transported, on ice, to the surgical pathology laboratory. Once fresh tissue has been secured, a representative tissue block will be submitted for formalin fixation, paraffin embedding, and routine hematoxylin and eosin (H&E) staining.

In addition to conventional histopathology and immunohistochemistry, many other specialized procedures may be necessary for accurate diagnosis, prognostic subgrouping, and patient protocol eligibility. Immunophenotyping by flow cytometry is indicated for suspected lymphomas and classification of leukemias. Cytogentic analysis is critical in many tumors, including lymphoid malignancies, neuroblastoma, rhabdomyosarcoma, Ewing's sarcoma, and nonlymphoid leukemias. DNA ploidy is important prognostially in leukemias and neuroblastoma. Oncogene amplification studies are critical in neuroblastoma. New molecular genetic methods (fluorescent *in situ* hybridization (FISH), *in situ* hybridization, and reverse transcriptase–polymerase chain reaction (rt–PCR) are also available for optimal diagnostic evaluation.[11]

EVALUATION

Once an accurate pathologic diagnosis has been made, it is critical to establish the correct stage of a tumor. Combination therapy protocols are based on the stage of the tumor, which determines such factors in treatment as use and intent of radiotherapy and intensity of chemotherapy. Noninvasive imaging techniques may include plain films, computed tomography (CT), and/or magnetic resonance imaging (MRI) of the primary tumor. The preferred imaging study is generally based on the presumed tumor site, factoring the relative strengths of each imaging modality (Chapter 7). CT evaluation of the chest and abdomen and radionuclide bone scans are often necessary to detect metastatic disease. Cerebrospinal fluid must be examined for tumor cells if there is invasion of tumor through the base of the skull and in cases of parmeningeal rhabdomyosarcoma lymphomas and leukemias. Bone marrow examination is necessary for specific tumors with potential for bone marrow metastases such as soft tissue sarcomas, leukemias, and lymphomas. Identification of extracellular tumor markers such as catecholamines, serum ferritin, and lactate dehydrogenase (LDH) may be helpful in establishing the diagnosis, defining prognostic subgroups, or permitting tumor monitoring.

TREATMENT

A multimodality treatment approach, which integrates surgery and radiotherapy to control local disease with combination chemotherapy to eradicate systemic disease, has become the standard approach to treating most childhood cancers with the goal of curing the patient of his or her cancer.

Surgical considerations are site and tumor specific. Biopsy is required of tumors in all locations, but improvement in response to chemotherapy and radiotherapy has obviated the need in most cases for immediate surgical resection. Occasionally, complete resection of the malignancy with pathologic margins that are free of tumor is possible. However, many head and neck tumors are difficult to approach surgically or are impossible to resect completely without major surgical sequelae. In others, the tumor has metastasized at the time of diagnosis, precluding surgical cure. In many cases, surgical extirpation is not sufficient for cure because of micrometastatic disease.[12,13]

Conventional front-line treatment regimens for most childhood cancers use combination chemotherapy, i.e., multiple anticancer drugs administered in combination regimens at their maximum tolerated dose intensity. Compared with single-agent therapy, combination chemotherapy has achieved much higher complete remission rates as well as long-term remissions and cures. Combination chemotherapy is most often administered in the adjuvant setting to patients without evidence of residual disease or with minimal residual disease after local therapy with surgery or radiation who are at high risk to relapse at metastatic sites.

It is important that adjuvant chemotherapy begin as soon as possible after definitive local therapy; delays may compromise long-term outcome. One strategy to avoid delays is the administration of chemotherapy before definitive local therapy. This approach, called neoadjuvant chemotherapy, may be advantageous in preserving organ function and cosmesis and may improve local control by shrinking the primary tumor, thus making it potentially more amenable to surgical resection or radiotherapy. It may also provide earlier therapy for micrometastases.[4,14–16]

Radiation therapy is also a highly effective treatment modality for many pediatric malignancies. The total dose of radiation for tumor control is tumor specific and depends on target volume. Table 13.5 shows general radiation doses for specific tumors.

COMPLICATIONS

Acute Side Effects

Myelosuppression

An acute toxicity common to many chemotherapy drugs is myelosuppression with the development of severe neutropenia, anemia, and thrombocytopenia. Growth factors such as granulocyte-colony stimulating factor and, less commonly, erythropoietin are integrated in chemotherapy protocols to minimize these toxicities. Despite the use of growth factors, blood product support is frequently required with intensive chemotherapy regimens. In order to prevent transfusion-related graft vs. host disease, which is commonly lethal, all blood products must be irradiated. Leukofiltration is also employed to reduce cytomegalovirus transmission and febrile transfusion reactions.

Epistaxis

A potential complication of myelosuppression in these children is intermittent epistaxis, particularly with platelet counts less than 20,000 per cubic millimeter. This disconcerting sequela can be problematic to manage because any additional mucosal manipulation may induce additional or ongoing bleeding. Most management protocols for myelosuppressive-related epistaxis use minimal tissue trauma with the application of topical decongestants and various organic or manufactured soft material as intranasal packing, if necessary. The best treatment, however, remains the correction of the underlying thrombocytopenia.

TABLE 13.5
General Radiation Doses for Specific Tumors

Tumor	Radiation dose (GY)
Hodgkin's disease	
Radiation therapy alone	36–40
Combined modality	15–25
Rhaddomyosarcoma	40–55
Neuroblastoma	
<12 Months	15
>12 Months	20–5
Histiocytosis	4.5–10.0
Acute lymphoblastic leukemia (central nervous system treatment)	18–24
Medulloblastoma	
Craniospinal	23–40
Posterior fossa	54–55
Nasopharyngeal carcinoma	60–70

Nausea and Vomiting

Chemotherapy-related nausea and vomiting are experienced by almost all cancer patients and should be anticipated. Several effective antiemetics now available, including, among others, ondansetron, dexamethasone, and granisetoron, are routinely employed. Although complete elimination of symptoms may not be possible in all patients, a substantial reduction in symptoms can usually be achieved.

Other Toxicities

Alopecia, orointenstinal mucositis, and allergic and cutaneous reaction are also acute chemotherapy and/or radiation toxicities. Alopecia nearly always completely resolves several months after completion of therapy. Further delays in hair regeneration may be related to radiation location, volume, and dose. Gastrointesinal cell damage from therapy can cause ulcerations in the mucosal lining of the oral cavity extending down into the esophagus. The lesions appear as edematous, erythematous, eroded lesions that are often exquisitely painful. Prevention of infection and treatment of pain are the main objectives in treating digestive tract mucocitis until the ulcerations heal, usually with resolution of the severe neutropenia.

Specific Drug Toxicities

Many drugs have unique toxicities affecting specific organs and tissues. Examples include ototoxitiy from cisplatin, which mandates monitoring baseline and serial audiologic assessments; cardiotoxicity associated with the anthracyclines, which require baseline and serial cardiac function evaluations; neuropathies associated with vincristine and cisplatin requiring routine neurologic assessments; and hemorrhagic cystitis associated with cyclophosphamide and ifosfamide, which is followed by serial urine analysis.

Infections

Infections cause significant morbidity and mortality in children with cancer.[17] Many chemotherapy drugs, in addition to being myelosuppressive, are toxic to the mucosal epithelium, increasing the risk for bacterial and fungal infection. Radiation therapy also contributes to local tissue breakdown and provides potential sites of infection. The otolaryngologist is often asked to provide consultation for head- and neck-related infectious complications. Otitis media in the neutropenic patient may be caused by the usual pathogens, *S. pneumoniae* and *H. influenza*; however, these patients are also susceptible to Gram-positive and Gram-negative bacteria that may have colonized the nasopharynx and oropharynx and require broad spectrum antibiotic coverage.

Immunocompromised patients, — particularly those with an anatomic abnormality of the middle ear or mastoid from radiation sequelae — are at risk for development of mastoiditis. The severely neutropenic patient is at risk for the usual bacterial pathogens as well as the fungal mastoiditis that often requires surgical management for cure. Acute sinusitis in the immunocompromised, severely neutropenic patient remains a therapeutic challenge. A high index of clinical suspicion must be maintained because these patients may lack the classic symptoms. They may present only with prolonged fever, unresponsiveness to broad spectrum antibiotics, and minimal complaints of sinus tenderness or nasal stuffiness.

In addition to bacterial pathogens, fungal pathogens are particularly worrisome in the neutropenic, immunocompromised host. A CT scan and detailed nasopharyngeal examination by the otolaryngologist are critical. Fungal sinusitis caused by Aspergillus or Rhizopus sp. can progress with invasion through the cribriform plate and into the central nervous system. Early tissue sampling and aggressive and repeat surgical debridement of involved tissue is often required in addition to early institution of antifungal therapy. Hyperbaric oxygen therapy has also been reported as effective adjuvant therapy.[18] In addition to these aggressive therapeutic modalities, adequate recovery of the granulocte count is critical for a successful outcome in this group of patients.

LONG-TERM EFFECTS

Because of a child's life expectancy and the particular issues confronting a growing organism, late effects must be of great concern. The tumor may cause significant anatomic abnormalities. Surgical extirpation may cause long-term sequelae, including potential disfigurement in addition to functional deficits.

Chermotherapeutic agents have relatively few direct long-term effects on the head and neck. Vincristine may cause motor nerve problems, but these usually resolve within months. Second malignant neoplasms, particularly nonlymphoid leukemias, are associated with several agents, particularly VM-26, VP16, and the anthracyclines.

Radiation therapy to the head or neck can cause significant problems. Xerostomia is common after oral/pharyngeal radiation. Bone tumors and sarcomas are seen 10 to 20 years after high-dose radiation and occur in the involved field.[19] Patients with bilateral retinoblastoma are at very increased risk for sarcomas within and outside the radiation fields. Developing bone will fail to grow normally after high-dose radiation. The risk for external auditory canal stenosis increases if surgery is followed by radiation therapy.[20]

Most pediatric cancer centers have developed specific clinics to optimize long-term follow-up effects. Referral for such care can be of great benefit to enhance the child's physical and emotional recovery. The goal today must be a child not only medically cured, but also able to assume normal roles in society.

FAMILY ISSUES

The consequences of cancer and its treatment may pose long-term issues for patients and their families. These may include physical, emotional, educational, financial, and insurance problems. In addition, the diagnosis, treatment, and follow-up may cause or exacerbate family problems and have consequences for the siblings. These potential issues must be recognized and are best addressed through a multidisciplinary team approach involving physicians, nurses, social workers, psychologists, clergy, educational professionals, dieticians, and other selected disciplines. These services should be available to all patients and are regularly available in pediatric cancer centers.

Availability of Internet-based information can be a mixed blessing. Excellent resources are available through sites such as The National Cancer Institute (http://www.cancer.gov) and The American Cancer Society (http://www.cancer.org). Unfortunately, many other sites are far less accurate and reputable. In addition, it may be difficult for families to assess accurately how specific approaches or data may apply to their child. The physician should be able to provide guidance for these issues.

It should be recognized that managing pediatric cancer may result in sequelae determined by the specific diagnosis and site of the lesion, the specific therapy required (surgery, chemotherapy, radiation therapy), and the age of the patient. Young children and infants will typically sustain more toxicity from radiation than older children and adolescents because of the growth arrest caused by high-dose radiation. The young, less myelinated brain is also more affected by radiation than more developed brains. The adolescent, on the other hand, may have significant problems dealing with changes in appearance during developmental stages of identification and sexual identity — especially when they live in a society that stresses physical appearance. Sensitivity and awareness of family and cultural concerns is needed to support the child and family optimally through these difficult issues.[21]

CONCLUSIONS

Dramatic improvements in the survival of pediatric patients with cancer rely on the systematic use of therapeutic clinical trials designed through cooperative group, multi-institutional trials. It has been well documented that children on therapeutic protocols in pediatric oncology centers have far better survival and disease-free survival than children treated outside these centers. Today, there are very few indications for making management decisions without, or at least in consultation with, one of these centers. Through it all, the underlying philosophy of caring for children with cancer remains unchanged: remain sensitive to the whole needs of the patient, including his or her family. Diagnostic and management algorithms will undoubtedly continue to evolve. Nonetheless, despite all of the medical advances, pediatric oncology will never cease to remind us, often equally and at once, of our human fragility and our indomitable emotional resilience. The words of a 15th century French folk saying ring as true today as they did over 500 years ago: "To cure sometimes. To relieve often. To comfort always."

REFERENCES

1. Smith, M.A. and Gloeckler Ries, L.A. Childhood cancer: incidence, survival, and mortality. In Pizzo, P., Ed. *Principles and Practice of Pediatric Oncology*, 4th ed. Philadelphia: Lippincott Williams & Wilkins, 2000, 1, 1–12.
2. Josephson, G.D. and Wohl, D. Malignant tumors of the head and neck in children. *Curr. Opin. Otorhinolaryngol. Head Neck Surg.*, 1999, 7(2), 61–67.
3. Cunningham, M.J., Meyers, E.N., and Bluestone, C.D. Malignant tumors of the head and neck in children: a twenty year review. *Int. J. Pediatr. Otorhinolaryngol.*, 1987, 13, 279–292.
4. Green, D.M., Tarbell, N.J., and Shamberger, R.C. Solid tumors of childhood. In DeVita, V.T., Hellman, S., and Rosenburg, S.A., Eds. *Cancer, Principles and Practices of Oncology.* 5th ed. Philadelphia: Lippincott, 1997, 2091–2130.
5. Gadwal, S.R., Gannon, F.H., Fanburg–Smith, J.C., Becoskie, E.M., and Thompson, L.D.R. Primary osteosarcoma of the head and neck in pediatric patients. *Cancer*, 2001, 91(3), 598–605.
6. Vaccani, J.P., Forte, V., de Jong, A.L., and Taylor, G. Ewing's sarcoma of the head and neck in children. Int. *J. Pediatr. Otorhinolaryngol.*, 1999, 48(3), 209–216.
7. Uzel, O., Yoruk, S.O., Sahinler, I., Turkan, S., and Okkan, S. Nasopharyngeal carcinoma in childhood: long-term results of 32 patients. *Radiother. Oncol.*, 2001, 58(2), 137–141.
8. Bentz, B.G., Hughes, A., Ludemann, J.P., and Maddalozzo, J. Masses of the salivary gland region in children. *Arch. Otolaryngol. Head Neck Surg.*, 2000, 126, 1435–1439.

9. Vietti, T.J. and Steuber, C.P. Clinical assessment and differential diagnosis of the child with suspected cancer. In Pizzo, P., Ed. *Principles and Practice of Pediatric Oncology*, 4th ed. Philadelphia: Lippincott Williams & Wilkins, 2000, 7, 149–159.

10. Bain, G., Bearcroft, P.W.P., Berman, L.H., and Grant, J.W. The use of ultrasound-guided cutting-needle biopsy in paediatric neck masses. *Eur. Radiol.*, 2000, 19, 512–515.

11. Triche, T.J. and Sorenson, P.H. Molecular pathology of pediatric malignancies. In Pizzo, P., Ed. *Principles and Practice of Pediatric Oncology*, 4th ed. Philadelphia: Lippincott Williams & Wilkins, 2000, 8, 161–204.

12. Daya, H., Chan, H.S.L., Sirkin, W., and Forte, V. Pediatric rhabdomyosarcoma of the head and neck. Is there a place for surgical management? *Arch. Otolaryngol. Head Neck Surg.*, 2000, 126(4), 468–472.

13. Andrassy, R.J. and Hays, D.M. General principles of surgery. In Pizzo, P., Ed. *Principles and Practice of Pediatric Oncology*, 4th ed. Philadelphia: Lippincott Williams & Wilkins, 2000, 10, 273–287.

14. Raney, R.B., Asmar, L., Vassilopoulou-Sellin, R. et al. Late complications of therapy in 213 children with localized, nonorbital soft-tissue sarcoma of the head and neck: a descriptive report from the Intergroup Rhabdomyosarcoma Studies (IRS) — II and III. IRS Group of the Children's Cancer Group and the Pediatric Oncology Group. *Med. Pediatr. Oncol.*, 1999, 33(4), 362–371.

15. Berg, S.L., Grisell, D.L., Delaney, T.F., and Balis, F.M. Principles of treatment of pediatric solid tumors. *Pediatr. Clin. North Am.*, 1991, 38, 249.

16. Martin, D.S. The scientific basis for adjuvant chemotherapy. *Chemo. Treat. Rev.*, 1981, 8, 169.

17. Alexander, S.W., Walsh, T.J., Freifeld, A.G., and Pizzo, P.A. Infectious complications in pediatric cancer patients. In Pizzo, P., Ed. *Principles and Practice of Pediatric Oncology*, 4th ed. Philadelphia: Lippincott Williams & Wilkins, 2000, 1237–1283.

18. Garcia-Covarrubias, L., Barratt, D.M., Bartlett, R., Metzinger, S., and VanMeter, K. Invasive Aspergillosis treated with adjuctive hyperbaric oxygenation: a retrospective clinical series at a single institution. *South Med. J.*, 2002, 95(4), 450–456.

19. Dreyer, Z.E., Blatt, J., and Bleyer, A. Late effects of childhood cancer and its treatment. In Pizzo, P., Ed. *Principles and Practice of Pediatric Oncology*, 4th ed. Philadelphia: Lippincott Williams & Wilkins, 2000, 49, 1431–1461.

20. Carls, J.L., Mendenhall, W.M., Morris, C.G., and Antonelli, P.J. External auditory canal stenosis after radiation therapy. *Laryngoscope*, 2002, 112(11), 1975–1978.

21. Hersh, S.P. and Weiner, L.S. Psychiatric and psychosocial support for the child and family. In Pizzo, P., Ed. *Principles and Practice of Pediatric Oncology*, 4th ed. Philadelphia: Lippincott Williams & Wilkins, 2000, 46, 1365–1392.

Section IV

Head and Neck

14 Obstructive Sleep Apnea Syndrome

David E. Tunkel and Laura M. Sterni

...the stupid-looking lazy child who frequently suffers from headache at school, breathes through his mouth instead of his nose, snores and is restless at night...is well worthy of the solicitory attention of the school medical officer.

W. Hill, *British Medical Journal*, **1899**

CONTENTS

INTRODUCTION

The obstructive sleep apnea syndrome (OSAS) is now recognized as being common in children. Complications of OSAS can occur without proper diagnosis and expeditious treatment. Although adenotonsillar hyperplasia is the leading risk factor in children with OSAS, factors other than tonsillar size, such as neuromotor tone and craniofacial anatomy, play a role in the pathophysiology of this disease. OSAS causes a variety of daytime and nighttime symptoms in affected children. This chapter discusses the complications of OSAS in children, emphasizing the risks of delayed or missed diagnosis. It also discusses the complications of the surgical treatment of OSAS in children, with emphasis on defining the high-risk patient before surgery and suggestions for perioperative management to avoid complications.

CLASSIFICATION OF CHILDHOOD OBSTRUCTIVE SLEEP DISORDERS

Approximately 10% of children snore on most or all nights, and most of these children have *primary snoring* (PS), [1-3] which is snoring that occurs without associated hypoventilation, apnea, hypoxemia, or excessive arousals.[4] Children with PS have no associated sleep disturbance and no daytime symptoms referable to sleep-associated breathing difficulties. The natural history of snoring in children is unclear. Ali et al. found that snoring resolved in half of their 4- to 5-year-old patients with habitual snoring within 2 years.[5] In another study, older children with PS continued to snore but did not develop OSAS over the course of several years.[6]

Children with upper airway resistance syndrome (UARS) snore and have daytime symptoms similar to those seen with OSAS, but have no evidence of apnea, hypopnea, or gas exchange abnormalities on polysomnography.[7] Affected children do have repetitive episodes of increased respiratory effort, secondary to partial upper airway obstruction, which end in arousals. The incidence of UARS in children is unknown and the criteria for diagnosis remain controversial. Currently, the diagnosis is made using polysomnography with esophageal pressure measurements to assess respiratory effort-related arousals. When polysomnography is performed without eso-phogeal pressure monitoring, snoring with marked paradoxical breathing movements or repetitive arousals may suggest UARS treatment options. UARS is identical to those for OSAS.

Approximately 3% of all children, and as many as 40% of snoring children referred to a sleep clinic or to an otolaryngologist will have *obstructive sleep apnea syndrome*.[8-10] Childhood OSAS is characterized by sleep-related upper airway obstruction, usually associated with a reduction in oxyhemoglobin saturation or hypercarbia or both.[11] Sleep-related upper airway obstruction in children can manifest as complete obstructive apnea or partial obstruction with hypoventilation.[12] Obstructive hypoventilation results from continuous partial airway obstruction, which leads to paradoxical respiratory efforts, hypercarbia, and often hypoxemia. Diagnosis of obstructive hypoventilation requires end-tidal CO_2 monitoring during polysomnography. Even without complete apneas, children with obstructive hypoventilation are at risk for all of the reported complications of OSAS.

Obstructive hypoventilation is not usually seen in adults with OSAS. Other important differences between adult and childhood OSAS are displayed in Table 14.1.

SYMPTOMS OF CHILDHOOD OSAS

OSAS can cause a variety of daytime and nighttime symptoms in children. Almost all children with OSAS snore and have increased inspiratory effort during sleep.[10,13,14] Parents often report nighttime sweating, restless sleep, and unusual sleeping positions. Enuresis has been associated with OSAS in children.[14-17] Resolution of enuresis has been reported following adenotonsillectomy in children with symptoms of nocturnal upper airway obstruction or polysomnography diagnostic for OSAS.[17-19]

Daytime symptoms associated with OSAS include mouth breathing, nasal obstruction, and hyponasal speech. Although the hallmark of adult OSAS is excessive daytime sleepiness, this symptom is unusual in children with OSAS. Children are less likely than adults to terminate an obstructive episode with an arousal.[20] Unlike their adult counterparts, pediatric OSAS patients also generally have normal sleep efficiency and sleep architecture.[10-16] This preservation of sleep quality in children with OSAS may explain why excessive daytime sleepiness is rarely seen in these patients.

DIAGNOSIS OF CHILDHOOD OSAS

In children, the definitive diagnosis of OSAS is made using polysomnography. A number of studies have shown that OSAS cannot be distinguished from primary snoring on the basis of clinical history and physical examination alone.[8,10,21-24] In one report, 89% of parents of children with

TABLE 14.1
Comparison of OSAS in Adults and Children

Presentation	Adult	Child
Excessive daytime sleepiness	Main presenting complaint	Infrequent complaint
Associated obesity	Majority of patients	Minority of patients
Underweight/failure to thrive	Not seen	Frequent finding
Daytime mouth breathing	Not seen	Frequent finding
Gender	Males 2× > Female	Male = Female
Enlarged tonsils and adenoids	Not seen	Frequent finding
Sleep		
Obstructive pattern	Obstructive apnea	Obstructive apnea or obstructive hypoventilation
Arousal with obstruction	Usually	Not often seen
Disrupted sleep pattern	Usually	Not often seen
Treatment		
Surgical	In minority of cases	Definitive therapy in most cases
Medical (CPAP,[a] BiPAP[b])	Most common treatment	Only in selected cases

[a] Continuous positive airway pressure.

[b] Bilevel positive airway pressure.

Source: From Carroll, J.L. and Loughlin, G.M. *Pediatr. Pulmonol.*, 1992, 14, 71–74. With permission.

polysomnogram-proven OSAS observed their child struggling to breathe during sleep, as did 58% of parents of children with snoring and normal polysomnography. The majority of caregivers of OSAS and primary snoring patients were frightened by their child's nighttime breathing.[10] Goldstein et al. evaluated 30 snoring children referred to a pediatric otolaryngology clinic using a focused history and examination and a review of an audiotape of breathing during sleep. Only half of the 18 children thought to have definite OSAS based on clinical grounds had polysomnography diagnostic for OSAS.[8]

Polysomnography remains the gold standard for diagnosing OSAS in children because clinical assessment alone is sensitive but not specific for OSAS. The use of routine preoperative polysomnography is most controversial in healthy children with obstructive adenotonsillar hypertrophy and no other indication for adenotonsillectomy.[25] Historically, adenotonsillectomy has been used to treat obstructive symptoms in healthy children without preoperative polysomnography. This practice may allow children without OSAS, but with primary snoring, to undergo adenotonsillectomy.

Polysomnography for the diagnosis of OSAS in children should involve clinicians with expertise in pediatric respiratory and sleep disorders. Overnight studies are recommended because negative nap studies do not exclude the possibility of finding OSAS on an overnight study.[26] The use of sedatives and sleep deprivation is not recommended because they may artifactually increase upper airway obstruction.[27,28] End-tidal CO_2 should be monitored to detect obstructive hypoventilation. A consensus statement adopted by the American Thoracic Society, *Standards and Indications for Cardiopulmonary Sleep Studies in Children,* also recommends measurement of

- Respiratory effort as assessed by chest wall and abdominal movement
- Airflow at the nose, mouth, or both
- Arterial oxygen saturation
- Electrocardiography to monitor heart rate and rhythm
- Electromyography in the anterior tibial region to monitor arousals
- Electroencephalography, electrooculography, and electromyography for sleep staging purposes[29]

Achondroplasia	Klippel-Feil syndrome
Apert syndrome	Mucopolysaccharidosid
Beckwith-Wiedemann syndrome	Obesity
Cerebral palsy	Osteopetrosis
Choanal stenosis	Papillomatosis (oropharyngeal)
Crouzon syndrome	Pierre Robin sequence
Cystic hygroma	Pfeiffer syndrome
Down syndrome	Prader-Willi syndrome
Hallermann-Streiff syndrome	Sickle cell disease
Hypothyroidism	Treacher-Collins syndrome

FIGURE 14.1 Medical conditions associated with OSAS in children. Other conditions, not listed, may be associated with OSAS. (From Marcus, C.L. and Carroll, J.L. In Loughlin, G.M. and Eigen, H., Eds. *Respiratory Disease in Children: Diagnosis and Management*. Baltimore: Williams and Wilkens, 1994, 475–499. With permission.)

Because full polysomnography in children may be difficult to obtain, expensive, or inconvenient, in-home screening methods to diagnose OSAS are being investigated. Videotapes, audiotapes, and continuous pulse oximetry have been helpful in predicting OSAS when positive, but do not rule out OSAS when negative.[30–32] Screening tests also provide minimal assessment of the severity of OSAS. Preliminary studies suggest that evaluation of nighttime breathing difficulties may be accomplished in the home using a combination of video and cardiorespiratory recordings with extended oximetry.[33,34] Currently, these studies are not widely available, and additional validation of unattended home studies is needed.

The diagnosis of OSAS in children requires recognition of the aforementioned signs and symptoms by caregivers and primary care providers. A recent study by Richards and Ferdman found that the mean period of time between onset of symptoms and treatment of OSAS in a group of 45 children was 3.3 years.[35] Of these children, 40% self-referred to an otolaryngologist even when the primary care providers were thought to be aware of the problem. Delays in treatment were related to physician issues, parental issues, and third-party payer factors. Continued efforts to increase awareness of childhood OSAS is necessary to avoid complications related to delayed diagnosis and treatment.

OSAS is associated with a number of childhood medical conditions that affect neuromotor control of the upper airway, reduce airway caliber, or increase collapsibility of the upper airway. Children with these conditions (Figure 14.1) need to be followed closely for signs of sleep-related airway obstruction.

COMPLICATIONS AND CONSEQUENCES OF CHILDHOOD OSAS

GROWTH

Early reports of children with OSAS often described children with failure to thrive.[13,14,21] Although overt failure to thrive is now seen less frequently because of early diagnosis and treatment of OSAS, children with OSAS often grow poorly. Improved growth has been reported after treatment of childhood OSAS with adenotonsillectomy.[36–38] Marcus et al. reported decreased growth in children with even mild OSAS, which appeared to be related to increased work of breathing during sleep.[36] After adenotonsillectomy, improved growth and decreased energy expenditure during sleep were documented. OSAS should be included in the differential diagnosis of the child with growth impairment unexplained by other medical conditions.

CARDIOPULMONARY

Severe untreated OSAS can lead to pulmonary hypertension and cor pulmonale.[13,14] Pulmonary hypertension results from the recurrent severe nocturnal hypoxemia, hypercarbia, and acidosis. With increased awareness of this condition in even young children, these complications are now rarely seen. Cor pulmonale is readily reversible by treatment of OSAS, but children with this complication require perioperative precautions detailed later in this chapter.[39–41] Systemic hypertension has also been documented in children with OSAS.[14,17,42,43] Chest radiographs, electrocardiograms, and echocardiography should be considered for any child with OSAS and signs or symptoms of cardiopulmonary disease. Children with severe OSAS on polysomnography may require cardiopulmonary evaluation as well. Children with cardiovascular complications of OSAS should have repeat polysomnography after therapy to confirm resolution of OSAS.

BEHAVIORAL/LEARNING

Sleep-related upper airway obstruction may have significant neurocognitive and behavioral consequences. Developmental delay has been described in association with severe OSAS in children,[13] and behavioral problems, such as hyperactivity and aggression, have been linked to OSAS.[13–16] One study of 12 children with moderate to severe OSAS showed resolution of behavioral disturbances after treatment, with a significant reduction in inattention, aggression, and hyperactivity as assessed by the Conners' Parent Rating Scale and an improvement in vigilance on a continuous performance task.[44]

Obese children with OSAS have deficits in memory, vocabulary, and learning as assessed by standardized tests when compared with obese children without OSAS.[45] Additional evidence of learning difficulties in children with OSAS was provided by Gozal, who demonstrated an increased incidence of snoring with nocturnal gas exchange abnormalities in a large group of children who were in the lowest 10th percentile of their first-grade class.[46] The children with sleep-associated gas exchange abnormalities who underwent adenotonsillectomy showed improvement in academic performance in the second grade, but no such improvement was seen in affected children who did not pursue therapy. Although a causal relationship between neurocognitive function and sleep-related breathing obstruction is not established, the diagnosis of OSAS should be considered in children with learning and behavioral disorders.

TREATMENT OF CHILDHOOD OSAS

Surgical and nonsurgical methods of treatment have been used successfully for children with OSAS. Adenotonsillectomy remains the mainstay of treatment of OSAS in otherwise healthy children. Children with more complex, multifactorial forms of OSAS associated with neuromotor disease or craniofacial abnormalities can be treated with other forms of surgery, such as uvulopalatopharyngoplasty (UPPP), craniofacial advancement, or tracheotomy. Nasal continuous (CPAP) or bilevel (BiPAP) positive airway pressure, the most common nonsurgical treatments of children with OSAS, is usually used for children with contraindications for surgery or for children with persistent OSAS after surgery.

COMPLICATIONS OF SURGERY FOR OSAS

The complications of adenotonsillectomy are addressed in this chapter of the textbook. The unique, and most severe, complication of adenotonsillectomy (and other pharyngeal surgery) when performed for childhood OSAS is perioperative respiratory compromise. Upper airway obstruction can occur on induction of general anesthesia, upon emergence from anesthesia, and during the immediate perioperative period. High-risk children can be identified preoperatively and then monitored aggressively for the need for respiratory support.

OSAS may persist after surgical treatment. Suen et al. reported that children with severe OSAS on preoperative polysomnography were likely to have residual OSAS after surgery.[22] A respiratory disturbance index of less than 19.1 on preoperative polysomnography predicted cure of OSAS by adenotonsillectomy in this study. Helfaer et al. performed polysomnography on otherwise healthy children with mild OSAS on the first night after adenotonsillectomy.[47] The number of apnea events decreased and oxygen saturation during sleep improved immediately after surgery in these children. Rapid relief of obstructive symptoms after adenotonsillectomy can be expected in children with mild OSAS, but OSAS may persist in severe cases.

IDENTIFICATION OF THE HIGH-RISK CHILD

Recent reports have analyzed the risk factors for postoperative respiratory compromise after adenotonsillectomy for OSAS. McColley et al. retrospectively reviewed the records of 69 children who had had adenotonsillectomy performed for sleep study–proven OSAS, 23% of whom had had respiratory difficulties after surgery.[48] They found that children younger than 3 years and children with obstructive apnea indices greater than 10 had the greatest risk for postoperative respiratory compromise requiring intervention. Rosen et al. studied 37 children with sleep study–proven OSAS, and 27% had respiratory difficulties after surgery. Risk factors for respiratory compromise in this group included age less than 2 years, severe OSAS on preoperative polysomnography, cor pulmonale, morbid obesity, failure to thrive, neuromotor disease, and craniofacial anomalies.[49]

Biavati et al. reviewed 355 children who had had adenotonsillectomy for clinical evidence of nocturnal breathing obstruction (not sleep study–proven OSAS) and identified five conditions associated with postoperative respiratory complications: age less than 3 years, cerebral palsy, seizures, congenital heart disease, and history of prematurity.[50] A similar analysis by Gerber et al. identified neuromuscular disorders, chromosomal abnormalities, clinical symptoms of sleep-disordered breathing (snoring, restlessness, and apnea on history), and recent upper respiratory infection as risk factors for respiratory compromise after adenotonsillectomy.[51]

Most children at risk for respiratory compromise after adenotonsillectomy can be identified preoperatively based on clinical grounds. Children with severe OSAS, children with complex issues of upper airway tone or craniofacial anatomy (cerebral palsy, syndromic craniofacial disease, etc.), and very young children are at increased risk for respiratory compromise or prolonged recovery after adenotonsillectomy. The use of preoperative polysomnography can quantify the severity of OSAS and (1) predict the likelihood of perioperative respiratory compromise, and (2) provide a baseline for assessment of postoperative respiratory indicators during sleep.

PERIOPERATIVE PRECAUTIONS

The preoperative management of children with severe OSAS centers on risk assessment for general anesthesia and for respiratory compromise. High-risk children may require clinical evaluation of cardiopulmonary status, looking for signs of right ventricular hypertrophy. Clinical evaluation may be supplemented with chest radiographs, electrocardiograms, and even echocardiograms. The anesthesia and surgical team must be prepared for the possibility of airway obstruction from preoperative sedation or on induction of general anesthesia. Finally, parents of children with complex OSAS from craniofacial or neuromotor issues should be counseled that relief of OSAS may be incomplete after adenotonsillectomy. Additional surgical therapy or CPAP may be necessary if OSAS persists.

Adenotonsillectomy is performed using standard techniques, with attention to minimizing postoperative pharyngeal edema in high-risk children. Steroids are often administered, and nasopharyngeal airways may be placed during the procedure to provide airway support during emergence from anesthesia.

Postoperative management is dictated by the severity of OSAS as assessed preoperatively based on clinical and polysomnographic information. High-risk children, as discussed previously, require in-patient monitoring after surgery with careful attention to cardiopulmonary status. Recovery should occur in an area in which signs of respiratory depression and airway swelling can be recognized and prompt intervention can occur. Narcotic analgesics and other sedating medications should be used judiciously, and postoperative oxygen supplementation should be monitored carefully for signs of depressed ventilatory drive.

Brown et al. suggest several days of endotracheal intubation and mechanical ventilation after adentonsillectomy in the unusual child with severe OSAS who presents with cor pulmonale.[52] Nasal bilevel positive airway pressure has been used successfully for airway support immediately after pharyngeal surgery in children with complex severe OSAS from neuromotor disease or obesity.[53]

UVULOPALATOPHARYNGOPLASTY

Uvulopalatopharyngoplasty (UPPP) is not widely used in children with OSAS. Although this procedure is commonly used to treat snoring or mild OSAS in adults, UPPP is generally reserved for children at high risk for persistent obstruction after adenotonsillectomy. UPPP has been performed in children at the time of adenotonsillectomy and as a second procedure for persistent symptoms. UPPP has been used for children with neuromotor disease such as cerebral palsy or with craniofacial anomalies such as those seen in Down syndrome.

Kosko and Derkay performed UPPP to treat 15 children with cerebral palsy and OSAS.[54] Twelve patients were clinically improved, and the two patients who had postoperative polysomnography showed marked improvement in apnea scores. Jacobs et al. used plication of the tonsillar pillars combined with adenotonsillectomy to treat upper airway obstruction successfully in eight patients with Down syndrome.[55] These authors note residual obstruction in three of four children with Down syndrome treated with UPPP. Bower and Gungor have recommended the use of UPPP in children with severe OSAS, particularly when the palate is abnormal or the tonsils and adenoids are small, and in children with neuromotor or craniofacial issues.[56]

The major concern about the use of UPPP in children is the possible increased incidence of two complications: nasopharyngeal stenosis and velopharyngeal incompetence (VPI). These conditions are also rare complications of adenotonsillectomy. Although it is very difficult to establish whether UPPP in children can cause VPI or nasopharyngeal stenosis, the more extensive mucosal dissection and excision certainly would predispose to cicatrix formation or poor velar closure. Children who are candidates for UPPP may have craniofacial features (narrow skull base, etc.) that increase the risk of nasopharyngeal stenosis. Similarly, children with OSAS and pharyngeal hypotonia may be at increased risk of VPI after adenotonsillectomy and/or UPPP because of pre-existing neuromotor issues inhibiting velopharyngeal closure.

Nasopharyngeal stenosis after UPPP has been associated with several factors:

- Postoperative bleeding treated with packing and electrocautery
- Performance of adenoidectomy at the time of UPPP
- Excessive excision or cautery of the posterior tonsillar pillars
- Wound infection or dehiscence of suture lines
- Tendency for keloid formation[57]

Nasopharyngeal stenosis after adenoidectomy or adenotonsillectomy has been associated with the preceding factors, as well as overzealous removal of lateral adenoid tissue with or without damage to the posterior tonsillar pillars, excessive cautery use, or use of the KTP laser.[58]

Bower and Gungor suggest leaving a longer mucosal surface on the nasopharyngeal side of the palate during UPPP to prevent nasopharyngeal stenosis.[56] Dissection to minimize denuded surface areas, along with judicious removal of lateral adenoid bands and posterior tonsillar pillars, should reduce the rate of nasopharyngeal stenosis. Nasopharyngeal stenosis has been treated successfully with submucosal resection of scar and coverage with mucosal rotation flaps and with CO_2 laser excision followed by obturator placement.[57,58]

Because children who have UPPP performed represent complex severe OSAS, it is not surprising that persistent OSAS has been reported after this procedure. Magardino and Tom performed UPPP as a secondary procedure after adenotonsillectomy in two children with cerebral palsy.[59] Although both patients appeared to have improved OSAS, they required tracheotomy for pulmonary issues. Sculerati performed UPPP in three patients with syndromic craniofacial anomalies and tracheotomy, two of whom required additional pharyngeal surgery and midfacial advancement before decannulation.[60] When they are considering UPPP for treatment of OSAS in children with neuromotor or craniofacial issues, parents should be counseled about the need for follow-up polysomnography, as well as the need for additional treatment such as tracheotomy or nasal positive airway pressure if OSAS persists.

NONSURGICAL TREATMENT OF OSAS

Although the majority of children with OSAS can be treated with adenotonsillectomy, some will require additional or alternative therapies. Steroid therapy has been used successfully to treat obstructive symptoms in conditions, such as infectious mononucleosis, that acutely increase adenoid and tonsillar size. However, a recent study found that a 5-day course of oral prednisone was not effective in treating children with OSAS from adenotonsillar hypertrophy.[61]

CPAP and BiPAP have been successfully used to treat children with OSAS who had failed surgery or who were not candidates for surgery.[62–65] CPAP or BiPAP may help avoid tracheotomy in the child with OSAS related to craniofacial or neuromotor abnormalities. CPAP can be used to stabilize children with severe OSAS until surgery can be performed safely.[64,66] The level of positive pressure required to eliminate sleep-related obstruction is determined in the sleep laboratory, and serial evaluation and adjustments may be necessary because pressure requirements will change in growing children.[63,65]

Complications of CPAP or BiPAP include local discomfort or irritation to the eyes and facial skin from improper mask fit. Close follow-up is necessary to reassess mask fit in growing children. Nasal congestion and rhinorrhea are common with this therapy, and humidification and nasal steroid sprays may be helpful. Some children on CPAP have increased central apneas with hypoventilation, and bilevel ventilation with a "back-up rate" may be necessary to ensure adequate ventilation.[67] Cardiopulmonary complications of CPAP or BiPAP, such as reduction of cardiac output or pneumothorax, have not been reported in children treated for OSAS. Midfacial hypoplasia has been reported in association with long-term use of nasal mask CPAP.[68] Long-term use of a nasal mask in children requires serial evaluation of facial development.

The greatest limitation to CPAP or BiPAP use in children is poor acceptance of the mask or poor compliance with use. Compliance with this therapy has been estimated between 50 and 100% in children, with adolescent patients being the least compliant.[63] Patients may find BiPAP use more acceptable than CPAP because the pressure delivered during exhalation can be reduced to improve comfort. J.C. Rains improved compliance with CPAP therapy in four developmentally delayed children with OSAS by using intensive behavioral interventions including modeling, parent training, and desensitization.[69] In general, careful training and close follow-up with aggressive treatment of minor side effects will optimize compliance with CPAP/BiPAP in children with OSAS.

Nocturnal oxygen supplementation has been studied as a temporary treatment for children with hypoxemia associated with OSAS until definitive therapy occurs.[70,71] Supplemental oxygen may suppress hypoxic ventilatory drive, decrease upper airway tone, and worsen OSAS.[72] Aljadeff et al. administered supplemental oxygen to 16 children with mild or moderate OSAS from adenotonsillar hyperplasia; they found a decrease in apneic events, lessened paradoxical breathing, increased rapid-eye-movement sleep, and decreased arousals during sleep, without hypoventilation or increased central apneas.[71] Marcus et al., however, noted significant hypercarbia in 2 of 23 children with OSAS when they breathed supplemental oxygen.[70] Nocturnal oxygen therapy for children with OSAS should be initiated in a monitored setting.

CONCLUSIONS

The complications of OSAS in children can be divided into problems from inaccurate diagnosis; perioperative complications, usually involving respiratory compromise; and sequelae of long-term untreated OSAS. Increasing knowledge of the pathophysiology of OSAS in children, with increased awareness of the signs and symptoms of this disease, has led to earlier diagnosis. Groups of children who are at high risk for development of OSAS have been identified in order to avoid the cardiopulmonary, cognitive, and other late complications of untreated disease. Indications for polysomnography in children have been established, and standards for performance of such tests have been outlined. This polysomnography facilitates accurate diagnosis of OSAS in children with assessment of disease severity and perioperative risk. Most importantly, clinical factors to identify children at risk for perioperative respiratory morbidity and persistent OSAS have been described. These children require careful monitoring around the time of surgery to avoid complications.

REFERENCES

1. Ali, N.J., Pitson, D., and Stradling, J.R. The prevalence of snoring, sleep disturbance and sleep related breathing disorders and their relation to daytime sleepiness in 4- to 5-year-old children. *Am. Rev. Respir. Dis.*, 1991, 143, A381.
2. Corbo, G.M., Fuciarelli, F., Foresi, A., and De Benedetto, F. Snoring in children: association with respiratory symptoms and passive smoking [published erratum appears in *Br. Med. J.*, 1990, Jan 27, 300(6719), 226]. *Br. Med. J.*, 1989, 299, 1491–1494.
3. Owen, G.O. and Canter, R.J. Overnight pulse oximetry in normal children and in children undergoing adenotonsillectomy. *Clin. Otolaryngol.*, 1996, 21, 59–65.
4. Diagnostic Classification Steering Committee of the American Sleep Disorders Association MJTMDC. *The International Classification of Sleep Disorders*. Rochester, MN: American Sleep Disorders Association, 1997.
5. Ali, N.J., Pitson, D., and Stradling, J.R. Natural history of snoring and related behaviour problems between the ages of 4 and 7 years. *Arch. Dis. Child*, 1994, 71, 74–76.
6. Marcus, C.L., Hamer, A., and Loughlin, G.M. Natural history of primary snoring in children. *Pediatr. Pulmonol.*, 1998, 26, 6–11.
7. Guilleminault, C., Pelayo, R., Leger, D., Clerk, A., and Bocian, R.C. Recognition of sleep-disordered breathing in children. *Pediatrics*, 1996, 98, 871–882.
8. Goldstein, N.A., Sculerati, N., Walsleben, J.A., Bhatia, N., Friedman, D.M., and Rapoport, D.M. Clinical diagnosis of pediatric obstructive sleep apnea validated by polysomnography. *Otolaryngol. Head Neck Surg.*, 1994, 111, 611–617.
9. Gislason, T. and Benediktsdottir, B. Snoring, apneic episodes, and nocturnal hypoxemia among children 6 months to 6 years old. An epidemiologic study of lower limit of prevalence. *Chest*, 1995, 107, 963–966.
10. Carroll, J.L., McColley, S.A., Marcus, C.L., Curtis, S., and Loughlin, G.M. Inability of clinical history to distinguish primary snoring from obstructive sleep apnea syndrome in children. *Chest*, 1995, 108, 610–618.
11. Carroll, J.L. and Loughlin, G.M. Obstructive sleep apnea syndrome in infants and children: clinical features and pathophysiology. In Ferber, R. and Kryger, M.H., Eds. *Principles and Practice of Sleep Medicine in the Child*. Philadelphia: Saunders, 1995, 163–191.

12. Rosen, C.L., D'Andrea, L., and Haddad, G.G. Adult criteria for obstructive sleep apnea do not identify children with serious obstruction. *Am. Rev. Respir. Dis.*, 1992, 146, 1231–1234.

13. Brouillette, R.T., Fernbach, S.K., Hunt, C.E. Obstructive sleep apnea in infants and children. *J. Pediatr.*, 1982, 100, 31–40.

14. Guilleminault, C., Korobkin, R., and Winkle, R. A review of 50 children with obstructive sleep apnea syndrome. *Lung*, 1981, 159, 275–287.

15. Brouilette, R., Hanson, D., David, R., Klemka, L., Szatkowski, A., Fernbach, S. et al. A diagnostic approach to suspected obstructive sleep apnea in children. *J. Pediatr.*, 1984, 105, 10–14.

16. Frank, Y., Kravath, R.E., Pollak, C.P., and Weitzman, E.D. Obstructive sleep apnea and its therapy: clinical and polysomnographic manifestations. *Pediatrics*, 1983, 71, 737–742.

17. Guilleminault, C., Eldridge, F.L., Simmons, F.B., and Dement, W.C. Sleep apnea in eight children. *Pediatrics*, 1976, 58, 23–30.

18. Weider, D.J. and Hauri, P.J. Nocturnal enuresis in children with upper airway obstruction. *Int. J. Pediatr. Otorhinolaryngol.*, 1985, 9, 173–182.

19. Weider, D.J., Sateia, M.J., and West, R.P. Nocturnal enuresis in children with upper airway obstruction. *Otolaryngol. Head Neck Surg.*, 1991, 105, 427–432.

20. McGrath–Morrow, S.A., Carroll, J.L., McColley, S.A., Pyzik, P., and Loughlin, G.M. Termination of obstructive apnea in children is not associated with arousal. *Am. Rev. Respir. Dis.*, 1990, 141, A195.

21. Leach, J., Olson, J., Hermann, J., and Manning, S. Polysomnographic and clinical findings in children with obstructive sleep apnea. *Arch. Otolaryngol. Head Neck Surg.*, 1992, 118, 741–744.

22. Suen, J.S., Arnold, J.E., and Brooks, L.J. Adenotonsillectomy for treatment of obstructive sleep apnea in children. *Arch. Otolaryngol. Head Neck Surg.*, 1995, 121, 525–530.

23. Nieminen, P., Tolonen, U., and Lopponen, H. Snoring and obstructive sleep apnea in children: a 6-month follow-up study. *Arch. Otolaryngol. Head Neck Surg.*, 2000, 126, 481–486.

24. Wang, R.C., Elkins, T.P., Keech, D., Wauquier, A., and Hubbard, D. Accuracy of clinical evaluation in pediatric obstructive sleep apnea. *Otolaryngol. Head Neck Surg.*, 1998, 118, 69–73.

25. Messner, A.H. Evaluation of obstructive sleep apnea by polysomnography prior to pediatric adenotonsillectomy. *Arch. Otolaryngol. Head Neck Surg.*, 1999, 125, 353–356.

26. Marcus, C.L., Keens, T.G., and Ward, S.L. Comparison of nap and overnight polysomnography in children. *Pediatr. Pulmonol.*, 1992, 13, 16–21.

27. Canet, E., Gaultier, C., d'Allest, A.M., and Dehan, M. Effects of sleep deprivation on respiratory events during sleep in healthy infants. *J. Appl. Physiol.*, 1989, 66, 1158–1163.

28. Hershenson, M., Brouillette, R.T., Olsen, E., and Hunt, C.E. The effect of chloral hydrate on genioglossus and diaphragmatic activity. *Pediatr. Res.*, 1984, 18, 516–519.

29. American Thoracic Society. Standards and indications for cardiopulmonary sleep studies in children. *Am. J. Respir. Crit. Care Med.*, 1996, 153, 866–878.

30. Sivan, Y., Kornecki, A., and Schonfeld, T. Screening obstructive sleep apnea syndrome by home videotape recording in children. *Eur. Respir. J.*, 1996, 9, 2127–2131.

31. Lamm, C., Mandeli, J., and Kattan, M. Evaluation of home audiotapes as an abbreviated test for obstructive sleep apnea syndrome (OSAS) in children. *Pediatr. Pulmonol.*, 1999, 27, 267–272.

32. Brouillette, R.T., Morielli, A., Leimanis, A., Waters, K.A., Luciano, R., and Ducharme, F.M. Nocturnal pulse oximetry as an abbreviated testing modality for pediatric obstructive sleep apnea. *Pediatrics*, 2000, 105(2), 405–412.

33. Morielli, A., Ladan, S., Ducharme, F.M., and Brouillette, R.T. Can sleep and wakefulness be distinguished in children by cardiorespiratory and videotape recordings? *Chest*, 1996, 109, 680–687.

34. Jacob, S.V., Morielli, A., Mograss, M.A., Ducharme, F.M., Schloss, M.D., and Brouillette, R.T. Home testing for pediatric obstructive sleep apnea syndrome secondary to adenotonsillar hypertrophy. *Pediatr. Pulmonol.*, 1995, 20, 241–252.

35. Richards, W. and Ferdman, R.M. Prolonged morbidity due to delays in the diagnosis and treatment of obstructive sleep apnea in children. *Clin. Pediatr.*, 2000, 39, 103–108.

36. Marcus, C.L., Carroll, J.L., Koerner, C.B., Hamer, A., Lutz, J., and Loughlin, G.M. Determinants of growth in children with the obstructive sleep apnea syndrome. *J. Pediatr.*, 1994, 125, 556–562.

37. Stradling, J.R., Thomas, G., Warley, A.R., Williams, P., and Freeland, A. Effect of adenotonsillectomy on nocturnal hypoxaemia, sleep disturbance, and symptoms in snoring children. *Lancet*, 1990, 335, 249–253.

38. Williams, E.F., Woo, P., Miller, R., and Kellman, R.M. The effects of adenotonsillectomy on growth in young children. *Otolaryngol. Head Neck Surg.*, 1991, 104, 509–516.

39. Hunt, C.E. and Brouillette, R.T. Abnormalities of breathing control and airway maintenance in infants and children as a cause of cor pulmonale. *Pediatr. Cardiol.*, 1982, 3, 249–256.

40. Brown, O.E., Manning, S.C., and Ridenour, B. Cor pulmonale secondary to tonsillar and adenoidal hypertrophy: management considerations. *Int. J. Pediatr. Otorhinolaryngol.*, 1988, 16, 131–139.

41. Tal, A., Leiberman, A., Margulis, G., and Sofer, S. Ventricular dysfunction in children with obstructive sleep apnea: radionuclide assessment. *Pediatr. Pulmonol.*, 1988, 4, 139–143.

42. Serratto, M., Harris, V.J., and Carr, I. Upper airways obstruction. Presentation with systemic hypertension. *Arch. Dis. Child*, 1981, 56, 153–155.

43. Marcus, C.L., Greene, M.G., and Carroll, J.L. Blood pressure in children with obstructive sleep apnea. *Am. J. Respir. Crit. Care Med.*, 1998, 157, 1098–1103.

44. Ali, N.J., Pitson, D., and Stradling, J.R. Sleep disordered breathing: effects of adenotonsillectomy on behaviour and psychological functioning. *Eur. J. Pediatr.*, 1996, 155, 56–62.

45. Rhodes, S.K., Shimoda, K.C., Waid, L.R., O'Neil, P.M., Oexmann, M.J., Collop, N.A. et al. Neurocognitive deficits in morbidly obese children with obstructive sleep apnea. *J. Pediatr.*, 1995, 127, 741–744.

46. Gozal, D. Sleep-disordered breathing and school performance in children. *Pediatrics*, 1998, 102, 616–620.

47. Helfaer, M.A., McColley, S.A,. Pyzik, P.L., Tunkel, D.E., Nichols, D.G., Baroody, F.M. et al. Polysomnography after adenotonsillectomy in mild pediatric obstructive sleep apnea. *Crit. Care Med.*, 1996, 24, 1323–1327.

48. McColley, S.A., April, M.M., Carroll, J.L., Naclerio, R.M., and Loughlin, G.M. Respiratory compromise after adenotonsillectomy in children with obstructive sleep apnea. *Arch. Otolaryngol. Head Neck Surg.*, 1992, 118, 940–943.

49. Rosen, G.M., Muckle, R.P., Mahowald, M.W., Goding, G.S., and Ullevig, C. Postoperative respiratory compromise in children with obstructive sleep apnea syndrome: can it be anticipated? *Pediatrics*, 1994, 93, 784–788.

50. Biavati, M.J., Manning, S.C., and Phillips, D.L. Predictive factors for respiratory complications after tonsillectomy and adenoidectomy in children. *Arch. Otolaryngol. Head Neck Surg.*, 1997, 123, 517–521.

51. Gerber, M.E., O'Connor, D.M., Adler, E., and Myer, C.M. Selected risk factors in pediatric adenotonsillectomy. *Arch. Otolaryngol. Head Neck Surg.*, 1996, 122, 811–814.

52. Brown, O.E., Manning, S.C., and Ridenour, B. Cor pulmonale secondary to tonsillar and adenoidal hypertrophy: management considerations. *Int. J. Pediatr. Otorhinolaryngol.*, 1988, 16, 131–139.

53. Friedman, O., Chidekel, A., Lawless, S.T., and Cook, S.P. Postoperative bilevel positive airway pressure ventilation after tonsillectomy and adenoidectomy in children — a preliminary report. *Int. J. Pediatr. Otorhinolaryngol.*, 1999, 51, 177–180.

54. Kosko, J.R. and Derkay, C.S. Uvulopalatopharyngoplasty: treatment of obstructive sleep apnea in neurologically impaired pediatric patients. *Int. J. Pediatr. Otorhinolaryngol.*, 1995, 32, 241–246.

55. Jacobs, I.N., Gray, R.F., and Todd, N.W. Upper airway obstruction in children with Down syndrome. *Arch. Otolaryngol. Head Neck Surg.*, 1996, 122, 945–950.

56. Bower, C.M. and Gungor, A. Pediatric obstructive sleep apnea syndrome. *Otolaryngol. Clin. North Am.*, 2000, 33(1), 49–75.

57. Krespi, Y.P. and Kacker, A. Management of nasopharyngeal stenosis after uvulopalatoplasty. *Otolaryngol. Head Neck Surg.*, 2000, 123, 692–695.

58. McLaughlin, K.E., Jacobs, I.N., Todd, N.W., Gussack, G.S., and Carlson, G. Management of nasopharyngeal and oropharyngeal stenosis in children. *Laryngoscope*, 1997, 107, 1322–1331.

59. Magardino, T.M. and Tom, L.W. Surgical management of obstructive sleep apnea in children with cerebral palsy. *Laryngoscope*, 1999, 109, 1611–1615.

60. Sculerati, N., Gottlieb, M.D., Zimbler, M.S., Chibbaro, P.D., and McCarthy, J.G. Airway management in children with major craniofacial anomalies. *Laryngoscope*, 1998, 108, 1806–1812.

61. Al–Ghamdi, S.A., Manoukian, J.J., Morielli, A., Oudjhane, K., Ducharme, F.M., and Brouillette, R.T. Do systemic corticosteroids effectively treat obstructive sleep apnea secondary to adenotonsillar hypertrophy? *Laryngoscope*, 1997, 107, 1382–1387.

62. Waters, K.A., Everett, F.M., Bruderer, J.W., and Sullivan, C.E. Obstructive sleep apnea: the use of nasal CPAP in 80 children. *Am. J. Respir. Crit. Care Med.*, 1995, 152, 780–785.

63. Marcus, C.L., Ward, S.L., Mallory, G.B., Rosen, C.L., Beckerman, R.C., Weese–Mayer, D.E. et al. Use of nasal continuous positive airway pressure as treatment of childhood obstructive sleep apnea. *J. Pediatr.*, 1995, 127, 88–94.

64. Guilleminault, C., Pelayo, R., Clerk, A., Leger, D., and Bocian, R.C. Home nasal continuous positive airway pressure in infants with sleep-disordered breathing. *J. Pediatr.*, 1995, 127, 905–912.

65. Downey, R., Perkin, R.M., and MacQuarrie, J. Nasal continuous positive airway pressure use in children with obstructive sleep apnea younger than 2 years of age. *Chest*, 2000, 117(6), 1608–1612.

66. McNamara, F. and Sullivan, C.E. Effects of nasal CPAP therapy on respiratory and spontaneous arousals in infants with OSA. *J. Appl. Physiol.*, 1999, 87, 889–896.

67. Waters, K.A., Everett, F., Bruderer, J., MacNamara, F., and Sullivan, C.E. The use of nasal CPAP in children. *Pediatr. Pulmonol. Suppl.*, 1995, 11, 91–93.

68. Li, K.K., Riley, R.W., and Guilleminault, C. An unreported risk in the use of home nasal continuous positive airway pressure and home nasal ventilation in children: mid-face hypoplasia. *Chest*, 2000, 117(3), 916–918.

69. Rains, J.C. Treatment of obstructive sleep apnea in pediatric patients. Behavioral intervention for compliance with nasal continuous positive airway pressure. *Clin. Pediatr. (Phila.)*, 1995, 34, 535–541.

70. Marcus, C.L., Carroll, J.L., Bamford, O., Pyzik, P., and Loughlin, G.M. Supplemental oxygen during sleep in children with sleep-disordered breathing. *Am. J. Respir. Crit. Care Med.*, 1995, 152, 1297–1301.

71. Aljadeff, G., Gozal, D., Bailey–Wahl, S.L., Burrell, B., Keens, T.G., and Ward, S.L. Effects of overnight supplemental oxygen in obstructive sleep apnea in children. *Am. J. Respir. Crit. Care Med.*, 1996, 153, 51–55.

72. Gauda, E.B., Carroll, J.L., McColley, S., and Smith, P.L. Effect of oxygenation on breath-by-breath response of the genioglossus muscle during occlusion. *J. Appl. Physiol.*, 1991, 71, 1231–1236.

15 Tonsillectomy and Adenoidectomy

Michael J. Cunningham and Charles M. Myers III

The invariable mark of wisdom is to see the miraculous in the common.

Ralph Waldo Emerson

CONTENTS

INTRODUCTION

Tonsillectomy and adenoidectomy, whether individually or jointly, are two of the most common pediatric operative procedures. Approximately 340,000 adenotonsillectomies are performed yearly in the United States, for infectious and obstructive indications, in children of all ages and in a wide variety of operative settings.[1] As with any operative procedure, tonsillectomy and adenoidectomy are associated with a myriad of potential major and minor complications. Some of these complications occur intraoperatively and others immediately postoperatively; some may be delayed for days to weeks after surgery. Although this procedure may be associated with morbidity, because of improved anesthetic and surgical techniques, mortality due to adenotonsillar surgery should be avoidable. Mortality rates associated with adenotonsillar surgery have decreased to approximate those of general anesthesia alone, ranging from 1 in 16,000 to 1 in 35,000 cases.[2]

HEMORRHAGE

One of the most common and potentially life-threatening complications of adenotonsillectomy is hemorrhage. Estimates of the incidence of adenotonsillar hemorrhage in the pediatric population vary greatly, ranging from 0.1 to 8%.[3-6] The variability in this incidence is attributable to different definitions as to what constitutes reportable bleeding. The risk of requiring transfusion after adenotonsillectomy is estimated at 0.04% with a bleeding mortality of approximately 0.002%.[2,7] Children and adolescents in general have a decreased risk of adenotonsillar hemorrhage compared with adults.[8]

INTRAOPERATIVE HEMORRHAGE

The volume of intraoperative blood loss is of particular importance in the young child. Total blood volume is best estimated at 7.5 cc per 100 g of body weight. Intraoperative blood loss exceeding 10% of total blood volume has been associated with a complicated postoperative course.[9] The surgeon should keep in mind the maximal allowable blood loss (MABL). This is calculated by the following formula:

$$MABL = [estimated\ blood\ volume\ (EBV) \times (hematocrit - 25)] \div hematocrit$$

Estimated blood volume (EBV) is calculated as 80 to 90 mL/kg in newborns, 70 to 80 mL/kg in infants, and 70 mL/kg in children.

Intraoperative adenoidectomy bleeding is most frequently due to too superficial an adenoidectomy with residual or retained adenoid tissue or too deep an adenoidectomy with surgical trauma to the posterior pharyngeal wall musculature. Complete adenoid removal in the plane immediately superficial to the posterior pharyngeal wall musculature is advocated. Bleeding can further be controlled by cauterization of the adenoid bed or by the application of topical pressure with gauze packing; such packing can be dry or coated with a topical vasoconstrictor or other hemostatic agent. Persistent nasopharyngeal bleeding despite such measures may require posterior nasal pack placement. The adenoid receives its blood supply from the ascending pharyngeal, vidian, and spheno-palatine arteries.[10] Injury to these specific arterial branches is very infrequent; therefore, recalcitrant postadenoidectomy hemorrhage rarely dictates arteriography evaluation.

Intraoperative tonsillar bleeding also commonly results from residual lymphoid tissue remnants or disruption of the lateral pharyngeal wall. Careful dissection in the plane between the tonsil capsule and the pharyngeal musculature comprising the tonsillar fossa limits such bleeding. There is considerable controversy as to the ideal operative technique to perform this dissection. Options include standard cold knife technique with subsequent selective vessel cauterization or suture ligature placement;[11] electrosurgery techniques using monopolar blade, monopolar suction, bipolar and microscopy-assisted procedures;[12] laser techniques using the carbon dioxide, KTP532, or Nd:YAG laser;[13] or use of the ultrasonic scalpel.[14] Alternatively, an intracapsular "tonsillotomy" approach can be performed using radiofrequency electrosurgery,[15] powered instrumentation microdebrider resection,[16] or laser.[17]

Electrosurgery techniques tend to have a shorter operative time with a correspondingly reduced intraoperative blood loss; this appears to be true regardless of the electrosurgery device used. Cold knife technique with associated prophylactic cautery also limits intraoperative hemorrhage compared with an approach in which only actively bleeding sites are cauterized; suture ligature techniques are associated with increased intraoperative blood loss and a greater potential for delayed catastrophic bleeding.[11] The additional operative time and expense associated with the use of laser instruments brings into question their benefit in clinical practice for routine adenotonsillectomy.[13]

As in the case of adenoidectomy, the application of topical pressure with gauze packing with or without topical vasoconstrictors or other hemostatic agents proves helpful in limiting intraoperative blood loss during tonsillectomy. Suturing a pack into the tonsillar fossa is considered hazardous because of the risk of arterial injury and the potential for later pack displacement with aspiration.

Vessel disruption with arterial bleeding is more common during tonsillectomy than adenoidectomy due to the larger caliber blood supply to the tonsils. The superior tonsillar pole is supplied by the descending palatine artery, the middle fossa region by the ascending pharyngeal artery, and the inferior pole by the tonsillar and ascending palatine branches of the facial artery and the tonsillar branches of the lingual artery.[18]

When major arterial bleeding persists and remains uncontrollable by local methods, two potential therapeutic options are available.[19] The surgical option is an ipsilateral external carotid artery ligation. The external carotid artery is distinguished from the internal carotid artery during neck exploration by its cervical branches. A minimum of two arterial branches should be identified before ligation is performed. The nonsurgical option is a diagnostic and therapeutic angiography. Angiography is an absolute need when external carotid artery ligation fails to control tonsillar hemorrhage, suggesting possible internal carotid artery injury.[20] The internal carotid artery lies just deep to the pharyngeal musculature; it is at particular risk in children.[21] Pseudoaneurysm formation of the external or internal carotid artery may also occur after tonsillectomy with subsequent late-onset hemorrhage.[22,23] This diagnosis requires MRI or angiographic confirmation.

POSTOPERATIVE HEMORRHAGE

Postoperative hemorrhage is typically defined as primary or immediate if it occurs within the first 24 hours; it is referred to as secondary or delayed if it occurs any time after the first postoperative day. One of the more extensive reviews of adenotonsillectomy patients suggests an incidence of approximately 1.0% for primary hemorrhage and approximately 3.0% for secondary hemorrhage.[3] Primary or immediate hemorrhage can often be attributed to technical error or less frequently to an underlying bleeding diathesis.[24] Most secondary or delayed hemorrhage occurs 5 to 12 days after surgery and is uncommon beyond the 14th postoperative day.[25,26] Secondary or delayed bleeding is influenced by a multitude of perioperative and postoperative factors.

Various severity criteria have been applied to classify postoperative bleeding. One example is the following classification:

- Immediate major bleeding requiring return to the operating room
- Immediate minor bleeding requiring hospital admission
- Delayed major bleeding requiring hospital admission
- Delayed minor bleeding occurring at home but not requiring hospital admission

Classification criteria are important in defining the incidence of postoperative bleeding and in dictating therapeutic interventions.[27,28] A return to the operating room for hemostatic control is often advised for children with postadenotonsillectomy hemorrhage who are actively bleeding or who have a clot in the tonsillar fossa that cannot be removed by nonoperative means. Children who have lost significant blood volume must be monitored closely for hemodynamic instability. If necessary, the administration of plasma expanders and judicious surgical intervention is preferable to blood transfusions. Children with a positive history of bleeding but a negative examination should be observed in the emergency department or on the hospital floor for a specific period of time. If no additional bleeding occurs, discharge to home without surgical intervention is safe for the majority of these children.

AIRWAY OBSTRUCTION AND INPATIENT/OUTPATIENT RELEVANCE

Although bleeding issues are always a concern, outpatient (ambulatory) surgery is safe for the majority of children undergoing adenotonsillectomy. Guidelines exist to assist physicians in determining which pediatric patients are suitable candidates for ambulatory tonsillectomy.[29,30] Relative contraindications include children younger than 3 years of age,[31,32] children with polysomnography-confirmed obstructive sleep apnea,[33,34] and children with systemic disorders that place them at increased cardiopulmonary, metabolic, or general medical risk.[35] Other pediatric patients in whom outpatient surgery is contraindicated are those with syndromic disorders or other airway abnormalities such as Down syndrome, Pierre Robin anomalad, mucopolysaccaridoses, craniofacial abnormalities, and neurologically impaired children who increase their risk of airway obstruction. In one large prospective study using preoperative parental questionnaires and perioperative respiratory status documentation, postoperative respiratory compromise was significantly increased in children under 3 years of age and those with neuromuscular disorders, chromosomal abnormalities, difficulty in breathing during sleep, restless sleep, loud snoring with apnea, and with a respiratory infection within 4 weeks prior to surgery.[36]

HEMATOLOGIC PREOPERATIVE EVALUATION

The utility of preoperative hematologic assessment in adenotonsillectomy patients is controversial.[37] In the vast majority of patients, bleeding associated with adenotonsillectomy is due primarily to local hemostatic and surgical factors, rather than to underlying systemic hematologic disorders. Congenital bleeding disorders are so rarely the source of unexpected postadenotonsillectomy bleeding that the American Academy of Otolaryngology–Head and Neck Surgery recommends the performance of coagulation studies only in patients whose clinical history, family history, or physical examination suggests a possible bleeding diathesis.[38]

A personal or familial history of multiple or frequent bruising, bruising often greater than 5 cm in diameter, hematoma development under bruises, or epistaxis lasting longer than 20 minutes should raise concern, as should a history of excessive bleeding following surgery or dental extractions. Medications — including over-the-counter drugs — that may increase the incidence of hemorrhage need to be known. Some nutritional supplements can also adversely effect coagulation. Aspirin and aspirin-containing products should be discontinued 2 weeks preoperatively. Nonsteroidal anti-inflammatory drugs should be discontinued at least 3 to 4 days prior to surgery.

The potential advantage of a detailed preoperative history and physical examination lies in the detection of an inherited or acquired bleeding disorder that might result in severe perioperative bleeding.[39] Children may not have had sufficient time to develop a bleeding history that would be a clue to an underlying hemostatic disorder. The planned adenotonsillectomy may be the child's first surgical procedure. Advocates of preoperative screening argue that a coagulation profile can identify children with bleeding diatheses that would not be detected by clinical evaluation alone.[40–42] In contrast, several studies have shown that preoperative screening provides no additional information beyond a thorough bleeding history for the general pediatric population undergoing adenotonsillectomy surgery.[43–45]

One of the better designed studies prospectively evaluated laboratory and bleeding histories of 1603 children undergoing tonsillectomy.[46] All patients had preoperative laboratory screening with a complete blood count (CBC); prothrombin time (PT); activated partial thromboplastin time (PTT); and bleeding time (BT). Laboratory abnormalities that persisted on repeat testing 1 week after the initial screening were investigated further by a standardized schema. A subset of 129 patients, including all those who bled perioperatively or had laboratory abnormalities, completed a standard historical questionnaire. In predicting perioperative bleeding, history and laboratory screening had a high specificity but a very low positive predictive value due to poor sensitivity and a low prevalence of bleeding.

Some children with bleeding disorders are indeed identified by routine perioperative coagulation testing. Delay or cancellation of surgery and proper hematologic management may reduce or prevent perioperative hemorrhage in these patients. However, the comparatively high number of false positive laboratory tests, coupled with the relative rarity of inherited and acquired coagulopathies, raises doubts as to the overall value of routine hematologic screening. Screening tests such as the PTT and bleeding time can notably be normal in patients with certain subtypes of von Willebrand's disease. The use of a bleeding time as a hematologic screen is even more severely criticized because it is felt by many hematologists to be an inaccurate predictor of surgical bleeding.[47]

A frequent false-positive screening abnormality in asymptomatic patients who undergo preoperative testing is prolongation of the PTT secondary to a lupus anticoagulant.[45,46] The lupus anticoagulant is an antibody against phospholipids that interferes with the PTT assay but does truly influence clotting capability. Lupus anticoagulants can be induced by infection and are therefore frequently present in children undergoing adenotonsillectomy for infectious indications. Because these lupus anticoagulants are usually transient, until the PTT returns to normal, this approach prevents occult coagulopathies from being overlooked. Alternatively, surgery in the presence of a documented lupus anticoagulant is not necessarily contraindicated because there is no true associated risk of increased bleeding.

SPECIAL HEMATOLOGIC CIRCUMSTANCES

VON WILLEBRAND'S DISEASE

With a prevalence of 0.8%, von Willebrand's disease (VWD) is the most common hereditary bleeding disorder.[48,49] Individuals with VWD are at risk for bleeding due to a quantitative or qualitative deficiency of von Willebrand's factor (VWF). VWF causes platelets to adhere to vascular subendothelium and acts as a carrier for factor VIII. VWD is subclassified into three categories:

- Type 1 occurs in 75% of VWD patients and is due to a quantitative decrease in VWF.
- Type 2 (A,B,N) disease affects 20% of VWD patients and is associated with qualitative and quantitative abnormalities of VWF. Subtypes 2A and 2B occur commonly; type 2N is exceedingly rare.
- Type 3 disease is also rare, accounting for just 5% of VWD. These patients have an absence of VWF and ristocetin cofactor as well as a very low factor VIII level.

Patients with VWD Type 1 or Type 2A respond to desmopressin (DDAVP), which is given intravenously at a dose of 0.3 mcg/kg in 50 mL normal saline, starting 30 to 60 minutes before adenotonsillectomy. Another dose of DDAVP is given 24 hours after the procedure. DDAVP serves to release preformed VWF from storage sites and increases the number of larger, more functionally active VFW multimers in plasma. Patients with Type 3 or Type 2B VWD are unresponsive to DDAVP and alternatively require preoperative treatment with factor VIII concentrate, which is rich in VWF. Donor-designated cryoprecipitate, rich in all VWF multimers, can also be used but carries a slightly greater risk of transmitting HIV and hepatitis B and C.

DDAVP (desmopressin) is a synthetic analogue of naturally occurring antidiuretic hormone. This agent stimulates the resorption of free water by the kidney. The most important potentially adverse side effect of desmopressin use is hyponatremia, which, if severe, can cause seizures and even death. Predisposing factors to DDAVP-induced hyponatremia include young age with weight less than 10 kg, postoperative administration of hypotonic intravenous fluids, recurrent emesis, and administration of multiple doses of desmopressin. Even single doses of DDAVP may lead to substantial hyponatremia if accompanied by aggressive intravenous hydration and poor oral intake.

Amicar (epsilon-aminocaproic acid) can be used postoperatively in all VWD patients to inhibit fibrinolysis and inactivate proteolytic enzymes in saliva, thus enhancing hemostasis. The initial dose of Amicar is administered intravenously at a rate of 400 mg/kg/day given either by bolus every 6 hours or by continuous infusion. At discharge, Amicar can be given orally to complete 10 to 14 days of total therapy. For patients who cannot tolerate oral Amicar, a long-term access line may be placed for home intravenous therapy. Failure to use Amicar in one clinical study may have accounted for an increased risk of delayed adenotonsillectomy bleeding in children with von Willebrand's disease (13%) compared with adenotonsillectomy patients without known coagulopathy (3.6%).[50]

Hemophilia and Christmas Disease

Hemophilia (factor VIII deficiency) and Christmas disease (factor IX deficiency) are bleeding diatheses inherited as sex-linked recessive traits. The incidence of factor VIII deficiency is approximately 1 per 10,000 males whereas factor IX deficiency is 1 per 40,000 males.

Factor VIII and factor IX concentrates are commercially available. A loading dose of concentrate is administered preoperatively to attain a factor level 100% of normal; half the loading dose (maintenance dose) is then given at the end of the procedure.[51,52] For 3 to 5 days postoperatively, the maintenance dose is infused every 8 hours for factor VIII or every 12 hours for factor IX to keep trough factor levels above 50%. When the trough level approaches 75%, the dosing interval is increased to every 12 and 24 hours for factor VIII and factor IX, respectively. After the third to fifth postoperative day, concentrate is given once a day for 1 week and then once every other day for an additional week. Pharmacologic agents that enhance hemostasis such as DDAVP and Amicar may be used as adjuncts to factor replacement therapy.

Jehovah's Witnesses

Children of families of the Jehovah's Witness faith pose a particular problem relative to adenotonsillectomy.[53] Such families generally seek medical attention and refuse only one facet of medical care: the transfusion of blood or blood products. A consistent approach to the surgical treatment of children of Jehovah's Witness families is advocated.

This approach should ideally be outlined in an institutional policy that acknowledges Jehovah's Witnesses' beliefs and respects the fact that competent adults may exercise these beliefs by rejecting specific treatments. The policy, however, should also state that the courts and the hospital do not allow such beliefs to serve as a basis for withholding medical treatment for minor children when death or serious disability might otherwise occur. It should clearly outline that if the physicians and parents are unable to agree on a course of treatment and the physicians believe that such treatment is necessary for the child, legal intervention may be requested. In such circumstances the parents will be given adequate notice to participate fully in the judicial proceedings.

A document outlining the policy should be signed by the physician, with a copy placed in the patient's chart and a copy given to the parents or guardian. It is not a formal signed consent for the transfusion of blood or blood products. However, it does provide medical record documentation that the family has been informed of the physicians' and hospital's policy toward transfusion of dependent children and that the parents wish to proceed with their child's planned surgery.

KETOROLAC ADMINISTRATION

Ketorolac tromethamine (Toradol) is a peripherally acting, nonsteroidal, anti-inflammatory drug. It has gained popularity in ambulatory surgical anesthesia management because of its pain relief efficacy combined with its lack of respiratory depression in comparison with more traditional opioid analgesics. Unfortunately, ketorolac, like other nonsteroidal, anti-inflammatory drugs, prolongs bleeding time by inhibiting platelet aggregation and thromboxane A2 production. This potentially increases the risk of postoperative bleeding in adenotonsillectomy patients.

Such increased risk has been documented in one combined adult and pediatric series in which 17% of the ketorolac group compared with 4.4% of the nonketerolac group experienced postoperative bleeding.[54] An additional study demonstrated a similar higher rate of postadenotonsillectomy bleeding in adults (16%) but not in children (6.5%).[55] This differential bleeding rate was attributed to differences in the pharmacokinetics of ketorolac between children and adults; plasma clearance of ketorolac is higher in children. This may explain why a more recent study restricted solely to pediatric patients did not demonstrate an increased incidence of postadenotonsillectomy hemorrhage in children who received ketorolac compared with those who did not. This latter study also identified no difference between patients receiving high-dose (greater than 0.6 ml/kg) or low-dose (less than or equal to 0.6 mg/kg) ketorolac.[56]

EMESIS AND POOR FLUID INTAKE

Two of the more common postoperative problems in children following adenotonsillectomy are emesis and poor fluid intake. A certain degree of emesis is expected secondary to anesthesia. However, recurrent or protracted emesis is of significant concern because of the risk of dehydration. Estimates of the incidence of severe postadenotonsillectomy emesis in the pediatric population range from 0.7 to 7.5%, with reported dehydration rates of 0.3 to 1.9%.[30]

The role of required oral fluid intake after adenotonsillectomy is being reconsidered.[57] Offering small amounts of clear liquids to ensure that the child is able and willing to drink is appropriate, but forcing fluids to establish resumption of normal oral fluid intake does not appear to be beneficial. The alternative administration of adequate intraoperative and postoperative intravenous fluids is crucial. Delayed oral intake necessitating prolonged intravenous hydration is reported in up to 9 to 16% of children after adenotonsillectomy. Such intravenous hydration should replace cumulative fluid deficits related to the length of preoperative NPO status, the volume of intraoperative blood loss, and anticipated deficits based on the duration of limited postoperative fluid intake. Such intraoperative and postoperative intravenous hydration should always be with isotonic solutions.[58]

In the pediatric population, maintenance as well as replacement rates of intravenous hydration are based upon the child's weight. The maintenance rate is the summation of 4 cc/kg/h for the first 10 kg of body weight; 2 cc/kg/h for the next 10 kg of body weight; and an additional 1 cc/kg/h for each kilogram over 20 kg.

The preoperative deficit is determined by multiplying the number of fasting hours times the maintenance rate as calculated previously. This deficit should be corrected over the first 3 postoperative hours, with one half of the deficit returned during the first hour and one quarter of the deficit returned during each of the next 2 hours. If oral intake is established before the deficit has been fully corrected, the patient's intrinsic thirst mechanism will complete the job and further IV fluid administration may be curtailed.

The third factor to be considered in fluid replacement is blood loss. This loss can certainly be replaced with an equivalent volume of blood or plasma expander. However, in the setting of routine adenotonsillectomy, blood volume loss is preferably replaced with isotonic solutions in a 3-cc isotonic solution to 1-cc blood loss ratio. For example, 50 cc of blood loss requires replacement with 150 cc isotonic fluid. Nonhematologic fluid losses, such as vomiting, are replaced in 1 cc to 1 cc fashion.

In addition to intravenous fluid administration, pharmacologic methods are also used to decrease the morbidity related to postoperative nausea and vomiting (PONV). Such methods include peri-operative protocols incorporating metaclopramide,[59] antiemetic agents such as ondansetron,[60] and dexamethasone or other steroid preparations.[61–64]

Of the three, the beneficial effect of dexamethasone is perhaps most debated.[65,66] The effect of preoperative dexamethasone (1 mg/kg to a maximum dose of 25 mg) on PONV in children undergoing electrocautery tonsillectomy has been compared with saline placebo with standardiza-tion of other anesthetic and nonanesthetic factors.[67] The dose of IV dexamethasone recommended is greater than that reported in previous studies assessing the effect of steroid treatment in patients undergoing adenotonsillectomy, but is equivalent to treatment dosages recommended for use in children with airway obstruction. The incidence of PONV, need for rescue antiemetics, quantity of oral intake, and analgesic requirements did not differ between the two groups prior to home discharge. However, during the 24 hours after discharge, more patients in the control group experienced PONV (62% compared with 25% in the steroid treated group), and more children in the control group (8% compared with 0% in the steroid treated group) returned to the hospital for intravenous hydration. This delayed efficacy of dexamethasone in decreasing the incidence of late PONV is consistent with its biological half-life of 36 to 48 hours as well as its established prolonged antiemetic effect in chemotherapy patients.

Complications from steroid therapy are typically related to long-term use, and the risk of significant adverse side effects when steroids are administered for less than a 24-hour duration is negligible.

RISK POPULATIONS

Down Syndrome

Down syndrome (DS) occurs in 1 in 800 live births and is one of the most common autosomal chromosomal disorders. Adenotonsillectomy may be required in children with Down syndrome for obstructive as well as infectious indications. Upper airway obstruction and obstructive sleep apnea syndrome (OSAS) are commonly recognized problems in these children. Predisposing factors include midfacial hypoplasia, micrognathia, narrow nasopharyngeal and oropharyngeal dimensions, macroglossia, hypotonia, associated laryngotracheal abnormalities, and a tendency toward systemic obesity in addition to relative adenotonsillar hypertrophy.[68]

Down syndrome children should be assessed preoperatively for atlantoaxial instability known to be potentially present at a higher incidence in this population.[69] These children also have smaller tracheal airways than do non-DS children and should be intubated with an endotracheal tube two sizes smaller than that typically chosen; the fit of the tube should always be confirmed by an air leak test.[70] Such safe intubation practices will help decrease postintubation airway complications in this population.

Down syndrome children have a greater likelihood of underlying medical problems, particularly cardiac disease and neurodevelopmental delay. These contribute to an increased rate of postoperative respiratory complications and a more protracted recovery course in Down syndrome children compared with age- and sex-matched controls.[71,72] Inpatient hospitalization with overnight cardio-respiratory and pulse oximetry monitoring, as well as intravenous hydration until the resumption of adequate postoperative oral intake, is necessary in all DS children. Those with confirmed or suspected OSAS are at particularly high risk for postoperative upper airway obstruction, arterial oxygen desaturation, and respiratory failure, and should be observed in an intensive care setting with the ready capability for cardiopulmonary resuscitation and intubation.

CHILDREN WITH NEUROMUSCULAR DISEASE

When children with neuromuscular disease undergo adenotonsillectomy, their parents must be made aware of the potential postoperative complications.[35,36] Low oxygen saturation levels are seen for a prolonged period of time following surgery in many patients. The use of a nasopharyngeal airway may be valuable, and it is often inserted immediately following surgery before anesthesia has been reversed. Underlying lung disease and gastroesophageal reflux disease should be treated aggressively to lessen postoperative problems. Additionally, postoperative risk can be diminished by extubating patients only when they are fully awake, avoiding narcotics, and using steroids intraoperatively.

Once patients leave the postanesthesia care unit, they should be fully monitored in order to follow the oxygen saturation levels. Oxygen administration should be minimized in order to avoid depression of the hypoxic respiratory drive. Narcotics and sedative agents should be administered with careful consideration because of their potential for respiratory compromise. Nursing care is critical, including aggressive physiotherapy, regular suctioning, and appropriate positioning. Parents must always be aware that a tracheotomy may be necessary in some neurologically impaired children with severe airway obstruction and adenotonsillar hypertrophy. However, the adenotonsillectomy is certainly justified when there is hypertrophy with obstruction in an attempt to avoid a tracheotomy in these patients.

MUCOPOLYSACCHARIDOSES

The mucopolysaccharidoses (MPSs) are six closely related genetically determined lysosomal storage diseases. Each is characterized by a specific enzymatic defect that results in the accumulation of incompletely degraded mucopolysaccharides within cell lysosomes. Depending on the particular mucopolysaccharide by product and the affected organs, a wide range of clinical manifestations can occur.

All MPSs are inherited in an autosomal recessive pattern except for Hunter syndrome, which is X-chromosome sex-linked. MPSs occur in all ethnic groups and have a combined incidence of 1 in 30,000 to 1 in 150,000 live births. Airway obstruction in MPS patients is multifactorial due to a combination of narrow tracheobronchial airway dimensions, supraglottic and glottic anatomical abnormalities, macroglossia, short neck with small pharyngeal dimensions, tempomandibular joint problems, and characteristic copious pulmonary and nasal secretions in addition to relative adenotonsillar hypertrophy.[73,74]

Adenotonsillectomy is commonly necessary in MPS children as the initial procedural attempt to improve their marginal airway status. Their perioperative care can be very difficult. Maintenance of the upper airway during anesthetic induction and laryngotracheal intubation is often challenging. Atlantoaxial instability is also common in specific mucopolysaccharidoses. Postoperatively, they pose the same airway and general management risks as DS children.

SICKLE CELL DISEASE

Sickle cell anemia is a major disorder of beta chain hemoglobin function. This autosomal recessive inherited disease largely affects blacks, 8% of whom carry the sickle cell gene, as well as certain Mediterranean ethnic groups. Clinically, sickle cell disease is characterized by a chronic hemolytic anemia and vaso-occlusive complications due to the presence of abnormal hemoglobin. Children with sickle cell disease and obstructive sleep apnea secondary to adenotonsillar hypertrophy are at particular risk because repeated oxygen desaturation during periods of obstructive apnea may precipitate recurrent vaso-occulsive crises.[75]

Polysomnography is invaluable in this population for diagnostic purposes and to identify severely affected individuals. Established obstructive sleep apnea with elevated end-tidal carbon dioxide levels during sleep, hemoglobin S ratio greater than 40%, and age less than 4 years are all associated with increased postoperative risk in sickle cell disease children undergoing adenoton-sillectomy. The preoperative treatment of children with sickle cell disease before general anesthesia is primarily designed to minimize the potential dangers of hypoxia and hypoperfusion.[76] Such children are admitted 24 hours before surgery for preoperative hydration and packed red blood cell transfusion. The goal of transfusion is to decrease the hemoglobin S ratio to less than 40% total blood volume. Preoperative intravenous hydration is designed to maximize capillary blood flow.

INTRAOPERATIVE COMPLICATIONS

During the performance of an adenotonsillectomy, the surgeon and the anesthesiologist share the same anatomical region for airway maintenance and the operative field. Manipulations of the mouth gag put the endotracheal tube at risk for deleterious movement, kinking, or accidental dislodgement.

The surgeon and the anesthesiologist should assess the condition of the patient's teeth. Loose teeth can be inadvertently dislodged and aspirated during intubation or operative manipulation. Permission should be obtained preoperatively for extraction of extremely loose teeth. Careful mouth gag placement helps to avoid dental damage. Intraoperative chest radiographs should be obtained to rule out aspiration if a tooth or portion of a tooth is noted to be missing and cannot be accounted for at the completion of the case.

The potential for soft tissue injury to the face, mouth, and throat during operative intervention also exists. Surgical instruments, cautery, and lasers all pose a risk. Proper draping is essential. Red rubber catheters can be used to protect electrocautery devices that do not come commercially shielded, particularly at the junction where the spatula or needle tip inserts into the hand-piece. Mouth gags should be properly insulated with no exposed metal intraoral components, especially at the corners of the mouth. The eyes always should be covered. Penetrating towel clips are hazardous when securing the head drape; care must be taken to avoid orbit, auricle, or skin perforation.

Certain precautions are indicated to reduce the risk of electrocautery-induced fire, given the potentially flammable endotracheal tube when performing an electrodissection tonsillectomy.[77] The inspired oxygen concentration should be reduced with an oxygen–air ratio of 50% or less if possible. Although a standard endotracheal tube can still burn at this oxygen concentration, flame ignition is unlikely. The patient should be allowed to ventilate spontaneously whenever possible, because this prevents expired gases from flowing retrograde around the endotracheal tube in large quantities. Prophylactic measures from a surgical standpoint include using moist pharyngeal packs, maximizing the distance between the endotracheal tube and electrocautery tip, and setting the electrosurgical unit power as low as possible to minimize arcing.

The use of phenylephrine as a vasoconstrictive agent during adenotonsillectomy is contraindicated. There have been several reports of hypertension, pulmonary edema, and in some cases, death resulting from phenylephrine's intraoperative use. Phenylephrine is an alpha-selective agonist, which causes vasoconstriction, thus increasing systemic vascular resistance and potentially decreasing left-sided ventricular performance and cardiac output. The latter can lead to increased pulmonary capillary pressure and promote pulmonary edema, particularly in an anesthetic setting in which the concomitant use of a beta blocker or calcium channel blocker may further limit cardiac output by decreasing heart rate and cardiac contractility.

Recommendations have been published regarding the use of phenylephrine and other vasoconstrictive agents in the operating room.[78] These include

- The initial dose of phenylephrine should not exceed 0.5 mg (four drops of a 0.25% solution).
- The minimal amount of phenylephrine needed to achieve vasoconstriction should be administered.
- The blood pressure and pulse should be closely monitored.

- The dose of phenylephrine should be administered in a calibrated syringe and should be verified by the physician.
- The concomitant use of beta blockers and calcium channel blockers should be avoided.
- The potential for cumulative effects of other vasoconstrictive agents such as oxymetazoline, cocaine, and lidocaine with epinephrine commonly used in the operating room must be considered.

Laryngospasm is a potential immediate complication following adenotonsillectomy. Such acute forceful contraction of the laryngeal musculature can be precipitated by glottic stimulation secondary to the hypopharyngeal pooling of secretions and blood or an undesired level of anesthesia at the time of extubation. Laryngospasm results in a complete glottic block to inspiration and expiration, causing life-threatening hypoxia and hypercarbia. Careful surgical hemostasis, thorough suctioning of blood and secretions from the oropharynx and hypopharynx at the completion of the procedure, evacuation of stomach contents by passage of an orogastric tube, and extubation under a deep or very light anesthesia level are important preventative measures. The "tonsil position," with the head placed slightly dependent and the patient lying on the side during transport to the recovery room, further reduces aspiration risk in somnolent patients.

The perioperative use of topical or intravenous lidocaine is an additional method that may prevent immediate postoperative laryngospasm.[79,80] Both are safe methods as indicated by plasma lidocaine levels. Intravenous lidocaine has a higher incidence of deep sedation, suggesting that topical lidocaine may be the more preferable of the two methods.[81]

SHORT-TERM POSTOPERATIVE COMPLICATIONS

POSTOBSTRUCTIVE PULMONARY EDEMA

Patients with long-standing upper airway obstruction from adenotonsillar hypertrophy may develop a compensated state secondary to expiration against partial obstruction. This results in increased intrathoracic pressure with their resultant baseline pressure set at a higher level. Acute postoperative pulmonary edema may develop for several reasons in this situation.[82] If obstruction is suddenly relieved, intrathoracic pressure may rapidly decrease, with a corresponding increase in venous return, increased pulmonary blood volume, and increased pulmonary hydrostatic pressure; this leads to transudation of fluid from the capillary bed to the pulmonary interstitium. A similar cascade can occur from inspiration against obstruction such as that which occurs with laryngospasm following extubation.

When respiratory compromise occurs immediately following adenotonsillectomy, one should consider the development of acute postobstructive pulmonary edema if frothy secretions and a suggestive chest radiograph are seen.[83] Once this has been identified, the patient should be monitored carefully with the expectation that mechanical respiratory support may be necessary, including the use of positive end expiratory pressure or continuous positive airway pressure. The use of intravenous crystalloids should be restricted and colloids administered preferentially. Diuretic use may be necessary.

FEVER

The postoperative recovery from adenotonsillectomy is often protracted and characterized by throat and ear pain, intermittent fever, and foul odor from the oral cavity. Fever not only contributes to generalized morbidity but also increases insensible fluid losses promoting dehydration. Fever is particularly common within the first 36 hours, most likely secondary to a combination of factors including anesthetic effects, pulmonary atelectasis, and transient bacteremia.[84] In one prospective study of 32 children undergoing adenotonsillectomy for obstructive as well as infectious indications, greater than one third of perioperative blood cultures were positive.[85] *Hemophilus influenzae* was the most common cultured organism; the *Hemophilus influenzae* strains isolated from the blood were the same as those isolated from the tonsillar tissue in all cases.

Fever and halitosis may also reflect secondary bacterial infection or colonization of the operative site. These areas are left open to heal by secondary intention and become covered with a fibrinous inflammatory exudate postoperatively. Pharyngeal bacterial colonization is common. The organisms most frequently cultured from the tonsillar fossae in children are *Streptococcus viridans* and *Streptococcus pneumoniae*; nontypable *Hemophilus influenzae*, *Staphylococcus aureus*, and *Streptococcus pyogenes* also can be present. Does such bacteria colonization of the area result in clinically significant additional local and systemic inflammation or infection? If so, does antibiotic therapy prevent or suppress this process? Do the potential benefits of perioperative antibiotic therapy outweigh the risks and cost?

These questions appear to have been answered by well-designed, prospective, randomized, double-blind studies demonstrating a significant benefit from the routine administration of prophylactic antibiotic therapy in comparison with placebo.[86–88] Perioperative antibiotic therapy resulted in a statistically significant lower overall incidence of fever, a shorter duration of fever, and fewer high fevers. Children receiving antibiotics also had an earlier return to baseline diet and activities, a shorter duration of subjective pain, and a shorter duration and lesser severity of mouth odor.

Although antibiotic sensitivity and resistance patterns of oropharyngeal bacteriologic data suggest that broad spectrum antibiotic therapy might be more efficacious as perioperative adenotonsillectomy prophylaxis,[87] no increased benefit was achieved by broadening such therapy from a combination of ampicillin and amoxicillin to a combination of cefazolin and cefaclor.[88] Broader spectrum antibiotic therapy should probably be reserved for children who, despite standard ampicillin/amoxicillin treatment, demonstrate a protracted or difficult recovery course. Alternative antibiotic therapy is obviously also necessary in penicillin-allergic children.

The optimal duration of perioperative antibiotic therapy remains uncertain. Most studies support the use of an initial intravenous dose of antibiotic administration at the time of surgery. Historically, intravenous therapy would then be continued for 12 to 24 hours postoperatively. In the present context of ambulatory adenotonsillectomy, a switch is made to oral antibiotic therapy almost immediately as soon as oral intake is sufficient to allow discharge. A total of 5 to 7 days of antibiotic coverage is generally advocated.

THROAT PAIN

Sore throat (odynophagia) occurs in almost all patients following adenotonsillectomy surgery. Associated almost universally with tonsillectomy, it is a much less severe and much more transient complaint in children following adenoidectomy alone. The control of such throat pain is a crucial issue from a general morbidity standpoint as well as to promote maintenance of postoperative oral intake and avoidance of dehydration. Multiple intraoperative and postoperative efforts have been made to prevent or lessen the severity of sore throat following adenotonsillectomy.

Intraoperative measures have included alterations in surgical technique, infiltration of analgesic agents into the tonsillar bed, and systemic administration of intravenous or intramuscular analgesics with a prolonged postoperative effect. Postoperative measures also include the initial administration of intravenous and intramuscular analgesics, followed by the eventual use of a wide array of oral analgesics. Included in the latter group are acetaminophen, nonsteroidal anti-inflammatory agents, and narcotics such as codeine or oxycodone combinations. Topical medications such as sucralfate also have been tried. Aspirin and aspirin-based products are purposely avoided due to their potential bleeding risk. Perioperative antibiotic and steroid therapy also appears to lessen postoperative pain and discomfort as outlined in previous sections.

Measuring or assessing postoperative pain can be a difficult undertaking, particularly in young children.[89] Typical subjective and objective assessments are the use of pain scores by adult observers and documentation of analgesic intake regimens. Pediatric quality of life questionnaires also have been developed to assess the pain experienced by children following adenotonsillectomy.[90] Such questionnaires are only applicable to children old enough to verbalize their experiences; no equivalent assessment tool for younger, nonverbal children is available. Additional measures of post-tonsillectomy pain in children have included the total time it takes a child to drink a specific volume of liquid (the so-called deglutition time) and careful monitoring of a child's oral intake.

Clearly, any agent given intraoperatively to promote postoperative analgesia without sedation would be an ideal adjunct to adenotonsillar surgery. Bupivacaine hydrochloride, a commonly used local anesthetic for oral surgical procedures, is one such agent. Its half-life of 4 to 7 hours provides for short-term duration of action, and a period of analgesia theoretically persists even after the return of sensation, potentially further reducing the need for additional postoperative pain medication. Various studies have investigated the effectiveness of the intraoperative infiltration of bupivacaine hydrochloride on postoperative throat pain in pediatric adenotonsillectomy patients, with disparate results.[91–95]

In one prospective, randomized, double-blind study involving 50 children and adolescents 3 to 16 years of age who underwent tonsil resection by electrocautery dissection technique, 0.5% bupivacaine (1 mg/kg up to a maximum of 9 mg per tonsillar fossa and 18 mg total) or saline equivalent was infiltrated into the superior and inferior poles of both tonsillar fossae.[96] No parenteral narcotics were administered intraoperatively or in the recovery room. No steroids, antibiotics, or other agents were used during surgery or within the first 10 hours after surgery. This study demonstrated no improvement in pain control from bupivacaine use. Perceived pain levels between bupivacaine and saline groups at 2, 6, or 10 hours postoperatively did not differ. Oral intake levels over the first 10 hours were similar. Although bupivacaine group patients received fewer doses of oral acetaminophen, the difference between the groups was not statistically significant.

Another study similarly assigned 22 patients 8 to 18 years of age in double-blind, randomized fashion to receive 0.25% bupivacaine hydrochloride with epinephrine (1:200,000) or 0.9% saline with epinephrine as a peritonsillar infiltration prior to tonsillectomy by standard electrocautery technique.[97] Both patient groups did receive a standard postoperative pain protocol including morphine sulfate in the recovery room, acetominophin with codeine elixir over the first 72 hours postoperatively, and acetominophin elixir alone over the subsequent 72 hours postoperatively. Intensity of postoperative pain, constant baseline pain as well as pain with swallowing, were assessed using a visual analog self-rating method. An objective pain measurement was also used consisting of the total time to swallow 100 cc of water. This study suggested that bupivicaine infiltration was beneficial. Objective and subjective pain reductions reached statistical significance for postoperative days 0 through 5 and were marginally significant through postoperative day 10.

Bupicicaine injections do have potential complications; these appear to be associated more with the concurrent injection of epinephrine-containing solutions rather than due to the local anesthetic. Epinephrine-containing solutions administered at the time of general inhalational anesthesia can potentially precipitate cardiac ectopy. There is a reported case of brainstem stroke following bupivacaine with epinephrine injection into the tonsillar fossae and adenoid bed in a patient who was eventually determined to have anomalous neurovascular circulation.[98] Injections into the adenoid bed have additionally been associated with the subsequent development of meningitis.[99] Local anesthetic injections are probably best limited to the tonsillar fossae and are most safely administered without accompanying epinephrine.

Postoperatively, two analgesic sprays have been shown to be potentially effective in reducing postadenotonsillectomy pain (10% lidocaine and benzydamine hydrochloride).[100] However, their use is poorly tolerated and attempting to spray the tonsillar fossae in the post-tonsillectomy pediatric patient can be a technical challenge.

Sucralfate, a basic amino salt of sucrose octasulfate, binds to the matrix protein of mucosal ulcerations. Within the stomach, it creates a barrier that protects gastric ulcers from the irritating effects of gastric acid and pepsin. Sucralfate has been used postopertively in tonsillectomy patients to coat the raw mucosal surface overlying the pharyngeal musculature in an attempt to prevent muscle spasm and neural irritation.[101,102] Studies performed to date have been limited to adolescents and adults because this postoperative treatment regimen requires the patient to swish and swallow the sucralfate solution three to four times daily. Sucralfate has been shown to significantly reduce throat and ear pain and subsequent analgesic requirement by the second postoperative day; it does not, however, provide complete analgesia.

Nonsteriodal anti-inflammatory drugs (NSAIDs) are known to be efficacious in relieving postoperative pain. Pain control is most probably achieved by inhibition of the release of pain-mediating prostaglandins from injured tissues. Numerous studies have confirmed that ibuprofen and other NSAIDs are more effective than acetaminophen with codeine, hydrocodone, and even opiates in the relief of pain after oral surgery procedures. NSAIDs have no central nervous system side effects, no respiratory depression, and no alteration in airway protective reflexes — all of which make these drugs potentially useful in adenotonsillectomy patients.

The concern is that NSAIDs can potentiate postadenotonsillectomy hemorrhage due to their effect on platelet function. NSAIDs reversibly inhibit platelet aggregation while the drug is in circulation. In adult tonsillectomy patients, indomethacin has been shown to be as effective as intramuscular narcotics for lessening pain, but with an associated increased incidence of postoperative bleeding. In pediatric patients, ibuprofen has been compared with acetaminophen with codeine for pain management in 110 children undergoing tonsillectomy.[103] The only statistically significant difference between the groups was less nausea in patients receiving ibuprofen. No difference was found in postoperative bleeding, pain, or temperature control in this study.

Another prospective, randomized, double-blind study also assessed the efficacy and safety of ibuprofen compared with acetaminophen with codeine in pediatric adenotonsillectomy patients.[104] Acetaminophen with codeine was more effective in controlling pain on days 1 and 3; however, the treatment groups showed no difference with regard to pain control on day 5. The groups were not significantly statistically different with regard to return to normal diet or return to normal sleep pattern. The postoperative hemorrhage rate was 0% in the acetaminophen with codeine group and 12.5% in the ibuprofen group. The increased bleeding risk in the ibuprofen group could not be correlated with any documented significant difference in bleeding time, PT, or PTT between the two groups.

Acetaminophen alone at a maximum dose of 15 mg/kg every 4 hours, not exceeding 90 mg/kg in one 24-hour period, has been shown to be as efficacious as acetominophen with codeine in controlling postadenotonsillectomy pain in children.[105] Postoperative oral intake was significantly higher in the children treated solely with acetominophen. This is attributed to the absence of codeine-related side effects.

OTALGIA

Otalgia frequently accompanies sore throat, most commonly as a referred pain mediated via the glossopharyngeal nerve. Such referred otalgia is typically episodic and of brief duration, often induced by chewing, yawning, or other maneuvers that promote palatal motion. Nasopharyngeal edema or eustachian tube injury secondary to adenoidectomy may induce postoperative middle ear effusion or otitis media. A formal otologic examination should be performed to rule out middle ear disease if ear pain is persistent.

LONG-TERM POSTOPERATIVE COMPLICATIONS

VELOPHARYNGEAL INSUFFICIENCY

Velopharyngeal insufficiency (VPI) may result from adenotonsillectomy. Hypernasal speech (rhinolalia aperta) and nasal regurgitation constitute the main symptoms of VPI. Sometimes the hypernasality is only present on the pronunciation of those fricative and affricative consonants that require the greatest degree of sustained velopharyngeal sphincter closure. Adenoidectomy is the primary cause, but tonsillectomy can also potentially contribute to VPI. Postoperative transient VPI lasting only a few weeks to months is quite common. The incidence of more prolonged or permanent VPI varies widely with quoted figures between 1 in 1500 to 1 in 3000 adenotonsillectomies.[106–108] This discrepancy in the incidence of VPI is attributable to multiple reasons, including an absence of uniform duration of postoperative follow-up, variability in the formality of postoperative speech evaluation, and differences in the timing of speech evaluation in those who have been formally assessed.

One review of 137 patients with clinically significant hypernasality following adenoidectomy or adenotonsillectomy revealed one third of these patients to have preoperative findings on history or physical examination indicative of increased postoperative VPI risk.[108] These factors include a history of feeding problems with nasal regurgitation in infancy, a family history of VPI or palatal clefting, a pre-existing speech abnormality consisting of mixed nasality or difficulty distinguishing between hyponasal or hypernasal speech, and physical examination findings suggestive of submucous palatal clefting.

Submucous cleft palate occurs in 1 in 1200 patients.[109] Physical examination findings in such patients include a bifid uvula, a zona pellucida or attenuated medium raphe of the soft palate, and a V-shape notching of the hard palate.[110] Additional children at risk for postoperative VPI include those with overt cleft palate, those with orofacial anomalies such as Treacher–Collins syndrome or Pierre–Robin sequence, and those with neuromuscular disorders that impair palatal function.

In a patient with no clinical risk factors, the role of preoperative documentation of the velopharyngeal function — directly by fiberoptic nasopharyngoscopy or radiographically by videofluoroscopy — is controversial. Such documentation is definitely indicated, along with a careful preoperative evaluation by a speech therapist, in children at risk for VPI based on history or physical examination.[111] In the child with a submucous cleft palate or preoperative hypernasality, the indications for adenoidectomy or adenotonsillectomy need to be assessed carefully and discussed with the family from a "benefit to risk" ratio.[112] A modified surgical approach can be performed safely and effectively in such children when operative intervention is a necessity.

In a review of 22 children at high risk for velopharyngeal insufficiency who underwent modified adenoidectomy with standard instrumentation technique, none developed hypernasality or permanent nasal regurgitation of fluids.[113] The use of powered instrumentation or suction electrocautery provides alternative means of performing modified adenoidectomy. An endoscopic shaver system with a bendable blade appears to be of significant utility for this purpose.

Even in children whose formal speech evaluation confirms VPI following adenoidectomy or adenotonsillectomy, spontaneous improvement in hypernasal speech may occur, sometimes over quite a significant length of postoperative time. In one study, 13% of patients with confirmed postoperative VPI improved without treatment, and another 37% required only speech therapy — all with subsequent return of normal nasal resonance.[108] Such data support a conservative approach of delaying surgical intervention for at least 6 to 12 months postoperatively. The approximately 50% of patients with truly persistent VPI who do require surgical intervention are typically managed with palatal pushback or pharyngoplasty procedures. Palatal obturators may be tried but are uncomfortable and often difficult to fit, particularly in young children.

As mentioned earlier, adenoidectomy appears to be the primary cause of postoperative VPI. Tonsillectomy alone does not appear to pose a similar risk unless secondary palatal scarring is significant. Even in a group of children at risk for VPI due to palatal clefting, tonsillectomy alone did not show postoperative deterioration in velopharyngeal function as measured by three evaluation methods interpreted collectively: perceptual speech characteristics, aerodynamic measures, and fiberoptic nasopharyngoscopy.[114] In some cases, tonsillectomy actually improves speech quality in terms of decreased hypernasal resonance and decreased nasal air emission.

Nasopharyngeal and Oropharyngeal Stenosis

Nasopharyngeal stenosis (NPS) and oropharyngeal stenosis (OPS) are severe complications of adenotonsillectomy that result when circumferentially denuded surfaces heal in close proximity. NPS results in an obliteration of the normal communication between the nasopharynx and oropharynx due to fusion of the posterior tonsillar pillars and soft palate to the posterior pharyngeal wall. This complication is attributed to the overzealous removal of the inferior and lateral aspects of the adenoid, typically in combination with removal or severe damage to the posterior tonsillar pillars.

OPS obliterates the oropharynx due to adhesion of the anterior tonsillar pillars and inferior tonsillar fossae to the base of tongue. OPS occurs secondary to extensive dissection of the lower poles of the tonsils and removal of adjacent lingual tonsil tissue. The obstruction in both situations can vary from a partially obstructive thin diaphragm to a thick cicatrix with complete lumen obliteration.

An increased incidence of NPS and OPS has been associated with extensive cautery use necessitated by excessive bleeding, aggressive mucosa removal, failure to preserve normal pharyngeal anatomy, surgery in the presence of active infection, removal of exceptionally large lateral lymphoid pharyngeal bands, revision surgery, and surgery in patients with keloid tendency. NPS specifically has also been associated with potassium titanyl phosphate laser (KTP) adenoidectomy and other alternative means of thermal adenoidectomy; choanal stenosis can occur in such cases as well.[115]

The symptoms of NPS and OPS vary from mild complaints such as difficulty blowing the nose or handling pharyngeal secretions to symptoms suggestive of complete nasal obstruction such as requisite oral breathing, constant hyponasal speech resonance, chronic rhinorrhea, dysphagia, and obstructive sleep apnea.

Fortunately, NPS and OPS are rare complications because they are very difficult to reconstruct successfully. There is no uniformly successful treatment. The fundamental principle of NPS and OPS correction is adequate scar removal and coverage of denuded areas with viable mucosal flaps. Management options include lysis of thin adhesions, scar resection with rotational and advancement mucosal flaps, and in cases of obliterative cicatrix, jejunal or alternative free flap reconstruction.[116] Associated choanal stenosis may require endoscopic or transpalatal correction.

Adjuvant therapies include corticosteroid injections and topical mitomycin C application in an attempt to retard scar reformation, periodic postoperative dilatation, and prolonged palatal obturator use. Symptom relief, as opposed to normal restoration of oropharyngeal/nasopharyngeal anatomy, is the surgical goal.

Eagle Stylohyoid Syndrome

Eagle first reported the association of radiographic evidence of an elongated stylohyoid process in patients with pharyngeal pain symptoms related to swallowing. He described two distinct syndromes of pain associated with this anomalous stylohyoid process.[117] The classic syndrome occurs predominantly after tonsillectomy as a persistent painful sensation in the throat somewhat similar to chronic pharyngitis. The pain may radiate to the middle ear or mastoid region; frequently, a foreign body sensation is noted. There may be difficulty in swallowing. Patients often believe that they have not properly healed from their tonsillectomy.

All these symptoms are considered a form of pharyngeal neurological irritation, presumably due to postoperative scarring and fibrotic contraction of the tonsillar fossa over an elongated styloid process.[118] The pain may be transmitted through the trigeminal nerve, facial nerve, glossopharyngeal nerve, or vagus nerve, all of which provide sensory innervation to the pharyngeal mucosa.

Diagnosing Eagle syndrome requires a high degree of clinical suspicion. On physical examination, palpation of the tonsillar fossa should reveal a firm mass beneath the mucosa representing the distal portion of the elongated styloid process. The symptoms should be reproduced, sometimes to even greater severity, by palpation. Radiographic confirmation of the elongated styloid is typically suggested on a lateral projection plain film.

The nonoperative management of stylohyoid syndrome includes reassurance, nonsteroidal anti-inflammatory medications, and steroid injections. Many patients require surgical intervention for pain relief. Eagle described and advocated a transpharyngeal approach to remove the elongated portion of the styloid process. Alternatively, an external cervical approach offers less risk of secondary deep space neck infection as well as better anatomic visualization of the surgical field.

ATLANTOAXIAL SUBLUXATION (GRISEL SYNDROME)

Transient neck pain is common following adenoidectomy or adenotonsillectomy. This pain is attributed to spasm of the paraspinal cervical musculature due to inflammation of adjacent pharyngeal tissue planes. Persistent neck pain with secondary limitation of spontaneous neck motion should raise concern of potential atlantoaxial subluxation due to spontaneous dislocation of the first cervical vertebra (C-1) on the second cervical vertebra (C-2). This condition is known as Grisel syndrome and was first described in two young girls with nasopharyngitis by P. Grisel, a French otolaryngologist, in 1930.[119]

Grisel syndrome occurs most commonly in children 5 to 12 years of age in association with head and neck infections or otolaryngological procedures, including adenotonsillectomy.[120] The pathogenic mechanism is generally believed to be tissue hyperemia following infection or adjacent surgery, with resultant decalcification of the anterior arch of the atlas and laxity of the anterior transverse ligament between the first and second cervical vertebrae. Patients with atlantoaxial subluxation usually complain of a stiff neck and present with spasm of the sternocleidomastoid or deep cervical muscles. The patient will hold his or her head in fixed position, typically tilted to one side, with slight rotation toward the opposite side. Local tenderness can often be appreciated on palpation over the atlantoaxial joint posteriorly, and occasionally the spinous process of the axis is palpable away from the midline toward the affected side.

Radiographic evaluation should include anteroposterior and lateral cervical spine films with an open mouth view. If these are normal, then flexion and extension views should be performed in seeking evidence of mild subluxation. Computed tomography is useful in defining bony destruction and more accurately determining the severity of malalignment. Treatment of radiologically confirmed atlantoaxial subluxation is recommended to reduce the risk of permanent restriction of cervical motion or neurologic sequelae. Such treatment should be individualized depending on the degree and duration of the subluxation. If the anterior transverse ligament is intact, cervical traction with a hard cervical collar for 6 to 8 weeks is usually sufficient. If the ligament is deficient, cervical skeletal traction with Gardner–Wells tongs implanted in the skull may be required to effect reduction; immobilization of the cervical spine with a Minerva cast and halo vest is recommended to allow the ligaments to heal.

Systemic antibiotic therapy effective against oropharyngeal aerobic and anaerobic pathogens should be instituted in all cases of suspected atlantoaxial subluxation. Some authors advocate treating any patient presenting with postoperative neck pain following adenoidectomy or adenotonsillectomy with broad spectrum oral antibiotic therapy for a minimum of 7 days in the hope of eradicating a potential nasopharyngitis that may contribute to such adverse cervical spine sequelae.[121]

UNUSUAL COMPLICATIONS

In addition to the more common intraoperative and postoperative complications previously discussed, a variety of miscellaneous and unusual complications of adenotonsillectomy have been reported.[122–126] Some of these are listed in Figure 15.1.

Necrotizing fasciitis

Retropharyngeal abscess

Tracheitis

Osteomyelitis

Meningitis

Trismus secondary to mandible condyle fracture

Pneumomediastinum with subcutaneous emphysema

Pneumoperitoneum

Depression

FIGURE 15.1 Unusual complications following adenotonsillectomy.

- Avoid or minimize the use of sutures during adenotonsillectomy. If they are used, document their superficial placement and the inability of other means to control hemorrhage. If there is recurrent hemorrhage following the use of sutures, consider the performance of angiography due to the suspicion of carotid artery injury.

- If dehydration is a concern, encourage families to bring the patient in for intravenous fluids. Document these discussions.

- Use appropriate doses of narcotics based on patient weight.

- Minimize tissue trauma, especially to the nasal surface of the palate, to lessen the chances of development of nasopharyngeal and oropharyngeal stenosis.

FIGURE 15.2 Suggestions to avoid litigation.

CONCLUSION

Adenotonsillectomy typically is performed safely and uneventfully with gratifying results for the patient as well as the patient's family. Informed preoperative consent and attentive, comprehensive perioperative care will mitigate parental concern in most situations in which adverse intraoperative or postoperative sequelae do occur. Unfortunately, some adenotonsillectomy complications may still precipitate litigation. Experience from review of such cases yields the guidelines provided in Figure 15.2; it is to be hoped that they can help practitioners avoid such legal intervention.

REFERENCES

1. Derkay, C.S. Pediatric otolaryngology procedures in the United States: 1977–1987. *Int. J. Pediatr. Otorhinolaryngol.*, 1993, 25, 1–12.
2. Randall, D.A. and Hoffer, M.E. Complications of tonsillectomy and adenoidectomy. *Otolaryngol. Head Neck Surg.*, 1998, 118, 61–68.
3. Handler, S.D., Miller, L., Richmond, K.H., and Baranack, C.C. Post-tonsillectomy hemorrhage: incidence, prevention, and management. *Laryngoscope*, 1966, 96, 1243–1247.
4. Carithers, J.S., Gerhardt, D.E., and Williams, J.R. Postoperative risks of pediatric tonsilloadenoidectomy. *Laryngoscope*, 1987, 97, 422–429.
5. Maniglia, A.J., Kushner, H., and Cozzi, L. Adenotonsillectomy: a safe outpatient procedure. *Arch. Otolaryngol. Head Neck Surg.*, 1989, 115, 92–94.

6. Pratt, L. and Gallagher, R. Tonsillectomy and adenoidectomy: incidence and mortality, 1968–1972. *Otolaryngol. Head Neck Surg.,* 1979, 87, 159–166.
7. Szeremeta, W., Novelly, N.J., and Benninger, M. Postoperative bleeding in tonsillectomy patients. *Ear Nose Throat J.,* 1996, 75, 373–376.
8. Collison, P.J. and Mettler, B. Factors associated with post-tonsillectomy hemorrhage. *Ear Nose Throat J.,* 2000, 79, 640–649.
9. Berkowitz, R.G. and Zalzal, G.H. Tonsillectomy in children under 3 years of age. *Arch. Otolaryngol. Head Neck Surg.,* 1990, 116, 685–686.
10. Janfaza, P. and Fabian, R.L. Pharynx. In Janfaza, P., Nadol, J.B., Jr., Galla, R.J., Fabian, R.L., and Montgomery, W.W. *Surgical Anatomy of the Head and Neck.* Philadelphia, PA: Lippencott, Williams and Wilkins, 2001, p. 371.
11. Younis, R.T. and Lazar, R.H. History and current practice of tonsillectomy. *Laryngoscope,* 2002, 112, S3–S5.
12. Maddern, B.R. Electrosurgery for tonsillectomy. *Laryngoscope,* 2002, 112, S11–S13.
13. Laser tonsillectomy — a committee statement. *AAO-HNS Bull.,* 1992, 11, 18.
14. Wiatrak, B.J. and Willging, J.P. Harmonic scalpel for tonsillectomy. *Laryngoscopy,* 2002, 112, S14–S16.
15. Plant, R.L. Radiofrequency treatment of tonsillar hypertrophy. *Laryngoscope,* 2002, 112, S20–S22.
16. Koltai, P.J., Solares, A., Mascha, E.J., and Xu, M. Intracapsular partial tonsillectomy for tonsillar hypertrophy. *Laryngoscope,* 2002, 112, S17–S19.
17. Linder, A., Markstrom, A., and Hulcrantz, E. Using the carbon dioxide laser for tonsillectomy in children. *Int. J. Pediatr. Otorhinolaryngol.,* 1999, 50, 31–36.
18. Janfaza, P. and Fabian, R.L. Pharynx. In Janfaza, P., Nadol, J.B., Jr., Galla, R.J., Fabian, R.L., and Montgomery, W.W. *Surgical Anatomy of the Head and Neck.* Philadelphia. Lippencott Williams and Wilkins, 2001, p. 379–380.
19. Franco, K. and Wallace, R. Management of postoperative bleeding after tonsillectomy. *Otolaryngol. Clin. North Am.,* 1987, 20, 391–397.
20. Osgothorpe, J.D., Adkins, W.Y., Putney, F.J., and Hungerford, S.D. Internal carotid artery as a source of tonsillectomy and adenoidectomy hemorrhage. *Otolaryngol. Head Neck Surg.,* 1981, 89, 758–762.
21. Deutsch, M., Kriss, V.M., and Willging, J.P. Distance between the tonsillar fossa and internal carotid artery in children. *Arch. Otolaryngol. Head Neck Surg.,* 1995, 121, 1410–1412.
22. Tovi, F., Leiberman, A., Hertzanu, Y., and Goldman, L. Pseudoaneurysm of the internal carotid artery secondary to tonsillectomy. *Int. J. Pediatr. Otorhinolaryngol.,* 1987, 13, 69–75.
23. Karas, D.E., Sawin, R.S., and Sie, K.C.Y. Pseudoaneurysm of the external carotid artery after tonsillectomy: A rare complication. *Arch. Otolaryngol. Head Neck Surg.,* 1997, 123, 345–347.
24. Conley, S.F. and Ellison, M.D. Avoidance of primary post-tonsillectomy hemorrhage in a teaching program. *Arch. Otolaryngol. Head Neck Surg.,* 1999, 125, 330–333.
25. Wei, J.L., Beatty, C.W., and Gustafson, R.O. Evaluation of post-tonsillectomy hemorrhage and risk factors. *Otolaryngol. Head Neck Surg.,* 2000, 123, 229–235.
26. Irani, D.B. and Berkowitz, R.G. Management of secondary hemorrhage following pediatric adenotonsillectomy. *Int. J. Pediatr. Otorhinolaryngol.,* 1997, 40, 115–124.
27. Liu, J.H., Anderson, K.E., Willging, J.P., Myer, C.M., III, Shott, S.R., Bratcher, G.O., and Cotton, R.T. Post-tonsillectomy hemorrhage: what is it and what should be recorded? *Arch. Otolaryngol. Head Neck Surg.,* 2001, 127, 1271–1275.
28. Cressman, W.R. and Myer, C.M., III. Management of tonsillectomy hemorrhage: results of a survey of pediatric otolaryngology fellowship programs. *Am. J. Otorhinolaryngol.,* 1995, 16, 29–32.
29. Tonsillectomy and adenoidectomy inpatient guidelines: recommendations of the AAO-HNS Pediatric Otolaryngology Committee. *AAO-HNS Bull.,* 1996, 15, 13–15.
30. Cunningham, M.J. Guidelines for inpatient versus outpatient adenotonsillectomy in children. *Adv. Otolaryngol. Head Neck Surg.,* 1998, 12, 41–43.
31. Tom, L.W.C., DeDio, R.M., Cohen, D.E., Wetmore, R.F., Handler, S.D., and Potsic, W.P. Is outpatient tonsillectomy appropriate for young children? *Laryngoscope,* 1992, 102, 277–280.
32. Wiatrak, B.J., Myer, C.M., III, and Andrew, T.M. Complications of adenotonsillectomy in children under three years of age. *Am. J. Otorhinolaryngol.,* 1991, 12, 170–172.

33. McColley, S.A., April, M.M., Carroll, J.L., Naclerio, R.M., and Loughlin, G.M. Respiratory compromise after adenotonsillectomy in children with obstructive sleep apnea. *Arch. Otolaryngol. Head Neck Surg.,* 1992, 118, 940–943.
34. Rothschild, M.A., Catalano, P., and Biller, H.F. Ambulatory pediatric tonsillectomy and the identification of high-risk subgroups. *Otolaryngol. Head Neck Surg.,* 1994, 110, 203–210.
35. Biavatti, M.J., Manning, S.C., and Philips, D.L. Predictive factors for respiratory complications after tonsillectomy and adenoidectomy in children. *Arch. Otolaryngol. Head Neck Surg.,* 1997, 123, 517–521.
36. Gerber, M.E., O'Connor, D.M., Adler, E., and Myer, C.M., III. Selected risk factors in pediatric adenotonsillectomy. *Arch. Otolaryngol. Head Neck Surg.,* 1996, 122, 811–814.
37. Hartnick, C.J. and Ruben, R.J. Preoperative coagulation studies prior to tonsillectomy. *Arch. Otolaryngol. Head Neck Surg.,* 2000, 126, 684–685.
38. The American Academy of Otolaryngology–Head and Neck Surgery Clinical Indicators Compendium. Alexandria, VA: American Academy of Otolaryngology–Head and Neck Surgery Inc., 1999.
39. Derkay, C.S. A cost-effective approach for preoperative hemostatic assessment in children undergoing adenotonsillectomy. *Arch. Otolaryngol. Head Neck Surg,.* 2000, 126, 688.
40. Tami, T.A., Parker, G.S., and Taylor, R.E. Post-tonsillectomy bleeding: an evaluation of risk factors. *Laryngoscope,* 1987, 9, 1307–1311.
41. Bolger, W.E., Parsons, D.S., and Potempa, L. Preoperative hemostatic assessment of the adenotonsillectomy patient. *Otolaryngol. Head Neck Surg.,* 1990, 103, 396–405.
42. Kang, J., Brodsky, L., Danzinger, I., Volk, M., and Stanievich, J. Coagulation profile as a predictor for post-tonsillectomy and adenoidectomy hemorrhage. *Int. J. Pediatr. Otorhinolaryngol.,* 1994, 28, 157–165.
43. Manning, S.C., Beste, D., McBride, T., and Goldberg, A. An assessment of preoperative coagulation screening for tonsillectomy and adenoidectomy. *Int. J. Pediatr. Otorhinolaryngol.,* 1997, 39, 67–76.
44. Close, H.L., Kryzer, T.C., Nowlin, J.H., and Alving, B.M. Hemostatic assessment of patients before tonsillectomy: a prospective study. *Otolaryngol. Head Neck Surg.,* 1994, 111, 733–738.
45. Zwack, G.C. and Derkay, C.S. The utility of preoperative hemostatic assessment in adenotonsillectomy. *Int. J. Pediatr. Otorhinolaryngol.,* 1997, 39, 67–76.
46. Burk, C.D., Miller, S.D., and Cohen, A.R. Preoperative history and coagulation screening in children undergoing tonsillectomy. *Pediatrics,* 1992, 89, 691–695.
47. Lind, S.E. The bleeding time does not predict surgical bleeding. *Blood,* 1991, 77, 2547–2552.
48. Shah, S.B., Lalwani, A.K., and Koerper, M.A. Perioperative management of von Willebrand's disease in otolaryngologic surgery. *Laryngoscope,* 1998, 108, 326–36.
49. Derkay, C.S., Werner, E., and Plotnick, E. Management of children with von Willebrand's disease undergoing adenotonsillectomy. *Am. J. Otorhinolaryngol.,* 1996, 17, 172–177.
50. Allen, G.C., Armfield, D.R., Bontempo, F.A., Kingsley, L.A., Goldstein, N.A., and Post, J.C. Adenotonsillectomy in children with von Willebrand's disease. *Arch. Otolaryngol. Head Neck Surg.,* 1999, 125, 547–551.
51. Prinsley, P., Wood, M., and Lee, C.A. Adenotonsillectomy in patients with inherited bleeding disorders. *Clin. Otolaryngol.,* 1993, 18, 206–208.
52. Scott, T.A., Jackler, R.K., and Kuerper, M.A. Management of hemophilia in otolaryngologic surgery: a contemporary protocol. *Arch. Otolaryngol. Head Neck Surg.,* 1988, 114, 1445–1448.
53. Morrison, J.E., Jr., Lane, G., Kelly, S., and Stool, S. The Jehovah's Witness family, transfusions and pediatric day surgery. *Int. J. Pediatr. Otorhinolaryngol.,* 1997, 38, 197–2050.
54. Judkins, J.H., Dray, T.G., and Hubbell, R.N. Intraoperative ketorolac and post-tonsillectomy bleeding. *Arch. Otolaryngol. Head Neck Surg.,* 1996, 122, 937–940.
55. Gallagher, J.E., Blauth, J., and Fornadley, J.A. Perioperative ketorolac tromethamine and postoperative hemorrhage in cases of tonsillectomy and adenoidectomy. *Laryngoscope,* 1995, 105, 606–609.
56. Agrawal, A., Gerson, C.R., Seligman, J., and Dsida, R.M. Postoperative hemorrhage after tonsillectomy: use of ketorolac tromethamine. *Otolaryngol. Head Neck Surg.,* 1999, 120, 335–339.
57. Messner, A.H. and Barbita, J.A. Oral fluid intake following tonsillectomy. *Int. J. Pediatr. Otorhinolaryngol.,* 1997, 39, 19–24.
58. McRea, R.G., Weissburg, A.J., and Chang, K.W. Iatrogenic hyponatremia: A cause of dealth following pediatric tonsillectomy. *Int. J. Pediatr. Otorhinolaryngol.,* 1994, 30, 227–232.

59. Ferrari, L.R. and Donlon, J.V. Metaclopramide reduces the incidence of vomiting after tonsillectomy in children. *Anesthesia Analg.,* 1992, 75, 351–354.

60. Lawhorn, C.D., Bower, C., Brown, R.E., Jr., Schmitz, M.L., Kymer, P.J., Stoner, J., Vollers, J.M., and Shirey, R. Odansetron decreases postoperative vomiting in pediatric patients undergoing tonsillectomy and adenoidectomy, *Int. J. Pediatr. Otolaryngol.,* 1996, 36, 99–108.

61. Heatley, D.G. Perioperative intravenous steroid treatment and tonsillectomy. *Arch. Otolaryngol. Head Neck Surg.,* 2001, 127, 1007–1008.

62. Shott, S.R. Tonsillectomy and postoperative vomiting: do steroids really work? *Arch. Otolaryngol. Head Neck Surg.,* 2001, 127, 1009–1010.

63. Hengerer, A.S. Do intravenous steroids play a role for tonsillectomy patients? *Arch. Otolaryngol. Head Neck Surg.,* 2001, 127, 1010.

64. Palme, C.E., Tomasevic, P., and Pohl, D.V. Evaluating the effects of oral prednisolone on recovery after tonsillectomy: a prospective, double blind, randomized trial. *Laryngoscope,* 2000, 110, 2000–2004.

65. Steward, D.L., Welge, J.A., and Myer, C.M. Do steroids reduce morbidity of tonsillectomy? Meta-analysis of randomized trials. *Laryngoscope,* 2001, 111, 1712–1718.

66. Goldman, A.C., Govindarat, S., and Rosenfeld, R.M. A meta-analysis of dexamethasone use with tonsillectomy. *Otolaryngol. Head Neck Surg.,* 2000, 123, 682–686.

67. Pappas, A.L.S., Sukhani, R., Hotaling, A.J., Mikat–Stevens, M., Javorski, J.J., Donzelli, J., and Shenoy, K. The effect of preoperative dexamethasone on the immediate and delayed postoperative morbidity in children undergoing adenotonsillectomy. *Anesthesia Analg.,* 1998, 87, 57–61.

68. Jacobs, I.N., Gray, R.F., and Todd, N.W. Upper airway obstruction in children with Down syndrome. *Arch. Otolaryngol. Head Neck Surg.,* 1996, 122, 945–950.

69. Harley, E.H. and Collins, M.D. Neurologic sequelae secondary to atlantoaxial instability in Down syndrome: implications in otolaryngologic surgery. *Arch. Otolaryngol. Head Neck Surg.,* 1994, 120, 159–165.

70. Shott, S.R. Down syndrome: analysis of airway size and a guide for appropriate intubation. *Laryngoscope,* 2000, 110, 585–592.

71. Goldstein, N.A., Armfield, D.R., Kingsley, L.A., Bobland, L.M., Allen, G.C., and Post, J.C. Postoperative complications after tonsillectomy and adenoidectomy in children with Down syndrome. *Arch. Otolaryngol. Head Neck Surg.,* 1998, 124, 171–176.

72. Bower, C.M. and Richmond, D. Tonsillectomy and adenoidectomy in patients with Down syndrome. *Int. J. Pediatr. Otorhinolaryngol.,* 1995, 33, 141–148.

73. Bredenkamp, J.K., Smith, M.S., Dudley, J.P., Williams, J.C., Crumley, R.L., and Crockett, D.M. Otolaryngologic manifestations of the mucopolysaccharidoses. *Ann. Otol., Rhinol. Laryngol.,* 1992, 101, 472–478.

74. Leighton, S.E.J., Papsin, B., Vellodi, A., Dinwiddie, R., and Lane, R. Disordered breathing during sleep in patients with mucopolysaccharidoses. *Int. J. Pediatr. Otorhinolaryngol.,* 2001, 58, 127–138.

75. Maddern, B.R., Reed, H.T., Ohene–Frempong, K., and Beckerman, R.C. Obstructive sleep apnea syndrome in sickle cell disease. *Ann. Otol., Rhinol. Laryngol.,* 1989, 98, 174–178.

76. Halvorson, D.J., McKie, K., Ashmore, P.E., and Porubsky, E.S. Sickle cell disease and tonsillectomy: preoperative management and postoperative complications. *Arch. Otolaryngol. Head Neck Surg.,* 1997, 689–692.

77. Keller, C., Elliott, W., and Hubbell, R.N. Endotracheal tube safety during electrodissection tonsillectomy. *Arch. Otolaryngol. Head Neck Surg.,* 1992, 118, 643–645.

78. Jones, J., Greenberg, L., Groudine, S., Guertin, S., Hoffman, R., Hollinger, I., Mokhiber, L., Rosen, M., Ruben, R., and Schall, D. Phenylphrine advisory panel report. *Int. J. Pediatr. Otorhinolaryngol.,* 1998, 45, 97–99.

79. Gefke, K., Anderson, W., and Frissel, E. Lidocaine given intravenously as a suppressant of cough and laryngospasm in connection with extubation after tonsillectomy. *Acta Anesthesiol. Scan.,* 1983, 27, 111–112.

80. Staffel, J.G., Weissler, M.C., and Tyler, E.P. The prevention of postoperative stridor and laryngospasm with lidocaine. *Arch. Otolaryngol. Head Neck Surg.,* 1991, 117, 1123–1128.

81. Koc, C., Kocaman, F., Aygenc, E., Ozdem, C., and Cekic, A. The use of preoperative lidocaine to prevent stridor and laryngospasm after tonsillectomy and adenoidectomy. *Otolaryngol. Head Neck Surg.,* 1998, 118, 880–882.

82. DeDio, R.M. and Hendrix, R.A. Postoperative pulmonary edema. *Otolaryngol. Head Neck Surg.,* 1989, 101, 698–700.
83. Feinberg, A.N. and Shabino, C.L. Acute pulmonary edema complicating tonsillectomy and adenoidectomy. *Pediatrics,* 1985, 75, 112–114.
84. Krygusuz, I., Gok, U., Yalcin, S., Keles, E., Kizirgil, A., and Demirbag, E. Bacteremia during tonsillectomy. *Int. J. Pediatr. Otorhinolaryngol.,* 2001, 58, 69–73.
85. Francois, M., Bingen, E.H., Lambert–Zechovsky, N.Y., Mariana–Kurkdgian, P., Nottet, J-B., and Narcy, P. Bacteremia during tonsillectomy. *Arch. Otolaryngol. Head Neck Surg.,* 1992, 118, 1229–1231.
86. Telian, S.A., Handler, S.D., Fleisher, G.R., Baranak, C.G., Wetmore, R.F., and Potsic, W.P. The effect of antibiotic therapy on recovery after tonsillectomy in children: a controlled study. *Arch. Otolaryngol. Head Neck Surg.,* 1986, 112, 610–615.
87. Colreavy, M.P., Nanan, D., Benamer, M., Donnelly, M., Blaney, A.W., O'Dwyer, T.P., and Cafferkey, M. Antibiotic prophylaxis post-tonsillectomy: is it of benefit? *Int. J. Pediatr. Otorhinolaryngol.,* 1999, 50, 15–22.
88. Jones, J., Handler, S.D., Guttenplan, M., Potsic, W., Wetmore, R., Tom, L.W.C., and Marsh, R. The efficacy of cefaclor vs. amoxicillin on recovery after tonsillectomy in children. *Arch. Otolaryngol. Head Neck Surg.,* 1990, 116, 590–593.
89. Lavy, J.A. Post-tonsillectomy pain: the difference between younger and older patients. *Int. J. Pediatr. Otorhinolaryngol.,* 1997, 42, 11–15.
90. Myatt, H.M. and Myatt, R.A. The development of a pediatric quality of life questionnaire to measure post-operative pain following tonsillectomy. *Int. J. Pediatr. Otorhinolaryngol.,* 1998, 44, 115–123.
91. Ohlms, L.A. Injection of local anesthetic in tonsillectomy. *Arch Otolaryngol. Head Neck Surg.,* 2001, 127, 1276–1278.
92. Cook, S.P. Bupivicaine injection to control tonsillectomy pain. *Arch. Otolaryngol. Head Neck Surg.,* 2001, 127, 1279.
93. Gibson, W.S., Jr., Concerns with bupivicaine injection. *Arch. Otolaryngol. Head Neck Surg.,* 2001, 127, 1280.
94. Vasan, N.R., Stevenson, S., and Ward, M. Preincisional bupivicaine in post-tonsillectomy pain relief. *Arch. Otolaryngol. Head Neck Surg.,* 2002, 128, 145–149.
95. Goldsher, M., Podoshin, L., Fradis, M., Malatskey S., Gertsel, R., Vaida, S., and Gritani, L. Effects of peritonsillar infiltration on post-tonsillectomy pain. A double-blind study. *Ann. Otol., Rhinol. Laryngol.,* 1996, 105, 868–870.
96. Schoem, S.R., Watkins, G.L., Kuhn, J.J., and Thompson, D.H. Control of early postoperative pain with bupivacaine in pediatric tonsillectomy. *Ear Nose Throat J.,* 1993, 25, 149–154.
97. Jebeles, J.A., Reilly, J.S., Gutierrez, J.F., Bradley, E.L., Jr., and Kissin, I. Tonsillectomy and adenoidectomy pain reduction by local buivicaine infiltration in children. *Int. J. Pediatr. Otorhinolaryngol.,* 1993, 25, 149–154.
98. Alsarraf, R. and Sie, K.C.Y. Brainstem stroke associated with bupivicaine injection for adenotonsillectomy. *Otolaryngol. Head Neck Surg.,* 2000, 122, 572–573.
99. Isaacson, G. and Parke, W.W. Meningitis after adenoidectomy: an anatomic explanation. *Ann. Otol., Rhinol. Laryngol.,* 1996, 105, 684–688.
100. Raj, B. and Wickham, M.H. The effect of benzydamine hydrochloride spray on post-tonsillectomy symptoms. *J. Laryngol. Otol.,* 1988, 102, 813–814.
101. Freeman, S.B. and Markwell, J.K. Sucralfate in alleviating post-tonsillectomy pain. *Laryngoscope,* 1992, 102, 1242–1246.
102. Ozcan, M., Altuntas, A., Unal, A., Nalca, Y., and Aslan, A. Sucralfate for post-tonsillectomy analgesia. *Otolaryngol. Head Neck Surg.,* 1998, 119, 700–704.
103. St. Charles, C.S., Matt, B.H., Hamilton, M.M., and Katz, B.P. A comparison of ibuprofen versus acetominophen with codeine in the young tonsillectomy patient. *Otolaryngol. Head Neck Surg.,* 1997, 117, 76–82.
104. Harley, E.H. and Dattolo, R.A. Ibuprofen for tonsillectomy pain in children: efficacy and complications. *Otolaryngol. Head Neck Surg.,* 1998, 119, 492–496.
105. Moir, M.S., Brir, E., Shinnick, P., and Messner, A. Acetaminophen versus acetaminophen with codeine after pediatric tonsillectomy. *Laryngoscope,* 2000, 110, 1824–1827.

106. Fernandes, D.B., Grobbelaar, A.O., Hudson, D.A., and Lentin, R. Velopharyngeal incompetence after adenotonsillectomy in non-cleft patients. *Br. J. Maxillofacial Surg.,* 1996, 34, 364–367.
107. Ren, Y.F., Isberg, A., and Henningsson, G. Velopharyngeal incompetence and persistent hypernasality after adenoidectomy in children without palatal defect. *Cleft Palate Craniofacial J.,* 1995, 32, 476–482.
108. Witzel, M.A., Rich, R.H., Margar–Bacal, F., and Cox, C. Velopharyngeal insufficiency after adenoidectomy: an 8-year review. *Int. J. Pediatr. Otorhinolaryngol.,* 1986, 11, 15–20.
109. Croft, C.B., Shprintzen, R.J., Daniller, A., and Lewin, M.L. The occult submucous cleft palate and the musculus uvulae. *Cleft Palate J.,* 1978, 15, 150–154.
110. Sphrintzen, R.J., Schwartz, R.H., Daniller, A., and Hoch, L. Morphologic significance of bifid uvula. *Pediatrics,* 1985, 75, 553–561.
111. Willing, J.P, Velopharyngeal insufficiency. *Int. J. Pediatr. Otorhinolaryngol.,* 1999, 49, Suppl. 1, 5307–5309.
112. Krueger, L.J., Morris, H.L., and Bumsted, R.M. Indications of congenital palatal incompetence before diagnosis. *Ann. Otol.,* 1982, 91, 115–118.
113. Kakani, R.S., Callan, N.D., and April, M.M. Superior adenoidectomy in children with palatal abnormalities. *Ear Nose Throat J.,* 2000, 79, 300–305.
114. D'Antonio, L.L., Snyder, L.S., and Samadani, S. Tonsillectomy in children with or at risk for velopharyngeal insufficiency: effects on speech. *Otolaryngol. Head Neck Surg.,* 1996, 115, 319–323.
115. Giannoni, C., Sucek, M., Friedman, E.M., and Duncan, N.O., III. Acquired nasopharyngeal stenosis: a warning and review. *Arch. Otolaryngol. Head Neck Surg.,* 1998, 124, 163–167.
116. McLaughlin, K.E., Jacobs, I.N., Todd, N.W., Gussack, G.S., and Carlson, G. Management of nasopharyngeal and oropharyngeal stenosis in children. *Laryngoscope,* 1997, 107, 1322–1331.
117. Brugh, R.F. and Stocks, R.M. Eagle's syndrome: a reappraisal. *Ear Nose Throat J.,* 1993, 72, 341–344.
118. Rechtwey, J.S. and Way, M.K. Eagle's syndrome: a review. *Am. J. Otolaryngol.,* 1998, 19, 316–321.
119. Grobman, L.R. and Stricker, S. Grisel's syndrome. *Ear Nose Throat J.,* 1990, 69, 799–801.
120. Wilson, B.C., Jarvis, B.L., and Haydon, R.C., III. Nontraumatic sublumation of the atlantoaxial joint: Grisel's syndrome. *Ann. Otol., Rhinol. Laryngol.,* 1987, 96, 705–708.
121. Baker, L.L., Bower, C.M., and Glasier, C.M. Atlantoaxial subluxation and cervical osteomyelitis: two unusual complications of adenoidectomy. *Ann. Otol., Rhinol. Laryngol.,* 1966, 105, 295–299.
122. Feinerman, I.L., Tan, H.K.K., Roberson, D.W., Malley, R., and Kenna, M.A. Necrotizing fasciitis of the pharynx following adenotonsillectomy. *Int. J. Pediatr. Otorhinolaryngol.,* 1999, 48, 1–7.
123. Guiruis, M. and Berkowitz, R.G. Meningococcal septicemia post adenotonsillectomy in a child: case report. *Int. J. Pediatr. Otorhinolaryngol.,* 2001, 57, 161–164.
124. Miman, M.C., Ozturan, O., Durmas, M., Kalcioglu, M.T., and Geoik, E. Cervical subcutaneous emphysema: an unusual complication of adenotonsillectomy. *Pediatr. Anesth.,* 2001, 11, 491–493.
125. Klausner, R.D., Tom, L.W.C., Schindler, P.D., and Potsic, W.P. Depression in children after tonsillectomy. *Arch. Otolaryngol. Head Neck Surg.,* 1995, 121, 105–08.
126. Tami, T.A., Burkus, J.K., and Strom, C.G. Cervical osteomyelitis: an unusual complication of tonsillectomy. *Arch. Otolaryngol. Head Neck Surg.,* 1987, 113, 992–994.

16 Head and Neck Infections

Earl H. Harley and Samir Midani

General Washington was attacked with an inflammatory affection of the upper part of the windpipe, called in technical language *Cynache trachealis*. The disease commenced with a violent ague, accompanied with some pain in the upper and forepart of the throat, a sense of stricture in the same part, a cough, and a difficult, rather than painful deglutition, which was soon succeeded by a fever and a laborious respiration ... he expired without a struggle.

> **James Craik, attending physician**
> **Elisha C. Dick, consulting physician**
> *The Virginia Herald*, **December 21, 1799**

CONTENTS

INTRODUCTION

Head and neck infections represent a diverse grouping of disease processes with various manifestations despite their similarities due to progressive soft tissue inflammation. Accurate and prompt diagnosis of these inflammatory disorders is as essential as any systemic or major organ disease in that the natural sequelae and potential complications can, at times, become life threatening.[1] A broad potential range of etiologic agents depends, in part, on the location of the infection, age of the patient, immunization status, presence of an underlying illness, and other predisposing factors such as travel history.

BACTERIAL MILIEU

The human oral cavity provides an environment favorable to the growth of microorganisms, with bacterial counts in the range of 10^8 to 10^{11} organisms per milliter of saliva.[2,3] Age, diet, oral hygiene, prior antibiotic therapy, systemic disease, cancer chemotherapy,[4] and hospitalization can modify the microbial population. The most frequently isolated pathogens from orofacial infections[5,6] include *Streptococcus milleri*, Peptostreptoccus specie, bacteroides (Prevotella), and fusobacterium. *Staphylococcus aureus*, part of the normal human flora, is a major cause of infections in the head and neck region. Other important organisms include Group A beta-hemolytic streptococcus (GABHS), *Streptococcus pneumoniae*, *Hemophilus influenzae*, and actinomyces.

Staphylococcus infections may be transmitted by multiple routes, including contact with infected persons, contact with asymptomatic carriers, airborne spread, and contact with contaminated objects. GABHS epidemiological studies[7] of patients with streptococcal pharyngitis indicate that the airborne route of spread and environmental contamination play little, if any, role in spreading GABHS. Close contact is required for transmission of streptococcal pharyngitis to occur; fomites and household pets are not vectors. Pneumococci are ubiquitous and colonize many persons in the upper respiratory tract.[8] Of young children who acquire a new pneumococcal stereotype in the nasopharynx, 15% develop an illness, usually within 1 month of acquiring the stereotype. The rate of colonization depends on a number of variables including age, race, exposure to young children, and the population studied. Results of studies of healthy children conducted at regular intervals indicate that approximately one third of throat and nasopharyngeal cultures are positive for *S. pneumoniae*.[9,10]

H. influenzae type B (HIB) colonization begins early in life; most infants are colonized before 1 month of age.[11] Since the widespread availability of HIB vaccine, infection due to this organism has become rare, although nontypeable *H. influenzae* strains are readily colonized within the upper mucosal lined cavities of the ear, sinonasal region, and upper aerodigestive tract.

ANTIBIOTIC TREATMENT CONSIDERATIONS

Empiric treatment — antibiotic therapy begun before culture results are available — is directed toward the most common expected offending agents and is crucial to ensuring a favorable outcome.

This therapy is based on multiple factors, including the site of infection, age of the patient, immunization status, and bacterial resistance pattern in certain geographic areas.

Tonsillopharyngitis is usually caused by a viral infection. Bacteria responsible for pharyngitis include *Streptococcus pyogenes* (GABHS), *Corynebacterium diphtheriae*, *Arcanobacterium haemolyticm*, *Neisseria gonorrhea*, group C streptococci, *Chlamydia pneumoniae*, and *Mycoplasma pnemoniae*.

Empiric antimicrobial treatment for pharyngitis is unlikely to be needed because most cases are caused by group A streptococcus or viruses, which is self-limiting; treatment begun within 9 days of the onset of an acute streptococcal pharyngititis is highly effective in preventing acute rheumatic fever — the main aim of treatment.[12] Despite the widespread use of penicillin to treat streptococcal pharyngitis, no GABHS resistance to penicillin has developed over the past 20 years.[13]

Cervical adenitis, when bacterial in origin, is most likely to be caused by a species that normally inhabits the nose, mouth, pharynx, and skin. In neonates, *S. aureus* and group B streptoccci are the most common pathogens. Some studies[14–16] indicate that *S. aureus* is the most common bacterial pathogen in infancy, whereas in childhood, *S. aureus* and group A streptococcus account for 65 to 89% of consecutive cases in prospectively evaluated series.[14,16,17] Based on these data, empiric therapy for cervical lymphadenitis includes clindamycin, naficillin, cefazolin, cefuroxime, cephalexin, or dicloxacillin.

Deep neck abscesses (peritonsillar, retropharyngeal, and parapharyngeal) are usually polymicrobial infections with an average number of five isolates.[18–23] Predominant organisms include GABHS, *S. aureus*, *H. influenzae*, and anaerobes (prevotella, fusarium, peptostreptococcus, and others). Currently, more than two thirds of deep neck infections contain organisms that produce B-lactamase.[21–24] A retropharyngeal abscess in young children is more likely to have aerobic isolates (group A streptococcus and *S. aureus*) alone or in a mixed culture.[25] Fusobacterium necrophorum infections are especially associated with deep neck infections that cause thrombophlebitis (Lemierre disease).[25,26] Empiric treatment for deep neck abscesses consists of clindamycin and cefotaxime; the combination antibiotic ampicillin–sulbactam is an acceptable alternative.

Epiglottitis (supraglottitis) is primarily a bacterial inflammatory disorder that is no longer caused predominantly by *H. influenzae* type B, except in children with purified polysaccharide vaccine failures. In immunocompetent and immunized children, therapy should be directed against *H. influenzae* type B and *S. aureus*.

Croup (laryngotracheobronchitis) is a viral inflammatory disorder that does not require antibiotic treatment. Bacterial tracheitis, however, appears to be an old disease that is becoming more prevalent.[27] *S. aureus*, *H. influenzae*, or *S. pneumoniae* most often cause it. Empiric treatment includes nafcillin and third-generation cephalosporins such as cefotaxime. Alternatively, cefuroxime can be used.

ANTIBIOTIC RESISTANCE

The microbial resistance that invariably follows broad clinical use of antibiotics gradually erodes the therapeutic value of every class of anti-infective agent.[28–30] Some strains of *S. aureus* have emerged as resistant to methicillin/oxacillin (MRSA/ORSA) and, recently, *S. aureus* with intermediate or full resistance to vancomycin (VISA and VRSA) has been documented.

S. pneumoniae resistant to penicillin (SPRP) has become a significant problem, accounting for 15 to 85% of pneumococcus isolates depending on geographic area. Beta-lactam antibiotics such as penicillin inhibit bacteria by binding covalently to the penicillin-binding proteins (PBP) on the outer bacterial membrane. Alteration of PBP can lead to beta-lactam antibiotic resistance.[31] In Gram-positive bacteria such as *S. pneumoniae*, resistance to beta-lactam antibiotics may be associated with a decrease in the affinity of the PBP for the antibiotics[32] or with a change in the amount of PBP produced by the bacterium.[33]

Other mechanisms of antibiotic resistance include enzymatic inhibition such as that caused by bacterial beta-lactame production, which inhibits some antibiotics, such as nafcillin, by splitting the amide bond of the beta-lactame ring. Staphylococci are the major pathogens that produce beta-lactame. This enzyme also contributes to the resistance of some anaerobic bacteria.[34,35] Resistance to erythromycin and other macrolides is frequently the result of alteration in the cytoplasmic ribosomal target site or inactivation by the enzyme erythromycin esterase.

CERVICAL INFECTIONS

GENERAL CONSIDERATIONS

Cervical infections and infections of the spaces of the neck are frequent in the pediatric age group. Unfortunately, complications can occur even if appropriate intervention has been implemented. Adenoiditis, tonsillitis, and pharyngitis, for example, are common infections that are readily treated and usually resolve without complications in most children. Without prompt and appropriate treatment, however, serious sequelae such as retropharyngeal abscess, peritonsillar abscess, and other deep neck infections may develop.

Occasionally, an infectious cervical complication is the result of an uncommon infectious problem. In these cases, awareness of the potential for these disease processes, and their prompt recognition, may be critical in their management. Examples may include the various granulomatous cervical infections. Other inflammatory processes, such as Kawasaki's disease, may present with enlarged cervical lymph nodes. Even though there is usually a constellation of other associated features, the incidence is uncommon and the multiple presentation variable enough to result potentially in a delay in diagnosis.

FASCIAL SPACES

Any understanding of the complexity and severity of severe infections in the head and neck requires a working knowledge of the spaces of the neck. The fascia of the head and neck is divided into the superficial and deep layers. The superficial cervical fascia is essentially the subcutaneous tissue. The platysma in the neck and the muscles of expression in the face lie within this layer of fascia. The deep cervical fascia is divided into superficial, middle (pretracheal), and deep cervical layers.

Below the level of the hyoid bone, the superficial layer of the deep cervical fascia encircles the neck and invests the trapezius, sternocleidomastoid, omohyoid, and strap muscles. When the fascia of the strap muscles is traced superiorly, it attaches to the hyoid bone. When traced inferiorly, the fascia becomes two layers at the level of the sternum to form the spaces of Burns, with the leaves attaching anteriorly and posteriorly to the sternum. Above the hyoid bone, this layer splits anteriorly to attach anterior and posterior to the mandible. More posteriorly, it splits to form the capsule of the submandibular gland. Further back, it splits to enclose the masseter and medial pterygoid muscles. The masseteric portion continues to insert on the zygomatic arch and the other portion following the internal portion of the medial pterygoid muscle to the pterygoid place. Behind the angle of the mandible, the fascia encloses the parotid and continues as the parotid fascia as it attaches to the zygomatic arch.

The middle or pretrachael layer of the deep cervical fascia encircles the trachea, esophagus, and thyroid gland. Superiorly, it attaches to the thyroid cartilage and hyoid bone. Inferiorly, the fascia follows the strap muscles to their attachment behind the sternum and eventually fuses with the fibrous pericardium as it extends along the great vessels of the mediastinum.

The prevertebral or deep layer of the deep cervical fascia has two components that are normally in contact with each other. The alar layer, anteriorly, extends from the base of the skull to the diaphragmatic musculature; the true prevertebral fascia, posteriorly, extends from the skull base to the coccyx. Therefore, a potential space exists between these two layers. Infections that extend into these retrovisceral spaces have the potential to spread inferiorly between the "valveless" fascial layers into distant regions within the body.

LYMPHATICS OF THE HEAD AND NECK

The lymphatics of the head and neck are divided into two groups. The superficial cervical lymph nodes are divided into the superficial and deep groups. The deep cervical lymph nodes are divided into the superior deep cervical group, or jugulo-digastric nodes, and the inferior deep cervical group, or jugulo-omohyoid nodes. Knowledge of their respective drainage regions can be helpful in determining the location of an occult infection.

IMAGING STUDIES

With cervical infections, it is important to remain mindful of the potential for airway compromise from progressive soft tissue edema. Sophisticated imaging studies are often requested during the evaluative process to help determine the diagnosis and whether a medical or surgical treatment course is the better option. However, other than for plain films or possible ultrasound examination, some type of sedation may be required, which may exacerbate the already compromised airway; these children should not be left unattended. The current generation of scanners requires patients to be perfectly still for many minutes. Newer generation scanners, however, will have much improved acquisition time so that motion will not be a factor and sedation will not be necessary in most cases. For now, when maintenance of airway patency is of concern, it is reasonable and appropriate to request an anesthesia team be on standby, or to move directly to intubation. In some circumstances, controlling the airway with intubation before obtaining the imaging studies may prove to be the safest and most secure course of action.

Currently, a computer tomography (CT) scan with contrast is the study of choice in the diagnosis of pediatric deep space infections because it offers the greatest specificity.[36] Intravenous contrast adds to the clarity because the rim of an abscess will enhance, although it may still be difficult to differentiate edema from purulence. The use of contrast will also improve the ability to distinguish between an abscess and surrounding adenopathy. When soft tissue fullness without rim enhancement is present, the process most likely represents the presence of a phlegmon and cellulitis, rather than an abscess.

Sometimes, the diagnosis remains in question, even after obtaining a CT scan with contrast. In such cases, obtaining a magnetic resonance imaging (MRI) study with contrast may be helpful. It offers the advantage of no radiation and may help in distinguishing cellulitis vs. abscess. MRI, however, has the disadvantages of being more time consuming and more costly and is often less readily available than a CT scan.[37] Ultrasound studies are far less useful in the diagnosis of deep neck infections and can have a high false-negative rate.

COMPLICATIONS

GENERAL CONSIDERATIONS

Most complications of head and neck infections are related to inflammatory and/or purulent progression and extension of the most common infections such as tonsillitis, adenoiditis, and pharyngitis. Peritonsillar, retropharyngeal, and parapharyngeal abscesses can lead to significant negative local, regional, and systemic physiological sequelae secondary to pus trapped within or extending to vital regions such as the mediastinum or the highly vascular cervical tissue planes. Progressive airway obstruction from cervical infections may result from edema secondary to inflammatory extension. Complete occlusion of the airway is rare; however, breathing difficulties can be especially notable in the very young child. Promptly obtaining an accurate diagnosis, therefore, is crucial to implementing an appropriate management plan.

AIRWAY CONTROL

If the breathing difficulty is determined to be clinically significant and the child is being observed prior to a decision on surgical intervention, then airway precautions are appropriate. The most crucial management aspect of infectious complications in the head and neck is the potential for compromise of the airway. The several avenues of obstruction include

- Involvement of the fascial spaces
- Edema of hollow viscera with obstruction of the airway
- Rupture of purulent material into the airway

The first step in the decision tree is to decide who is at risk for airway obstruction and what level of precaution to exercise. Factors to consider include

- One's level of comfort
- The availability and expertise of intensivists trained in the management of critically ill children
- The adequacy and capability of the nursing personnel
- Availability and adequacy of ancillary staff such as respiratory therapy
- The adequacy of the physical plant
- Access to the operating room
- For the child who needs to be sedated or anesthetized for an imaging procedure, 24-hour anesthesia coverage for urgent needs for surgical intervention or for airway control
- In-house 24-hours-a-day physician house staff coverage, which can be helpful, but is not always available

Even under ideal circumstances, complications may occur. In general, one should attempt to anticipate potential problems and avoid them as much as possible. This may involve transporting the patient to a children's or university hospital if he or she is in a facility without adequate and appropriate resources and/or personnel. At times, the most reasonable option is to transfer the patient's care to an otolaryngologist, who is more skilled in the care of pediatric airway problems.

If a child's airway is at risk, the level of observation and the level of intervention should be determined early. Any level of concern warrants consideration of closer nursing attention and monitoring, including pulse rate, respiratory rate, temperature, and pulse oximetry. The levels of intervention may include supplemental oxygen, nasal airway, endotracheal intubation, or even urgent tracheotomy. Other airway interventions such as high-frequency ventilation and the use helium–oxygen mixture may be helpful in certain circumstances; one should consult with an intensivist about the need for such techniques.

With head and neck infections in which the airway is compromised or at risk, one should consider ordering a tracheotomy set to the bedside. Such an order should only be rendered with the full awareness that "bedside trachs" and other emergency surgical airways in such noncontrolled environments are very difficult — even risky, particularly in children. Therefore, if a surgical airway is required, it is preferable to perform this with an anesthesiologist in the operating room or a procedure room in the intensive care unit designed for minor operations.

Prophylatic placement of a nasal airway may be helpful with nasopharyngeal obstruction from adenoiditis, but is not advised with a retropharyngeal abscess because of the possibility of rupturing the abscess and subsequent aspiration of purulent material. Endotracheal intubation in the intensive care unit carries the same potential risk. Use of corticosteroids is not advised early in the course of management of head and neck infections with secondary airway edema because of the potentially deleterious effect on untreated infections. After an infection has been drained and adequate serum levels of antibiotics achieved, the surgeon, often in consultation with a pediatric infectious disease specialist, may consider the judicious use of several doses of an intravenous steroid such as dexamethasone or methylprednisolone.

MEDIASTINITIS

Mediastinitis is one of the most feared and potentially lethal complications of head and neck infections. As the infection extends into deeper fascial planes, progressively developing mucopurulence may descend into the mediastinum. If unrecognized, mediastinitis has a high mortality rate. The diagnosis is sometimes able to be made on physical examination; a supportive prodromal history plus progressive fever and tachycardia will be present. Occasionally, a characteristic "knock" or "crunch" can be heard with chest auscultation. Plain chest x-ray may show widening of the mediastinum. A CT scan with contrast of the chest will be conclusive. Treatment requires high-dose intravenous antibiotics and drainage of the mediastinum, which may require a thoracotomy.[38]

VASCULAR COMPLICATIONS

Vascular complications of deep neck infections in children are, fortunately, rare. Erosion of the great vessels, with tragic consequences, and septic emboli from thrombosis of major vessels may occur.[39] Among the recognized and potentially lethal bearers of these complications is Lemierres's syndrome,[25,26] usually seen with parapharyngeal space infections. In the early part of the 20th century, a French physician by the name of Lemierre described a condition characterized by facial swelling, thrombosis of the internal jugular vein, and septic emboli to the chest. The fatality rate is very high if the disorder goes undetected or when diagnosis is delayed. Treatment requires anticoagulation and antibiotic therapy. Rarely is removal of the venous thrombus recommended.

NEURAL COMPLICATIONS

Primary neural complications due to head and neck infections generally do not occur because the neural structures are usually within soft tissue planes and neuropraxic injury from stretching or mass effect pressure is not likely to occur. However, secondary neural complications from inflammatory spread to regional structures, such as the cranial nerves within the tongue, sinuses, orbit, cavernous sinus, and temporal bone, are sequelae with potentially serious consequences unless identified and treated promptly. Generalized or focal pain transmitted by regional somatosensory nerves is so common with infections that it is often not considered a true complication unless deemed excessive; in children, this may make compliance with therapy problematic. Other infections with the potential for neural complications include viral infections that result in inflammation of the facial nerve within the bony fallopian canal or those with a predilection for ganglia, such as varicella-zoster.

CERVICAL ADENITIS

Cervical adenitis is common in children. It is a natural immunologic response and normal, healthy children should be expected to manifest periodic cervical adenopathy as their bodies adapt and mature throughout childhood. Resolution of the adenopathy, however, may often occur gradually, so prominent cervical nodes will be identifiable after the acute, precipitating infectious process has resolved. Although cervical adenitis may result from a primary bacterial process, the infection is most often secondary to a viral tonsillopharyngeal infection. It is important, therefore, to be able to distinguish clinically between the relatively normal and expected cyclical periods of cervical adenopathy in children, whose natural history is for expectant spontaneous resolution, from more serious infectious pathology requiring directed therapeutic intervention. Acute cervical adenitis may progress to regional cellulitis or to an abscess. Chronic cervical adenitis is less common and several notable infections should be considered.

BACTERIAL DISEASE

Diphtheria,[40,41] caused by *Cornybacterium diphtheriae*, should be considered in the differential diagnosis with children who are unlikely to be appropriately immunized or who might be immuno-compromised. The pharyngeal form may be associated with cervical adenopathy. The membrane that covers the tonsillopharyngeal area may extend inferiorly to the larynx and result in airway obstruction. Of the various forms of diptheria, this one is most likely to be complicated with myocarditis and peripheral neuritis. Treatment requires early administration of antitoxin and erythromycin.

Caused by *Francisella tularensis*, tularemia results from contact with wild rabbits or tick or deer-fly bite. There are multiple forms: ulceroglandular, oropharyngeal, glandular, oculoglandular, and typhoidal. The ulceroglandular form is most likely to affect the head and neck and occurs when contact is made with the eyes. Patients experience ulcers and tender regional lymphadenopathy.[42,43] Treatment is with gentamicin or streptomycin.

Plague is caused by *Yersinia pestis* and has two forms: bubonic and pneumonic. Fever, hemoptysis, and mucopurulent or watery sputum occur in the pneumonic variety; fever and tender lymph nodes are present in the bubonic condition.[44,45] The treatment is with streptomycin, gentamicin, or doxycycline.

GRANULOMATOUS DISEASE

In general, granulomatous lesions are self-limiting, but they may spontaneously drain and result in less than ideal scarring when compared with controlled surgical management. Cat scratch disease[46] is caused by the bacteria *Bartonella henslae*. Usually, there is a history of exposure to cats or kittens. The diagnosis is made by elevated titer or polymerase chain reaction. For histologic confirmation, a Wharthin Starry stain is used. In the absence of a frank abscess, interventional treatment may not be necessary. Several antibiotics exhibit some degree of activity against the offending bacteria. These include quinolones, sulfmethoazole/trimethoprim, azithromycin, clarithromycin, rifampin, and cefotaxime. Ciprofloxacin has been used in adult patients.

Mycobacterial infections in the neck (scrofula) are sometimes confused with other disorders. *Mycobacterium tuberculois* is the etiology of tuberculosis (TB).[47] Tuberculosis is usually transmitted by fomites and causes primarily pulmonary symptoms. Most patients with cervical TB have pulmonary disease. In contrast, atypical or nontuberculosis mycobacterial (NTM) infections are rarely associated with pulmonary disease. In the United States, the recovered organisms are usually *M. avium-intracellulare*, *M. scrofulaceum*, and *M. kansasii*,[48] although *M. fortuitum* and *M. haemophilum* have also been recovered.

The two disease processes have other differences. True TB may present with bilateral lymphadenopathy, sometimes large enough to require airway support. NTM is usually unilateral, often affecting the submandibular and parotid areas. The purified protein derivative (PPD) skin test is positive in true TB, but negative or weakly positive in NTM disease. The chest x-ray is negative with NTM, but many show active lesions in true tuberculosis. The Ziel–Nielson stain may reveal the organisms, but the gold standard for diagnosis is culture. However, at best, bacteria may be recovered only about 50% of the time, and culture results may take from 3 to 8 weeks for isolation. More recently, polymerase chain reaction has shown some promise in earlier diagnosis of these disorders.[49,50]

Treatment of the two diseases varies. True TB is a medical disease and triple and quadruple drug therapy may be recommended. NTB disease is a surgical disease in that the organisms are frequently resistant to antibacterial chemotherapy. However, some of the newer macrolides have some efficacy with NTM infections. Classically, a thorough surgical extirpation is the treatment of choice because of a decreased revision rate.[51] However, proximity to facial nerve branches may limit the dissection and the wisdom of "chasing" nodes that would most likely remain subclinical and resolve spontaneously has been challenged. Curettage[52] and repeated aspirations,[53] often in combination with macrolides, have been advanced as a less aggressive surgical plan with equal, if not better, cosmestic results.

VIRAL DISEASE

Several common viral illnesses, including Epstein–Barr virus (EBV), cytomegalovirus (CMV), adenovirus, and human immunodeficiency virus (HIV) can result in cervical adenopathy. The patterns of adenopathy and the potential for complications in the head and neck vary for these disorders.

Epstein–Barr Virus

Epstein–Barr virus (EBV) causes infectious mononucleosis (IM) and may be associated with significant cervical infection with or without involvement of Waldeyer's ring. The clinical presentation may be indistinguishable from an acute bacterial tonsillopharyngitis, especially GABHS infections, when Waldeyer's ring is involved. In fact, the two infections may coexist to the point that many children with IM are treated with antibiotics.[54] Beware, however, because about a third of patients with EBV–IM will develop a nonallergic rash when treated with ampicillin.

Infectious mononucleosis is diagnosed by serologic methods. The monospot test is based on the presence of serum heterophile antibodies, an IgM protein. They are present in 70% of IM patients by the first weeks of illness but can be found in 95% of IM patients by the third week; detectable levels may persist for months. In children less than 4 years old, the monospot test can be very unreliable because of their low rate of heterophile antibody production. Newly acquired IM is best diagnosed by the VCA–IgM — the IgM antibody directed against the EBV capsid antigen that peaks at 1 to 2 weeks after infection. IgG antibodies directed against the EBV capsid antigen also develop acutely and may remain positive for life. Antibodies to EBV nuclear antigens are not detectable until several weeks to months later.[55]

Epstein–Barr viral illnesses may result in significant airway compromise from the increase in the mass of hyperplastic lymphoid tissue in Waldeyer's ring or from diffuse pharyngeal soft tissue edema.[55] If the airway obstruction is severe enough, the patient may require admission to the hospital for monitoring of the airway. Generally, intravenous corticosteroids are recommended when the airway is severely affected. Placement of a nasal airway may be beneficial; in the most severe cases, intubation may be required. For severe obstruction due to palatine tonsillar hyperplasia, acute tonsillectomy may be helpful.

Cytomegalovirus

Cytomegalovirus is responsible for most of the heterophile negative infectious mononucleosis cases (CVM–IM).[56] Patients affected by CMV–IM tend to be older[18–30] and tend to have less severe cervical adenopathy and tonsillopharyngitis. Patients with CMV–IM may also develop an ampicillin-induced rash. Cytomegalovirus may cause cervical and generalized adenopathy, but the mediastinum and abdomen are not affected. Cytomegalovirus disease can be diagnosed by detection of the antigen or CMV-specific antibodies or with polymerase chain reaction.

Other Viral Infections

Adenoviral infections[57,58] cause cervical, abdominal, and generalized lymphadenopathy, but spare the mediastinum. Human immunodeficiency virus may cause varying degrees of cervical and generalized adenopathy,[59] but little abdominal or mediastinal disease.

OTHER

Kawasaki's disease,[60] also referred to as mucocutaneous lymph node syndrome, is generally considered an autoimmune vasculitis. Characteristic erythematous changes in the skin and mucous membranes may occur several days after fever and cervical adenopathy. Distinguishing head and neck manifestations include nonexudative conjunctivitis, oral cavity erythema, fissured lips, "strawberry tongue," and nonsuppurative adenitis with fever unresponsive to antibiotic therapy. Definitive treatment should include prompt institution of gamma-globulin. Severe cardiac sequelae may develop; once suspected, all affected children should be promptly evaluated for coronary artery dilation and pericardial effusion.

DEEP SPACE ABSCESSES

Progressive inflammation in the cervical tissue planes may occur if local lymph nodes are unable to effectively eliminate draining infections. On occasion, the overwhelmed node(s) will suppurate and a localized abscess may develop. Three generalized regions may be affected, each with the potential for variable presentation and clinical risk based on anatomic location and relation to cervical fascial planes (Figure 16.1).

PERITONSILLAR ABSCESS

Peritonsillar abscess (PTA) or "quinsy" is relatively rare in a young child. The peak age range is 16 to 20 years, but PTA has been seen in toddlers and infants.[61] The infection is a complication of bacterial tonsillitis with secondary inflammation and the progressive development of a purulent collection within the space between the tonsil and the lateral pharyngeal wall, usually beginning in the superior pole. An abscess in the actual parenchyma of the tonsil is very rare. Cases of multiple abscess pockets and bilateral peritonsillar abscesses are rare but do occur. Although peritonsillar abscess does not occur in children who have had a complete tonsillectomy, a clinical peritonsillar abscess-like presentation can occur in post-tonsillectomy patients due to infections involving (Weber's) glands in the superior tonsillar fossa.[62]

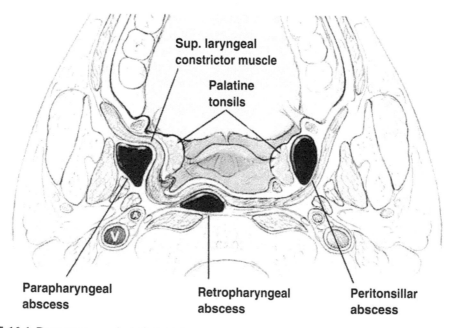

FIGURE 16.1 Deep space cervical abscesses.

PTA usually arises as a complication of a severe case of acute tonsillopharyngitis due, initially, to a viral process; it frequently occurs in association with a more generalized viral upper respiratory tract infection and secondary bacterial tonsillitis may then develop. When acute bacterial tonsillitis evolves into an abscess, it is not unusual to have a mixed bacterial flora collection, including GABHS, staphylococcal species, and anaerobic bacteria. GABHS infection is a serious bacterial pharyngeal infection that, if untreated, may lead to sequelae such as rheumatic fever and rheumatic heart disease.[54] As discussed earlier, other microbes, such as Eptstein–Barr virus, mycoplasma, and Chlamydia, may be the etiology of an acute sore throat.

In general, tonsillopharyngitis begins as a sore throat and quickly evolves. Low- to moderate-level fevers may be seen. Drooling, trismus, hot potato or muffled voice, earache, and neck swelling are the common presenting symptoms. Swelling of the tonsillar faucial area creates painful swallowing and difficulty handling normal oral secretions. Hot potato voice is characterized by muffled speech produced by swelling of the oropharyngeal tissue. Trismus — painful and difficult opening of the mouth — is produced by spasm of the medial pterygoid muscles; examination of the oropharynx may be difficult when trismus is severe. Earache caused by referred pain from the oropharyngeal area may be bilateral with a generalized throat infection, but is often unilateral on the side of a peritonsillar abscess, mediated by branches of cranial nerves V, VII, IX, and X. Neck swelling secondary to cervical adenitis is common with PTAs, but spasm of the cervical muscles is unusual.

The hallmark of PTA is unilateral tonsillar and faucial swelling with deviation of the uvula to the contralateral side. The mucosa is usually inflamed and overlying exudates may be present. The symptoms and physical findings are usually sufficient to make the diagnosis. However, in certain situations, there may be uncertainty. Early in the disease process, a peritonsillar cellulitis may be the presenting finding, which may mimic a true PTA to many observers; antibiotics alone may be sufficient. Imaging studies are not often requested, but CT scanning with contrast is the most accurate. Ultrasound is advocated by some, but sensitivity and specificity are low with this modality. MRI has high sensitivity and specificity, but is usually not as readily available as CT.[36]

When an abscess occurs, the primary mode of treatment is drainage. The simplest method of drainage is via needle aspiration; however, this may be difficult in the office or emergency department without sedation in very young children and some older nervous children, or with nervous parents around. The second method of drainage is to use a formal incision of the abscess and drainage of the cavity. Many otolaryngologists will use needle aspiration to locate the abscess cavity and obtain good cultures and then perform a wide incision and drainage. The depth of penetration with either of these methods must be controlled to prevent further spread of purulence to deeper tissue planes and to avoid injury to vital neural and vascular structures.

A third, infrequently employed technique of drainage is performing an "abscess tonsillectomy." This procedure is known by several other names, including hot tonsillectomy, tonsillectomy à chaud, and Quinsy tonsillectomy. Circumstances in which a Quinsy tonsillectomy is necessary are rare; the most common indication is failure to improve after incision and drainage or instances of multiple recurrences. In the past, it was recommended to eliminate the possibility of recurrent abscess. However, it is now recognized that the recurrence rate of PTA is much lower than suspected.[63] Most authors rate the chance of recurrence below 20%, and some think that the recurrence rate is in the range of 5 to 10%. Thus, there is no rationale for routinely recommending tonsillectomy for children who have had one episode of peritonsillar abscess.

RETROPHARYNGEAL ABSCESS

The retropharyngeal space extends from the skull base to the mediastinum. Infections in this space usually occur in young children and should be taken very seriously because they may result in progressive airway obstruction and significant inflammatory extension. The retropharyngeal space is rich with lymphoid tissue and lies behind (deep to) the posterior pharyngeal musculature. If the infection has not spread into the alar or prevertebral spaces, a characteristic unilateral bulging to the oropharyngeal tissues will occur because the vertically oriented muscular median raphe separating the left and right pharyngeal constrictors will limit the edematous spread. This single physical examination feature can help distinguish retropharyngeal abscess (RPA) from the more commonly encountered retropharyngeal cellulitis (RPC) due to a respiratory viral infection, which typically exhibits panpharyngeal edema associated with fever and leukocytosis.

Soft tissue lateral neck x-rays may suggest inflammation in the retropharyngeal tissue planes, but obtaining consistent and appropriate neck extension may be difficult in young children. If an RPA is clinically suspected, CT with contrast enhancement will be the most reliable imaging study for distinguishing cellulitis (medical management) from abscess (usually surgical management).

A retropharyngeal abscess is usually drained through an intraoral approach. On occasion, parapharyngeal space extension may dictate an external incision or a combined approach.[64] If a small RPA is identified early in the disease progression, it may be acceptable in some cases without airway symptomatology to admit the child and treat with intravenous antibiotics. In such circumstances, airway monitoring and precautions are maintained, and surgery is reserved for children who do not respond within an adequate time frame, typically between 12 and 48 hours.

If the child undergoes surgical intervention, adequate drainage is achieved when the dissection extends deep to the muscle plane in the posterior oropharynx and when adjacent loculated purulent "pockets" are bluntly opened into the drainage incision. Drains are generally not necessary and would pose an airway foreign body risk if not secured. Significant airway obstruction risk is still present from tissue edema and increased secretions, however, and (continued) postoperative care in an intensive care unit is considered appropriate.

Parapharyngeal Abscess

The parapharyngeal space is described as an inverted pyramid whose base extends from the base of the skull to the hyoid bone. Infections in this region may result from the extension of a pharyngeal infection or may be the result of a dental infection. The parapharyngeal space is not as predisposed to infections as the retropharyngeal area because the lymphatic supply is not as rich. The progression of parapharyngeal cellulitis to parapharyngeal abscess (PPA) is similar to that encountered with PTAs and RPAs.

PPAs generally do not cause airway symptoms unless they have extended to the tip of the inverted pyramid; in such cases, the hypopharyngeal airway may be compressed from extensive edema. Parapharyngeal space infections may present with odynophagia, drooling, referred ear pain, torticollis, trismus, and swelling of the lateral pharyngeal wall, often pushing the tonsil medial in such a fashion as to create some confusion with a possible PTA.[64] Cervical adenitis — especially on the involved side — is to be expected. Laboratory findings are similar to those for other pharyngeal infections.

Plain x-rays are not very useful in distinguishing an RPA from an RPC; computed tomography with intravenous contrast enhancement is the study of choice. The CT scan is also valuable in localizing the abscess collection relative to the carotid and jugular vascular structures. If the abscess is medial to the great vessels, an intraoral approach is usually preferred. However, if the abscess is lateral to the great vessels, an external approach is usually more appropriate. A CT scan will also be useful in determining the relative location of adjacent loculated "pockets" of purulence, in addition to the main abscess cavity.

Similarly to PTAs and RPAs, if a developing PPA is identified early and the airway is deemed stable and discomfort is limited, an initial clinical trial with intravenous antibiotics may prove sufficient and the child may not need to go to operating room.[64] Within a relatively short period of time, however, most PPAs will develop extensively and become multiloculated. In such cases, it is important to be certain that each pocket is opened and (usually) drained into a common abscess cavity. This process is best accomplished bluntly to avoid blind dissection with sharp instruments into potentially major anatomic structures within the neck. The placement of a postincision and drainage-dependent drain and/or packing is an essential step in assuring that the abscess cavity closes from inside to outside, thus reducing the potential for a new purulent collection to develop before resolution is complete.

SALIVARY GLAND INFECTIONS

Salivary gland infections[65] occur mainly in the large parotid and submandibular glands, although any aerodigestive tract gland, no matter the size, is a potential medium for entrapped mucus with secondary development of mucopurulence. Treatment of acute sialoadenitis includes hydration, sialogugues, and antibiotics. Coagulases-positive *S. aureus* is the usual bacterial culprit and, as such, antistaphylococcal antibiotics such as oxacillin, clindamycin, and certain cephalosporins are useful.

Salivary gland infections may be secondary to acute or chronic sialolithiasis. Onset is often painful and abrupt and may be exacerbated by eating. Although relatively uncommon in children, salivary gland stones occur more frequently in the submandibular glands for two primary reasons. First, the saliva is more viscous than in other glands; second, saliva can pool in the more dependent location within the submandibular triangle rather than exiting through the natural duct and punctae within the floor of the mouth. When a sialolith (stone) is in the submandibular duct, it may be palpable along the floor of the mouth in cooperative children. Most salivary stones are radiopaque and may be imaged in plain film or a CT scan.

Submandibular stones can often be removed by opening the duct along the floor of the mouth; careful dissection should minimize the potential for postoperative stricture formation. When the stone occurs in the hilum of the gland, an excision of the gland may be necessary if conservative measures fail. Infection in the parotid gland is treated in a similar fashion. Although parotid stones are far less common, on occasion extraction may be required. When operating on either major salivary gland, the surgeon should maintain standard head and neck surgery precautions for minimizing potential injury to the facial nerve and facial artery and veins (Chapter 17).

Relapsing juvenile sialoadenitis is a rare disease secondary to sialectasis. Multiple recurrences may occur over several years, but gradual spontaneous resolution should be anticipated. *S. aureas* is the usual bacterial culprit and acute treatment is the same as other forms of sialoadenitis.[65] Other salivary gland diseases that may be encountered in children include nontuberculous (atypical) mycobacterial disease, cat-scratch disease, sarcoidosis, and HIV/AIDS. These clinical entities are relatively uncommon in children and, therefore, may not initially be considered. A fine needle aspirate may be potentially helpful in ascertaining an accurate diagnosis without surgery.

EPIGLOTTITIS AND CROUP

Epiglottitis (Supraglottitis)

Epiglottitis was rightly considered one of the most feared infectious disorders because of its propensity for precipitous severe airway obstruction. A significant delay in diagnosis or a delay in safe implementation of appropriate therapy could prove fatal. More accurately called supraglottitis, rapid soft tissue inflammatory expansion of the supraglottic structures, including the lingual surface of the epiglottis, results in ball-valving of swollen tissue into an edematous laryngeal inlet. During inhalation effort, in particular, potential for complete glottic obstruction is increased. The vocal fold epithelium adheres more tightly than the supraglottic structures and, therefore, is generally spared from inflammatory edema; true hoarseness is not typical with epiglottitis. Inflammatory extension below the glottis is exceptionally rare.[66]

Hemophilus influenzae type B has historically been the offending bacteria. Prior to the introduction of the HIB vaccine in the late 1980s, epiglottitis was considered a disease of childhood. Since that time, the number of cases in children has been reduced dramatically. Today, pediatric physicians may not even see a true pediatric bacterial epiglottitis case. Vigilance is still necessary, however, because nonimmunized children, especially those who have recently migrated to this country, are still at risk. Furthermore, teenagers and others who may have missed the introduction of the HIB vaccine will remain susceptible. Even with the vaccine, bacterial epiglottitis may occur with a change in the inciting flora, including staphylococcal species.[67]

Epiglottitis presents with abrupt onset of stridor and a high fever. Drooling and painful swallowing are common. Air hunger is such that the child classically positions himself to open the laryngeal airway with the neck flexed and head extended — the "snifter position." Prompt recognition, control of the airway with intubation or ICU monitoring in selected cases, and treatment with systemic antibiotics are necessary to prevent a potentially disastrous outcome.

In earlier times, securing a stable airway meant a tracheotomy, previously the mainstay of treatment. It has been postulated that George Washington died from epiglottitis and that he could have survived his bout of "*Cyanache trachealis*" if an urgent surgical airway had been created. Unfortunately, tracheotomy as a planned technical procedure was only newly introduced into the "modern" surgical armamentarium at that time and had not been performed in the new continent; his treating physicians elected to perform repeated phlebotomy, a current standard of care then.[68]

A fiberoptic examination should *not* be used to verify a clinically suspected case of obstructing epiglottitis; the move should be to intubation under controlled circumstances. However, on occasion, the controlled and skilled use of a fiberoptic examination should not precipitate an airway crisis and may be helpful in ruling out a diagnosis of epiglottitis. With a somewhat similar argument, obtaining plain cervical x-rays may be helpful, but is not necessarily the best and safest option. Not only might the child be placed in a supine position, further stressing the supraglottic airway, but he would also be away from the ER or ICU setting in which skilled intubation personnel and equipment are readily available.

Epiglottitis in adolescents may have a presentation more similar to adults.[69] A severe sore throat may be the initial clinical symptom, and airway embarrassment may be a late finding. In some cases, securing the airway with intubation may not initially be necessary. However, close observation in a monitored setting such as an intensive care unit or step-down unit is to be considered a mandatory requirement because the need for urgent intubation will remain present until the inflammatory process subsides.

CROUP (LARYNGOTRACHEOBRONCHITIS)

Laryngotracheobronchitis (LTB) is a common inflammatory disorder of the upper conductive airway in children that is characterized by low-grade fever, hoarseness, a "barky" cough, and progressive respiratory difficulty of varying severity. The etiology is usually viral. The diagnosis and management are typically handled by the primary care physician and/or a pediatric-trained intensivist. The otolaryngologist–head and neck surgeon can be helpful with airway management.

As the longer name suggests, croup results from inflammation spanning the larynx into the trachea and bronchi. In contrast to epiglottitis, symptomatic onset is more gradual; fever is generally lower; hoarseness is present; and the child with progressive airway restriction is more often supine and tired from the prolonged increase in the work of breathing. Management must be directed at maintaining an airway and reducing edema; intubation is avoided as much as possible because of the potentially greater risk of internal trauma to the upper conductive airway from prolonged intubation through an inflamed lumen.

Young children and children with an underlying disorder or abnormality predisposing to upper conductive airway compromise are at more risk for croup or croup-like symptoms secondary to a decreased margin of airway reserve. It is uncommon to be affected by more than one true episode of viral LTB per season. Children with a history of intermittent upper conductive airway obstruction, often characterized as recurrent croup, should be considered for an evaluation to assess for the potential of intrinsic or extrinsic airway- or aerodigestive tract-related pathology.[70]

FACIAL SKIN INFECTIONS

The face is a highly vascularized region of the body. The venous drainage of the central region has extensive collateral connections with the intracerebral venous system via the cavernous sinus. Under normal circumstances, the venous pressure gradient is such that flow is from inside to outside through this valveless network. However, if an infection is within the "danger triangle," roughly defined by the nose and surrounding midfacial skin from the glabella to the upper lip, there is potential for intracranial spread of the infection. This can occur when a pressure dressing is applied over a wound in this region or, more classically, when a teenager's repeated action to "pop" an infected acne gland forces bacteria internally through the venous channels.[39]

OTHER INFECTIONS

Almost any systemic or topical infection may develop head and neck manifestations or secondarily develop complications affecting head and neck physiology. The reader is referred to comprehensive textbooks on pediatric infectious diseases for in-depth information. Several notable infectious disease processes have received a fair amount of recent popular attention, three of which are briefly discussed next.

BOTULISM

Botulism, caused by *Clostridium botulinum*, is a neurotoxic infection caused by preformed endo-toxin in contaminated food. In the head and neck, this produces muscular weakness and cranial neuropathies. Diagnosis is by serum analysis for the toxin. In contrast, infant botulism[71,72] is a rare endemic infection caused by the ingestion of spores that then grow in the poorly colonized gut and elaborate toxin. The treatment for botulism, in either form, is airway support and antitoxin.

ANTHRAX

Anthrax is a noncontagious acute disorder caused by the Gram-positive spore forming *Bacillus anthracis*. It may occur as pulmonary, cutaneous, or gastrointestinal infections. Pulmonary, the most serious form, begins as a flu-like syndrome. The diagnosis needs to be made early in the disease process for therapy to be effective. The infections respond to penicillin, but ciprofloxacin or doxcyline should be considered, even in children.[73]

SMALLPOX

Smallpox infection is caused by the variola virus and is acquired by inhalation of respiratory droplets or contact with secretions or skin lesions. It has been eradicated worldwide and currently survives only in government-controlled research facilities. The symptoms include high fever, head-ache, and a muculopapular rash beginning on the face and spreading to the trunk and legs. It is a highly fatal disorder that may be treated by vaccination within 3 days of exposure; beyond this period, vaccination and immune globulin are required.[73]

CONCLUSION

MANAGED CARE INFLUENCES

Managed care has spurred a change in the method of treating and managing most children with head and neck infections. In earlier times, a child would be admitted for any required surgical intervention and/or a prolonged course of postoperative intravenous antibiotics. Children would often be transitioned to an oral antibiotic and observed for 1 to 2 days to assess for clinical efficacy or relapse. Now, in the era of managed care — and managed costs — most children with head and

Complications in Pediatric Otolaryngology

neck infections can be safely treated for shorter periods in the hospital, followed by continued out-patient treatment and observation at home.

The use of home infusion services has made this a very practical and cost-saving approach with the potential for no reduction in quality of care — recognizing, however, that out-patient care operates within a less regulated environment than in-patient care. The goal, then, is to identify promptly and appropriately children whose infections and clinical sequelae demand monitoring and hospital observation by medically trained nurses, respiratory therapists, physicians, and other support staff members of an integrated pediatric care team.

REFERENCES

1. Chow, A.W. Life-threatening infections of the head and neck. *Clin. Infect. Dis.*, 1992, 14(5), 991–1002.
2. Barlett, J.G. and Gorbach, S.L. Anaerobic infections of the head and neck. *Otolaryngol. Clin. North Am.*, 1976, 9, 655–678.
3. Busch, D.E. Anaerobes in infections of the head and neck and ear, nose and throat. *Rev. Infect. Dis.*, 1984, 6, S115–S122.
4. O'Sullivan, E.A., Duggal, M.S., Bailey, C.C. et al. Changes in the oral microflora during cytotoxic chemotherapy in children being treated for acute leukemia. *Oral Surg.*, 1993, 76, 161–168.
5. Heimdahl, A., Von Konow, L., Satoh, T. et al. Clinical appearance of orofacial infections of odontogenic origin in relation to microbiological findings. *J. Clin. Microbiol.*, 1985, 22, 299–302.
6. Lewis, M.A.O., MacFarlane, T.W., and McGowan, D.A. Quantitative bacteriology of acute dento-alveolar abscesses. *J. Med. Microbiol.*, 1986, 21, 101–104.
7. Rammelkamp, C.H., Jr. Epidemiology of streptococcal infections. *Harvey Lectures*, 1957, 51, 113–142.
8. Gwaltney, J.M.J., Sande, M.A., Austriaur, R. et al. Spread of *Streptococcus pneumoniae* in families. *J. Infect. Dis.*, 1975, 132, 62–68.
9. Hendley, J.O., Sande, M.A., Stewart, P.M. et al. Spread of *Streptococcus pneumoniae* in families. I. Carriage rate and distribution of type. *J. Infect. Dis.*, 1975, 132, 55–68.
10. Dowling, J.N., Sheehe, P.R., and Feldman, H.A. Pharyngeal pneumococcal acquisitions in normal families: a longitudinal study. *J. Infect. Dis.*, 1971, 124, 9–17.
11. St. Geme, J.W., III. Nontypeable *Hemophilius influenzae* disease: epidemiology, pathogenesis, and prospects for prevention. *Infect. Agents Dis.*, 1993, 2, 1.
12. Catanzaro, F.J., Stetson, C.A., Morris, L.J. et al. Symposium on rheumatic heart disease. *Am. J. Med.*, 1954, 17, 749–756.
13. Denny, F.W. Current problems in managing streptococcal pharyngitis. *J. Pediatr.*, 1987, 111, 797–806.
14. Dajani, A., Garcia, R., and Wolinsky, E. Etiology of cervical lymphadenitis in children. *New Engl. J. Med.*, 1963, 268, 1329–1333.
15. Sundaresh, H.P., Kumar, A., Hokanson, J.T. et al. Etiology of cervical lymphadenitis in children. *Am. Fam. Phys.*, 1981, 24, 147–151.
16. Yamauchi, T., Ferrieri, P., and Anthony, B.F. The aetiology of acute cervical adenitis in children: serological and bacteriological studies. *J. Med. Microbiol.*, 1980, 13, 37–43.
17. Barton, L.L. and Feigin, R.D. Childhood cervical lymphadenitis: a reappraisal. *J. Pediatr.*, 1974, 84, 846–852.
18. Finegold, S.M. *Anaerobic Bacteria in Human Diseases*. New York: Academy Press, 1977.
19. Brook, I. Aerobic and anaerobic bacteriology of peritonsillar abscess in children. *Acta Pediatr. Scand.*, 1981, 70, 831–838.
20. Brook, I. Microbiology of retropharyngeal abscess in children. *Am. J. Dis. Child*, 1987, 141, 202–204.
21. Brook, I. Microbiology of abscess of the head and neck in children. *Am. Otol. Rhinol. Laryngol.*, 1987, 96, 429–433.
22. Floodstrom, A. and Hallander, H.O. Microbiology aspects of peritonsillar abscesses. *Scand. J. Infect. Dis.*, 1976, 8, 157–160.
23. Dodds, B. and Maniglia, A.J. Peritonsillar and neck abscesses in the pediatric age group. *Laryngoscope*, 1988, 98, 956–959.

24. Asmar, B.I. Bacteriology of retropharyngeal abscess in children. *Pediatr. Infect. Dis. J.*, 1990, 9, 595–596.
25. Hughes, C.E., Spear, R.K., Shinabarger, C.E. et al. Septic pulmonary emboli complicating mastoiditis: Lemierre's syndrome. *Clin. Infect. Dis.*, 1994, 18, 633–635.
26. Moreno, S., Altonzano, J.G., Pinilla, B. et al. Lemierrre's disease: postanginal bacteremia and pulmonary involvement caused by fusobacterium necrophorum. *Rev. Infect. Dis.*, 1989, 2, 319–324.
27. Safer, S., Duncan, P., and Cuernick, V. Bacterial tracheitis: an old disease rediscovered. *Clin. Pediatr.*, 1983, 22, 407–411.
28. Parry, M.F. Epidemiology and mechanisms of antimicrobial resistance. *Am. J. Infect. Control*, 1989, 17, 286–294.
29. Cohen, M.L. Epidemiology of drug resistance: implications for a post antimicrobial era. *Science*, 1992, 257, 1050–1055.
30. Levy, S.B. Confronting multidrug resistance: a role for each of us. *JAMA*, 1993, 269, 1840–1842.
31. Malouin, F. and Bryan, L.E. Modification of penicillin — binding proteins as mechanisms of B-lactum resistance. *Antimicrob. Agents Chemo. Ther.*, 1986, 30, 1–5.
32. Williamson, R. Resistance of cclostridium perfringes to beta-lactum antibiotics mediated by a decreased affinity of a single essential penicillin-binding protein. *J. Gen. Microbiol.*, 1983, 129, 2339–2342.
33. Giles, A.F. and Reynolds, R.E. *Bacillus megaterium* resistance to clexacillin accompanied by a compensatory change in penicillin-binding proteins. *Nature*, 1979, 280, 167–167.
34. Nord, C.E. Mechanisms of beta-lactum resistance in anoerobic bacteria. *Rev. Infect. Dis.*, 1986, 8 (Suppl. 5), S543–S548.
35. Appelbaum, P.C. Patterns of resistance and resistance mechanisms in anoerobes. *Clin. Microbiol. Newslett.*, 1995, 14, 49–53.
36. Weber, A.L. CT and MR imaging evaluation of neck infections with clinical correlations. *Radiol. Clin. North Am.*, 2000, 38(5), 941–968.
37. Nagy, M. Comparison of the sensitivity of lateral neck radiographs and computed tomography scanning in pediatric deep-neck infections. *Laryngoscope*, 1999, 109(5), 775–779.
38. Tan, P.T. Deep neck infections in children. *J. Microbiol. Immunol. Infect.*, 2001, 34(4), 287–292.
39. Gradon, J.D. Space-occupying and life-threatening infections of the head, neck, and thorax. *Infect. Dis. Clin. North Am.*, 1996, 10(4), 857–878.
40. Bisgard, K.M., Hardy, I.R., Popovic, T., Strebel, P.M., Wharton, M., Chen, R.T., and Hadler, S.C. Respiratory diptheria in the United States, 1980 through 1995. *Am. J. Public Health*, 1998, 88(5), 787–791.
41. Izurieta, H.S., Strebel, P.M., Youngblood, T., Hollis, D.G., and Popovic, T. Exudative pharyngitis possibly due to *Corynebacterium pseuododiphtheriticum*, a new challenge in the differential diagnosis of diphtheria. *Emerg. Infect. Dis.*, 1997, 3(1), 65–68.
42. Nordahl, S.H., Hoel, T., Scheel, O., and Olofsson, J. Tularemia: a differential diagnosis in oto–rhino–laryngology. *J. Laryngol. Otol.*, 1993, 107(2), 127–129.
43. Ellis, J., Oyston, P.C., Green, M., and Titball, R.W. Tularemia. *Clin. Microbiol. Rev.*, 2002, 15(4), 631–646.
44. Bottone, E.J. *Yersinia enterocolitica*: overview and epidemiologic correlates. *Microbes Infect.*, 1999, 1(4), 323–333.
45. Titball, R.W. and Leary, S.E. Plague. *Br. Med. Bull.*, 1998, 54(3), 625–633.
46. Schutze, G.E. Diagnosis and treatment of *Bartonella henselae* infections. *Pediatr. Infect. Dis. J.*, 2000, 19(12), 1185–1187.
47. Merino, J.M. Microbiology of pediatric primary pulmonary tuberculosis. *Chest*, 2001, 119(5), 1434–1438.
48. Fageeh, N.A. and Lamothe, A. Tuberculosis of the retropharyngeal space. *J. Otolaryngol.*, 1998, 27, 43–45.
49. Chesney, P.J. Nontuberculous mycobacteria. *Pediatr. Rev.*, 2002, 23(9), 300–309.
50. Peterson, L.R. Use of the clinical microbiology laboratory for the diagnosis and management of infectious diseases related to the oral cavity. *Infect. Dis. Clin. North Am.*, 1999, 13(4), 775–795.
51. Flint, D., Mahadevan, M., Barber, C. et al. Cervical lymphadenitis due to nontuberculous mycobacteria. *Int. J. Pediatr. Otorhinolaryngol.*, 2000, 53, 187–194.

52. Olson, N.R. Nontuberculous myobacterial infections of the face and neck — practical considerations. *Laryngoscope*, 1981, 91(10), 1714–1726.
53. Tunkel, D.E. Fine-needle aspiration biopsy of cervicofacial masses in children. *Arch. Otolaryngol. Head Neck Surg.*, 1995, 121(5), 533–536.
54. Richardson, M.A. Sore throat, tonsillitis, and adenoiditis. *Med. Clin. North Am.*, 83(1), 75–83, viii.
55. Wohl, D.L. and Isaacson, J.E. Airway obstruction in children with infectious mononucleosis. *ENT J.*, 1995, 74(9), 630–638.
56. Khoshnevis, M. Cytomegalovirus infections. *Dermatol. Clin.*, 2002, 20(2), 291–299.
57. American Academy of Pediatrics. Summaries of infectious diseases: adenovirus infections. In Pickering, L.K., Ed. *2000 Red Book: Report of the Committee on Infectious Diseases*, 25th ed. Elk Grove Village, IL: American Academy of Pediatrics, 2000, 162–163.
58. McIntosh, K. Adenovirus. Behrman, R.E., Kliegman, R.M., and Jenson, H.B., Eds. *Nelson Textbook of Pediatrics*, 16th ed. Philadelphia: W.B. Saunders, 2000, 994–995.
59. Truitt, T.O. and Tami, T.A. Otolaryngologic manifestations of human immunodeficiency virus infection. *Med. Clin. North Am.*, 1999, 83(1), 303–315, xii.
60. Rowley, A.H. Kawasaki syndrome. *Pediatr. Clin. North Am.*, 1999, 46(2), 313–329.
61. Szuhay, G. Peritonsillar abscess or cellulitis? A clinical comparative paediatric study. *J. Otolaryngol.*, 1998, 27(4), 206–212.
62. Kraitrakul, S. Distribution of minor salivary glands in the peritonsillar space. *J. Med. Assoc. Thai.*, 2001, 84(3), 371–378.
63. Paradise, J.L. Tonsillectomy and adenotonsillectomy for recurrent throat infection in moderately affected children. *Pediatrics,* 2002, 110(1 Pt. 1), 7–15.
64. Nagy, M. Deep neck infections in children: a new approach to diagnosis and treatment. *Laryngoscope,* 1997, 107(12 Pt. 1), 1627–1634.
65. McQuone, S.J. Acute viral and bacterial infections of the salivary glands. *Otolaryngol. Clin. North Am.,* 1999, 32(5), 793–811.
66. Healy, G.B. Paraglottic laryngitis in association with epiglottitis. *Ann. Otol. Rhinol. Laryngol.,* 1985, 94(6 Pt. 1), 618–621.
67. González Valdepeña, H. Epiglottitis and *Haemophilus influenzae* immunization: the Pittsburgh experience — a 5-year review. *Pediatrics,* 1995, 96(3 Pt. 1), 424–427.
68. Stavrakis, P. Heroic medicine, bloodletting, and the sad fate of George Washington. *MD Med. J.,* 1997, 46(10), 539–540.
69. Carey, M.J. Epiglottitis in adults. *Am. J. Emerg. Med.,* 1996, 14(4), 421–424.
70. Farmer, T.L. and Wohl, D.L. Diagnosis of recurrent intermittent airway obstruction ("recurrent croup") in children. *Ann. Otol. Rhinol. Laryngol.,* 2001, 110(7), 600–605.
71. Wohl, D.L. and Tucker, J.A. Infant botulism: considerations for airway management. *Laryngoscope,* 1992, 102(11), 1251–1254.
72. Anderson, T.D., Shah, U.K., Schreiner, M.S., and Jacobs, I.N. Airway complications of infant botulism: ten-year experience with 60 cases. *Otolaryngol. Head Neck Surg.,* 2002, 126(3), 234–239.
73. Patt, H.A. Diagnosis and management of suspected cases of bioterrorism: a pediatric perspective. *Pediatrics,* 2002, 109(4), 685–692.

17 Managing Head and Neck Lesions

Laurence J. DiNardo, Scott R. Schoem,
and James E. Arnold

The wise man solves the problem. The genius avoids it.

Albert Einstein

CONTENTS

INTRODUCTION

Agreeing to surgery for a child is never a simple decision for a parent. By the very nature of their location, head and neck lesions present parents with the additional potential consideration of visible life-long scarring or disfigurement. If the lesion is a tumor, there is the additional concern to patients and their families as a result of the fear of cancer.

THE NATURE OF COMPLICATIONS IN HEAD AND NECK SURGERY

GENERAL CONSIDERATIONS

Complications in head and neck surgery can and do occur; therefore, they must be anticipated and properly managed. They may arise as a consequence of the course of the disease process or surgical or medical intervention, or as part of healing and recovery. Complications may occur beyond the head and neck region and underscore the need to communicate with pediatricians and other pediatric specialists involved with the patient.

Complications related to head and neck masses take many forms. They may involve the airway, interfere with swallowing and nutrition, or impair vital functions such as hearing or sight. Secondary infections related to mucosal involvement can occur, as well as local or regional growth disturbances secondary to surgical scarring or radiation therapy. Systemic effects must be considered, such as those related to chemotherapy or the bleeding diathesis secondary to platelet sequestration as seen with hemangiomas that cause Kassabach–Merrit syndrome.

Mortality from childhood cancer — the most extreme complication — ranks second in incidence only to trauma. Of pediatric malignancies, 5% arise in the head and neck region, and it is estimated that 25% of all pediatric malignancies will eventually involve the head and neck. Early recognition and accurate diagnosis, therefore, are critically important to maximize the potential benefit(s) of the selected management protocol.[1]

AIRWAY MANAGEMENT AND ANESTHESIA

Congenital airway anomalies, tumors, and infections may compromise a child's airway and are often worsened with the administration of anesthesia. The anesthesia, nursing, and surgical teams must communicate and cooperate closely. The surgeon's impression of the airway should be discussed as well as the results of the radiologic studies and clinical examinations, including office endoscopies. The surgeon should be present at induction and emergence from anesthesia and, if needed, be available to assist the anesthesiologist or to provide immediate airway intervention.

COMMUNICATION WITH OTHER SUBSPECIALISTS

Experienced pathologists familiar with the wide variety of tumors that may occur in the head and neck of a child must be available for consultation, if needed, to assure the proper handling of tissue. It is often important to provide fresh tissue for processing. Extra tissue requiring proper fixative may be needed for special studies such as flow cytometry, genetic studies, or electron microscopy. If a malignancy is anticipated, it is necessary to consult with a pediatric oncologist and consider coordination of staging procedures such as bone marrow studies, a spinal tap, or establishing central venous access.

Multiple specialists, even those within a closely integrated team, will place their own perspective on the treatment approach used for a child. Consequently, some degree of confusion is *always* perceived by patients and their families. This is important to recognize and address. The specialists should develop a mutually agreed upon treatment plan that is regularly reviewed and modified as conditions change. In complicated cases, one person should be identified as the "captain of the ship."

In cases of malignancy, a pediatric oncologist is often best suited for coordinating the team efforts. Multimodality treatment, often by protocol, is the norm for a variety of pediatric tumors; long-term induction and maintenance chemotherapy, frequently in conjunction with radiation therapy, is commonly employed. The oncologist can usually best monitor the systemic consequences of the disease as well as its treatment. Radiation therapy, some chemotherapy, and the presence of a previous malignancy are risk factors for the subsequent development of a secondary malignancy. Long-term follow-up, therefore, is mandatory, and tumor registries should be used as important tools for data collection and patient tracking.

COMMUNICATION WITH PARENTS AND FAMILY

Open communication and guidance for parents is especially important in the "information age." Families may receive information from parent support groups; regional, national, and international meetings; and the Internet. Much of this unedited information is not accurate or balanced and needs to be addressed and placed in appropriate context for the child's condition. Parents often have a great deal of knowledge and insight related to their child's problems and must be thought of as members of the team. At times, parents become the primary care givers for their child, particularly when medical problems are associated with a chronic or protracted treatment course. Potential complications should be anticipated in advance and discussed with the patient and the families. As a result, their occurrence will cause far less anxiety and may serve to enhance trust and communication between the family and the treating physicians.

EMBRYONIC LESIONS

The key to successful management of a congenital or embryonic lesion is a thorough understanding of the differential diagnosis and natural history of each potential etiologic factor. A head and neck mass warrants timely evaluation, but not necessarily urgent surgical intervention. For example, if a child has a presumed neck lymphangioma or branchial cleft cyst based on history, physical examination, and computed tomography, the next step should be the education of the family and primary care provider rather than urgent surgery. Congenital lesions not physically apparent at birth may arise at any time, even in adulthood. Witness the occasional case report of a branchial cleft cyst misdiagnosed and mistreated as a squamous cell carcinoma based on frozen section diagnosis.[2]

PREAURICULAR SINUS TRACTS AND ACROCHORDONS

A preauricular sinus tract or acrochordon ("skin tag") results from the improper fusion of the first and second branchial arches leaving an epithelium-lined tract or a mound of tissue (accessory hillock). Acrochordons are familial and may contain vestigial cartilaginous elements; cosmetic surgical removal may be considered by the family. True fistulas to the external ear canal or middle ear are rare. Sinus tracts are usually isolated; however, they may arise as part of first arch syndromes. Because of an associated risk of kidney malformations, ultrasound to detect kidney abnormalities has been suggested.[3]

Management

Most tracts are asymptomatic and do not require therapy. Parents and primary care providers need to be educated that the occasional discharge does not represent infection. However, once infection occurs, the chance of recurrent infection, and possible abscess formation, increases and removal is warranted (Figure 17.1). During an acute infection with abscess formation, oral antibiotics and needle aspiration are usually sufficient. Incision and drainage should be avoided if possible to minimize facial scarring.

With sinus tracts, the choice for the parent is often whether to trade a pit for a scar. Therefore, if the main issue is cosmetic, this needs to be discussed as part of informed consent. Some debate has taken place as to the best method of removal. An elliptical incision with dissection around the tract to the auricular cartilage may leave a small remnant behind. Including a small portion of the

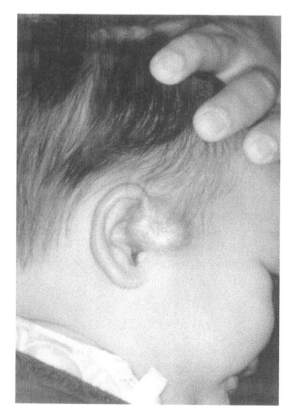

FIGURE 17.1 An infected preauricular cyst. This may be treated with needle aspiration and oral antibiotics rather than incision and drainage, followed by interval surgical excision. By avoiding incision and drainage, the ultimate result may be improved.

cartilage increases the likelihood that the entire tract is removed. The superior access approach has also been described. Although it results in a longer scar, it may reduce the recurrence rate[4] and may be especially useful in revision cases.

Branchial Cleft Anomalies

Evaluation and General Considerations

Branchial cleft anomalies (BCA) include brachial cleft cysts, sinus tracts, and fistulae. The surgical definitions of cyst, sinus, and fistula are not always fully considered in these neck abnormalities. To review, a cyst is a self-contained endodermal epithelial-lined mass sometimes containing lymphoid tissue deposits. It is a remnant of the pharyngeal pouch from which it arises. Sinus tracts may have internal or external openings. Fistulas have both internal and external openings. The occasional aberrant skin and cartilage rest may also represent a vestigial remnant. Excellent texts on embryology depict the pouchs and clefts.[5]

The adjective *branchial* comes from the Greek word *branchia*, meaning gill. The head and neck regions of a 4-week-old human embryo resemble those of a developing fish embryo. Although embryologists now use the term *pharyngeal* rather than *branchial*, common usage persists. There are four main branchial (pharyngeal) arches, five internal pouches, and five external grooves (clefts). The arches have their own nerves, muscles, and skeletal structures. The small sixth arch fuses with the fourth arch. The fifth arch is absent or rudimentary with no recognizable cartilage.

Branchial cysts do not often become apparent until the second decade of life. They enlarge by slow accumulation of fluid and debris from the desquamation of their epithelial lining. Usually, the cyst gradually enlarges with some degree of fluctuation. Often, there is a sense of fullness and mild dysphagia. They may become acutely infected causing great alarm for the primary care provider or parent. If no acute respiratory difficulty is present, an orderly evaluation should take place.

On CT scan with contrast, the cyst is unilocular, well circumscribed, round, or ovoid. There is no "pseudopod" infiltration as seen with lymphangiomas. If a CT scan does not show significant surrounding lymphadenopathy and the clinical course is consistent with a branchial cyst rather than an abscess, incision and drainage should be avoided. If necessary, needle aspiration to decompress the mass or differentiate between purulence and straw-colored, milky, or mucoid contents should be performed instead. Recurrent neck "abscesses" that undergo repeated incision and drainage procedures usually result in an eventual diagnosis of a branchial anomaly.

Second cleft defects are most common and arise along the anterior border of the sternocleidomastoid muscle. As embryological advances have led to a greater understanding of specific arch abnormalities, many masses thought to be isolated second arch cysts are now thought to fit within the classification of first, third, or fourth branchial arch anomalies.[6-8] Branchial anomalies may also be embryologically associated with other congenital cervical or mediastinal pathology, such as DiGeorge anomaly,[9] which should be considered when evaluating and managing these children.

Furthermore, any mass that arises around the ear, lower face, mandible, or upper lateral neck should have a first branchial arch abnormality in the differential diagnosis. One author removed a large, nontender, noninfected "parotid cyst" present for over a year in an 11-year-old boy (Figure 17.2). Although there was no stalk to the external auditory canal, perhaps this, nevertheless, represented a first branchial arch anomaly.

Management

- The first step in successful treatment is to rely on one's knowledge of embryology and resist the temptation to intervene prematurely.
- Arrive at an accurate diagnosis. Check for other anomalies.

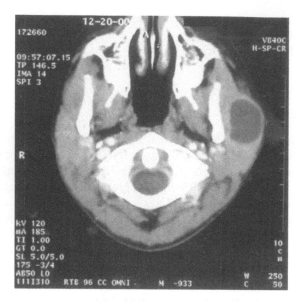

FIGURE 17.2 CT scan demonstrating a uniloculated, cystic mass within the region of the parotid gland. At surgery, the facial nerve was wrapped around the mass, but not adherent to the mass. The pathologist read the specimen as a cuboidal-epithelium lined cyst. This may represent a first branchial cyst rather than a "parotid cyst."

- Recurrent neck abscesses are branchial cleft anomalies until proven otherwise. CT scan with contrast may help to delineate an inflamed internal sinus tract. Surgical cure will require dissection to the point of internal origin.
- If the mass seems pulsatile, a preoperative imaging study is necessary to rule out a vascular growth or malformation.
- For some sinuses and all suspected fistulas, fistula dye studies may be helpful in determining the degree of surgical resection, type and number of necessary external incisions, and whether endoscopy at the time of surgery may be helpful to locate and treat the internal tract. This affords the surgeon and parent maximal preoperative information, reduces the number of "surprise" findings at surgery, and avoids potentially uncomfortable postoperative discussions.
- If recommending radiographic studies, insist that the study be performed at a radiology center that routinely cares for children, inserts intravenous lines to administer contrast, and can perform safe and adequate sedation protocols. An inadequately performed study provides no useful information for the clinical providers and may endanger the health of the child.
- When bilateral sinus tracts are present, a family history to rule out branchio-oto-renal syndrome is important. Regardless, the child requires a hearing test and kidney ultrasound.
- To minimize recurrence and secondary complications, the surgeon should carefully dissect the lesion — whether it is a sinus tract, cyst, or complete fistula — to assure complete removal of the abnormality. Some cysts have vestigial endothelial lined tracts going to or emanating from the lesion, which must be identified and included in the surgical specimen. If a complete fistula or sinus tract with an internal ostium is being dissected, careful ligation or complete removal of the medial segment close to the internal entrance into the oral cavity or hypopharynx is essential.
- Stepladder incisions using the pull-through technique avoid extensive skin incisions and unnecessary dissection.

- Revision surgery is made more difficult because of fibrosis from the previous violation of tissue planes. In these cases, excising a wider cuff of tissue around a presumed tract and/or cyst remnant is essential.
- Passive drains are usually sufficient for most BCA dissections.

THYROGLOSSAL DUCT ANOMALIES

Evaluation and General Considerations

The most common midline cervical mass in a child is the thyroglossal duct cyst (TDC).[10] Most become apparent in the first decade of life and arise with upper respiratory symptoms. Although a collection of embryologically migrating thyroid tissue may be found anywhere from the base of the tongue to above and around the thyroid gland, the most frequent site is just below the hyoid bone. If the cyst ruptures *in utero* or after birth, a sinus tract may ensue. Most lesions are sporadic; however, familial cases have been reported.[11]

Sometimes, a TDC may be differentiated on physical examination from a dermoid cyst or lymph node by having the patient swallow. Because the thyroglossal cyst is fixed to the hyoid bone, it will rise with the hyoid bone on swallowing; a dermoid or lymph node should remain in the same position and a dermoid is often found to be fixed to the overlying skin on palpation.

Previously, radioisotope scanning was performed to ensure that the cyst did not contain all of the patient's functioning thyroid tissue. Today, this is rarely necessary. Noninvasive ultrasound examination clearly delineates if functioning thyroid tissue is present in the proper location[12] and should be considered if the surgeon is uncertain whether a palpably normal thyroid gland is present in the normal location in an otherwise normal child. Also, screening blood tests are rarely needed. If a patient exhibits any signs of hypothyroidism, such as growth delay, chronic constipation, low energy, or sleep apnea, then preoperative testing should be considered.

Papillary carcinoma arising in a TDC is rare, occurring in less than 1% of adults with a TDC.[13] Therefore, in counseling the parent of a child with a TDC, a few points should be considered:

- It should be made clear that the only treatment is surgery. Because the hyoid bone is intimately involved, to reduce the chance of recurrence, the midportion of the hyoid bone must be resected.
- Because the risk of developing cancer is very small, surgery is not needed immediately.
- If the cyst becomes infected, it usually causes minimal scarring and has little impact on eventual outcome, but it is recommended that the acute infection be addressed before elective resection.

Management

- Intraoperatively, the surgeon may not be able to distinguish between a TDC and a dermoid. In this situation, the surgeon may puncture the cyst to examine the contents. If the cyst contains mucoid fluid (TDC) rather than epithelial contents (dermoid), the midhyoid bone should be removed. Occasionally, parents wish to have preoperative confirmation. If so, the surgeon may perform an office-based needle aspiration.
- On occasion, a resectable cyst is not present but the clinical history is supportive of a thryoglossal duct anomaly or a repeat resection is necessary because of clinical occurrence. In such cases, an "anterior neck dissection" is advocated.[14] The inferior portion of the specimen should include a small portion of thyroid tissue (often a pyramidal lobe extension of the thyroid isthmus). With an initial resection, dissection of a duct or limited central tissue resection to the hyoid bone is sufficient.

- With revision surgery, the central anterior neck dissection should encompass a broader region to include previous scar tissue.
- The central portion of the hyoid bone should be completely resected. Occasionally, during revision surgery, a significant portion of the central hyoid bone is identified and needs to be more thoroughly removed. Staying adjacent and medial to the junction of the greater and lesser horns will minimize inadvertent dissection, which could potentially compromise the hypoglossal nerve. Moderate bleeding may occur in this region, more so if active marrow space is within the hyoid in older children.
- An ongoing debate concerns the necessity of dissection superior to the hyoid bone. Some surgeons include tissue only if there is an obvious extension. Others advocate taking a cuff of 1 cm of tongue muscle to excise any small, nonvisible sinus tract diverticula. Others recommend further dissection to include the tongue base up to the level of the foramen cecum, followed by oversewing the small hypopharyngeal defect. To minimize the chance of recurrence, it is recommended to include at least some cuff of tissue above the hyoid bone in the specimen.
- Most surgeons use dependent drains overnight after surgery. Even with meticulous hemostasis, a small seroma may develop without the advantage of a drain.

ANGIOMAS

Angiomas are growths composed of blood vessel or lymph vessel origin. They fit into the broad category of hamartomas from the Greek word *hemartia* meaning "to err" or "defect." They represent an abnormal mixture and amount of tissues belonging in that specific site of the body. Current thought is that, during embryogenesis, failure to establish appropriate vessel linkage of merging mesodermal tissues leads to these defects.

Hemangiomas

Hemangiomas are very common. Females are more likely than males to develop hemangiomas by a 3:1 ratio.[15] The vast majority are simple cutaneous lesions of no consequence. However, subcutaneous and visceral growths may expand rapidly with severe consequences. Head and neck growths may ulcerate the skin, deform vision, weaken ear or nasal cartilages, or interfere with swallowing or respiration. In extreme, rare circumstances, platelet trapping may occur with a thrombocytopenic coagulopathy (Kasalbach–Merritt syndrome).[16]

A typical and disturbing scenario starts with a normal, healthy baby with a noticeable small hemangioma at birth or within the first month after birth. The lesion undergoes a rapid proliferative phase because the microvessels of hemangiomas are lined with mitotically active endothelial cells and pericytes. This important distinction differentiates hemangiomas from true vascular malformations, which are present at birth and do not undergo a proliferative and involution stage. Recently, growth factors and inhibiting factors, including proliferating cell nuclear antigen (PCNA) and tissue inhibitors of metalloproteinases (TIMP), have been identified.[17] These may provide useful clinical tools in predicting when the growth reaches its zenith and the involution phase begins.

Management

- Treatment depends on site, rapidity of growth, and functional disturbance.
- Medical therapy to retard proliferation consists of intralesional steroid injection, oral steroids, and interferon alfa-2a.
- Traditionally, surgery has been advocated for resection of remaining fibrofatty tissue once it has been determined that involution has not achieved full resolution.
- More recent approaches advocate aggressive early use of copper vapor laser[18] or combined laser, embolization, and surgery with emphasis on maintaining acceptable cosmesis.

- Subglottic hemangiomas represent a small but significant subclass. Early diagnosis leads to successful laser or surgical treatment without the need for tracheotomy. Therefore, progressive, worsening stridor in the young infant with normal flexible laryngoscopy warrants timely evaluation to rule out subglottic hemangioma. This may be achieved by imaging techniques or via endoscopic examination.
- Parental concerns often drive the management scheme. It is the responsibility of the clinician to discuss all options for treatment with their attendant risks. Often, multiple conversations and close follow-up are necessary. Primary care providers may be uncomfortable advising parents on management. In this situation, review and discussion with parents of sequential digital photos via electronic mail, with copies to the medical chart, offers a time-saving tool for long-distance families. If no functional deficit of breathing, swallowing, speech, or vision is present, the clinician may elect to observe the natural history of most hemangiomas.

Lymphatic Malformations (Lymphangiomas)

In contrast to hemangiomas, lymphangiomas have a single layer of endothelial lining[19] and a low rate of cell turnover. They are characterized as capillary, cystic, cavernous, and combined lymphangio-hemangioma. Cervical lymphangiomas are thought to arise due to incomplete development and linkage of the jugular lymph sacs with main lymphatic channels. Some postulate that the neck webbing seen in Turner's syndrome is the result of fetal cervical lymphangiomas with incomplete resolution leading to excess lateral neck skin.

Painless, distensible, lymph-filled sacs, most lesions are present at birth or become apparent by 2 years of age. Although cosmetically disturbing, they usually do not cause significant dysphagia, respiratory obstruction, or organ dysfunction unless they expand rapidly due to acute infection. Involvement of the floor of the mouth may lead to tongue mobility and control problems affecting speech and swallowing. Rare individuals require tracheotomy for extensive cervical involvement. Most lesions are multiloculated with "pseudopod" extensions along and around important structures. Differential diagnosis includes branchial cleft cysts, teratomas, neck abscess, and hemangiomas.

Clinical presentation should distinguish a lymphangioma from a lymphoma or other rapidly expanding neoplastic growth. Needle aspiration should reveal clear, watery fluid. CT scan with contrast or MRI is helpful to confirm the diagnosis, count the number of sacs, and determine the extent of growth. Intracystic hemorrhage may confuse the clinician into falsely believing that a hemangioma component exists. The main issue is that the inherent nature of lymphangiomas, with their extensive infiltration of tissues via natural tissue planes and along neurovascular bundles, renders complete surgical excision unlikely.

Management

- As with hemangiomas, communication with patients and the parents of these children is very time intensive. They and their primary care providers require extensive education and proper planning. Because there is no biologically mediated growth phase as with hemangiomas, primary care providers must understand that steroids and interferons are not useful.
- Although spontaneous resolution has been reported, some degree of waxing and waning is the norm.
- If the management plan is for observation alone, acute swelling may be managed by needle aspiration to alleviate breathing or swallowing problems.
- Nonsurgical therapy has not been useful. Sclerotherapy has been attempted with a variety of agents with little success. However, one promising agent, OK-432, which is a lyophilized mixture of a low-virulent strain of *Streptococcus pyogenes* of human origin, has

been used extensively in Japan with good results.[20] The agent induces an inflammatory response that results in cyst sclerosis. However, it does not seem to cause inflammatory scarring outside the cyst. Therefore, salvage surgery would not be more difficult. A multi-institutional trial is underway in the United States to further determine efficacy.[21] Another sclerotherapy modality being investigated is the use of intralesional sotradecol instillation (a "detergent" agent) and aspiration followed by dehydrated ethanol instillation and aspiration with preliminarily excellent results (information from personal communication).

ARTERIOVENOUS MALFORMATIONS

Treatment of arteriovenous malformations (AVMs) has been characterized as challenging, frustrating, and potentially life threatening.[22] These lesions contain significant communications between arterial and venous systems, which may result from trauma, and can grow during puberty. Soft tissue as well as intraosseous AVMs has been described. Complete excision is the preferred treatment. Preoperative embolization should be performed within 24 to 48 h of surgery and must be planned to preserve feeder vessels for possible local, regional, or free-flap reconstructions. Preoperative speech therapy and prosthetic consultations should be considered with intraosseous lesions, particularly of the mandible and maxilla. During surgery, use of a cell saver should be considered.

Management

- Several alternative treatments are available for lesions not suitable for resection. Venous embolization for control of bleeding with unresectable AVMs has been described.[23] Injection with synthetic polymers, steel coils, and even silk suture has been employed.[18]
- More recently, frameless stereotactic radiosurgery has been advocated for the treatment of extracranial ateriovenous malformations.[19]

TERATOMAS

Teratomas are congenital masses derived from pluripotential cells at locations where they are not normally found. They may contain only primitive elements or more differentiated tissues including gastrointestinal lining, cartilage, hair, and teeth. Most head and neck teratomas in children are benign, whereas in adults most are malignant.[24] The most common sites are the nasopharynx and neck. CT scan and MRI will distinguish between the solid nature of a teratoma and the cystic nature of lymphangioma or branchial cleft cyst and determine the extent of the lesion.

Management

- Surgery is the only curative treatment. It is exceedingly important that the pathologist be comfortable reading head and neck specimens and soft tissue tumors in children.
- Immature elements may be inappropriately determined to be malignant, thus leading to unwarranted chemotherapy. One should not hesitate to request a review of the pathologic specimen at a major national referral center.

STERNOCLEIDOMASTOID MUSCLE TUMOR OF INFANCY

Congenital fibrosis of the sternocleidomastoid muscle (SCM) occurs occasionally with contracture and shortening of the muscle fibers. At or shortly after birth, a palpable mass, the etiology of which is unclear, is present in the muscle. Ultrasound, CT scan, or MRI will reveal this condition and help to rule out other masses. Fine needle aspiration to confirm a benign fibrotic nature may be useful.

Management

- By 1 month, maximal fibrosis occurs and then slowly regresses. The contracted muscle forces the head to tilt toward the affected side with the chin pointing away.
- Intensive physical therapy alone is usually effective in alleviating this condition.
- Biopsy of the fibrotic portion should be performed only if potential malignancy is a concern.
- Because the natural history is resolution of the problem, the clinician should avoid recommending surgery except in unusual circumstances. Only occasionally will lysing the sternal and clavicular heads of the SCM be necessary to resolve the torticollis.

OTHER NECK MASSES

Other rare congenital masses of the neck include heterotopic salivary gland tissue, cervical thymic cysts, and bronchogenic cysts. Masses located in anatomic zones IV and VI of the neck require preoperative imaging to assess possible mediastinal extension. Most masses are benign; malignancy is occasionally reported.[25]

NASAL DERMOIDS AND ENCEPHALOCELES

At birth, dermoids may arise or they may become apparent soon after birth. They may occur anywhere from the junction of the septal cartilage and nasal bones in the midline superiorly to the glabella. A dermoid should not enlarge on crying as does an encephalocele. Often, a pit may be present over the mass. On CT scan, if the crista galli is bifid, then there is an increased chance of communication intracranially to the frontal lobe rather than only a fibrous stalk remnant.[26] In this case, an MRI may help delineate the degree of extension. In addition, preoperative neurosurgical consultation helps to reduce potential "surprises" at the time of surgery. A combined approach from above and below may be necessary for complete resection.

Management

- The traditional surgical approach is directly through the midline to the lesion and then following the tract superiorly. However, an external rhinoplasty approach with or without endoscopic guidance may provide adequate exposure.
- If it has been determined preoperatively that the tract extends or may extend superiorly, the consulting neurosurgeon must be available for a combined operative approach. This avoids a staged surgical approach for the patient, as well as confusion for the parent as to why this was not known prior to the operation.

Encephaloceles are usually recognized at or soon after birth; they need to be distinguished from gliomas. Encephaloceles should pulsate and compress whereas gliomas should not. The most common type is the frontoethmoidal encephalocele, followed by nasopharyngeal and orbital lesions. CT scan and MRI are justified preoperatively to assess for bony defects and soft tissue extension intracranially. Because 15% of gliomas have a fibrous stalk connection with the dura, no preoperative imaging technique is foolproof. Therefore, preoperative counseling for gliomas must include the chance of finding an intracranial extension during surgery with the need for a neurosurgeon. For encephalocoles, neurosurgical consultation is mandatory.

- Some encephaloceles may be removed via direct "open sky" approaches.

- Rarely are intranasal approaches with endoscopic guidance sufficient if the lesion extends into the frontal lobe. The resulting bony defect may be substantial and requires reconstruction with calvarial bone and/or plating techniques.
- Postoperative CSF leak may occur in up to 20% of cases and should be discussed preoperatively with the family and evaluated for postoperatively.

NONEMBRYONIC CONGENITAL/NONCONGENITAL MASSES

The presentation of pediatric head and neck tumors is similar to adult counterparts. The low frequency of occurrence and variable behavior, however, often result in diagnostic and therapeutic dilemmas. In addition, the effect of treatment on growth and development is of significant concern. As a result, the management of these lesions contains numerous challenges and pitfalls.

SALIVARY GLAND TUMORS

Evaluation and General Considerations

Parotid and submandibular tumors are unusual in children. Jaques et al. reported that 124 of 10,000 parotid tumors reviewed at the Armed Forces Institute of Pathology occurred in children less than 15 years of age.[27] Most of these lesions presented in late childhood or adolescence. Benign lesions predominated and were typically hemangiomas and benign mixed tumors; malignancy occurred in 27%, most commonly mucoepedermoid and acinic cell carcinoma. Consequently, excision of solid parotid tumors in children is advised.

Preoperative evaluation should not include open biopsy or aspiration with greater than a 22-gauge needle for fear of tumor seeding. Fine needle aspiration (FNA) is useful but not definitive. An accuracy rate of between 60 to 80% has been reported.[28] The extent of resection, and particularly sacrifice of the facial nerve, should not be based only on the FNA. Imaging studies are typically not helpful if the lesion is mobile, well circumscribed, and benign on FNA.

Facial Nerve Preservation

Avoiding facial nerve injury is of obvious importance in parotid gland surgery. The patient should be draped to allow visualization of the full half-face during the operation. A facial nerve monitor should be employed whenever possible. A facial nerve stimulator should be used at a low setting (0.5 mamp) and repetitive stimulation is to be avoided to prevent transient neuropraxia. Use of the facial nerve stimulator is no substitute for knowledge of facial nerve anatomy, especially because thick connective tissue and perineurium may shield the proximal nerve from external stimulation.

One of the recognized approaches to the facial nerve should be used. Identification of the tympanomastiod suture line appears to be the most accurate. An operative microscope is best employed for revision parotid surgery or procedures on small children. Loops may also be helpful in avoiding facial nerve injury. Hemostasis is best achieved with careful bipolar cautery, suture, and epinephrine-soaked pledgets. Monopolar cautery is to be avoided.

At the conclusion of the procedure, the integrity of all dissected facial nerve branches is ascertained and repairs are made as necessary. In the event that eye closure is temporarily compromised due to neuropraxia, artificial tears and eye ointment are used. A bubble may be placed over the eye while the patient is sleeping. Occlusive eye patches are not used because corneal irritation or abrasions may result from such dressings. If long-term paresis is anticipated, gold weight placement and/or tarsorrhaphy along with ophthalmologic consultation are recommended.

Hematoma

Perioperative hematoma is best avoided through meticulous hemostasis and valsalva maneuver to search for uncontrolled vessels prior to wound closure. Placement of a suction drain and the use of a pressure dressing are also helpful. Prompt recognition and drainage of a hematoma are important to prevent skin flap necrosis.

Frey's Syndrome (Gustatory Sweating)

Frey's syndrome results from auriculotemporal innervation of cholinergic mediated sweat glands. Although frequently demonstrated by the Minor's starch test, it is not usually symptomatic.[29] It is, however, more commonly seen in children. The best treatment is avoidance. Development of a thick skin flap with adipose left on the undersurface provides some protection. Remnant superficial parotid fascia may also be secured onto the parotid bed. Various autografts and synthetic materials have been interposed between the parotid bed and skin with varying success and complications. Tympanic neurectomy has been advocated for troublesome cases.[30] Applying clear antiperspirant to the affected skin twice daily is a simple measure used to control the problem.

Salivary Sialocele and Fistula

Remnant parotid gland may produce enough saliva to collect under the skin surface (sialocele) or drain to the surface (fistula). Removing as much parotid gland as is reasonable at the time of surgery may prevent this complication. The maintenance of a suction drain until output is less than 15 cc/24 h and placement of a pressure dressing are also useful measures. Treatment of a sialocele includes repeated needle aspirations and placement of a pressure dressing until resolution. Similarly, fistulas are treated conservatively with a pressure dressing. Drains should not be replaced. The oral administration of glycopyrrolate may also decrease the secretion of saliva. Anticholinergic side effects must be considered with the use of this medication. Most sialoceles and fistulas resolve over time with conservative treatment. Excision of a fistula tract is rarely required. Planned postoperative radiation therapy for malignancy will also assist in resolution of these problems.

THYROID GLAND TUMORS

Evaluation and General Considerations

The majority of thyroid neoplasms in children affect adolescents. Differentiated thyroid neoplasms in this age group are associated with early regional metastasis. Nevertheless, long-term survival is greater than 90% with appropriate treatment.[31] Fine needle aspiration (FNA) is of significant value in diagnosing thyroid tumors, but is typically unable to classify follicular lesions as carcinoma or adenoma. This distinction relies on the demonstrable presence or absence of capsular invasion. Moreover, the extent of thyroidectomy for well-differentiated thyroid cancer remains the subject of much debate. Despite these uncertainties, general guidelines for the extent of gland removal will be outlined with respect to the avoidance and treatment of surgical complications.

Prior to surgical intervention, it is important for children with medullary carcinoma to receive screening for multiple endocrine neoplasia, Type 11b (MEN IIb) and patients with Grave's disease to be rendered euthyroid.[32,33] Suppression of hyperthyroidism may involve the administration of propylthiouracil and propanolol. Some surgeons administer Lugol's solution for 2 weeks prior to surgery to decrease the vascularity of the thyroid gland in patients with Grave's disease.[34]

Recurrent Laryngeal Nerve Preservation

The identification and preservation of the recurrent laryngeal nerve(s) is important to avoiding debilitating complications from a thyroidectomy. Unilateral nerve paresis may result in permanent voice damage, and bilateral injury can induce airway compromise. As with adults, the nerve should first be identified low in the neck in the triangle created by the clavicle, trachea, and common carotid artery. While searching for the nerve, care should be taken to avoid disruption of the inferior thyroid artery and accompanying vein proximal to their supply of the parathyroid glands.

Bipolar cautery is used with precision and at a low setting. Monopolar cautery is avoided. Vessel clamping and tying are performed with the nerve under direct vision. Epinephrine-soaked pledgets are used to control oozing well enough to afford adequate visualization of the surgical field. Loops and, occasionally, an operating microscope may prove valuable in nerve identification and dissection. The surgeon must be aware that the recurrent laryngeal nerve typically bifurcates 0.5 cm or more inferior to the cricoid cartilage and that all branches are to be preserved. Occasionally, a nonrecurrent right-sided nerve exists and may be inadvertently and unexpectedly damaged. Postoperative fiberoptic examination of the larynx in the recovery room avoids unrecognized vocal fold paresis, which, if bilateral, can result in immediate or delayed airway compromise.

Parathyroid Gland Preservation

The preservation of parathyroid function requires maintenance of venous and arterial blood supplies. Although disruption of venous blood flow often results in a dusky to jet-black appearance of the gland, arterial compromise affords no such immediately recognizable change. Vasculature division as close to the thyroid capsule as possible yields the best protection of the parathyroid glands. This is particularly true for the inferior thyroid artery, which provides 85% of the blood supply to the parathyroid glands. The superior vascular pedicle is also divided close to the thyroid gland in an effort to avoid injury to the superior laryngeal nerve.

Occasional reports of parathyroid glands found within the thyroid capsule should prompt the surgeon to examine the specimen prior to delivery from the surgical field. If parathyroid tissue is identified by frozen section, it should be sliced into 0.5- to 1.0-mm sections and reimplanted in the sternocleidomastoid muscle. A metal clip is used to close the muscle pocket, which should be free of active bleeding. The clip reveals the location of the reimplanted tissue if later excision becomes necessary. This maneuver is also recommended for *in situ* parathyroid tissue that appears devascularized or does not bleed on incision.

Hematoma

Hematoma is best avoided by suture ligature of substantial arteries and the anterior jugular veins, if their division proves necessary. Avoidance of strap muscle division, whenever possible, may also prove preventative. A valsalva maneuver is preformed prior to wound closure. A suction drain may also be placed, but this is controversial. The timely recognition of a wound hematoma is imperative. Immediate wound exploration is needed to avoid potential airway compromise. For this reason, the wound should not be covered.

Extent of Thyroidectomy

The extent of thyroidectomy required for a patient with well-differentiated thyroid carcinoma remains controversial. In general, patients with small tumors without extracapsular invasion and in a low-risk demographic should undergo at least a subtotal thyroidectomy. Individuals with extensive or multicentric disease, with metastases, or in a high-risk group should receive a total thyroidectomy. Occasionally, a subtotal thyroidectomy is performed on these patients to avoid complications. When the parathyroid glands or the recurrent laryngeal nerve is damaged during resection of the involved lobe, a subtotal resection of the contralateral lobe is advisable, if possible, to avoid the risk of hypoparathyroidism or bilateral vocal fold paresis. Consequently, the thyroid lobe involved with tumor should be removed first.

Postoperative Considerations

Patients receiving a total or subtotal thyroidectomy require postoperative calcium monitoring. It is important to understand that although parathyroid hormone (PTH) levels decline immediately upon parathyroid gland devascularization, the associated lowering of serum calcium levels may be delayed. In fact, serum calcium levels often reach a nadir 48 to 72 h postoperatively. Patients and their families should be made aware of the symptoms of hypoparathyroidism; provisions should be in place for outpatient calcium monitoring because most patients are discharged on the day of surgery or the following morning.

Although thyroid replacement is required after total thyroidectomy, long-term monitoring of thyroid function is important after hemithyroidectomy. A gradual decline in thyroid function may occur over years and remain undetected. This is especially important to the growth and development of children.

RHABDOMYOSARCOMA

Rhabdomyosarcoma is the most common soft tissue malignancy in the pediatric age group, accounting for 70% of such tumors in children under the age of 12 years. It most commonly affects the orbit followed by the nasopharynx, middle ear, and sinonasal tract; hematogenous as well as lymphatic metastases occur. The Intergroup Rhabdomyosarcoma Studies I and II have established superior survival rates with multimodality therapy. Treatment typically consists of chemotherapy, radiation therapy, and when appropriate, surgery.

Even with medical treatment alone, the otolaryngologist–head and neck surgeon is often responsible for the diagnosis and avoidance of treatment complications. Airway impairment may become obstruction with advancing tumor or during radiation therapy. Paranasal sinus obstruction secondary to tumor can lead to sinus infection with serious implications for a child receiving chemotherapy. Early recognition and prompt surgical management of these conditions are imperative.

Surgical resection of tumor is a reasonable addition to primary medical therapy if complete removal can be accomplished with minimal morbidity. Surgical salvage is considered for incomplete tumor response to chemotherapy and radiation treatment. Complications of surgery such as postoperative infection, wound breakdown, and fistula formation are accentuated in previously treated patients.

FIBROMATOSIS

Fibrous tumors may manifest in various forms, from the benign keloid to fibrosarcoma. Aggressive fibromatosis and desmoid tumor are locally destructive, sometimes multicentric lesions that fail to metastasize. These tumors are rare in childhood with the majority occurring in adults, primarily in the third through fifth decades of life.[35,36] The preferred treatment is excision with a 2-cm margin. Pitfalls in management include difficulty in judging margins and the inability to achieve clear margins with tumors greater than 5 cm in size without significant morbidity.

The use of preoperative CT scans and MRIs may assist in margin assessment. Additional therapies in the event of positive resection margins or unresectability include adjunctive radiation treatment and chemotherapy. The utility of these methods is controversial. A total radiation dose of 5000 cGy or more may achieve tumor regression but is detrimental to the growth of small children.[37] Chemotherapy with agents such as vinblastine and methotrexate has been advocated to control unresectable lesions to allow for further growth and development prior to definitive treatment.[38]

NASOPHARYNGEAL ANGIOFIBROMA

The treatment of juvenile nasopharyngeal angiofibroma (JNA) presents challenges similar to those encountered with AVMs regarding hypervascularity. Additional concern exists due to the pitfalls encountered in accessing these tumors and their proximity to vital structures. Although they are benign lesions, intracranial extension occurs in 20 to 36% of patients and is typically extradural.[39]

Significant bleeding may occur if a biopsy is attempted. Therefore, if suspected, the diagnosis is confirmed by gadolinium-enhanced MRI and angiography at the time of preoperative embolization, which is usually performed within 24 hours of resection. Polyvinyl alcohol (PVA) particles measuring greater than 300 μm are used in an effort to decrease the risk of stroke, cranial nerve deficits, and visual loss associated with arterial embolization. If blood supply arises from the internal carotid artery, intratumoral embolization should be considered.

The location and size of the tumor dictate the surgical approach used for removal. Because most complications of treatment arise from the surgical approach, the surgeon must carefully consider the method used in each case. Small tumors without extension into the infratemporal fossa or cranial cavity may be removed endoscopically if well embolized.[40] The midfacial degloving approach is versatile, affords bilateral access, and is cosmetically superior to other external approaches.

For larger tumors, the malar-cheek-maxillary flap allows exposure to the lower clivus, petrous apex, eustachian tube, infratemporal fossa, and parapharyngeal space according to Danesi et al.[41] These authors have abandoned the lateral skull base approach due to associated permanent conductive hearing loss, temporomandibular discomfort, and trigeminal nerve hypoaesthesia. Nevertheless, Browne and Jacob describe a lateral preauricular temporal approach that preserves hearing and may prove useful for tumors extending lateral to the horizontal portion of the internal carotid artery.[42] Although JNAs with intracranial extension typically remain extradural, neurosurgical collaboration seems prudent for such tumors.

Recurrence rates have been reported between 17 and 86%.[39,43] To lessen the risk of residual tumor, Danesi et al. also advocate drilling out the pterygoid plate and, when involved with tumor, the clivus.[41] Follow-up MRI is recommended to monitor patients and re-resection advocated for extracranial recurrence. Recently, intensity-modulated radiation therapy (IMRT) has been reported to control recurrent JNAs.[44]

LANGERHANS' CELL HISTIOCYTOSIS

Langerhans' cell histiocytosis (LCH) is characterized by the proliferation of histiocytic cells in various tissues and organs. The precise etiology is unknown but may be the result of an undefined immunologic disturbance. Clinical manifestations can vary substantially, accounting for a variety of presentations ranging from the unifocal eosinophilic granuloma to the diffuse, and often fatal, Letterer–Siwe disease.

The otolaryngologist–head and neck surgeon should be aware that over 60% of patients present with complaints referable to the head and neck, and an additional 20% will develop lesions in the region.[45] Because the disease is extremely heterogeneous, a multitude of insidious manifestations may obscure the diagnosis. Hand–Shuller–Christian disease, for instance, manifests as a triad of irregular membranous bony defects, exophthalmos, and diabetes insipidus. Skin involvement, frequently the harbinger of diffuse disease, often begins as a vesiculopustular rash. Scalp lesions typically occur behind the ears or present as seborrhea-like involvement that resembles cradle cap. Mandibular and gingival lesions are mostly unifocal. They may present with jaw pain and swelling, inflamed gums, abnormal dentition with loss of alveolar bone, and floating teeth on radiographic evaluation. Temporal bone involvement with LCH can be confused with more common disorders, such as chronic suppurative otitis media with aural polyps not responsive to conservative therapy. In most cases, a friable gray to tan-pink external auditory canal mass is present, usually in conjunction with erosion of the posterior canal wall.

Treatment of Langerhans' cell histiocytosis must be appropriate for the extent of disease. Singular bony lesions of eosinophilic granuloma are initially treated with curettage or localized radiation of 600 to 1000 rads. Multifocal disease is usually treated with chemotherapy, especially when soft tissue disease predominates.

RARE TUMORS: DIAGNOSTIC AND TREATMENT PITFALLS

Several rare childhood tumors are difficult to diagnose or manifest protean behavior. Complications arising from inappropriate management of these lesions are all too possible. For example, nodular fasciitis, the most common pseudosarcoma of the soft tissues,[46] often presents a diagnostic dilemma. Clinically, the lesion is a rapidly growing subcutaneous mass that seldom exceeds 5 cm. Histologically, its high cellularity, significant mitotic activity, and infiltrative borders may be confused with sarcoma. In children, it is most commonly misinterpreted as malignant fibrous histiocytoma. Because local excision is curative for nodular fasciitis, the correct diagnosis is imperative to avoid unnecessary and harmful therapy. The otolaryngologist–head and neck surgeon's communication with the pathologist regarding the clinical history is the first step in avoiding such errors.

Melanotic neuroectodermal tumor of infancy (MNTI) represents a rare tumor with variable behavior. It is considered a benign lesion composed of epitheloid melanin-containing and neuroblastic cells with a prominent stroma.[47] It often occurs in the anterior maxilla but may present with orbital extension. Treatment includes local excision with preservation of vital structures. Nevertheless, recurrence has been documented in 15% and malignant behavior in 3% of cases.[48] Children presenting at less than 6 months of age are thought to be at greater risk. Consequently, the extent of resection and the use of adjuvant chemotherapy must be carefully considered without clear guidelines.

ANTENATAL DIAGNOSIS OF CONGENITAL MASSES

With the recent widespread use of fetal ultrasound in obstetrics, cervicofacial teratomas (Figure 17.3) and lymphangiomas are being discovered by 20 to 24 weeks' gestation. In the past, the diagnosis would occur at delivery, often with severe respiratory distress or death. Emergent attempts at tracheotomy would be heroic or futile. Now, early diagnosis allows for a team approach to the orderly management of these congenital tumors. Once these tumors are identified, a team is assembled consisting of the obstetrician, maternal–fetal specialist, neonatologist, pediatric anesthesiologist, otolaryngologist, pediatric surgeon, operating room support staff, intended primary

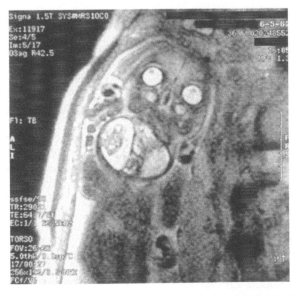

FIGURE 17.3 *In-utero* MRI demonstrating a solid mass in the cervical region at 28 weeks' gestation. This mother and child were successfully treated employing the EXIT procedure. Pathology was a benign teratoma.

care provider, and family support services. The maternal–fetal specialist carefully monitors for polyhydramnios until term or prior to term if further waiting is deemed too risky.

The EXIT (*ex utero* intrapartum treatment) procedure takes advantage of uninterrupted placental support and allows up to 60 minutes of continuous cord perfusion before uteroplacental gas exchange deteriorates. The sequence involves deep maternal–fetal anesthesia for uterine relaxation, a controlled hysterotomy, delivery of the fetal head and neck, and establishment of an airway while maintaining fetal–placental circulation.[49,50] Once a secure airway has been achieved, the baby is delivered through the hysterotomy and the umbilical cord divided. The otolaryngologist is prepared to perform laryngoscopy with intubation, bronchoscopy, and tracheotomy. Once the baby is stabilized, surgical resection commences.

The key to success is excellent communication with the parents and team members, as well as preparation and practice runs to identify any logistical problems. Numerous meetings with the parents prior to the event help to prepare them for potential risks and outcomes.

REFERENCES

1. Josephson, G.D. and Wohl, D.L. Malignant tumors of the head and neck in children. *Curr. Opin. Otolaryngol. Head Neck Surg.*, 1999, 7(2), 61–67.
2. Flanagan, P.M., Roland, N.J., and Jones, A.S. Cervical node metastases presenting with features of branchial cysts. *J. Laryngol. Otol.*, 1994, 108, 1068–1071.
3. Kohelet, D. and Arbel, E. A prospective search for urinary tract abnormalities in infants with isolated preauricular tags. *Pediatrics*, 2000, 105, E61.
4. Prasad, S., Grundfast, K., and Milmoe, G. Management of congenital preauricular pit and sinus tract in children. *Laryngoscope*, 1990, 100, 320–321.
5. Moore, K.L. and Persaud, T.V.N. *Before We Are Born,* 5th ed. Philadelphia: W.B. Saunders Company, 1998, 208–211.
6. Triglia, J.-M., Nicollas, R., Ducroz, V., Koltai, P.J., and Garabedian, E.-N. First branchial cleft anomalies. *Arch. Otolaryngol. Head Neck Surg.*, 1998, 124, 291–295.
7. Edmonds, J.L., Girod, D.A., Woodroof, J.M., and Bruegger, D.E. Third branchial anomalies. *Arch. Otolaryngol. Head Neck Surg.*, 1997, 123, 438–441.
8. Jordan, J.A., Graves, J.E., Manning, S.C., McClay, J.E., and Biavati, M.J. Endoscopic cauterization for treatment of fourth branchial cleft sinuses. *Arch. Otolaryngol. Head Neck Surg.*, 1998, 124, 1021–1024.
9. DiNardo, L.J. and Wohl, D.L. Partial DiGorge anomaly presenting as an enlarging third pharyngeal pouch cyst. *Otolaryngol. Head Neck Surg.*, 1995, 113, 785–787.
10. Josephson, G.D., Spencer, W.R., and Josephson, J.S. Thyroglossal duct cyst, the New York Eye and Ear Infirmary experience and a literature review. *ENT J.*, 1998, 77(8), 642–651.
11. Greinwald. J.H., Leichtman, L.G., and Simko, E.J. Hereditary thyroglossal duct cysts. *Arch. Otolaryngol. Head Neck Surg.*, 1996, 122, 1094–1096.
12. Tunkel, D.E., and Domenech, E.E. Radioisotope scanning of the thyroid gland prior to thyroglossal duct cyst excision. *Arch. Otolaryngol. Head Neck Surg.*, 1998, 124, 597–599.
13. Heshmati, H.M., Fatourechi, V., van Heerden, J.A., Hay, I.D., and Goellner, J.R. Thyroglossal duct carcinoma: report of 12 cases. *Mayo Clin. Proc.*, 1997, 72, 315–319.
14. Isaacson, G. Central neck dissection for infected or recurrent thyroglossal duct cysts. *Operative Tech. Otolaryngol. Head Neck Surg.*, 2001, 12(4), 225–238.
15. Bowers, R.E., Graham, E.A., and Tomlinson, K.M. The natural history of the strawberry nevus. *Arch. Dermatol.*, 1960, 82, 667–670.
16. Kasalbach, H.H., and Merritt, K.K. Capillary hemangioma with extensive purpura. *Am. J. Dis. Child*, 1940, 59, 1063–1070.
17. Takahashi, K., Mulliken, J.B., Kozakewich, H., Rogers, R.A., Folkman, J., and Ezekowitz, A.B. Cellular markers that distinguish the phases of hemangioma during infancy and childhood. *J. Clin. Invest.*, 1994, 93, 2357–2364.

18. Waner, M., Suen, J.Y., and Dinehart, S. Treatment of hemangiomas of the head and neck. *Laryngoscope*, 1992, 102, 1123–32.

19. Wenig, B.M. Neoplasms of the oral cavity, nasopharynx, tonsils, and neck. In Wenig, B.M. ed. *Atlas of Head and Neck Pathology*. Philadelphia: W.B. Saunders Company, 1993, 148.

20. Ogita, S., Tsuto, T., Nakamura, K., Deguchi, E., and Iwai, N. OK-432 therapy in 64 patients with lymphangioma. *J. Ped. Surg.*, 1994, 29, 784–5.

21. Greinwald, J.H., Burke, D.K., Sato, Y., Poust, R.I., Kimura, K., Bauman, N.M., and Smith, R.J.H. Treatment of lymphangiomas in children: an update of picibanil (OK-432) sclerotherapy. *Otolaryngol. Head Neck Surg.*, 1999, 121, 381–7.

22. Mulliken, J.B., Murray, J.E., and Castaneda, A.R. Management of vascular malformation of the face using total circulatory arrest. *Surg. Gynecol. Obstetr.*, 1978, 146, 168.

23. Stal, S., Hamilton, S., and Spira, M. Hemangiomas, lymphangiomas, and vascular malformations of the head and neck. *Otolaryngol. Clin. North Am.*, 1986, 19, 769–796.

24. Abemayor, E., Newman, A., and Dudley, J. Teratomas of the head and neck in childhood. *Laryngoscope*, 1984, 94, 1489–1492.

25. Graeber, G.M., Thompson, L.D., Cohen, D.J., Ronnigen, L.D., Jaffin, J., and Zajtchuk, R. Cystic lesion of the thymus: an occasionally malignant cervical and/or anterior mediastinal mass. *J. Thorac. Cardiovasc. Surg.*, 1984, 87, 295–300.

26. Posnick, J.C., Bortoluzzi, P., Armstrong, D.C., and Drake, J.M. Intracranial nasal dermoid sinus cysts: computed tomographic scan findings and surgical results. *Plast. Reconstr. Surg.*, 1994, 93, 745–754.

27. Jaques, D.A., Krolls, S.O., and Chambers, R.G. Parotid tumors in children. *Am. J. Surg.*, 1976, 132(4), 469–471.

28. Johns, M.E. Management of the primary site:salivary glands. In Pillsbury, H.A. and Goldsmith, M.M. eds. *Operative Challenges in Otolaryngology Head and Neck Surgery*. Chicago: Year Book Medical Publishers, Inc., 1990, 377–386.

29. Minor, V. Eines neues verfahren zu der klinischen untersuhung der schweissab-sonderung. *Dtsch. Z. Nervenheilkunge*, 1927, 101, 302.

30. Goldwin-Wood, P.H. Tympanic neurectomy. *J. Laryngol. Otol.*, 1962, 76, 683–693.

31. Newman, K.D., Black, T., Heller, G., Azizkhan, R.G., Holcomb, G.W., Sklar, C., Vlamis, V., Hasse, G.M., and La Quaglia, M.P. Differentiated thyroid cancer, determinants of disease progression in patients < 21 years of age at diagnosis: a report from the Surgical Discipline Committee of the Children's Cancer Group. *Ann. Surg.*, 1998, 227(4), 533–541.

32. Delius, R.E. and Thompson, N.W. Early total thyroidectomy in patients with multiple endocrine neoplasia IIb syndrome. *Surg. Gynecol. Obstetr.*, 1989, 169(5), 442–444.

33. Bryarly, R.C., Shockley, W.W., and Stucker, F.J. Method and management of thyroid surgery in the pediatric patient. *Laryngoscope*, 1985, 95, 1025–1028.

34. Young, A.E. and Marigold, J.M. Thyroidectomy: is Lugol's iodine necessary? [Letter]. *Ann. R. Coll. Surg. Engl.*, 1983, 65, 63.

35. Rock, M.G., Pritchard, D.J., and Reiman, H.M. Extra-abdominal desmoid tumors. *J. Bone Joint Surg. Am.*, 1984, 66, 1369–1374.

36. Enzinger, F.M. and Shiraki, M. Musculo-aponeurotic fibromatosis of the shoulder girdle (extra-abdominal desmoid): analysis of 30 cases followed up for ten or more years. *Cancer*, 1967, 20, 1131–1140.

37. Raney, R.B. Chemotherapy for children with aggressive fibromatosis and Langerhan's cell histiocytosis. *Clin. Orthop.*, 1991, 119(262), 58–63.

38. Skapek, S.X., Hawk, B.J., Hoffer, F.A., Dahl, G.V., Granowetter, L., Gebhardt, M.C., Ferguson, W.S., and Grier, H.E. Combination chemotherapy using vinblastine and methotrexate for the treatment of progressive desmoid tumor in children. *J. Clin. Oncol.*, 1998, 16(9), 3021–3027.

39. Kamel, R. Transnasal endoscopic surgery in juvenile nasopharyngeal angiofibroma. *J. Laryngol. Otol.*, 1996, 100, 962–968.

40. Khalifa, M.A. Endonasal endoscopic surgery for nasopharyngeal angiofibroma. *Otolaryngol. Head Neck Surg.*, 2001, 124, 336–337.

41. Danesi, G., Panizza, B., Mazzoni, A., and Calabrese, V. Anterior approaches in juvenile nasopharyngeal angiofibromas with intracranial extension. *Otolaryngol. Head Neck Surg.*, 2000, 122, 277–283.

42. Browne, J.D. and Jacob, S.L. Temporal approach for resection of juvenile nasopharyngeal angiofi-bromas. *Laryngoscope*, 2000, 110(8), 1287–1293.

43. Deschler, D.G., Kaplan, M., and Boles, R. Treatment of large juvenile nasopharyngeal angiofibroma. *Otolaryngol. Head Neck Surg.*, 1992, 106, 278–284.

44. Kuppersmith, R.B., Teh, B.S., Donovan, D.T., Mai, W.Y., Chiu, J.K., Woo, S.Y., and Butler, E.B. The use of intensity modulated radiotherapy for the treatment of extensive and recurrent juvenile angiofi-broma. *Int. J. Pediatr. Otorhinolaryngol.*, 2000, 52(3), 261–268.

45. DiNardo, L.J. and Wetmore, R.F. Head and neck manifestations of histiocytosis-X in children. *Laryngoscope*, 1989, 99, 721–724.

46. DiNardo, L.J., Wetmore, R.F., and Potsic, W.P. Nodular fasciitis of the head and neck in children. *Arch. Otolaryngol. Head Neck Surg.*, 1991, 117, 1001–1002.

47. Melissari, M., Tragni, G., Gaetti, L., Gabrielli, M., Bozzetti, A., and Raffiani, M. Melanotic neuro-ectodermal tumour of infancy (MNTI). Immunohistochemical and ultrastructural study of a case. *J. Craniomaxillofacial Surg.*, 1988, 16, 330.

48. Cutler. L.S., Chaudhrey, A.P., and Topazian, R. Melanotic neuroectodermal of infancy. An ultrastructural study, literature review and reevaluation. *Cancer*, 1981, 48, 257–270.

49. Mahapatra, A.K. and Suri, A. Anterior encephaloceles: a study of 92 cases. *Pediatr. Neurosurg.*, 2002, 36, 113–118.

50. Hubbard, A.M., Crombleholme, T.M., and Adzick, N.S. Prenatal MRI evaluation of giant neck masses in preparation for the fetal EXIT procedure. *Am. J. Perinatol.*, 1998, 15, 253–257.

18 Pediatric Swallowing Disorders

Jacqueline E. Jones, Chandra M. Ivey, and William F. McGuirt, Jr.

There is an objective reality, but we're nowhere near to grasping it in its totality … and if we did get to the truth, would we ever know it?

Michael Redhead

CONTENTS

INTRODUCTION

The goal of this chapter is to identify common abnormalities in anatomy, physiology, and functional development of the fundamental elements of swallowing that afflict children of different ages. In the neonate, congenital abnormalities of the oropharynx and esophagus cause difficulty swallowing. These abnormalities include vocal cord paralysis as well as anatomic and functional causes of stridor. In the infant, genetic syndromes, vascular rings, and neoplastic disease may initially present with feeding difficulties. Gastroesophageal reflux is a common cause for dysphagia at this age, and neurogenic problems at any level of the nervous system may severely compromise the development of feeding behaviors. As children age, they are more prone to accidents. Trauma and foreign body ingestion commonly present with dysphagia. Feeding disorders are common in early childhood, with minor feeding difficulties reported between 25 and 35% in healthy children and more severe problems in children with chronic medical conditions and in premature infants.[1-3]

ANATOMY AND DEVELOPMENTAL PHYSIOLOGY

Swallowing is defined as the "semiautomatic motor action of the muscles of the respiratory and gastrointestinal tracts that propels food from the oral cavity to the stomach ..."[4] It also clears salivary secretions and particles from the upper airway as a protective measure against aspiration. The swallowing process involves four main phases: pre-oral, oral, pharyngeal, and esophageal.[5]

- The *pre-oral* phase encompasses movements necessary to bring matter to the mouth; it may be affected by medications as well as the emotional state of the child. More generalized oral aversions may occur after a negative feeding experience or after long-term intubation or tube feeding. This oral defensiveness can persist long after the medical condition has stabilized.[6]
- The *oral* phase involves the creation of a proper food bolus. The lips, cheeks, and palate must be intact in order to maintain matter within the mouth. Adequate motor coordination of the tongue, maxilla, and mandible are necessary for bolus formation. Breathing continues during this phase due to the apposition of the soft palate and the posterior tongue. This phase initially consists of suckling, which occurs in bursts and reflexively initiates swallowing.[7]
- The *pharyngeal* phase involves the movement of food toward the posterior oropharynx for entry into the esophagus. As the food bolus is swept past the anterior tonsillar pillars, reflexive swallowing is activated. The larynx is moved anteriorly and superiorly into the tongue base as the tongue sweeps posteriorly, aiding in the descent of the epiglottis. The aryepiglottic folds and true and false cords reflexively appose and the pharyngeal constrictor muscles begin the primary peristaltic wave. This allows for the protection of the airway while matter is passed from the oropharynx into the esophagus.
- The *esophageal* phase occurs with the relaxation of the cricopharyngeal muscle as the larynx is elevated, and with the passage of the primary peristaltic wave to the esophagus. Secondary and, if necessary, tertiary, peristaltic waves originate within the esophageal musculature and continue down its length. The lower esophageal sphincter, a zone of relatively higher pressure, begins to relax as peristaltic activity reaches this level.[8]

Swallowing occurs in a coordinated pattern controlled through the cranial and cervical nerves. Problems with swallowing occur when any level of anatomic or neurologic function is compromised. It is also intricately tied to the respiratory system. Aspiration may occur if oral contents enter the posterior pharynx before the larynx elevates into its protected position, or if cricopharyngeus relaxation does not occur and contents are not emptied into the esophagus.[8]

Many important differences between infants and adults affect oral feeding and swallowing behavior. Many reflexes initially aid in suckling behavior. These include the phasic bite (rhythmic opening and closing of the jaws when the gums are stimulated), the tongue thrust (protrusion of the tongue with sensory input at its tip), and the rooting response.[5] In the infant, a cyclic, coordinated pattern of breathing, sucking, and swallowing is mainly controlled by reflex at birth. This is facilitated by obligate nasal breathing in the neonate. Neonatal tongue motion is mainly horizontal, and vertical motion is absent. Buccal fat pads are present within the masseter that aid in suckling by causing greater apposition. The posterior tongue, soft palate, pharynx, and larynx are in close proximity during this developmental stage, and the nasopharynx slopes into the oropharynx, creating a natural reservoir for air.

As descending inhibition increases, neonatal reflexes are suppressed and greater voluntary control of feeding behavior occurs. By approximately 4 months of age, the tongue thrust disappears, and horizontal and vertical tongue motions are soon present. By 6 to 8 months, secondary feeding patterns are initiated. Growth of the jaw and strengthening of the oral musculature occurs. With growth, the angle between the nasopharynx and oropharynx becomes more acute. As the larynx shifts downward with growth, the change in its proximity to the soft palate and tongue causes a transition from cyclic sucking, swallowing, and breathing to alternate breathing and feeding.

EVALUATION

The historical presentation of the child with feeding problems includes symptoms of food refusal, failure to thrive, oral aversion, recurrent pneumonias, chronic lung disease, or recurrent emesis. Swallowing and feeding disorders are complex and have multiple causes, as will be discussed in this chapter. The delay in the initiation of feeding caused by underlying disorders may affect the normal acquisition of feeding skills. An interdisciplinary evaluation facilitates integration of expertise from different disciplines to address the feeding issues as well as the overall health of the child.

A focused feeding history includes current diet, textures and route and time of administration, modifications, and feeding position. Prolonged length of meals may suggest ineffective feeding mechanics or possibly a behavioral problem in a healthy child. Specific food aversions may help to identify metabolic problems or food allergens. Medical comorbidities need to be addressed. Nutritional and psychological assessments need to be undertaken early and can elicit behaviorial and parental factors that may be contributing to the feeding disorder. Observation of a feeding session often provides insight into the feeding mechanics.

Physical examination begins with the observation of feeding as well as attention to articulation and voice quality. The examination includes observation of tone, posture, and position during feeding; oral structure and function; and patient interaction and motivation toward feeding. Structural or neurologic problems can be suggested by difficulties with oral secretions, escape of food, repetitive swallows to clear a bolus, discoordination of suck and swallow, noisy breathing after swallowing, gagging, coughing, or emesis. Oral anatomic abnormalities need to be excluded. The absence of obvious signs of a swallowing disorder does not rule out a disorder. The selection of further diagnostic tests is based on a developmental, feeding, and medical history followed by a thorough physical examination.

Radiographic studies can address anatomic or structural problems and allow evaluation of coordination of movement of a bolus through the upper digestive tract. The radiograph is often used to assess the base of the tongue, neck and esophagus, and trachea as they enter the mediastinum. Narrowing of these structures on x-ray may indicate edema or obstruction. AP and lateral films aid in the diagnosis of radiopaque foreign bodies in the airway or esophagus. Subcutaneous emphysema and structural displacement of structures can be documented.

CT and MRI are also useful in assessing structures in the head and neck region. Soft tissue structures are visualized in greater detail, and these tests are often used to evaluate speculative lesions and the extent of trauma. CT is also used frequently in the assessment of foreign body aspiration and ingestion, due to its ability to identify radiopaque and radiotranslucent objects.[9] MR imaging may be useful in those suspected of a central nervous system disorder such as Arnold–Chiari malformation or to evaluate a possible vascular ring/sling. Ultrasound may also be useful in the assessment of cystic and solid structures in the pharynx and neck.

Upper GI, barium, and gastrograffin swallows can be useful to show structural abnormalities. Videofluoroscopic swallowing studies (VSS) are often used in functional assessment of the pharynx and esophagus.[9] These studies offer functional imaging of bolus placement and muscle coordination in the mouth and pharynx, and of peristaltic action and bolus movement within the esophagus. Such studies may also offer direct evidence of aspiration during feeding or of loss of protective coordination between breathing and swallowing. Esophageal manometry studies are often added in conjunction with these exams to measure pressure along the esophagus at rest and during swallowing in an effort to document neuromuscular function.[10] The evaluation of gastroesophageal reflux disease (GERD) and the use of pH studies are discussed in Chapter 19.

Adjunctive testing or alternative testing involves the use of transnasal fiberoptic examination (FEES) of the pharyngeal and laryngeal structures during speech and swallowing. The management of the food bolus or secretions can be assessed by green food coloring on the tongue or with a colored applesauce bolus. Fiberoptic evaluation of swallowing does not assess oral preparation but is similar to the information obtained of the pharyngeal phase by VSS. Sensation in the pharynx can be evaluated by a calibrated puff of air onto the arytenoids or epiglottis.[11] FEES and sensory testing may be an alternative to VSS in difficult patients. Office-based fiberoptic examinations are not a substitute for rigid endoscopy for the complete anatomic evaluation.

Endoscopy is a necessary step in the evaluation of the anatomy of the larynx, trachea, and esophagus. Esophagoscopy may be useful in treatment and evaluation of webs, strictures, and inflammatory lesions. Laryngeal clefts or tracheal lesions are best inspected directly by endoscopy.

THE NEONATE

At birth, the neonate is an obligate nasal breather. This is aided by the anatomy of the head and neck, including the small oral cavity, higher suspension of the larynx, relative macroglossia, and anterior tongue placement due to a smaller mandible and the presence of buccal fat pads.[7,12,13] Suckling in the neonate involves precisely controlled sequential movements allowing for nasal breathing while feeding. Oral stimulation from the breast or bottle initiates the early reflexive tongue-thrusting motions needed for suckling. Suckling initially occurs in small bursts that reflexively initiate swallowing. The pharyngeal phase of swallowing reflexively inhibits respiration and is controlled in a precise fashion by subcortical structures at this age. This unique anatomic arrangement, as well as the precise synchronous control of suckling, breathing, and swallowing, helps to protect the airway during the first few months of life.

Congenital anomalies of any structures of the nasopharynx, oropharynx, lips, tongue, palate, cheeks, mandible, maxilla, larynx, or esophagus may cause difficulty in suckling or swallowing in the neonate. These include choanal stenosis or atresia; craniofacial anomalies, including cleft lip and cleft palate; congenital tracheoesophageal fistula and/or atresia; vocal chord paralysis; laryngomalacia; or other causes of tracheoesophageal obstruction.

CHOANAL STENOSIS AND ATRESIA

Choanal stenosis and atresia occur with the failure of the nasopharyngeal septum to rupture during development. Unilateral atresia is more common than bilateral.[14] Symptoms from unilateral atresia are milder and are usually not investigated until the older child presents with rhinorrhea in the setting of unilateral nasal obstruction.[15] Symptoms of bilateral atresia may begin as early as with the first feeding and include severe cyanosis with feedings.[16] Cyanosis is alleviated with crying and agitation. Evaluation of the posterior choanae for patency can be accomplished by passing catheters through the nasal passages, through the use of a flexible fiberoptic nasopharyngoscope, or with axial CT scan oriented parallel to the infraorbitomeatal line and posterior hard palate. Other causes of nasal obstruction without choanal atresia include deviated nasal septum, pyriform aperture stenosis, mucosal edema, trauma, adenoid hypertrophy, neonatal rhinitis, or congential mass lesion such as an encephalocele or neoplasm.

CRANIOFACIAL ANOMALIES

Craniofacial anomalies include mandibular hypoplasia, midface hypoplasia, cleft palate, and cleft lip. Abnormal position and coordination of the mandible and tongue in craniofacial anomalies are commonly associated with abnormalities of feeding. Mandibular hypoplasia may be seen as an isolated defect as in trisomy 18, but is frequently associated with the Pierre Robin sequence.[16,17] Mandibular hypoplasia with associated tongue displacement (glossoptosis) may cause stridor, respiratory obstruction and cyanosis, difficulty swallowing, and severe malnutrition. Tracheostomy and gastrostomy may be indicated in severely affected children. Otherwise, tube feedings and postural treatment are used to prevent aspiration and promote the outgrowth of the mandible.

Crouzon's disease, a severe form of craniofacial dystosis, can be associated with mid-face hypoplasia.[18] All cranial sutures are prematurely fused in this syndrome, leading to beaking deformity of the nose, maxillary hypoplasia, mandibular protrusion, and exophthalmos. Swallowing problems are common, due not only to hypoplasia of the jaw, but also to neurologic dysfunction in these patients. Apert's syndrome commonly displays bilateral coronal suture synostosis and syndactylism of hands and feet. Swallowing problems may present in the face of concomitant choanal atresia or stenosis, and stridor at rest may necessitate tracheotomy.[16]

CLEFT LIP AND PALATE

Cleft lip and palate are the most common craniofacial malformations, accounting for half of documented defects.[19–21] For embryologic reasons, clefts are characterized as primary if anterior to the incisive foramen, or secondary if posterior to it.[20] Submucous clefts, where intact mucous membranes cover a bony fissure, may be initially difficult to diagnose, but should be evaluated for when a bifid uvula is discovered. A submucous cleft palate may affect swallowing by allowing incomplete closure of the velopharyngeal orifice and resultant reflux. Swallowing problems and velopharyngeal incompetence occurring from cleft palate are very common. Even when surgically corrected, facial growth may be disordered, and orthodontic and speech problems may arise as the child develops.[20] Other craniofacial anomalies associated with swallowing dysfunction in the neonate include congenital macroglossia, lack of development of the lingual frenulum, and lingual thyroid.[20]

LARYNGEAL ABNORMALITIES

Laryngeal abnormalities impair the protective role of the larynx during swallowing and can lead to stridor or manifestations of respiratory distress. During the pharyngeal phase of swallowing, the larynx must elevate and move anteriorly and the laryngeal sphincter must close. This timed reflex, along with the downward displacement of the epiglottis and closure of the false and true chords, provides protection against oropharyngeal contents reaching the trachea and lungs. Laryngeal abnormalities may present as difficulty swallowing or coughing, or cyanosis with feeding. Problems presenting in this way include laryngeal or subglottic stenosis, laryngeal clefts, vocal cord paralysis, and laryngomalacia.[16,22]

Symptoms of *subglottic stenosis* include stridor at rest or with agitation, respiratory distress, recurrent infections, retractions, and difficulty feeding.[23,24] Placement of a gastrostomy tube may be necessary due to the increased work of breathing while feeding. Tracheotomy may be required for severe stenosis accompanied by respiratory distress.

Laryngeal clefts are a rare cause of dysphagia and are classified depending on the extent of laryngeal involvement.[22,25] Common symptoms include aspiration of milk or oral secretions; difficulties while feeding, including cyanosis and choking; or aspiration pneumonitis.[22] Endoscopy is necessary for diagnosis. Other anomalies such as a tracheoesophageal fistula should be searched for when a laryngeal cleft is diagnosed.[25] Although more extensive laryngeal clefts require surgical correction, the correction of a type I cleft is indicated only when severe aspiration occurs.

Vocal cord paralysis leads to a cord in a relaxed midline position with resultant partial obstruction of the passage of air into the trachea. Bilateral cord paralysis in the neonate is usually central in origin. Bilateral true vocal cord paralysis may resolve as cerebral edema subsides, but when present, it causes severe respiratory distress. Tracheotomy may be required. Unilateral paralysis or varied degrees of paresis most commonly present with mild respiratory compromise, but predispose to aspiration. Paresis, or weakening of vocal cord apposition, interferes with protection of the airway. This may present with symptoms of coughing, grunting, or stridor in the neonate. Laryngoscopy is required for diagnosis. Treatment should be aimed at relief of any primary disorder contributing to cord paralysis.

Laryngomalacia is the most common cause of neonatal stridor — a condition exacerbated by agitation as well as feeding.[25] Although the stridor is often worrisome to parents, symptoms usually resolve by 18 months of age. Complications are rare, but may include feeding difficulties, failure to thrive, or symptoms of apnea. Epiglottoplasty has been described for severe cases of laryngomalacia.[26]

Esophageal atresia presents in the neonatal period with the inability to swallow, cough with feeding, respiratory distress, and cyanosis. Isolated esophageal atresia occurs in about 7% of cases. Four other degrees of fistulae are recognized; the most common is esophageal atresia with distal tracheoesophageal fistula. Most cases of atresia are diagnosed very early in the neonatal period. The H-type, with fistulous communication but no atresia, often presents later in childhood with recurrent pneumonia or coughing spells with feeds. Down syndrome and low birth weight are found with increased frequency in neonates with tracheoesophageal atresia or fistula.[27] The incidence of other congenital anomalies is increased and includes the VACTERL syndrome.[28]

Atresia may be suspected *in utero* by the presence of polyhydramnios on ultrasound. Inability to pass a nasogastric tube or lack of gastric juice in the aspirate affirms the diagnosis of atresia. A chest x-ray demonstrates the lack of progression of the tube to the stomach. If large amounts of gas are demonstrated, a fistula is presumed. Isolated atresia may be implied by lack of air in the stomach, but this may be misleading if a mucous plug is preventing air from tracking in a fistulous passage. Bronchoscopy is recommended preoperatively to assess for the presence of or confirm location of the fistula. Ultrasound or CT to search for associated anomalies is also strongly recommended.

Immediate management of atresia includes continuous suction application to the proximal pouch in order to prevent aspiration and placement of the infant in an upright position to minimize any reflux of gastric secretions through the fistulous connection. Gastrostomy for decompression of the stomach may be indicated in children with severe reflux. This option should be used with caution in neonates on ventilators because gastrostomy may create a low-pressure alternative through the fistula and cause respiratory compromise.[29]

THE INFANT

The period of infancy begins after neonatal week 4. As the central nervous system of the infant matures in these first few months, early suckling patterns shift into a mature sucking pattern with increased muscular strength and multiplanar tongue thrusting. After about 3 months of age, there are distinct oral movements for solids vs. liquids; prior to this time, the infant makes a similar sucking motion regardless of the food presented. Swallowing acquires greater complexity and increased voluntary cortical control as the reflexive bursts of sucking as well as the tongue thrust are slowly extinguished with increasing age.[7,12,13] Coordination of the maxilla and mandible to accomplish bite is established by about 12 months of age.

Some of the common swallowing disorders seen during infancy may have been present from birth, but have delayed onset of symptoms. Neurogenic problems may be symptomatic from the outset or may not be diagnosed until an infant begins to lag behind in normal developmental milestones. Causes of pediatric dysphagia that may be seen in infancy include genetic disorders, neurogenic abnormalities, adenotonsillar hyperplasia, and obstruction due to benign cysts, congenital tumors, and vascular rings.

GENETIC SYNDROMES

Often genetic syndromes involve problems with feeding or swallowing within their symptom complex. This includes craniofacial syndromes that involve dysplastic development of facial structures. This affects feeding behavior in multiple ways. It may disrupt the normal suck–breathe–swallow cyclic reflex of the obligate nasal breather by causing obstruction or abnormal communication between nasopharynx and oropharynx. These syndromes may interfere with suction development among the lips, tongue, cheeks, and palate; may disrupt maxilla or mandible formation; or may disrupt proper tongue or pharyngeal motion.[30] Other genetic syndromes may have mild or no specific facial anomalies, but may still present with feeding or sucking difficulties. Some may have general hypotonia and developmental delay. Poor feeding and sucking then predisposes to failure to thrive for these infants. Often this prompts further evaluation and a genetic etiology is discovered. Genetic disorders with poor suck include Prader–Willi, Coffin–Siris, Smith–Lemli–Opitz syndrome, Cornelia de Lange syndrome, Dubowitz, Rubenstein–Taybi, Beckwith–Wiedemann, Trisomy 18, and Trisomy 21.[31]

CRANIAL NERVE DEFICITS

Cranial nerve deficits constitute a major abnormality and may account for feeding and sucking difficulties seen in infants with these specific cranial nerve palsies. These include Klippel–Feil and Mobius sequence.[31] Klippel–Feil is characterized by fusion of the cervical vertebrae. Syringomyelia may develop in children with this genetic disorder and, if rostral enough in the cord, can disrupt the cranial nerves and cause dysphagia. Mobius sequence involves multiple cranial nerve palsies from birth, including permanent paralysis of nerves VI and VII. Dysphagia may not occur unless there is wide involvement of other nerves important for oral motor and sensory innervation, such as cranial nerves V or XII.

NEUROGENIC DYSPHAGIA

Neurogenic dysphagia occurs when central nervous system or neuromuscular abnormalities interfere with normal feeding and swallowing skills. These neurologic difficulties are usually present at basic as well as higher functional levels and need comprehensive assessment and management to improve feeding and other behaviors. Neurogenic problems may be congenital or acquired.[13] Acquired deficits may be caused by infections or encephalopathies, as well as by polymyositis and dermatomyositis. These problems, along with intracranial hemorrhage and cerebral infarction, occur suddenly and can have deleterious effects on neurologic status and muscle coordination. They may resolve or may lead to permanent deficit and dysfunction in swallowing and sucking. Other causes of neurogenic dysphagia include cerebral palsy, kernicterus, neonatal withdrawal syndromes, Arnold–Chiari malformation, many genetic disorders, neoplastic disease, degenerative white and gray matter disease, infantile spinal muscular atrophy, or disorders of the peripheral nervous system.[13]

Cerebral palsy (CP) is the most common congenital neurologic deficit associated with neurogenic dysphagia. These problems lead to chronic growth, developmental, and feeding problems for these children and can also lead to significant morbidity and mortality secondary to aspiration and respiratory infection. CP causes abnormal oral–motor, fine, and gross motor movement, all of which may have an impact on feeding behavior in any stage. Often these children have significant food loss because they are unable to control their lips and tongue in order to create a proper food bolus and prevent expulsion of food through the lips. This is further complicated by persistent primitive reflexes that normally disappear with development of cortical inhibition.[32] These dysfunctional movements and a delayed or absent swallowing reflex increase the risk of aspiration.[33]

Children with CP often have concurrent abnormalities in other systems. Spasticity often prevents or impairs attempts at self-feeding. Motor dysfunction of the larynx may lead to aspiration. These children may have intolerance for their own secretions associated with silent aspiration and drooling. Learned avoidance of food and eating may occur in these children due to unpleasant and frequent episodes of coughing, choking, regurgitation, vomiting, aspiration, and hypoxemia associated with meal times.[25]

Understanding the origin of dysphagia in the child with CP is the first step toward optimizing feeding behavior and facilitating proper development, growth, and behavior. The basic phases of swallowing should be evaluated, and specific therapies implemented based on the child's individual issues. Proper positioning during meals may promote better tolerance of oral intake and prevent undesired reflexes and movements. Use of palatal plates and orthodontic appliances may assist oral movements and minimize food loss.[34] Bolus size and consistency of feeds may be modified to permit greater tolerance. It is important also to take into account the cognitive and general motor development of the child when developing appropriate goals and therapeutic plans. Supplemental nutrition by parenteral or gastrostomy feeds may also be necessary. Although these strategies can be time- and labor-intensive, many children have improved feeding outcomes when they are implemented.

Gastroesophageal Reflux

Gastroesophageal reflux (GER) is common in infancy, usually beginning when the child is between 1 and 4 months of age. Symptoms may be minimal or cause severe discomfort and long-term sequelae. Vomiting is the most common symptom in children, present in greater than 90% of cases.[35] This is often effortless emesis or "spitting up." More severe symptoms may include chest pain, hematemesis, esophagitis, anemia, Barrett's esophagus, and failure to thrive.[36] Respiratory symptoms may include wheezing, stridor, cough, or apnea. Reflux should also be considered in infants with increased irritability, poor appetite, weight loss, sore throat, or hoarseness.

Proper esophageal and gastric function is necessary for the prevention of GER. This includes proper lower esophageal sphincter pressure and location, as well as normal gastric emptying and acid clearance. Reflux is commonly classified as functional, pathogenic, or secondary. Functional reflux is common and includes nonregurgitant reflux or effortless vomiting. No associated abnormality in esophageal or gastric function and no neurologic condition predisposes to functional reflux. One possible contribution to the etiology of functional reflux may be an obtuse angle of His. In the normal newborn this angle is obtuse, but becomes more acute with growth and thus more effectively prevents retrograde reflux. This anatomic change may partially account for the frequency of reflux early in life that resolves over time. There seem to be no long-term sequelae; thus, in the absence of any other signs or symptoms, functional reflux need not be vigorously evaluated or treated. Functional GER is by far the most common type of reflux and usually resolves without treatment by 12 to 18 months of age.

Infants with pathogenic GER can suffer more severe symptoms of reflux such as hematemesis, esophagitis, failure to thrive, anemia, or Barrett's esophagus. These conditions require evaluation and intervention to treat or prevent long-term complications. The chronicity of this condition, as well as the caustic damage caused by gastric contents, creates irritation and inflammation, which may lead to esophagitis and bleeding. This may then cause esophageal dysmotility that exacerbates the original GER. Stricture formation also can occur after chronic reflux and can cause progressive dysphagia.

Many abnormalities of the GI system may contribute to pathogenic GER. Antral dysmotility has been shown to cause chronic vomiting.[37] Delayed gastric emptying may be an exacerbating factor, but clinical studies have been equivocal. Poor basal LES tone has been presumed to contribute to reflux as well; however, studies have shown that normal muscular tone is achieved early in infancy and no difference is recorded between infants with functional and pathogenic reflux.[38]

Transient LES relaxation is considered a major factor contributing to pathogenic GER in infancy; this has been found to account for up to 50% of reflux episodes in children up to 2 years, while increased abdominal pressure accounts for only 5%.[39]

Prematurity seems to pose a risk for GER in infants and is postulated to contribute to apneic events as well as sudden infant death syndrome. In one study, 63% of infants with a mean gestational age of 30 weeks were shown to have GER by esophageal pH measurement.[40] Of these infants, 98% had recurrent episodes of apnea and abnormal breathing cycles. Another study showed that surgical correction of GER in infants less than 6 months old with apneic attacks resolved the GER and improved the apnea, thus suggesting a causative role of GER in the apnea.[41] The mechanism by which GER may cause apnea may be a direct response to acid in the esophagus or by laryngospasm. Children with other anatomic defects or neurogenic syndromes, including hiatal hernia or central nervous system disorders such as disorders of dystonia, mental retardation, seizure activity, Sandifer's syndrome, and rumination syndromes, may have a predisposition for GER.[41]

Evaluation of gastroesophageal reflux and treatment are more thoroughly defined in Chapter 19. It is important to remember that functional GER is by far the most common type seen. Many infants who are diagnosed with pathologic reflux will also have resolution of symptoms by 2 years of age. Many children also respond well to conservative treatment. Secondary gastroesophageal reflux due to other treatable conditions must be evaluated for and the primary condition treated when possible. Surgical options, when necessary, reduce reflux in many patients, with a low failure rate.

ANATOMIC ANOMALIES OF THE GREAT VESSELS

Anatomic anomalies of the great vessels within the mediastinum may lead to compressive symptoms of the esophagus and trachea. These anomalies may cause symptoms very early in life or may cause more slowly developing symptoms of respiratory distress or dysphagia. Anomalies of the aortic arch and its branches are the most common vascular rings described.[42] The most frequently seen anomalies are double aortic arch and right-sided aortic arch with left ligamentum arteriosus, with or without an anomalous left subclavian artery. The most common anatomy is a left-sided arch lying anterior to the trachea with left carotid and subclavian arterial branches, and a right arch lying posterior to trachea and esophagus with right carotid and subclavian arterial branches. The posterior arch is most often the larger of the two, and the anterior arch may commonly have areas of stenosis or atresia between the left carotid and subclavian branches or distal to these branches. This anomaly creates a full vascular "ring" surrounding trachea and esophagus and often leads to early onset severe respiratory stridor, cough, and feeding difficulties, usually noticed in the first few months of life. These symptoms worsen with time, and reflex apnea may contribute to respiratory difficulties.

Another vascular anomaly consists of a right-sided aortic arch with persistence of a leftward ligamentum arteriosus. This incomplete vascular ring may at times be further complicated by the presence of an anomalous left subclavian artery at the base of which the left ligamentum originates. At times, a Kommerell diverticulum may also arise from the base of the improperly placed subclavian. The alternate position of this subclavian, especially with the inclusion of an enlarged diverticulum, may tighten the ring even more, causing greater respiratory and esophageal symptoms. These symptoms are similar to those of the double aortic arch; however, they are usually milder and are noticed after age 1, in part due to the partial obstruction of the incomplete vs. the complete ring. Surgical correction of these vascular rings is imperative to alleviate symptoms.

TUMORS OF THE HEAD AND NECK

Tumors of the head and neck are relatively rare in the pediatric population; at least 90% of lesions in this area are found to be benign on assessment.[43] These tumors enlarge and often obstruct or impinge on structures within the respiratory and digestive tracts, causing symptoms of stridor and dysphagia. Benign lesions that may cause dysphagia include hemangioma, lymphangioma, cysts, papilloma, leiomyoma, and neurofibroma.[25,43–45] Of specific interest, leiomyoma of the esophagus involves hyperplasia of smooth muscle with thickening of the distal esophagus.[25] This abnormality is found, concurrent with hereditary nephritis in Alport's syndrome. Thickening of the musculature leads to narrowing of the esophageal lumen, which can be diagnosed by barium swallow or CT. In severely symptomatic cases, esophagectomy, esophagogastrectomy, or esophagomyotomy may be performed for palliation.

THE OLDER CHILD

Oral exploration of the environment predisposes children to ingestion and aspiration of foreign bodies. The constant placement of objects in the mouth puts toddlers at risk for trauma to the oropharynx due to their uncoordinated walking. Children are prone to viral and bacterial infections that may cause dysphagia or pain with swallowing. Tumors of the head and neck may be diagnosed during childhood due to symptoms of acquired stridor and dysphagia. Finally, rare disorders such as myogenic disease or disease intrinsic to the esophagus may present during this time period.

FOREIGN BODIES

Oral exploration of the environment predisposes children to aspiration and ingestion of foreign bodies. Complications of foreign bodies and their management are discussed in detail in Chapter 21 and Chapter 23. However, it is briefly mentioned in this chapter because it relates to disorders with swallowing. Ingestions greatly outnumber aspirations, and the majority of ingestions pass without sequelae. Yet, there is still significant mortality (1 to 2%) from swallowed or inhaled objects.[46] The mortality figures for complete laryngeal obstruction approach 45%, with about 30% of surviving children suffering hypoxic encephalopathy. Usually, children between the ages of 1 and 3 years have the highest rate of ingestions and inhalations. If a child younger than 1 year presents with a foreign body, there may be suspicion of the object being fed to the child by an older sibling or family member.[46] Other risks for ingestion or aspiration of objects include mental retardation, seizure disorder or other neurologic dysfunction, and structural or functional abnormalities of the larynx or esophagus.[47]

Impaction of foreign bodies in the esophagus may occur at areas of physiologic narrowing. These include the cricopharyngeus muscle, the esophageal impressions of the aorta and the left mainstem bronchus, and at the cardioesophageal junction (lower esophageal sphincter, LES). If an object has impacted in the region of the cricopharyngeus muscle, the child may exhibit respiratory symptoms or stridor due to the proximity of the larynx. Other symptoms include gagging, choking, vomiting, odynophagia, dysphagia, drooling, anorexia, and weight loss.[46]

Esophageal impaction can be misdiagnosed as viral respiratory illness due to cough and "throat" pain or as a gastrointestinal illness. Impaction is more likely to occur in children with a history of esophageal abnormality. Chest radiograph is an important diagnostic tool for the evaluation of swallowed material. Objects naturally tend to orient in the coronal plane as they are swallowed, so PA and lateral films are needed to assess the specific location of the object. Failure of an ingested object to orient in the coronal plane usually indicates structural abnormality in the region and thus greater likelihood that the object will become impacted and need removal. Due to high utilization of plastic in toys, ingested foreign bodies are less likely to be radiopaque and be diagnosed by radiograph. Plastic objects often go undiagnosed until inflammation becomes severe enough to cause obstructive symptoms such as vomiting and dysphagia.[47] The physician must assess tracheal compression, esophageal narrowing due to edema, or air in the esophagus as evidence of a radiolucent foreign body impaction. Perforation can also be assessed with findings of retroesophageal air or fullness.

The rigid esophagoscope is used to evaluate for foreign bodies under direct visualization. Perforation may occur due to the impaction of the foreign body, or may occur by instrumentation of the esophagus during removal of the object. The risk of perforation increases during the procedure if sharp objects or facets are not protected when they are withdrawn. If large, sharp objects are impacted and carry high risk of tearing or perforation, esophagotomy may be considered. Postoperative gastrograffin study should always be performed in order to assess any perforations that may need drainage. Other complications of surgical intervention include accidental extubation, pulmonary complications, mucosal destruction, or edema.

TRAUMA

Minor trauma to the oral cavity is common in young children and may result in dysphagia. During the toddling years, children have less motor coordination; objects placed in the mouth while running may result in subsequent lacerations with a fall. These lacerations are usually minor in nature, but more severe injury may occur. Other types of penetrating and blunt trauma to the head and neck from external causes occur with less frequency in children. This is due, in part, to the lower incidence of motor vehicle accidents and interpersonal conflicts involving children. Also, the larynx is at a more elevated position in children, thus allowing greater protection behind the mandible. The cartilages in the larynx are also less ossified and thus protect against fractures. The esophagus can be damaged in blunt trauma by being compressed directly against the spinal column.

The most common types of injuries in children occur from intraoral trauma, usually from objects placed in the mouth or from falls onto objects. Lacerations, puncture wounds, and contusions of the mucosa are often caused by toothbrushes, utensils, toys, sticks, or pencils carried in the mouth.[48] Lacerations from self-inflicted bites after falls may also be serious. Most often these injuries need only evaluation; hemostasis; removal of the object, fragments of objects, or teeth that have become imbedded in the tissue; and oral antibiotics. Bleeding, soft tissue edema, cervical emphysema, or hematoma may develop. Penetrating or blunt injuries to the posterior pharynx may involve the retropharyngeal space or may directly involve the cervical spine. Any injury of the lateral tonsillar area or lateral soft palate should elevate suspicion for trauma to the carotid artery. Although uncommon, carotid artery involvement may include intimal disruption or thrombosis, causing acute neurologic symptoms and changes in level of arousal. If vascular injury of this type is evident, emergent treatment must ensue.

Blunt trauma to the esophagus and larynx is uncommon in children, but may cause significant mortality if not diagnosed in a timely fashion. Because its location between the trachea and the cervical spine predisposes to damage, esophageal injury should be assessed with the presence of any midline cervical injury. Common initial complaints include dysphagia, odynophagia, hoarseness, and shortness of breath. Voice changes and subcutaneous emphysema are hallmarks of injury to structures in this area.

CAUSTIC INGESTION

Caustic ingestion continues to be a source of morbidity in young children. The extent of esophageal damage tends to be related to the type of substance ingested more frequently than it is to the quantity of ingested material. Alkalis tend to cause greater damage than do acids because they cause liquefactive necrosis that allows diffusion of the substance deeper into the tissues.[49] Children ingest liquid bleach (Clorox) more frequently than any other type of caustic substance; however, this is a mild irritant and typically causes less damage.[50] Symptoms of caustic ingestion include oral burns, pain, drooling, dysphagia, cough, and abdominal pain.[50] Associated burns to the larynx, stomach, or duodenum may also be present in severe cases. The mortality rate for severe and complicated burns is high. Metabolic acid-base disturbance, airway obstruction, mediastinitis, and peritonitis may also occur.[49]

Because correlation between the presence of oral and esophageal burns is poor, esophagoscopy is diagnostic and should be performed whenever esophageal burns are suspected.[51] This procedure allows direct visualization of areas of trauma and is helpful is assessing the extent of esophageal damage. Endoscopy should be performed in the first 48 hours because the risk of esophageal perforation is highest at 72 hours. Long-term complications of caustic burns may also cause chronic swallowing problems and include chronic esophagitis, motor dysfunction, and stricture formation.[52]

In severe burns, nasogastric intubation has been suggested to maintain adequate nutrition while maintaining patency during healing. Some clinicians suggest gastrostomy with endless-loop string or bougienage to allow proper esophageal healing.[49,53] Follow-up with frequent esophagoscopy may be necessary to evaluate effective healing and acquired stricture formation in early stages. Dilation using balloons or bougienage may reduce acquired strictures. Surgical repair with direct end-to-end anastamosis, gastric pull-up, or esophagogastric or esophagocolic anastamosis may be necessary with severe stricture formation.[49]

INFECTIOUS ETIOLOGIES

In cases of acute onset of odynophagia or dysphagia without a history of trauma, infectious causes are suspected. Infectious pharyngitis and laryngitis are common in children and may lead to inflammation, swelling, pain, drooling, and decreased oral intake when severe. These episodes also commonly include fever, cervical lymphadenopathy, and tonsillar exudate.[25] Respiratory viruses are the most common cause of pharyngitis; the most common offenders are rhinovirus and coronavirus. Adenovirus and herpes virus may also cause a painful pharyngitis — as can Epstein–Barr virus, the cause of infectious mononucleosis.

Similarly, other illnesses such as measles (paramyxo virus); hand, foot, and mouth disease (coxsackie virus); and influenza (influenza viral strains) may have prominent pharyngitis within their symptom complexes.[54] Bacterial infection is found in up to 30% of diagnosed pharyngitis; the most common organism is group A beta-hemolytic streptococcus. These bacteria are also commonly found in cases of peritonsillar and retropharyngeal abscesses. Other commonly found bacteria include *Staphylococcus aureus*, *Streptococcus pneumoniae*, *Haemophilus influenzae*, *Moraxella catarrhalis*, and Bacteroides.[54] Chlamydia and *Mycoplasma pneumoniae* are less common causes of pharyngitis.[55]

Complications of bacterial pharyngitis include cellulitis or abscess formation, and cervical lymphadenitis. Severe inflammation of the oropharynx may lead to trismus, as well as dysphagia and severe drooling. Asymmetric pharyngeal swelling in the face of fever, irritability, and dysphagia or drooling may suggest abscess. Common locations for abscess formation include the peritonsillar area and retropharyngeal space.[25] Radiographs of the neck or CT scanning may be helpful in diagnosing this problem. Fine-needle aspiration and intravenous antibiotics have been recommended as effective treatment by some authors; surgical incision and drainage coupled with antibiotic therapy remain the most effective form of therapy.

Corynebacterium diphtheriae and *Neisseria gonorrhoeae*, although uncommon, may also cause pharyngitis.[54] Diphtheria should be suspected in nonimmunized children living in crowded, polluted conditions. When severe, this disease presents as a tough, grayish membranous covering on the tonsils, pharynx, uvula, or soft palate. Treatment with toxoid should begin based on clinical suspicion, not on culture results. Penicillin and erythromycin are effective antibiotic therapy. Gonococcal pharyngitis may be present in sexually abused children or in sexually active adolescents. Symptoms may be mild to absent, so culture is necessary to confirm the diagnosis. The incidence of gonorrhea is increasing, and it should be considered in cases of atypical or prolonged cases of pharyngitis. Treatment with penicillin is indicated in culture-positive children.

Fungal infection may occur in the oral cavity and esophagus, causing a thrush-like condition or esophagitis. These infections are more common in neonates or in immunocompromised children, including those with acquired and congenital immunodeficiencies or on immunosuppressive therapy for malignancies or other medical conditions.[54] The most common fungal infection of the oral cavity is *Candida albicans*, but other less common fungal infections, such as histoplasmosis, blastomycosis, actinomycosis, or mucormycosis, may be found in immunocompromised children.[56] Nystatin, ketoconazole, amphotericin, or fluconazole are commonly used to treat oral thrush as well as esophagitis in children.

ADENOTONSILLAR HYPERPLASIA

Adenotonsillar hyperplasia is the most common cause of upper airway respiratory obstruction in children.[57] Dysphagia may also be commonly seen in association with adenotonsillar hyperplasia. Children may exhibit selective eating, with avoidance of meats or other coarse foods. Many children may have hyperplasia but go unnoticed because the symptoms have not been reviewed in the pediatrician's office. Also, although some children may develop hyperplasia after chronic or recurrent episodes of pharyngotonsillitis, some have no history of infection. It is important to recognize this correctable cause of upper airway obstruction in children since surgical removal of the hypertrophied lymphoid tissue influences breathing patterns, growth, and psychosocial development. Care must be taken to assess for cleft palate, especially undiagnosed submucous cleft, prior to surgery; adenoidectomy when these conditions are present may lead to nasopharyngeal insufficiency with nasal regurgitation during feeding.[58]

MYOPATHIES

Myopathies are infrequently seen in children; however, they may be a cause of childhood swallowing problems. Myopathy may manifest as symmetric proximal muscle weakness with abnormal EMG patterns and muscle biopsies in the absence of sensory symptoms. Although myopathies are often congenital, a variety of acquired disorders may also be seen in the pediatric population. Myotonic dysfunction, or failure of muscle relaxation after contraction, may also be present. Congenital dystrophies include myotonic dystrophy and oculopharyngeal dystrophy. Conditions such as dermatomyositis and polymyositis as well as myasthenia gravis are acquired. Dysthyroid is a recognized cause of muscle weakness that may also present with oropharyngeal complaints. Dysphagia may be intrinsic to any of these disease processes, and thus myogenic disorders must be considered in the differential diagnosis of swallowing disorders when no other obvious cause is present.

Myotonic dystrophy is an autosomal dominant disorder that presents with progressive dysphagia and dysphonia, as well as bilateral facial and palatal weakness.[59] Symptoms may vary widely, from minor impairment of swallowing function to complete paralysis that predisposes to aspiration. Myotonic dystrophy involves impaired movement of the pharynx and esophagus, disallowing normal propulsive effort in the pharyngeal and esophageal phases of swallowing. The esophagus may become dilated, further contributing to regurgitation and aspiration of oral contents into the larynx and trachea.

Acquired myopathies include myasthenia gravis, progressive bulbar paralysis, polymyositis, dermatomyositis, systemic lupus erythematosus, and dysthyroid disease. Myasthenia gravis may present with varying degrees of laryngeal weakness, dysphagia, or dysphonia. Affected people, especially younger patients, usually exhibit ptosis and/or diplopia as well.[59] Swallowing worsens as the patient tires. Patients with bulbar paralysis exhibit many of the same oral, pharyngeal, and laryngeal complaints as do those with myasthenia gravis, but dysfunction originates from disease of the medulla instead of at the receptor level and is often progressive. Myopathic symptoms of polymyositis, dermatomyositis, and systemic lupus erythematosis are often due to acute inflammatory changes within the muscle that may lead to degeneration and dysfunction, causing abnormalities of swallowing.

Swallowing dysfunction in these syndromes may include shallow pharyngeal contractions and retention of food within the pharyngeal recesses.[59] Dysthyroid disease is characterized by generalized weakness and reflex abnormalities with resultant dysphagia. Quantitative thyroid hormone levels may help with diagnosis of dysphagia of thyroid origin.

FUNCTIONAL DISORDERS

Functional disorders of the esophagus are uncommon in children. Esophageal dysphagia may stem from a generalized motility dysfunction of the esophageal musculature, or from relaxation and coordination problems of the cricopharyngeus muscle or the lower esophageal sphincter.[59] Symptoms of dysphagia include problems with solids more than with liquids, feelings of food "sticking" in the throat, and the need to drink liquids to advance the bolus through the esophagus. When these symptoms occur, achalasia, esophageal spasm, and scleroderma should be ruled out.

Achalasia is usually diagnosed after the third decade, but cases have been reported in the pediatric population. This disorder is marked by esophageal dilation with symptoms of obstruction, frequently for liquids as well as solids. Decreased and uncoordinated esophageal muscle contractions are found on manometry studies. Esophageal spasm usually occurs in the older population and displays simultaneous and repetitive large amplitude contractions on manometry.[59] Spasm is usually accompanied by pain with swallowing. Esophageal dyssynergia occurs with failure of lower esophageal sphincter relaxation. Esophageal enlargement with regurgitant symptoms frequently occurs.

Scleroderma is a systemic disorder affecting blood vessels and connective tissues. There is fibrous degeneration of connective tissue with initial complaints usually stemming from tightness of the skin on the face and fingers. Eating becomes difficult because lip motion is decreased due to fibrosis. In scleroderma with concurrent Raynaud's, esophageal involvement seems to be more prevalent. In scleroderma, the smooth muscle of the esophagus is destroyed, while peristalsis is maintained in the striated muscle.[59] This causes difficulty in swallowing and clearing oral secretions. Along with concurrent gastroesophageal reflux from more extensive digestive system involvement, dysphagia in scleroderma can be severe.

TREATMENT

In children, the goal in treatment of feeding disorders should focus on recognition of treatable anatomic or inflammatory lesions. The specifics of these treatments have been described throughout this chapter. A child may still refuse to eat even after an underlying abnormality is corrected. Behavior therapy can address this learned aversion to eating with various therapeutic approaches.[60] Decisions regarding whether to allow oral feeding depend on balancing the risks for aspiration and lung disease with the emotional rewards and convenience of oral feeding. The amount of aspiration that is safe depends on the child's ability to clear secretions. Supplying nutritional needs by nasogastric or gastrostomy feeding may be necessary when aspiration is significant or when nutritional needs cannot be met by oral intake. Periodic evaluation of the child's medical status and overall development can help direct feeding recommendations. Families may need counseling to cope with these issues and a multidisciplinary team can help direct the child's care. Even if full oral feeding cannot be achieved, providing oral stimulation may help with later introduction of oral feeding and may help prevent oral aversion.

CONCLUSIONS

The causes of dysphagia in the pediatric population are myriad. The neonate, who is an obligate nasal breather, may have congenital or acquired disorders of the nasal cavity resulting in feeding abnormalities. In the infant, gastroesophageal reflux, infectious causes of dysphagia, and congenital abnormalities must be completely evaluated. From 1 year of age on, the most common cause for dysphagia is infections. The risk of foreign body and caustic ingestion must be evaluated in cases of unexplained or persistent dysphagia. The anatomic and physiologic differences between children and adults necessitate a thorough evaluation with an age-specific differential diagnosis in mind.

REFERENCES

1. Hawdon, J.M. et al. Identification of neonates at risk of developing feeding problems in infancy. *Dev. Med. Child Neurol.*, 2000, 42, 235–239.
2. Mackay, L.E., Morgan, A.S., and Bernstein, B.A. Swallowing disorders in severe brain injury: risk factors affecting return to oral intake. *Arch. Phys. Med. Rehabil.*, 1999, 80, 365–371.
3. Sullivan, P.B., Reilly, S., and Skuse, D. Characteristics and management of feeding problems of young children with cerebral palsy. *Dev. Med. Child Neurol.*, 1996, 34, 379–388.
4. Miller, A.J. Neurological basis of swallowing. *Dysphagia*, 1986, 1, 91–100.
5. Arvedson, J.C., Rogers, B., and Brodsky, L. Anatomy, embryology, and physiology. In Arvedson, J.C. and Brodsky, L., Eds. *Pediatric Swallowing and Feeding: Assessment and Management.* San Diego: Singular Publishing Group, Inc., 1993. 5–51.
6. DiScipio, W., Kaslon, K., and Ruben, R. Traumatically acquired conditioned dysphagia in children. *Ann. Otol. Rhinol. Laryngol.*, 1978, 87, 509–514.
7. Derkay, C.S. and Schechter, G.L. Anatomy and physiology of pediatric swallowing disorders. *Otolaryngol. Clin. North Am.*, 1998, 31(3), 397–404.
8. Schechter, G.L. and Derkay, C.S. Physiology of the mouth, pharynx, and esophagus. In Bluestone, C.D., Stool, S.E., and Kenna, M.A., Eds. *Pediatric Otolaryngology*, Vol. 2, 3rd ed. Philadelphia: W.B. Saunders Company, 1996. 939–944.
9. Potsic, W.P., Handler, S.D., and Tom, L.W. Methods of Examination. In Bluestone, C.D., Stool, S.E., and Kenna, M.A., Eds. *Pediatric Otolaryngology*, Vol. 2, 3rd ed. Philadelphia: W.B. Saunders Company, 1996. 945–957.
10. Tsou, V.M. and Bishop, P.R. Gastroesophageal reflux in children. *Otolaryngol. Clin. North Am.*, 1998, 31(3), 419–434.
11. Link, D.T. et al. Pediatric laryngopharyngeal sensory testing during flexible endoscopic evaluation of swallowing: feasible and correlative. *Ann. Otol. Rhinol. Laryngol.*, 2000, 109(10 Pt. 1), 899–905.
12. Logemann, J.A. Anatomy and physiology of normal deglutition. In Logemann, J.A. *Evaluation and Treatment of Swallowing Disorders.* San Diego: College-Hill Press, Inc., 1983. 9–31.
13. Arvedson, J.C. Dysphagia in pediatric patients with neurologic damage. *Semin. Neurol.*, 1996, 16(4), 371–386.
14. Lusk, R.P. Choanal atresia. In Healy, G.B., Ed. *Common Problems in Pediatric Otolaryngology.* Chicago: Year Book Medical Publishers, Inc., 1990. 171–177.
15. Myer, C.M., III and Cotton, R.T. Nasal obstruction. In Myer, C.M., III and Cotton, R.T. *A Practical Approach to Pediatric Otolaryngology.* Chicago: Year Book Medical Publishers, Inc., 1988. 84–104.
16. Brodsky, L. and Volk, M. The airway and swallowing. In Arvedson, J.C. and Brodsky, L., Eds. *Pediatric Swallowing and Feeding: Assessment and Management.* San Diego: Singular Publishing Group, Inc., 1993. 93–122.
17. Fraser, F.C., The branchial arch syndromes and cleft lip and cleft palate. In Avery, M.E. and Taeusch, H.W., Eds. *Schaffer's Diseases of the Newborn.* Philadelphia: W.B. Saunders Company, 1984. 816–819.
18. Menkes, J.H. Malformations of the central nervous system. In Avery, M.E. and Taeusch, H.W., Eds. *Schaffer's Diseases of the Newborn.* Philadelphia: W.B. Saunders Company, 1984. 680–702.
19. Anderson, K.N., Anderson, L.E., and Glanze, W.D. *Mosby's Medical Dictionary*, 4th ed. St. Louis: Mosby, 1994. 344–346.
20. Gray, S.D. and Parkin, J.L. Congenital malformations of the mouth and pharynx. In Bluestone, C.D., Stool, S.E., and Kenna, M.A., Eds. *Pediatric Otolaryngology*, Vol. 2, 3rd ed. Philadelphia: W.B. Saunders Company, 1996. 985–998.
21. Paradise, J.L. Primary care of infants and children with cleft palate. In Bluestone, C.D., Stool, S.E., and Kenna, M.A., Eds. *Pediatric Otolaryngology*, Vol. 2, 3rd ed. Philadelphia: W.B. Saunders Company, 1996. 999–1005.

22. Williams, D.J. and Mitchell, D.P. Pharyngoesophageal dysphagia in infancy. *Int. J. Pediatri. Otorhinolaryngol.*, 1980, 2, 231–242.

23. Avery, M.E. and Taeusch, H.W. Stridors in the newborn. In Avery, M.E. and Taeusch, H.W., Eds. *Schaffer's Diseases of the Newborn*. Philadelphia: W.B. Saunders Company, 1984. 122–128.

24. Willging, J.P. and Cotton, R.T. Subglottic stenosis in the pediatric patient. In Myer, C.M., III, Cotton, R.T, and Shott, S.R., Eds. *The Pediatric Airway: An Interdisciplinary Approach*. Philadelphia: J.B. Lippincott Company, 1995. 111–132.

25. Kosko, J.R., Moser, J.D., Erhart, N., and Tunkel, D.E. Differential diagnosis of dysphagia in children. *Otolaryngol. Clin. North Am.*, 1998, 31(3), 435–451.

26. Myer, C.M., III and Cotton, R.T. Airway obstruction. In Myer, C.M., III and Cotton, R.T. *A Practical Approach to Pediatric Otolaryngology*. Chicago: Year Book Medical Publishers, Inc., 1988. 169–205.

27. Morrow, S.E. and Nakayama, D.K. Congenital malformations of the esophagus. In Bluestone, C.D., Stool, S.E., and Kenna, M.A., Eds. *Pediatric Otolaryngology*, Vol. 2, 3rd ed. Philadelphia: W.B. Saunders Company, 1996. 1121–1130.

28. Holder, T.M. and Aschcraft, K.W. Esophageal atresia and tracheoesophageal fistula. *Curr. Probl. Surg.*, 1966, Aug., 1–68.

29. Templeton, J.M., Templeton, J.J., Scnaufer, L., Bishop, H.C., Ziegler, M.M., and Oneill, J.A., Jr. Management of esophageal atresia and tracheoesophageal fistula in the neonate with severe respiratory distress syndrome. *J. Pediatr. Surg.* 1985, 20(4), 394–397.

30. Cohen, M.M. Genetics, syndromology, and craniofacial anomalies. In Bluestone, C.D., Stool, S.E., and Kenna, M.A., Eds. *Pediatric Otolaryngology*, Vol. 2, 3rd ed. Philadelphia: W.B. Saunders Company, 1996. 33–61.

31. Rogers, B. and Campbell, J. Pediatric and neurodevelopmental evaluation. In Arvedson J.C. and Brodsky, L., Eds. *Pediatric Swallowing and Feeding: Assessment and Management*. San Diego: Singular Publishing Group, Inc., 1993. 53–91.

32. Christensen, J.R. Developmental approach to pediatric neurogenic dysphagia. *Dysphagia*, 1989, 3, 131–134.

33. Logemann, J.A. Swallowing disorders/neuromuscular disorders. In Logemann, J.A. *Evaluation and Treatment of Swallowing Disorders*. San Diego: College-Hill Press, Inc., 1983. 216–217.

34. Limbrock, G.J., Hoyer, H., and Scheying, H. Drooling, chewing and swallowing dysfunctions in children with cerebral palsy: treatment according to Castillo–Morales. *J. Dentistry Children*, 1990, 57(6), 445–451.

35. Rossi, T. Pediatric gastroenterology. In Arvedson, J.C. and Brodsky, L., Eds. *Pediatric Swallowing and Feeding: Assessment and Management*. San Diego: Singular Publishing Group, Inc., 1993. 123–156.

36. Tsou, V.M. and Bishop, P.R. Gastroesophageal reflux in children. *Otolaryngol. Clin. North Am.*, 1998, 31(3), 419–434.

37. Byrne, W.J., Kangarloo, H., Ament, M.E., Lo, C.W., Berquist, W., Foglia, R., and Fonkalsrud, E.W. Antral dysmotility: an unrecognized cause of chronic vomiting during infancy. *Ann. Surg.*, 1981, 193(4), 521–524.

38. Boix–Ochoa, J. and Canals, J. Maturation of the lower esophagus. *J. Pediatr. Surg.*, 1976, 11, 749–756.

39. Taminiau, J. Gastro-oesophageal reflux in children. *Scand. J. Gastroenterol.*, 1997, 32(Suppl. 223), 18–20.

40. Marino, A.J., Assing, E., Carbone, M.T., Hiatt, I.M., Hegyi, T., and Graff, M. The incidence of gastroesophageal reflux in preterm infants. *J. Perinatol.*, 1995, 15(5), 369–371.

41. Groben, P.A., Siegal, G.P., Shub, M.D., Ulshen, M.H., and Askin, F.B. Gastroesophageal reflux and esophagitis in infants and children. *Perspect. Pediatr. Pathol.*, 1987, 11, 124–151.

42. Andrews, T.M., Myer, C.M., III, Bailey, W.W., and Vester, S.R. Intrathoracic lesions involving the tracheobronchial tree. In Myer, C.M., III, Ed. *The Pediatric Airway*. Philadelphia: J.B. Lippincott Company, 1995. 223–245.

43. Gonzalez, C. Tumors of the mouth and pharynx. In Bluestone, C.D., Stool, S.E., and Kenna, M.A., Eds. *Pediatric Otolaryngology*, Vol. 2, 3rd ed. Philadelphia: W.B. Saunders Company, 1996. 1108–1119.

44. Ferlito, A., Rinaldo, A., and Marioni, G. Laryngeal malignant neoplasms in children and adolescents. *Int. J. Pediatr. Otorhinolaryngol.*, 1999, 49, 1–14.

45. Donaldson, S.S., Castro, J.R., Wilbur, J.R., and Jesse, R.H., Jr. Rhabdomyosarcoma of the head and neck in children: combination treatment by surgery, irradiation, and chemotherapy. *Cancer*, 1973, 31(1), 26–35.

46. Gibson, S.E. and Shott, S.R. Foreign bodies of the upper aerodigestive tract. In Myer, C.M., III, Ed. *The Pediatric Airway*. Philadelphia: J.B. Lippincott Company, 1995. 195–222.

47. Stool, S.E. and Manning, S.C. Foreign bodies of the pharynx and esophagus. In Bluestone, C.D., Stool, S.E., and Kenna, M.A., Eds. *Pediatric Otolaryngology*, Vol. 2, 3rd ed. Philadelphia: W.B. Saunders Company, 1996. 1169–1180.

48. Donat, T.L., Maisel, R.H., and Mathog, R.H. Injuries of the mouth, pharynx, and esophagus. In Bluestone, C.D., Stool, S.E., and Kenna, M.A., Eds. *Pediatric Otolaryngology*, Vol. 2, 3rd ed. Philadelphia: W.B. Saunders Company, 1996. 1181–1191.

49. Riding, K.H. and Bluestone, C.D. Burns and acquired strictures of the esophagus. In Bluestone, C.D., Stool, S.E., and Kenna, M.A., Eds. *Pediatric Otolaryngology*, Vol. 2, 3rd ed. Philadelphia: W.B. Saunders Company, 1996. 1157–1168.

50. Harley, E.H. and Collins, M.D. Liquid household bleach ingestion in children: a retrospective review. *Laryngoscope*, 1997, 107, 100–125.

51. Cardona, J.C. and Daly, J.F. Current management of corrosive esophagitis. *Ann. Otol., Rhinol., Laryngol.*, 1971, 80(4), 521–527.

52. Bautista, A., Varela, R., Villanueva, A., Estevez, E., Tojo, R., and Cadranel, S. Motor function of the esophagus after caustic burn. *Eur. J. Pediatri. Surg.*, 1996, 6(4), 204–207.

53. Okada, T., Ohnuma, N., Tanabe, M., Iwai, J., Yoshida, H., Kuroda, H., and Takahashi, H. Effective endless-loop bougienage through the oral cavity and esophagus to the gastrostomy in corrosive esophageal strictures in children. *Pediatr. Surg. Int.*, 1998, 13(7), 480–486.

54. Kenna, M. Sore throat in children: diagnosis and management. In Bluestone, C.D., Stool, S.E., and Kenna, M.A., Eds. *Pediatric Otolaryngology*, Vol. 2, 3rd ed. Philadelphia: W.B. Saunders Company, 1996. 958–964.

55. McMillan, J.A., Sandstrom, C., Weiner, L.B., Forbes, B.A., Woods, M., Howard, T., Poe, L., Keller, K., Corwin, R.M., and Winkelman, J.W. Viral and bacterial organisms associated with acute pharyngitis in a school-aged population. *J. Pediatr.*, 1986, 109(5), 747–752.

56. Derkay, C.S. and Schechter, G.L. Dysphagia. In Bluestone, C.D., Stool, S.E., and Kenna, M.A., Eds. *Pediatric Otolaryngology*, Vol. 2, 3rd ed. Philadelphia: W.B. Saunders Company, 1996. 965–973.

57. Maddern, B.R. Obstructive sleep disorders. In Bluestone, C.D., Stool, S.E., and Kenna, M.A., Eds. *Pediatric Otolaryngology*, Vol. 2, 3rd ed. Philadelphia: W.B. Saunders Company, 1996. 1067–1076.

58. Paradise, J.L. Tonsillectomy and adenoidectomy. In Bluestone, C.D., Stool, S.E., and Kenna, M.A., Eds. *Pediatric Otolaryngology*, Vol. 2, 3rd ed. Philadelphia: W.B. Saunders Company, 1996. 1054–1065.

59. Morrell, R.M. Neurologic disorders of swallowing. In Groher, M.E., Ed. *Dysphagia: Diagnosis and Management*. Boston: Butterworths, 1984. 37–59.

60. Khoshoo, V. et al. Benefits of thickened feeds in previously healthy infants with respiratory syncytial viral bronchiolitis. *Pediatr. Pulmonol.* 2001, 31, 301–302.

19 Gastroesophageal Reflux

William F. McGuirt, Jr. and Andrew J. Hotaling

Gentlemen, this is surely true, it is absolutely paradoxical; we cannot understand it, and we don't know what it means, but we have proved it, and therefore, we know it must be the truth.

Benjamin Peirce, Harvard mathematician

CONTENTS

INTRODUCTION

Pediatric extraesophageal reflux (EER) has gained increasing recognition over the past few years; it has been identified as a common pediatric disorder with symptoms ranging from benign postprandial vomiting in the first year of life to failure to thrive, esophagitis, and airway manifestations. Vandenplas and Sacre-Smith reported an estimated incidence of reflux in 18% of all infants.[1] In coexisting medical conditions such as tracheoesophageal fistula, neurologic impairment, or oral motor dysphagia, the incidence approaches 70% in some studies.[2,3] As early as 1884, William Osler postulated a direct effect of gastroesophageal reflux (GERD) on asthmatic patients.[4] In 1962, Kennedy described a close association between GERD and respiratory disease with only presentations related to respiratory pathophysiology.[5] The potential relationship of life-threatening airway complications associated with GERD was suggested by Koufman, in 1993, when he noted that "GER-related, life-threatening airway complications are higher in children; conversely, children rarely complain of heartburn and regurgitation."[6] It should not be surprising that no consensus exists in this area, yet in fact, even the nomenclature is confusing and contradictory.

CLASSIFICATION OF REFLUX

GERD in the child is generally defined in four categories:

- Physiologic reflux refers to infrequent emesis in children without any abnormalities on diagnostic studies. It is usually asymptomatic, rarely occurs during sleep, and is frequently in the upright position postprandially.[7]
- Functional GER is defined as silent or asymptomatic reflux and can be confirmed by intraesophageal pH monitoring.
- Pathologic GER is a more severe form of functional GER that can interfere with normal growth processes and cause complications of the gastrointestinal and/or respiratory tract. It can be quantitated diagnostically and/or pathologically.
- Secondary gastroesophageal disease is related to a secondary disorder such as neurologic deficits or anatomic abnormalities of the esophagus.[8]

A number of terms have been used to describe reflux in otolaryngology patients. These include laryngopharyngeal reflux (LPR), extraesophageal reflux (EER), chronic laryngitis, supraesophageal complications of gastroesophageal reflux, and gastroesophageal reflux disease (GERD). Because symptoms, physical findings, pathophysiology, and response to treatment of patients with otolaryngological complaints of reflux differ from those of patients with gastroesophageal reflux (GER), we do not believe that the use of GER or GERD to describe our patients is appropriate. We prefer LPR or EER and will use "extraesophageal reflux" in this chapter.

A clear difference in understanding the natural history of reflux in children is important in order to distinguish the manifestations and management of EER. This, in turn, is important to avoid unnecessary treatment, as well as to address unique concerns in the pediatric patient. In the majority of children, EER is usually a self-limited disease and children improve by the end of the first year of life when they begin a solid diet. Most symptomatic children require limited positional treatment. Almost all newborns during diagnostic testing with esophageal pH probes can be shown to have brief postprandial episodes of reflux.[9–11] However, children with persistent EER after the age of 3 are noted to have a higher rate of related complications and frequently require medical and surgical intervention.[12] Identification and treatment of these high-risk children may avoid delayed morbidity and mortality.

The infant is predisposed to GERD/EER due to a short intra-abdominal esophagus and an immature lower esophageal sphincter (LES). At the present time, there is still a disagreement in the literature concerning the role of gastric emptying in children with GERD/EER. However, gastric distention has been shown to trigger transient LES relaxations (TLESRs) with reflux.[13] Pediatric studies document that the majority of reflux episodes in children are caused by TLESRs and an otherwise normal LES.[1,14] These TLESRs appear to occur more frequently in the presence of esophagitis or in a postprandial state and may be triggered by vagal pathways, gastric distention, or respiration.[15,16] In addition, children are prone to excessive exposure of esophageal acid at night because they swallow less often while sleeping. Children with diagnosed esophagitis swallow less than children without GERD and have decreased response to reflux events, resulting in decreased esophageal acid clearance.[16] Traditional thinking also has blamed EER on abnormally low upper-esophageal pressure; however, recent investigation in children has failed to confirm this finding.[17]

MANIFESTATIONS

During the past decade, reports of EER's effects on the pharynx, larynx, and tracheobronchial tree have appeared more frequently. In the 1970s, Fearon and Brama recognized reflux as a cause of various upper respiratory symptoms in children.[18] Subsequently, additional authors have reported respiratory complications of reflux, including recurrent bronchitis, croup, and pneumonia, as well as chronic asthma.[19–25] Reflux has also been reported to be associated with, to complicate, or possibly to cause contact ulcers and granuloma.[26,27] Some of the reports of reflux and airway complications are anecdotal, but others represent a large number of patients followed over time. Virtually all of the studies have methodologic faults in their controls, selection of patients, or diagnosis of reflux disease.

Despite these limitations, patients with EER appear to complain of numerous symptoms leading them to an otolaryngologist in contrast to patients with GERD. Although many of these reports suggest an association between reflux and the development of these conditions, it remains difficult to demonstrate clinically a direct causal role due to the limitations of diagnosis and clarity of treatment modalities. The effect of EER in the pediatric airway is mediated through three mechanisms, which include (1) stimulation of the laryngeal protective reflex, (2) microaspiration with chemical pneumonitis, and (3) stimulation of esophageal receptor reflex responsible for causing bronchial constriction.

CHRONIC COUGH OR ASTHMA

A subset of infants and children with asthma or chronic cough refractory to standard medical therapy has been found to have EER.[19–21,28,29] Coughing can also lead to an increase in the intra-abdominal pressure that may promote EER, which in turns leads to more coughing. Unfortunately, many chronic cough and asthma patients have other coexisting medical problems that may complicate the diagnosis and management of reflux. In 1991, Andze et al. reported that 76% of 131 children with severe asthmatic disease had moderate to severe GERD by single-probe intraesophageal monitoring. Of those, 69% had a clinical improvement with medical therapy alone, while 88% had good to excellent results following surgical therapy.[28] Only a limited number of investigators and clinicians have measured the extent of pharyngeal reflux in children with respiratory disease.[30,31] Excluding infectious causes, EER is the third most common cause of chronic cough in pediatric patients overall and is the most common cause in the 0- to 18-month age group.[32]

HOARSENESS

The child with reflux laryngitis may present with dysphonia, chronic cough, globus sensation, or a wet sounding voice or cough.[33,34] Aggressive treatment of children with EER can avoid laryngeal sequelae. Direct reflux treatment related to dysphonia is mostly anecdotal, with no significant controlled trials of treatment and outcomes. In 1998, Gumpert et al. reported on 21 children with hoarseness; pH probes were found to be abnormal in two thirds of patients with posterior laryngitis. Although outcome results were not reported,[35] anecdotal evidence would suggest that treatment for reflux for these symptoms may result in improvement of patients' complaints.[36] Burton et al.[21] and Walner and Hollinger[37] have reported an association between GERD and supraglottic stenosis and granulomas.

LARYNGOMALACIA

Adherent to most respiratory diseases is increased respiratory effort, which leads to greater negative intrathoracic pressure and the possibility of EER because of this differential pressure. Variations in intrathoracic and intra-abdominal pressures have been shown to have an effect on reflux.[34] This may be very significant in patients with laryngomalacia. The association of EER with laryngomalacia has been well documented.[22,23] Also, anecdotal evidence is strong that the treatment of laryngomalacia patients with symptoms of failure to thrive or with apnea and bradycardia spells can be improved with aggressive reflux management. Children considered for supraglottoplasty should always have their reflux addressed and corrected prior to any surgical intervention.

In 1993, the first direct cause-and-effect relationship of stridor and GER was documented by Orenstein et al.[36] Contencin and Narcy were able to predict the presence of EER in children with stridor with a specificity of 83% and sensitivity of 100%, using a two-channel pH probe when the pharyngeal pH remained less than 6 for more than 1% of the study time.[31] This study has also been supported by work from Little et al.[30]

SUBGLOTTIC STENOSIS

The damaging effects of gastric acid on the larynx, leading to ulceration and granulation formation, and on the subglottic airway, causing subglottic stenosis, have been clearly demonstrated in animal models.[27,38] In the face of injury, reflux increases the risk of stenosis in animal models and is assumed to account for a significant number of patients failing laryngotracheal reconstruction. Antireflux therapy has been recommended and traditionally offered for all patients undergoing open laryngotracheal reconstruction.[39,40] Halstead has also suggested that antireflux therapy may increase the success of endoscopic repair of subglottic stenosis.[41] However, in 1996, Zalzal et al. reported their data on laryngotracheal reconstruction with regard to reflux management; they found no direct correlation between reflux treatment and outcome.[42] These studies are limited by an apparent lack of prospective control. This limitation is being addressed at the University of Cincinnati, where a prospective study of reflux control on laryngotracheal reconstruction results is currently underway.

APNEA/SUDDEN INFANT DEATH SYNDROME/APPARENT LIFE-THREATENING EVENT

The evaluation of a child in whom an apparent life-threatening event (ALTE) or apneic event is suspected starts with an exclusion of direct anatomic laryngeal or tracheal anomalies. Apnea may also arise from esophageal or laryngotracheal reflux events, which can occur from the presence of direct aspiration, altered gas exchange, or stimulation of the laryngeal chemoreceptor reflex.[43] Apnea can be a significant problem in preterm infants, and apnea frequency related to reflux events apparently increases 14-fold.[44] The chemoreceptor reflex is felt to be the cause of this; some evidence shows that arousal stimulation of the apnea may not occur in the presence of hypoxia resulting in airway obstruction.[45] This was noted by direct distal esophageal acid profusion in eight infants with resultant bradycardia and apnea.[46]

The reported incidence of pH probe-documented reflux in children evaluated for ALTE varies greatly (42 to 95%), depending on the series.[47,48] The incidences of reflux and sleep-related reflux is greater than any of the controls in each of these reports. Although a direct cause has not been illustrated between a reflux event and an ALTE, it is strongly recommended that any child presenting after an acute life-threatening event be evaluated for reflux.

In an animal model, Wetmore has demonstrated that laryngeal installation of acid causes obstructive apnea secondary to laryngospasm.[49] Duke et al. also confirmed these data in an immature canine model with evidence showing a probable vagal response from a chemoceptor that induced laryngospasm and arrest of diaphragmatic function in immature canine larynges.[50] Jolly et al. followed 499 children with reflux for 1 year and reported a 9.1% incidence of sudden infant death syndrome (SIDS) with a type I reflux pattern (a pH probe that demonstrates a high frequency of reflux episodes). In the group who underwent antireflux surgery, compared with those medically treated, no deaths were reported.[51]

OTHER CONSIDERATIONS

Relationships with EER and otitis media and sinusitis are under investigation, but anecdotal reports suggest that, occasionally, this may be a pathologic event leading to active disease in some patients.[52,53] At Wake Forest University, a small group of patients with otitis media have had pepsin identified in their middle ear fluid.

DIAGNOSIS

A complete history and physical should be undertaken, including an evaluation of the growth curve. Special attention should be paid to the child's birth and perinatal history, feeding, airway, and reflux history. Ornstein et al. has developed a 161-item questionnaire to aid in this task.[54] The presentation of EER may be atypical and a subset of children with reflux exists whose only presenting symptoms may be airway related. The history should also focus on the frequency of emesis or regurgitation, temporal relation to meals, associated respiratory symptoms, laryngeal associated neurologic disorders, and weight gain. Signs of neurologic impairment and of laryngeal inflammation or lesions can be detected by flexible fiberoptic nasopharyngoscopy.

The laryngeal examination may reveal a variety of findings. The most sought-after finding is that of laryngeal erythema or redness. In adults, attempts have even been made to quantify the degree of redness and its response to treatment.[55] Some authors refer to posterior laryngitis — swollen arytenoid mucosa with interarytenoid mucosal hypertrophy or edema.[56,57] Still others believe that infraglottic edema, as well as vocal fold and false vocal fold edema, is the hallmark of laryngopharyngeal acid exposure.[58,59] Few would doubt the probability of EER in individuals with chronic polypoid changes of the vocal folds or a diffusely swollen larynx with a granuloma. It is our belief that a broad spectrum of changes may occur and various findings can be seen in different individuals. Definitive laryngoscopy and bronchoscopy may be recommended to rule out lesions such as laryngotracheal esophageal cleft, foreign body, infection, or subglottic stenosis.

It should be apparent that GERD and EER are quite different. Several studies in adults have shown that GER and EER patients present with different symptoms.[57,60-65] Specifically, these show a low incidence of heartburn, indigestion, and regurgitation and a high incidence of hoarseness, globus, excessive throat clearing, chronic cough, exacerbations of reactive airway disease, and other otolaryngic complaints in EER patients. Heartburn is a symptom of esophagitis, and most EER patients do not have esophagitis. Wiener et al.[66] studied 32 EER adults with hoarseness and found that although pH-metry was abnormal in 78%, esophageal manometry was normal in 100% and esophagoscopy with biopsy was normal in 72%. Koufman found that only 18% (23/128) of EER adults had any findings of esophagitis on barium esophagography.[60]

The difference in incidence of esophagitis between EER and GER patients underscores the fact that the mechanisms of EER and GER differ significantly. EER and GER are caused by mucosal injury from acid and pepsin exposure. The esophagus has certain protective mechanisms that prevent mucosal injury (bicarbonate production, mucosal barrier, and volume clearance by peristalsis), but the pharynx and larynx do not.[60] Therefore, it takes much less acid/pepsin exposure to cause tissue damage in the pharynx and larynx than in the esophagus.[61] Thus, even if a patient does not have enough reflux to develop esophagitis (and its principal symptom, heartburn), he or she still may develop symptomatic EER. Examination of the esophagus for related pathology in adults with EER is commonly performed.[60,67] Whether all individuals with EER require esophagoscopy or radiologic imaging is not certain. A prospective trial of pediatric patients with airway complications is currently under way at the University of Cincinnati to address the utility of esophagoscopy with mucosal biopsies.

Although many diagnostic options are available, few are considered critical in the evaluation of EER. The sensitivity and specificity of a symptom-based diagnosis alone are low.[68] The sensitivity and specificity of common diagnostic tests in children are improved when the diagnosis is confirmed on two separate tests.[69]

BARIUM ESOPHAGRAM AND RADIONUCLEOTIDE REFLUX SCAN

Barium esophagram has the advantage of demonstrating anatomic abnormalities, such as esophageal stricture, hiatal hernia, gastric outlet obstruction, and gastrointestinal malrotation. It is recommended before the institution of any prokinetic agents or surgical consideration and should be considered in any child with significantly symptomatic EER. However, barium esophagram has limited sensitivity (20 to 60%) and specificity (64 to 90%).[34] The esophageal radionucleotide reflux scan may be beneficial in identifying reflux in the postprandial child, especially if it is of a higher pH that will not be identified on a pH probe. Scintiscan can also quantify the rate of gastric emptying. Looking at delayed imaging in a scintiscan may be advantageous for detection of patients with pulmonary aspiration.[70]

ESOPHAGOGASTRODUODENOSCOPY WITH BIOPSY

Esophagoscopy with biopsy allows for direct visualization of the mucosal lining; biopsy may show evidence of mucosal irritation, Barrett's metaplasia, or esophagitis. Direct examination of the larynx also allows for detection of increased supraglottic vascularity, laryngeal or subglottic edema, interarytenoid pachyemia, and small lymphoid aggregates in the wall of the trachea — all of which are suggestive of reflux disease. A bronchoalveolar lavage can also be taken during bronchoscopy. The presence of lipid-laden macrophages has approximately 85% sensitivity for GERD according to Nussbaum.[71] Lipid-laden macrophage score is quantitated after examining 100 macrophages on a bronchoalveolar lavage and a score greater than 70 is consistent with aspiration.

pH MONITORING STUDY

A great deal of work in adults has demonstrated that EER is best diagnosed by prolonged ambulatory double-probe pH monitoring. Barium esophagography, radionuclide scanning, the Bernstein acid-perfusion test, and esophagoscopy with biopsy are often negative in adults with EER.[61] This is probably because most EER adult patients do not develop the esophagitis typically observed in gastroenterology patients with GERD.[60,66] Although ambulatory 24-hour double-probe pH monitoring is considered the "gold standard" for reflux testing, in otolaryngology practice, there is no consensus concerning the number of sensors, their location, or the interpretation of the results.[72]

NEED FOR THE PHARYNGEAL SENSOR

Double-probe (simultaneous pharyngeal and esophageal sensor) pH monitoring is superior to diagnostic modalities such as barium swallow, endoscopy, and single-probe esophageal pH testing because it is highly sensitive as well as specific.[60,66,73–75] When the pharyngeal probe is positive, using appropriate criteria, it is diagnostic of EER. The importance of the pharyngeal sensor cannot be overestimated. Katz[76] showed in a small number of adults that relying solely on an esophageal probe would yield a number of falsely negative results regarding EER.

A recent review of pH-metry data at Wake Forest University demonstrated that 38% (126/334) of a consecutive series of adults with documented EER had normal upright, supine, and total esophageal acid exposure times in their esophagus; i.e., they had physiologic esophageal reflux. Therefore, in a highly select group of patients with otolaryngologic complaints, 38% of the patients would have been inappropriately assumed *not* to have EER if the pharyngeal sensor was not employed.[77] Similarly, in the pediatric population, Little et al.[30] have shown that the pharyngeal probe is important, demonstrating that 46% (78/168) of children with documented EER had normal esophageal acid exposure times. It is clear that measuring esophageal acid exposure does not allow one to make any assumptions concerning the presence or absence of EER.

It has been demonstrated that proximal esophageal reflux in normal patients is uncommon; its direct relationship to EER remains uncertain.[78–80] For example, measuring gastric pH and using it to extrapolate results regarding GER is a clearly invalid exercise. In a similar manner, using esophageal pH testing at any proximal location to prove the presence or absence of EER is questionable because the upper esophageal sphincter (UES) functions as the final barrier limiting EER. In addition, acid instillation into the esophagus increases the UES resting pressure, therefore enhancing its effectiveness as a barrier to EER.[81] Additional studies using two or three esophageal sensors with a pharyngeal sensor will be needed to evaluate this controversy further.

DEFINITION OF REFLUX EVENT

Early ambulatory pH-metry studies using a pharyngeal probe were occasionally flawed by the occurrence of "pseudoreflux" events.[60,82–85] This was believed to be due to placing the pharyngeal sensor high in the hypopharynx, thus allowing major changes in the impedance of the circuit depending on whether the sensor had dried or was in direct contact with the mucosa. This problem is now uncommon due to improved sensors, probe placement just above the UES, and using rigid criteria to define pharyngeal reflux episodes:

- pH drop < 4
- Pharyngeal pH drop during or immediately following distal esophageal acid exposure
- pH drop not occurring during eating or swallowing
- Rapid and sharp proximal sensor pH drop — not gradual

Applying these criteria and ensuring proper probe placement will result in few episodes of pseudoreflux.

Work regarding the function and stability of human pepsin shows it to be active at a pH of 5. Although controversial, using this pH level as a defining point for EER may be valid.[78,85] Using a pH of 5 as indicative of reflux in the proximal esophagus may also be valid because proximal acid exposure times are short and the dilutional and neutralizing factors present in saliva are greater at this level.[78]

WHAT IS NORMAL ACID EXPOSURE IN THE PHARYNX?

The natures of the larynx, pharynx, and upper airway make them highly susceptible to acid-induced injury. In contrast to the esophagus, the laryngopharynx does not have effective defense mechanisms to resist acid- and peptic-induced injury once the UES is breached.[65] It is clear that, in the setting of laryngeal or subglottic injury, a single EER event has great clinical significance. However, is occasional EER in an asymptomatic individual abnormal?

Due to work by Little et al. in the injured canine subglottis[38] and that of Delahunty,[27] it has been assumed that any extraesophageal acid contact was pathologic in nature. Testing 20 asymptomatic adult controls, Koufman also demonstrated no evidence of EER.[60] Eubanks et al. studied 10 healthy adult controls and found only a single episode of extraesophageal acid exposure in the entire group.[86] On the other hand, studies have shown laryngopharyngeal acid contact in entirely asymptomatic adults.[57,62,87,88] In fact, one study has documented pharyngeal acid reflux events in up to 20% of normal controls.[87] Smit et al. stated that perhaps as many as three EER events over 24 hours may be normal in adults.[89] However, this brief report did not mention laryngeal examinations or whether symptoms were present.

Individuals with asymptomatic EER may be at risk for upper airway damage in the event that the larynx or airway is traumatized. A "normal" individual with asymptomatic EER could undergo intubation or exhibit persistent vocally abusive behaviors that could more readily lead to the development of laryngeal or subglottic edema, granulation tissue, granuloma formation, posterior glottic, and/or subglottic stenosis. Prereflux inflammation or injury of the larynx may be the most important variable in these patients.[38] This mechanism may be at work in individuals undergoing brief periods of endotracheal intubation who then develop a subglottic or posterior glottic stenosis.[60,87]

In our opinion, judging whether a patient's EER found during pH monitoring is abnormal can be done only on an individual basis. In a patient with subglottic stenosis, laryngeal edema, or a recurrent granuloma, a single episode of EER would be considered highly significant and complete acid suppression warranted. One or two pharyngeal reflux events in an entirely asymptomatic person with a normal laryngeal examination may be of little importance — unless the patient is intubated, undergoes laryngeal surgery, or uses maladaptive vocal patterns.

pH-Metry Variability

EER is chronic/intermittent in nature, and therefore, the diagnosis may not be straightforward because a negative pH study does not rule out EER.[60,82] This difficulty in confirming the diagnosis of EER has been well demonstrated in a study by Vaezi et al.[80] On two occasions, 32 adults were studied using ambulatory double-probe pH monitoring with a distal sensor 5 cm above the LES and the proximal sensor just below the UES. Tests were done within 20 days of one another. Results showed significant day-to-day variability of acid exposure in the proximal esophagus. Healthy subjects had good intrasubject reproducibility (91 to 100%). Those with distal reflux (70 to 90%) and proximal reflux had poorer reproducibility (55%). This demonstrates good specificity but poor sensitivity for the detection of proximal reflux during any single 24-hour test period. Variability will also increase if testing periods of less than 20 to 24 hours are used.

Double-probe 24-hour pH study combined with symptom-based observation and/or respiratory monitoring is felt to be the current gold standard for reflux diagnosis in children. Reflux events are measured for 18 to 24 hours, and a diary is maintained to record symptoms, patient activity, and food consumption. The probe should be placed approximately 3 cm above the lower esophageal sphincter in infants and children and 5 cm above the lower esophageal sphincter in adolescents.[30] The proximal probe must be placed in the hypopharynx. One must be aware of the potential of pseudoreflux due to the drying of the probe or the consumption of acidic food substances.[30]

In a group of children screened for SIDS, values were abnormal when the reflux index is greater than 5% for noninfant patients and greater than 10% for infant patients.[1] There is still no consensus about normal pharyngeal pH values in children. Little et al. observed reflux in 76% of 225 children by double pH monitoring. Of note, 46% of these patients had EER without abnormal esophageal acid exposure. These patients tended to have more respiratory abnormalities. The authors have suggested that the pharyngeal probe allowed identification of an additional 46% of patients with EER.[30] The exact definitions of "normal" and "abnormal" continue to be debated. A recent article from Contencin and Narcy[31] notes a significant incidence of recurrent laryngotracheitis in patients with the number of pharyngeal episodes less than 6; Halstead suggests that episodes less than 10 were associated with respiratory difficulties.[90]

The final answer on the number of episodes to define abnormality of the proximal pharyngeal probe is not yet well established. Because of poor reproducibility and the lack of an established abnormal value for the proximal pharyngeal probe, we feel the use of empiric antireflux therapy may be indicated in patients with a high index of suspicion for EER. We are currently using pH probe testing for those who typically fail antireflux therapy to assess drug efficacy or in patients for whom the clinical picture is unclear.

THERAPY

The treatment of EER can be divided into phases; Silva and Hotaling describe phase 1 as lifestyle modification, phase 2 as pharmacologic treatment, and phase 3 as antireflux surgery.[91] The level of treatment is based on the severity of the reflux, and it is important to realize that many infants will respond to lifestyle and positional therapy. Many of the drugs used for EER are not approved by the FDA for use with infants — despite their widespread use — and establishing a diagnosis is important in these patients.

Generally, reflux treatment begins with conservative measures, including head of bed elevation, milk thickening, frequent but smaller feedings, avoidance of substances that may decrease lower esophageal sphincter (LES), and fasting before bedtime. With regard to sleep position, the postprandial prone position during sleep appears to decrease reflux; however, the supine position during sleep appears to reduce the occurrence of SIDS. The lateral position in infants can be maintained, which is a good alternative between these two positions in children typically less than 9 to 12 months of age. In addition, car seats should be avoided in postprandial infants who have demonstrated apnea or complications with reflux.

Phase 2 involves use of cytoprotective agents, H2 receptor blockers, prokinetic agents, or PPIs. Pharmacologic therapy for reflux is felt to be successful in 80% of cases. Mild reflux may be treated with a combination of conservative measures, antacids, and H2 antagonists, whereas prokinetic agents are recommended in the treatment of moderate to severe reflux, especially with dysmotility problems. Because of the lack of long-term experience with proton pump inhibitors in children, their use is limited to patients who typically fail a trial with H2 receptor blockers. Because many of these medications are not FDA approved for use in infants, the use of proton pump inhibitor therapy is controversial. It is our feeling that proton pump inhibitors are warranted, especially for severe or life-threatening symptoms.

Surgical intervention or phase-3 intervention is reserved for patients who fail aggressive medical therapy and continue to have life-threatening complications of reflux. The most common surgical procedure performed is the Nissen fundoplication, with its goal to restore the natural integrity of the lower esophageal sphincter and maintain normal deglutition. Nissen fundoplication has a 90% symptom control rate, with a 1% mortality rate.[92,93] Pennell et al. reported a better surgical success rate in esophageal reflux children without respiratory symptoms.[3]

A significant percentage of children with reflux may present with respiratory disorders. Treatment of the respiratory disorder may be unsuccessful until reflux is identified and treated. Close monitoring and follow-up of these patients is necessary to offer optimal outcome.

CONCLUSIONS

Extraesophageal reflux is a disorder commonly seen in otolaryngologic practice and differs from GERD in its clinical manifestations, pathophysiology, and response to treatment. Its association with numerous disorders in children should lead the otolaryngologist to consider this diagnosis in all patients with voice, airway, and swallowing complaints.

REFERENCES

1. Vandenplas, Y. and Sacre-Smith, L. Continuous 24-hour esophageal pH monitoring in 285 asymptomatic infants 0- to 15-months-old. *J. Pediatr. Gastroenerol. Nutr.*, 1987, 6, 220–224.
2. Harbovsky, E.E. and Mullett, M.D. Patterns of pediatric gastroesophageal reflux. *Am. Surg.*, 1985, 51, 212–216.
3. Pennell, R.C., Lewis, J.E., Cradock, T.V. et al. Management of severe gastroesophageal reflux in children. *Arch. Surg.*, 1984, 119, 553–557.
4. Osler, W. *The Principles and Practice of Medicine*. New York: Appleton, 1892.
5. Kennedy, J.H. "Silent" gastroesophageal reflux: an important but little known cause of pulmonary complications. *Dis. Chest*, 1962, 42, 42–45.
6. Koufman, J.A. The otolaryngologic manifestations of gastroesophageal reflux disease (GERD). In Myers, N., Buston, C.D., Breckman, D.E., and Krause, C.J., Eds. *Advances in Otolaryngology Head and Neck Surgery*, Vol 7. St. Louis: Mosby, 1993, 13–15.
7. Demester, T.R., Johnson, L.F., Joseph, G.J. et al. Patterns of gastroesophageal reflux in health and disease. *Ann. Surg.*, 1976, 184, 459–470.
8. Boyle, J.T. Gastroesophageal reflux disease in the pediatric patient. *Gastroenterol. Clin. North Am.*, 1989, 18, 315–337.
9. Orrstein, S.R. Invited review: controversies in pediatric gastroesophageal reflux. *J. Pediatr. Gastroenterol. Nutr.*, 1992, 14, 338–348.

10. Carre, I.J. The natural history of partial thoracic stomach hiatus hernias in children. *Arch. Dis. Child*, 1959, 34, 344–353.

11. Kibble, M.A. Gastroesophageal reflux and failure to thrive in infancy. In Gells, S.S., Ed. *Gastroesophageal Reflux 76th Ross Conference on Pediatric Research*. Columbus: Ross Laboratories, 1979, 39–42.

12. Treen, W.R., Davis, P.M., and Haynes, J.S. Gastroesophageal reflux in the older child: presentation, response to treatment and long-term follow-up. *Clin. Pediatr.*, 1991, 30, 435–440.

13. Cohen, R.M., Weintraub, A., Dimarino, A.J. et al. Gastroesophageal reflux during gastrostomy feedings. *Gastroenterology*, 1994, 106, 13–18.

14. Hebra, A. and Houfman, M.A. Gastroesophageal reflux in children. *Pediatr. Clin. North Am.*, 1993, 40, 1233–1256.

15. Boyle, J.T., Altschuler, S.M., Patterson, B.L. et al. Reflux inhibition of the lower esophageal sphincter (LES) following stimulation of pulmonary vagal afferent receptors. *Gastroenterology*, 1986, 90, 1353.

16. Sondheimer, J.M. Clearance of spontaneous gastroesophageal reflux in awake and sleeping infants. *Gastroenterology*, 1989, 97, 821–826.

17. Sondheimer, J.M. Upper esophageal sphincter and pharyngoesophageal motor function in infants with and without gastroesophageal reflux disease. *Gastroenterology*, 1983, 85, 301–305.

18. Fearon, B. and Brama, I. Esophageal hiatal hernia in infants and children. *Ann. Otol. Rhinol. Laryngol.*, 1981, 90, 387–391.

19. Euler, A.R., Byrne, W.J., Ament, M.E. et al. Recurrent pulmonary disease in children: a complication of gastroesophageal reflux. *Pediatrics*, 1979, 63, 47–51.

20. Malfroot, A., Vandenplas, Y., Vernlinden, M. et al. Gastroesophageal reflux and unexplained chronic respiratory disease in infants and children. *Pediatr. Pulmonol.*, 1987, 3, 208–213.

21. Burton, D.M., Pransky, S.M., Katz, R.M., Kearns, D.B., and Seid, A.B. Pediatric airway manifestations of gastroesophageal reflux disease. *Ann. Otol. Rhinol. Laryngol.*, 1992, 101, 742–749.

22. Belmont, J.R. and Grundfast, K. Congential laryngeal stridor (laryngomalacia): etiologic factors and associated disorders. *Ann. Otol. Rhinol. Laryngol.*, 1984, 93, 430–437.

23. Matthews, B.L., Little, J.P., McGuirt, W.F., Jr., and Koufman, J.A. Reflux in infants with laryngomalacia: results of 24-hour double-probe pH monitoring. *Otolaryngol. Head Neck Surg.*, 1999, 120, 860–864.

24. Bauman, N.M., Sandler, A.D., Schmidt, C., Maher, J.W., and Smith, R.J.H. Reflex laryngospasm induced by stimulation of distal esophageal afferents. *Laryngoscope*, 1994, 104, 209–214.

25. Boggs, D.F. and Bartlett, D. Chemical specificity of a laryngeal apneic reflex in puppies. *J. Appl. Physiol. Respir. Environ. Exerc. Physiol.*, 1982, 53, 455–462.

26. Koufman, J.A. Contact ulcer and granuloma of the larynx. In Gates, G., Ed. *Current Therapy in Otolaryngology–Head and Neck Surgery*. 5th ed. St. Louis: C.V. Mosby Publishers, 1993, 456–459.

27. Delahunty, J.E. and Cherry, J. Experimentally produced vocal cord granulomas. *Laryngoscope*, 1968, 78, 1941–1947.

28. Andze, G.O., Brandt, M.L., Dickens, S.V., Bensoussan, A.L., and Blanchard, H. Diagnosis and treatment of gastroesophageal reflux in 500 children with respiratory symptoms: the value of pH monitoring. *J. Pediatr. Surg.*, 1991, 26, 295–300.

29. Jolley, S.G., Herbst, J.J., Johnson, D.G., and Matlak, M.E. Esophageal pH monitoring during sleep identifies children with respiratory symptoms from gastroesophageal reflux. *Gastroenterology*, 1981, 80, 1501–1506.

30. Little, J.P., Matthews, B.L., Glock, M.S., Koufman, J.A., Reboussin, D.M., Loughlin, C.J., and McGuirt, W.F. Extraesophageal pediatric reflux: 24-hour double-probe pH monitoring in 222 children. *Ann. Otol. Rhinol. Laryngol.*, 1997, 106 (Suppl. 169), 1–16.

31. Contencin, P. and Narcy, P. Gastroesophageal reflux in infants and children: a pharyngeal pH monitoring study. *Arch. Otolarynol. Head Neck Surg.*, 1992, 118, 1028–1030.

32. Holinger, L.D. and Sanders, A.D. Chronic cough in infants and children: an update. *Laryngoscope*, 1991, 101, 596–605.

33. Contencin, P., Maurage, C., Ployet, M. et al. Symposium: gastroesophageal reflux and ENT disorders in childhood. *Int. J. Pediatr. Otorhinolaryngol.*, 1995, 32 (Suppl.), 135–144.

34. Orenstein, S.R. Gastroesophageal reflux. In Wyllie, R. and Hyams, J.S., Eds. *Pediatric Gastrointestinal Disease: Pathophysiology, Diagnosis, and Management*. Philadelphia: W.B. Saunders, 1993, 337–369.

35. Gumpert, L., Kalach, N., Dupont, C., and Contencin, P. Hoarseness and gastroesophageal reflux in children. *J. Laryngol. Otol.*, 1998, 112, 49–54.

36. Orenstein, S.R., Orenstein, D.M., and Whitington, P.F. Gastroesophageal reflux causing stridor. *Chest*, 1983, 84, 301–302.

37. Walner, D.L. and Hollinger, L.D. Supraglottic stenosis in infants and children. *Arch. Otolaryngol. Head Neck Surg.*, 1997, 123, 337–341.

38. Little, F.B., Koufman, J.A., Kohut, R.I. et al. Effects of gastric acid on the pathogenesis of subglottic stenosis. *Ann. Otol. Rhinol. Laryngol.*, 1985, 94, 516–519.

39. Gray, S., Miller, R., Myers, C.M., and Cotton, R.T. Adjunctive measures for successful laryngotracheal reconstruction. *Ann. Otol. Rhinol. Laryngol.*, 1987, 96, 509–513.

40. Bauman, N.M., Oyos, T.L., Murray, D.J., Kao, S.C.S., Biavati, M.J., and Smith, R.J.H. Post-operative protocol following single stage laryngotracheoplasty. *Ann. Otol. Rhinol. Laryngol.*, 1996, 1, 317–322.

41. Halstead, L.A. Gastroesophageal reflux: a critical factor in pediatric subglottic stenosis. *Otolaryngol. Head Neck Surg.*, 1999, 120, 683–688.

42. Zalzal, G.H., Choi, S.S., and Patel, K.M. The effect of gastroesophageal reflux on laryngotracheal reconstruction. *Arch. Otolaryngol. Head Neck Surg.*, 1996, 122, 297–300.

43. Wennergren, G., Bjure, J., Gertzberg, T. et al. Laryngeal reflex. *Acta Paediatr.*, 1993, 389 (Suppl. 82), 53–56.

44. Menon, A.P., Schlefft, G.L., and Thach, B.T. Apnea associated with regurgitation in infants. *J. Pediatr.*, 1985, 106, 625.

45. Lanier, B., Richardson, M.A., and Cummings, C. Effect of hypoxia on laryngeal reflux apnea-implications on sudden infant death. *Otolaryngol. Head Neck Surg.*, 1983, 91, 597–604.

46. Ramet, J., Egreteau, L., Cruzi–Dascaloval, L. et al. Cardiac, respiratory, and arousal responses to an esophageal acid infusion test in near-term infants during active sleep. *J. Pediatr. Gastroenterol. Nutr.*, 1992, 15, 135–140.

47. Newman, L.J., Russe, J., Glassman, M.S. et al. Patterns of gastroesophageal reflux (GER) in patients with apparent life threatening events. *J. Pediatr. Gastroenterol., Nutr.*, 1989, 8, 157–160.

48. Sacre, L. and Vandenplas, Y. Gastroesophageal reflux associated with respiratory abnormalities during sleep. *J. Pediatr., Gastroenterol. Nutr.*, 1989, 9, 28–33.

49. Wetmore, R.F. Effects of acid on the larynx of the maturing rabbit and the possible significance to the sudden infant death syndrome. *Laryngoscope*, 1993, 103, 1242–1254.

50. Duke, S.G., Postma, G.N., McGuirt, W.F., Jr. et al. Laryngospasm and diaphragmatic arrest in immature dogs after laryngeal acid exposure: a possible model for sudden infant death syndrome. *Ann. Otol. Rhinol. Laryngol.*, 2001, 110, 729–733.

51. Jolly, S.G., Halpern, L.M., and Tunell, W.P. The risk of sudden infant death from gastroesophageal reflux. *J. Pediatr. Surg.*, 1991, 26, 691–696.

52. Parsons, D.S. Chronic sinusitis a medical or surgical disease. *Otolaryngol. Clin. North Am.*, 1996, 29, 1–9.

53. Barbero, G.J. Gastroesophageal reflux and upper airway disease: a commentary. *Otolaryngol. Clin. North Am.*, 1996, 29, 27–36.

54. Orenstein, S.R., Cohen, J.A., Shalaby, T.M. et al. Reliability and validity of an infant gastroesophageal reflux questionnaire. *Clin. Pediatr.*, 1993, 32, 472–484.

55. Hanson, D.G., Jiang, J., and Chi, W. Quantitative color analysis of laryngeal erythema in chronic posterior laryngitis. *J. Voice*, 1998, 12(1), 78–83.

56. Ward, P.H. and Berci, G. Observations on the pathogenesis of chronic nonspecific pharyngitis and laryngitis. *Laryngoscope*, 1982, 92, 1377–1382.

57. Ulualp, S.O., Toohill, R.J., Hoffmann, R., and Shaker, R. Pharyngeal pH monitoring in patients with posterior laryngitis. *Otolaryngol. Head Neck Surg.*, 120, 5, 672–677.

58. Hickson, C., Simpson, C.B., and Falcon, R. Laryngeal pseudosulcus as a predictor of laryngopharyngeal reflux. *Laryngoscope*, 2001, 111, 1742.

59. Belafsky, P.C., Postma, G.N., and Koufman, J.K. The validity and reliability of the reflux finding score (RFS). *Laryngoscope*, 2001, 111, 1313–1317.

60. Koufman, J.A. The otolaryngologic manifestations of gastroesophageal reflux disease (GERD): a clinical investigation of 225 patients using ambulatory 24-hour pH monitoring and an experimental investigation of the role of acid and pepsin in the development of laryngeal injury. *Laryngoscope*, 1991, 101 (Suppl. 53), 1–78.

61. Koufman, J.K. and Amin, M. Laryngopharyngeal reflux and voice disorders. In Rubin, J.S., Sataloff, R.T., Korovin, G.S., and Gould, W.J., Eds. *Diagnosis and Treatment of Voice Disorders*, 2nd ed. New York–Tokyo: Igaku–Shoin Publishers. In press.

62. Koufman, J.A., Sataloff, R.T., and Toohill, R. Laryngopharyngeal reflux: consensus conference report. *J. Voice*, 1996, 10(3), 215–216.

63. Ossakow, S.J., Elta, G., Colturi, T., Bogdasarian, R., and Nostrant, T.T. Esophageal reflux and dysmotility as the basis for persistent cervical symptoms. *Ann. Otol. Rhinol. Laryngol.*, 1987, 96, 387–92.

64. Al Sabbagh, G. and Wo, J.M. Supraesophageal manifestations of gastroesophageal reflux disease. *Semin. Gastrointest. Dis.*, 1999, 10, 113–119.

65. Shaker, R., Milbrath, M., Ren, J., Toohill, R., Hogan, W.J., Li, Q., and Hofman, C.L. Esophagopharyngeal distribution of refluxed acid in patients with reflux laryngitis. *Gastroenterology*, 1995, 109, 1575–1582.

66. Wiener, G.J., Koufman, J.A., Wu, W.C. et al. Chronic hoarseness secondary to gastroesophageal reflux disease: documentation with 24-hour ambulatory pH monitoring. *Am. J. Gastroentrerol.*, 1989, 84, 1503–1508.

67. Ott, D.J. Gastroesophageal reflux disease. *Radiol. Clin. North Am.*, 1994, 32, 1147–1166.

68. Costantini, M., Crookes, P.F., Bremner, R.M. et al. Value of physiologic assessment of foregut symptoms in a surgical practice. *Surgery*, 1993, 114, 780–786.

69. Tolia, V., Calhoun, J.A., Kuhns, L.R. et al. Lack of correlation between extended pH monitoring and scintigraphy in the evaluation of infants with gastroesophageal reflux. *J. Lab. Clin. Med.*, 1990, 115, 559–563.

70. Fisher, R.S., Mamud, L.S., Roberts, G.S. et al. Gastroesophageal (GE) scintiscanning to detect and quantitate GE reflux. *Gastroenterology*, 1976, 70, 301–306.

71. Nussbaum, E., Maggi, J.C., Mathis, R. et al. Association of lipid-laden alveolar macrophages and gastroesophageal reflux in children. *J. Pediatr.*, 1987, 110, 190–194.

72. Postma, G.N. Ambulatory pH monitoring methodology. *Ann. Otol. Rhinol. Laryngol.*, 2000, 109 (Suppl. 184), 10–14.

73. Koufman, J.A. Laryngopharyngeal reflux (LPR) is different from classic gastroesophageal reflux disease (GERD): current concepts and a new paradigm. In Benninger, M., Ed. *Benign Disorders of Voice*, Alexandria, VA: American Academy of Otolaryngology–Head and Neck Surgery Foundation, 2002.

74. Bain, W.M., Harrington, J.W., Thomas, L.E. et al. Head and neck manifestations of gastroesophageal reflux. *Laryngoscope*, 1983, 93, 175–179.

75. Richter, J.E., Ed. *Ambulatory Esophageal pH Monitoring: Practical Approach and Clinical Applications*. 2nd ed., Baltimore: MD, William & Wilkins, 1997.

76. Katz, P.O. Ambulatory esophageal and hypopharyngeal pH monitoring in patients with hoarseness. *Am. J. Gastroenterol.*, 1990, 85, 38–40.

77. Johnson, P.E., Postma, G.N., Amin, M.A., Belafsky, P.C., and Koufman, J.A. pH monitoring in patients with laryngopharyngeal reflux (LPR): why the pharyngeal probe is essential. Submitted to *Laryngoscope*.

78. Dobhan, R. and Castell, D.O. Normal and abnormal proximal esophageal acid exposure: results of ambulatory dual-probe pH monitoring. *Am. J. Gastroenterol.*, 1993, 88, 25–29.

79. Kamel, P.L., Hanson, D., and Kahrilas, P.J. Omeprazole for the treatment of posterior laryngitis. *Am. J. Med.*, 1994, 96 (Apr.), 321–326.

80. Vaezi, M.F., Schroeder, P.L., and Richter, J.E. Reproducibility of proximal probe pH parameters in 24-hour ambulatory esophageal pH monitoring. *Am. J. Gastroenterol.*, 1997, 92, 825–829.

81. Gerhardt, D.C., Shuck, T.J., Bordeaux, R.A. et al. Human upper esophageal sphincter. Response to volume, osmotic, and acid stimuli. *Gastroenterology*, 1978, 75, 268–274.

82. Jacob, P., Kahrilas, P.J., and Herzon, G. Proximal esophageal pH-metry in patients with reflux laryngitis. *Gastroenterology*, 1991, 100, 305–310.

83. Richter, J.E. Ambulatory esophageal pH monitoring. *Am. J. Med.*, 1997, 103(5A), 130S–134S.

84. Ali, G.N. Detection of acid regurgitation with a pharyngeal pH sensor: validation of measurement criteria. *Gastroenterology*, 1998, 108(4), A258.

85. Panetti, M., ReVille, J., Clyne, S., Henszel, A., Doellgast, G., and Koufman, J. Clinical implications of the functional stability of pepsin. Presented at the annual meeting of the American Academy of Otolaryngology Head and Neck Surgery, September 1998, San Antonio, TX.

86. Eubanks, T.R., Omelanczuk, P.E. Maronian, N., Hillel, A., Pope II, C.E., and Pellegrini, C.A. Pharyngeal pH monitoring in 222 patients with suspected laryngeal reflux. *J. Gastrointest. Surg.*, 2001, 5, 183–191.

87. Toohill, R.T., Ulualp, S.O., and Shaker, R. Evaluation of gastroesophageal reflux in patients with laryngotracheal stenosis. *Ann. Otol. Rhinol. Laryngol.*, 1998, 107, 1010–1014.

88. Ylitalo, R., Lindestad, P.A., and Ramel, S. Symptoms, laryngeal findings, and 24-hour pH monitoring in patients with suspected gastroesophago-pharyngeal reflux. *Laryngoscope*, 2001, 111, 1735–1741.

89. Smit, C.F., Tan, J., Devriese, P.P., Mathus-Vliegen, L.M.H., Brandsen, M., and Schouwenburg, P.F. Ambulatory pH measurements at the upper esophageal sphincter. *Laryngoscope*, 1998, 108, 299–302.

90. Halstead, L. Role of gastroesophageal reflux in pediatric upper airway disorders. *Otolaryngol. Head Neck Surg.*, 1999, 120, 208–214.

91. Silva, A.B. and Hotaling, A.A. Pediatric gastroesophageal reflux disease. *Curr. Opin. Otolaryngol. Head Neck Surg.*, 1994, 2, 508.

92. Fung, K.P., Seagram, G., Pasieka, J. et al. Investigation and outcome of 121 infants and children requiring Nissen fundoplication for management of gastroesophageal reflux. *Invest. Med.*, 1990, 13, 237–240.

93. Little, A.G., Ferguson, M.K., and Skinner, D.B. Reoperation for failed antireflux operations. *J. Thorac. Cardiovasc. Surg.*, 1986, 91, 511–517.

Section V

General

20 Lasers in Otolaryngology

John P. Bent III and James S. Reilly

If you want to know the distance between two points, don't measure it before you've made sure your ruler is accurate.

Anonymous

CONTENTS

INTRODUCTION

Lasers no longer conjure images of high-tech, futuristic gadgetry. Because of lasers' ubiquity, most surgeons across all specialties have at least some laser experience. By cutting and/or coagulating in narrow, dark spaces into which conventional instruments do not easily reach, lasers continue to offer the surgical tool of choice for select head and neck procedures. Lasers have the ability to selectively photothermolyse certain cutaneous lesions that can provide unique advantages. In many

TABLE 20.1
Lasers Commonly Used by Pediatric Otolaryngologists

Laser	Wavelength (nm)	Penetration (mm)
Argon	514	0.8
Dye lasers	577	0.9
KTP	532	0.9
Nd: YAG	1,064	4.0
Ho: YAG	2,128	0.4
CO_2	10,060	0.03

other circumstances, lasers represent a controversial or secondary alternative line of therapy. Some lasers have become antiquated and replaced by tools that feature even less invasion and tissue trauma, such as flash scanners or microdebrider instrumentation.

Pediatric otolaryngology laser application occurs primarily, but not exclusively, in the airway. Other areas of common use include treatment of hemangiomata of the skin, primarily the face, and, more recently, to open the tympanic membrane for ventilation. This chapter will help the reader to apply different laser wavelengths and delivery systems appropriately. The discussion will focus on prevention of complications and proper management of those that do occur.

LASER PROPERTIES AND DELIVERY SYSTEMS

LASER represents an acronym for light amplification by the stimulated emission of radiation. This emission occurs when an exciting force such as light or electricity acts on a lasing medium (either a gas, such as CO_2, or solid, such as the ruby). As the excited molecules return to their native state, the laser harnesses the emitted light with the use of mirrors to produce a beam. This beam features monochromatic, coherent light with a synchronized wavelength. Table 20.1 lists lasers and their wavelengths commonly used by otolaryngologists.

Most pediatric otolaryngologists use lasers to ablate tissue via vaporization of water. The laser's wavelength and irradiance, as well as the properties of the target tissue, determine whether a laser cuts, coagulates, or ablates tissue. The term *irradiance* represents power density, which can be calculated by dividing intensity (watts) by beam area.[1] As the beam's diameter decreases, the irradiance increases. The surgeon can help minimize complication by being mindful that narrow laser beams have a greater ability to cut and penetrate. Many centers now have lasers with spot sizes as narrow as 50 μm ("microspot lasers"), which allow more precise lasering at reduced power settings.

The surgeon may deliver laser energy to the target tissue with a variety of hand pieces, or the laser may be linked to a microscope, bronchoscope, or other surgical instruments. Figure 20.1 through Figure 20.5 demonstrate some of the laser delivery systems. Most lasers can be introduced to the operative field via an optical fiber, which has advantages of light weight, small diameter, and flexibility. The CO_2 laser, probably the most popular laser in otolaryngology, remains without a fiberoptic delivery system and still relies on articulated arms that reflect the laser light down a series of tubes and mirrors. Because CO_2 light is not visible, a red helium–neon ("HeNe") beam is aligned with the laser beam to give the surgeon a visible target. The aiming beam may become misaligned from the laser beam through excessive use or frequently moving the microscope and should be tested by the surgeon or trained operating personnel prior to every case.

The laser light can be continuous or pulsed. The continuous wave gives a constant application of laser light to the target tissue and therefore has greater potential for thermal trauma. A pulsed beam generally gives a millisecond burst of laser light every second, using a much higher power

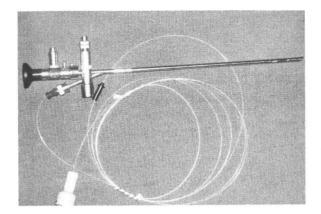

FIGURE 20.1 Rigid bronchoscope with 400-μm fiber in place, ready for use.

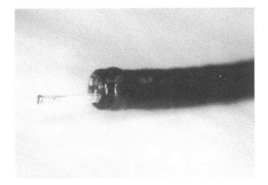

FIGURE 20.2 Many flexible bronchoscopes have a channel that can also be used for placement of a laser fiber.

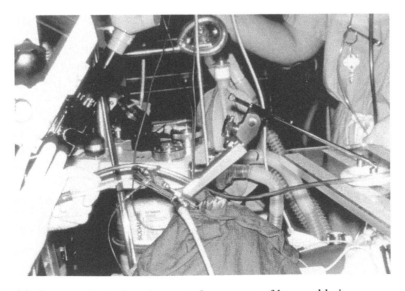

FIGURE 20.3 CO_2 laser coupled to the microscope for treatment of laryngeal lesions.

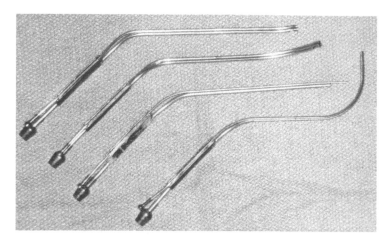

FIGURE 20.4 Handpieces for delivering fiberoptic laser cable to sinonasal lesions.

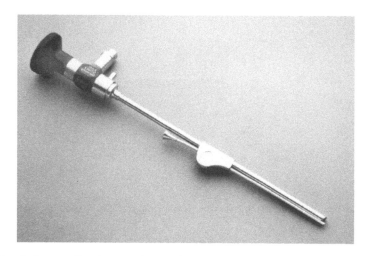

FIGURE 20.5 Sheath for coupling laser to sinus endoscope.

during this short duration than the continuous wave. Newer lasers offer "superpulse" options, in which the same laser power is delivered over an even shorter time interval. Not all lasers offer pulsing; however, if available, it is generally preferable because of its lower risk of lateral heating.

SAFETY CONSIDERATIONS

Hospitals certified by the Joint Commission of Accreditation of Hospital Organizations (JCAHO) have traditionally had to have a minimum of laser safety protocols in place, including creating a designated "laser safety officer." Most hospitals have maintained functioning laser safety committees as part of their administrative clinical oversight responsibilities even though the JCAHO (2002) does not currently require it. AORN, the Association of Operating Room Nurses, publishes a Recommended Practices and Guidelines handbook with specific information on laser safety to which the nursing team, and others, may refer.

PATIENT SAFETY

The patient's protection is the top priority. Most operation room circulating nurses are trained to provide protection for the patient, but the ultimate responsibility rests with the surgeon. In addition to routine operating room safety precautions, special care must be taken to avoid injury from inadvertent lasering. The skin, and eyes, in particular, must be shielded prior to initiating use of the laser. Taping the eyes closed or placing protective eye shields may accomplish optimal protection; covering exposed skin with moist towels is also beneficial. Flammable gels frequently placed as a precaution in the eyes should be eliminated in laser procedures. Adjacent facial skin and lips must be covered with moist towels. These steps are particularly important when the surgeon lasers via a hand piece or microscope because stray movements can injure an unprotected patient.

EQUIPMENT SAFETY

Perhaps no piece of equipment in the operating room is more prone to malfunction or capable of intimidating nursing personnel than the laser is. For these reasons alone, the laser should be turned on and tested before the patient enters the room. This allows all personnel a chance to gain comfort with the machine in a nonpressure situation, assure proper function, and in the case of the CO_2 laser, verify that the aiming beam is coaxial with the laser beam. These simple steps add a margin of safety and may even avert time delays from unrecognized equipment breakdown.

PERSONNEL SAFETY

Measures must be undertaken to protect the operating room personnel. The two steps generally advised involve eye protection and evacuation of the laser plume. Eyeglasses or clear shields serve as adequate protection for the CO_2 laser; specialized glasses are available for lasers with shorter wavelength and must be worn by all operating room personnel. The laser plume can be evacuated with routine suction in the operative field.

Evidence exists that viruses may transfer from patient to the laser plume.[2] When an elevated risk of infectious disease exists (e.g., recurrent respiratory papilloma [RRP] or human immunodeficiency virus [HIV]), more powerful suction can be employed near the site of lasering. In such circumstances, the operating personnel should wear specialized masks to reduce the risks of inhaling infectious laser smoke. Furthermore, there have been anecdotal reports of laryngologists acquiring RRP,[3] thus justifying the aforementioned precautions. The surgeon must also ensure, particularly when lasering via a microscope, that his or her fingers do not interfere with even a portion of the laser beam; otherwise, a painful and embarrassing fingertip burn may be sustained.

AERODIGESTIVE PROCEDURES

Laser procedures are commonly performed by otolaryngologists for laryngotracheal pathology. Other aerodigestive tract anatomic regions may also benefit from the adjunctive use of laser therapy.[4] Within the nasal vault and paranasal sinuses, laser therapy has been used for polyps, turbinate pathology, granulation tissue, posterior choanal pathology, and tear duct pathology. Within the oral cavity and oropharynx, laser therapy has been used for tonsillectomy, macroglossia, and soft palate surgery. Reports of success are therefore currently anecdotal. The potential usefulness of these relatively limited number of nonlaryngotracheal procedures has not been well studied with a large series of children, and none of these alternative applications of laser therapy has gained wide acceptance for use within the pediatric age group.

OXYGEN CONCENTRATION

The method of anesthesia affects safety of any laser procedure, especially when the laser is applied to the airway. The two factors that must be considered are the oxygen concentration and the means of maintaining the airway. By delivering higher oxygen concentration, the anesthesiologist directly increases the chance of fire. Most authorities recommend lowering the oxygen concentration below 40% during laser procedures, patient condition permitting. Most anesthesiologists know to lower

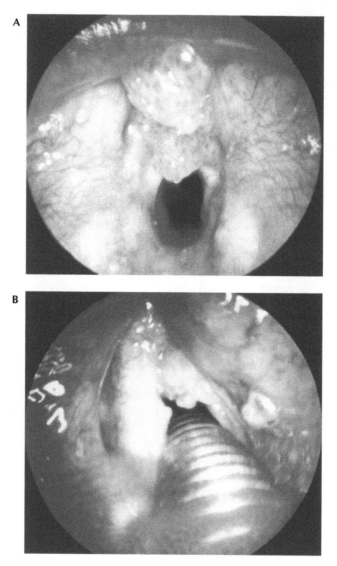

FIGURE 20.6 A. Laryngeal papillomas viewed during spontaneous ventilation. B. Flexible stainless steel endotracheal tube in place in preparation for lasering papillomas.

oxygen concentrations during laser procedures, but the surgeon shares responsibility for this rudimentary precaution. Although any oxygen concentration can be used, as oxygen levels increase, so do the risks. Continuous mode for laser use also increases the chance of fire.[5]

ANESTHETIC TECHNIQUE

Tubeless techniques (Figure 20.6A) include intermittent apnea during lasering, supraglottic or subglottic jet ventilation, or spontaneous ventilation. These techniques pose less of a fire hazard and provide greater exposure of the larynx, but theoretically expose operative personnel to forcibly exhaled gasses that would be more easily contained with the anesthesia circuit closed (Figure 20.6B). Vapors generated during airway lasering pose a health hazard from the unknown effect of repeated low-level exposure to anesthetic agents, as well as a potential infectious risk. Masks should be worn snugly. When work is done in the trachea or bronchoscope, the additional option of lasering and ventilating via a rigid bronchoscope exists (Figure 20.6).

INSTRUMENTATION

Working in small airways demands appropriate use of instrumentation to manipulate tissue gently for better visualization and accurate application of laser therapy. Metal conducts heat and laser-"blackened" instruments absorb less energy. A wide array of pediatric-compatible laryngeal micro-instrumentation is now available to minimize unwanted laser tissue effects, including angled and straight "spatulas" (with or without suction), straight and angled probes, reflective mirrors, atraumatic forceps, microsuction catheters, and vocal fold "rollers." Furthermore, various specialized straight and angled sinonasal instruments allow continuous suction with delivery of laser via a fiberoptic cable.

OTOLOGIC PROCEDURES

OSSICLES AND OVAL WINDOW

Laser application to the ear has had a limited role in children. It has been advocated for laser fenestration of the oval window (laser stapedotomy), primarily for otosclerosis in adult patients. These lasers are integrated into the microscope and have been used to open the appropriate size lumen to receive the prosthesis. No safety violations or injuries occur with this technique if proper technique is used. Appropriate selection of power settings avoids excessive transmission of thermal energy from the CO_2 laser to the perilymphatic fluid. Otosclerosis and middle ear adhesions infrequently present as a cause of conductive hearing loss in children; such cases may be managed with the laser. In theory, the CO_2 laser presents the greatest safety margin in the middle ear, especially near the oval window, because the shallow penetration protects the vestibule.[6] However, most surgeons choose a laser for middle ear work based on their comfort with the handpiece or delivery system.

TYMPANIC MEMBRANE

Lasers have been used for opening the tympanic membrane for almost two decades.[7] More recently, the introduction of laser frenestrations (e.g., myringotomies) by CO_2 laser integrated with small endoscopes connected to video images (Otolam) has a novel role; growing experience demonstrates no significant complications.[8] Current clinical trials are designed to elucidate the appropriate clinical indications for its consideration as a recommended treatment.

The safety value of the Otolam system is that the laser beam is completely enclosed within the ear canal when the image of the tympanic membrane is brought into focus. The beam is also controlled by a flash scanner that rapidly moves the laser beam across the tympanic membrane in a centripetal pattern, limiting the amount of heat created and dispensed to the tympanic membrane. The combination of (1) closed system, (2) rapid flash scanner, and (3) limited and controlled focal length protects the patient and medical personnel, the tympanic membrane, and most importantly, the ossicles and cochlea.

Experience with over 500 cases has not been associated with any permanent or unexplained damage to the child's ear or hearing, tympanic membrane, or patients and personnel.[8] The scan is set for a brief period (0.25 seconds) at short focal lengths of <2.4 cm, and pin-point accuracy and spot size (1.0 to 2.4 mm) creates a "nontouch" opening into the tympanic membrane with topical anesthesia. This allows longer and more complete drainage than is obtained with office myringotomy. Parents or other caretakers are permitted within the procedure room and do not need to wear safety glasses. The CO_2 laser is turned on only after the endoscope is in the child's ear, and the closed system and limited focal length enhance the experience for child and parent.

The safety features of this technique include prompt healing of the tympanic membrane with residual perforation in only 1 ear out of 500 (<0.005) at 60 days after the procedure. This opening lasts an average of 20 days when a myringotomy tube is not inserted. The limited amount of energy used with the pulse mode and the flash scanner protects the oval window and ossicles and limits the effect to the tympanic membrane only. Although this is a more expensive therapy, it is considered safer than using a myringotomy knife or placing a long spinal needle through the tympanic membrane for aspiration or tympanocentesis.[9]

External Auditory Canal

Lasering chronic otitis externa has been proposed but has never gained widespread application because of the real risk of external auditory canal stenosis. Medical treatments for otitis externa remain the mainstay of current therapy.

MANAGEMENT OF COMPLICATIONS

Healy and coworkers reviewed 4416 CO_2 laser cases in the aerodigestive tract for complications and found 0.2% incidents, with fire the most common.[10] In the airway, fire remains the most common and serious potential complication. Insufflation anesthesia with spontaneous ventilation ("tubeless anesthesia") via a rigid laryngoscope using a laser coupled to a microscope provides the greatest margin of safety because it eliminates the risk of an endotracheal tube or the fiberoptic cable igniting. When requesting this preferred technique in children, the endoscopist must be prepared to discuss anesthesia *in advance and prior to induction* in order to assure that an educated and experienced team will be safely sharing the airway.

Tracheotomy Tube Considerations

The potential hazards of laser surgery with a nearby indwelling endotracheal tube are more obvious than with a tracheostomy tube; an all too common scenario involves a tracheotomy-dependent patient being ventilated through a plastic tracheostomy tube while the surgeon lasers on the larynx or cervical trachea. Instead of ventilating through a rigid bronchoscope or a stainless steel tracheostomy tube, the surgeon instructs an assistant to withdraw the indwelling tracheostomy tube until the tip is flush with the tracheotomy stoma while lasering begins. The laser may then carry past its target and cause an explosion as it contacts the plastic tracheostomy tube. Nonmetal tracheostomy tubes should be removed or replaced with a stainless steel tube when lasering is performed in the vicinity of the tracheotomy stoma.

Fiberoptic Cable

Whenever lasering via a fiberoptic cable, the surgeon must also avoid charred residue on the cable tip, which can easily ignite. The YAG/KTP fiber, for example, can ignite and burn along its entire length, creating the very undesirable "blowtorch effect" with potentially significant injury to the mucosa of the larynx, trachea, nasal vault, nasopharynx, or oral cavity. It is important to prepare the fiber appropriately and to check throughout the procedure to ensure that the tip is free from charred debris; it may be necessary to prepare a fresh tip repeatedly.

Nonlaryngeal Head and Neck Procedures

When the laser procedure is primarily for the ear or skin, a plastic tube can be safely used if covered with moist towel and kept out of the surgical field. Even when lasering within the nose and nasopharynx, and all portions of the oral cavity, oropharynx, and hypopharynx, the endotracheal tube must be protected or a laser-compatible endotracheal tube should be employed for the case. In such cases, the anesthesiologist must intubate with a cuffed endotracheal tube that prevents oxygen leakage into the surgical air space. When cuffed, laser-safe metal-armored endotracheal tubes are used. If there is any chance of the laser striking the cuff, the endotracheal tube should be filled with water rather than air for added safety.

LARYNGEAL PROCEDURES

When lasering directly on the larynx and/or if the tube cannot be covered, the surgeon and anesthesiologist may decide to use tubeless "apnea" anesthesia or a wire-reinforced steel tube. Wire-reinforced steel endotracheal tubes have a larger outer-to-inner diameter ratio than standard endotracheal tubes and are generally not available for infants and neonates. In these very narrow airways, if no safe alternatives such as jet ventilation are possible, the surgeon may wrap a small rubber endotracheal tube with aluminum tape to protect the exposed tube surface area.

AIRWAY FIRES

For a fire to occur, a combustible substrate must be present. Plastic, particularly polyvinyl chloride (PVC), endotracheal or tracheostomy tubes are especially hazardous. Most laser fires occur when the laser strikes the oxygen-enriched environment around the tube used to maintain the airway. The surgeon may elect to take a shortcut and laser on the larynx with an endotracheal tube that is not laser compatible. It may be reasoned that "I don't need to use a metal tube .... protecting the tube with moist cottonoids is unnecessary and time consuming .... I know how to keep the laser beam out of trouble," but these casual assumptions may lead to disaster.

If an airway fire takes place, the surgeon should immediately take the following additional steps:

- Remove the flammable substrate,
- Discontinue lasering,
- Secure the airway,
- Irrigate the airway with sufficient quantities of cold sterile saline to stop the flames and quench the fire, and
- Administer parenteral steroids, such as high-dose dexamethasone.

The patient should also receive generous intravenous hydrated and humidified air postoperatively.

THERMAL INJURY

Thermal injury from excessive lasering can occur. Frequent cooling of ablated tissue surfaces throughout the procedure with chilled saline topically applied by cottonoid pledgets is recommended; these are available in multiple sizes and have a retrieval string attached. Thermal injury from laser therapy can also occur at the periphery of or outside the surgeon's view. For instance, a surgeon may be treating tracheal papillomas with a KTP 400-μm fiber; while he or she is focusing on the papilloma in the center of the monitor, it may be unapparent that the char of the fiber has created a diffuse beam with excessive lateral beam radiation, thus causing heating of the nondiseased tracheal walls. Similarly, the bronchoscope may become heated from defects in the laser fiber or beam alignment, causing thermal injury wherever the bronchoscope contacts tissue. Unfortunately, burns of the lip and tongue from overheated bronchoscopes have occurred. The surgeon should be immediately concerned if he or she senses increased temperature of the bronchoscope and should never use towels or any barriers besides routine surgical gloves to hold the bronchoscope.

EXCESSIVE TISSUE ABLATION

Excessive laser penetration may cause additional sites of injury throughout the head and neck. Unwanted scarring with primary or secondary negative effect on function and/or physiology may result. Good visualization, appropriate instrumentation, experience, and operator care must be applied to remove or dissect only that which is intended. The surgeon must also always be mindful that laser therapy may penetrate more deeply than intended and has the potential to injure vascular and other critical structures that lie immediately beneath the target lesion.

The nose and oral cavity are the portals of the aerodigestive tract and complications known to occur with laryngeal and tracheal lasering may also transpire with oral cavity/oropharyngeal or sinonasal lasering. Flammable gasses may leak into these regions, and the endotracheal tube, whether oral or nasal, may become jeopardized by being directly in the line of laser firing or by sliding into the nasophaynx. Thermal trauma represents the most likely risk in nasal or oral lasering. Giannoni et al.[11] noted a series of seven patients who developed nasopharyngeal stenosis after aggressive KTP laser adenoidectomy. Intranasal synechia, atrophic rhinitis, and velopharyngeal insufficiency represent additional problems attributable to injudicious laser application within the upper aerodigestive tract.

PNEUMOTHORAX

In the bronchi, penetration of the airway walls may cause a pneumothorax to develop. The occurrence of pneumothorax is less common with CO_2 lasers because they pose less risk of overpenetration than the KTP lasers, offering the "what you see is what you get" advantage. Particularly for lesions of the larynx, CO_2 lasers are most often indicated because of the reduced potential for injury from deeper penetration.[4] Careful auscultation and AP chest radiograph can establish the diagnosis. If the diagnosis of pneumothorax is confirmed intraoperatively and patient ventilation is compromised and unstable, the surgeon may elect to place an angiocatheter in the ipsilateral intercostal space along the lateral axillary line to decompress the tension pneumothorax until a chest tube can be placed.

CONTINUING EDUCATION

All residents currently completing U.S.-based programs approved by the Accreditation Council for Graduate Medical Education (ACGME) Residency Review Committee (RRC) gain broad exposure to laser application, most often in the airway. This surgical exposure generally consists of generous experiences with CO_2 lasers and significant additional experience with 532/1064/2128-nm wavelengths. Some training programs offer specialized experience in shorter wavelength lasers. Vigilance and safety concerns must never be neglected or trivialized because injury and danger can always occur if principles and correct procedures are not followed.

For recently trained residents, the primary issue at stake is maintenance of their technical skill and knowledge base. Most laser committees will certify a recently graduated resident for laser use if experience can be demonstrated in the requested frequencies. Generally, a letter from the residency director and an appropriate number of operative notes suffice for documentation for medical and surgical privileging. Obtaining laser privileges will be more difficult for surgeons removed from their residency. Additional requirements often include mentoring by a certified colleague for several cases and attendance at a postgraduate laser course, in addition to the requirements of recent resident graduates. Many laser committees require all their laser surgeons periodically to attend laser review courses of 4- to 8-hour duration.

Although safety requirements may appear as a frustrating nuisance for many experienced surgeons, these rules exist for good reason. Medical institutions demand high standards for laser surgery and often require documentation of ongoing continuing education in laser safety. Ideally, hospitals could provide the administrative support to facilitate credentialing upkeep, as well as concise annual laser review courses that would obviate the need to travel to courses in other cities.

TABLE 20.2
Pediatric Head and Neck Lesions/Procedures for Which Lasers Are Commonly Utilized

Lesion	Laser	Alternative
Subglottic hemangioma	CO_2; KTP	Steroids; interferon; tracheotomy; external excision
Recurrent respiratory papillomas (RRP)	CO_2	Microdebrider; interferon; cidofovir
Cutaneous hemangioma	Dye lasers	Steroids; observation
Photodynamic therapy	Dye lasers	See RRP
Nasal polyps	KTP	Microdebrider; forceps; steroids
Tympanostomy	CO_2	Steel
Laryngomalacia	CO_2	Antireflux; positioning; steel
Bilateral vocal fold paralysis — cordotomy or arytenoidectomy	CO_2	Tracheotomy; observation
Venous malformation	Nd; YAG	Resection; observation

CONCLUSIONS

Laser surgery has added a wonderful tool to the surgeon's armamentarium that with careful and thoughtful application, can be used safely and without complication. Table 20.2 lists pediatric head and neck lesions/procedures for which lasers are commonly used. Although the laser can provide a less traumatic alternative to the hammers and saws of previous generations, it can still injure tissue and result in potentially catastrophic complications. Consequently, as technology marches ahead, lasers may be replaced by microdebriders, modified radiofrequency generators, tissue coablators, and similar devices that offer less traumatic resection and more favorable tissue effects. The educated aerodigestive tract surgeon, therefore, needs to maintain his or her skills while keeping abreast of new clinical therapies.

REFERENCES

1. Reinish, L. Laser physics and tissue interaction. *Otol. Clin. North Am.*, 1996, 29, 893–914.
2. Kashima, H.K., Kessis, T., Mounts, P., and Shah, K. Polymerase chain reaction identification of human papillomavirus DNA in CO_2 laser plume from recurrent respiratory papillomatosis. *Otolaryngol. Head Neck Surg.*, 1991, 104, 191–195.
3. Hallmo, P. and Naess, O. Laryngeal papillomatosis with human papillomavirus DNA contracted by a laser surgeon. *Eur. Arch. Otorrhinolaryngol.*, 1991, 248, 425–427.
4. Ossoff, R.H., Coleman, J.A., Courey, R.S. et al. Clinical applications of lasers in otolaryngology — head and neck surgery. *Lasers Surg. Med.*, 1994, 15, 217–248.
5. Ossoff, R.H. Laser safety in otolaryngology — head and neck surgery: anesthetic and educational considerations for laryngeal surgery. *Laryngoscope*, 1989, 99(8 Pt. 2 Suppl. 48), 1–26.
6. Lesinski, S.G. Lasers for otosclerosis — which one if any and why? *Lasers Surg. Med.*, 1990, 10, 448–457.
7. Goode, R. CO_2 laser myringotomy. *Laryngoscope*, 1982, 92, 420–423.
8. Reilly, J.S., Deutsch, E.S., and Cook, S.P. Laser-assisted myringotomy for otitis media: a feasibility study with short-term follow-up. *Ear Nose Throat J.*, 2000, 79(8), 650–657.
9. Silverstein, H., Jackson, L.E., Rosenberg, S.I., and Conlon, W.C. Pediatric laser myringotomy. *Laryngoscope*, 2001, 111(5), 905–906.
10. Healy, G.B., Strong, M.S., Shapsay, S., Vaughan, C., and Jako, G. Complications of CO_2 laser surgery of the aerodiestive tract: experience of 4416 cases. *Otolaryngol. Head Neck Surg.*, 1984, 92, 13–18.
11. Giannoni, C., Sulek, M., Friedman, E.M., and Duncan, N.O. Acquired nasopharyngeal stenosis: a warning and review. *Arch. Otolaryngol. Head Neck Surg.*, 1998, 124, 163–167.

21 Foreign Bodies in Otolaryngology (Nontracheobronchial)

Jay N. Dolitsky and Amelia F. Drake

If there are two or more ways to do something, and one of those ways can result in a catastrophe, then someone will do it.

Edward A. Murphy, retired Air Force captain

CONTENTS

INTRODUCTION

Foreign bodies of the ear, nose, and upper aerodigestive tract are common among children, particularly those under 5 years of age. In 1998, aspiration and asphyxiation of a foreign body was the fourth leading cause of accidental death at home in children under 5 years.[1] Although this represents a significant reduction over the past 30 years, it still remains a substantial problem. Morbidity due to foreign body placement in the ear and nose also remains significant. As will be discussed, the alkaline disc battery presents a special situation, regardless of the site. When nonspecialists attempt extraction of foreign objects without the proper equipment and expertise, iatrogenic injuries are more likely to occur. Aspiration of airway foreign bodies is covered in another chapter; therefore, this chapter will cover esophageal foreign bodies and other foreign bodies of the ear, nose, and throat.

ESOPHAGEAL FOREIGN BODIES

More than half of the foreign bodies in children involve the esophagus, with the highest incidence occurring in the 14-month to 6-year age range.[2] Young children are curious and tend to explore objects orally. These objects are then swallowed intentionally or accidentally resulting from a startle. In the United States, coins are the most common foreign body to lodge in the esophagus.[3] In a recent review, coins were the most common esophageal foreign body in children under 10, and fish bones were the most frequent in children older than 10 years.[4]

There are four physiological areas of narrowing in the esophagus: the cricopharyngeal sphincter, the aortic arch, the area adjacent to the left mainstem bronchus, and the gastroesophageal sphincter. These areas correspond to the four most common sites of esophageal foreign body impaction. The cricopharyngeus is the most common and the aortic arch region the most dangerous.

PRESENTATION

A history of foreign body ingestion is often not obtained and many foreign bodies pass through the esophagus undetected. Those that have difficulty passing into the esophagus may irritate the larynx and stimulate coughing, gagging, or choking. Subsequent symptoms depend on the size, shape, composition, and site of the object. In young children, refusing to eat and drooling are typical symptoms. With complete esophageal obstruction, vomiting and choking occur.

Smaller foreign bodies, such as a small coin or fish or chicken bone, may pass through the esophagus with the main symptom related to mucosal injury. A foreign body sensation in the hypopharynx or esophagus may be the only symptom; the head and neck examination and laryngoscopy may be unremarkable. Vague, nonspecific pain on swallowing is usually a mucosal laceration or abrasion, whereas a specific, localized sensation is more indicative of an embedded object. Duration is a factor as well, because the longer an object remains lodged in the esophagus, the greater the local inflammation. This can lead to odynophagia, fever, and leukocytosis.

Radiographic diagnosis of esophageal foreign body supports the clinical impression and can be diagnostic if the foreign body is radiopaque (Figure 21.1). Edible foreign bodies, such as large pieces of meat, lodged in the esophagus may not be evident on a routine x-ray. Contrast studies are helpful for identifying nonradiopaque objects and demonstrating the degree and site of obstruction, if present. Water-soluble agents such as gastrograffin should be used when esophageal perforation is suspected because they are less noxious to the mediastinum.

MANAGEMENT

An esophageal foreign body does not require emergency measures but should be removed as soon as possible after proper evaluation and preparation.[5] Often, a child will have recently eaten and a an appropriate period of time should pass before he or she undergoes general anesthesia. If a foreign body is corrosive, such as an alkaline disc battery, it should be removed emergently to prevent severe inflammation and perforation of the esophageal wall.[6]

The method of removal depends upon the nature and location of the foreign body, the age of the patient, and the presence or absence of an associated complication. Flexible and rigid esophagoscopy have been reported with success and have their merits and risks. Flexible scopes are better tolerated in the sedated patient, while rigid endoscopy requires general anesthesia. The use of the rigid esophagoscope has been reported to cause such complications as esophageal tear and perforation; however, in a significantly impacted or sharp foreign body, the rigid scope may be more helpful in removal and in protecting the esophagus as the object is withdrawn. Also, when the object is too large to fit within the rigid esophagoscope, the scope should be withdrawn together with the foreign body. An assistant should hold the mouth wide open to prevent the foreign body from being stripped by the teeth, thus causing it to fall into the pharynx.

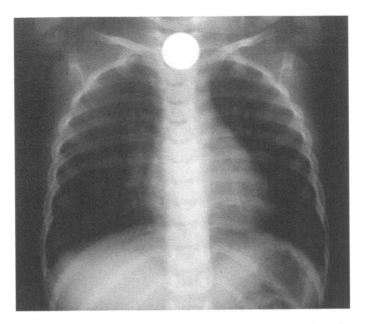

FIGURE 21.1 X-ray posterior-anterior view of chart with a metallic foreign body at the esophageal inlet.

Nonendoscopic techniques for removing an esophageal foreign body, such as the use of a Foley or Fogarty catheter, have been described.[7] The child is sedated and brought to the endoscopy or radiology suite. While the child is in steep Trendelenberg position, the catheter is placed beyond the foreign body and the balloon on the tip of the catheter is inflated and withdrawn. Because this method can lead to aspiration and airway obstruction if the foreign body is not carefully controlled as it exits the hypopharynx, it is not generally recommended.

COMPLICATIONS

Perforation of the esophagus can result from a sharp object such as a chicken bone or needle. It can also occur from the endoscopic procedure; therefore, rigid endoscopy should never be performed by unskilled persons. The esophagoscope should be advanced only when the esophageal lumen is visibly ahead and force should never be used. Following these rules will decrease the chance for iatrogenic esophageal injury.

When blood or purulent secretions are present in the esophagus, extra care must be taken because visualizing the lumen may be difficult. The symptoms of esophageal perforation and mediastinitis include fever, tachypnea, tachycardia, chest pain, and back pain, and must be recognized promptly. Confirmation is made with radiography using a water-soluble contrast study or CT scan. Treatment includes antimicrobial therapy to target Gram-negative rods and external drainage of a neck or mediastinal abscess, if necessary. The patient should not be allowed to feed orally; however, passing a nasogastric tube is also potentially dangerous because it may pass through the perforation. A large perforation may require surgical repair.

Erosion is more common when the foreign body contains an erosive substance such as the alkaline button type battery. As noted earlier, removal in this case is an emergency.

Retropharyngeal abscess has been reported as the most frequent complication of a sharp foreign body, such as a fish bone.[4] Objects that have been in the esophagus for an extended period of time may cause stricture formation. Although pseudodiverticulum is uncommon, it is also a recognized complication of a long-standing foreign body such as a coin (Figure 21.2).

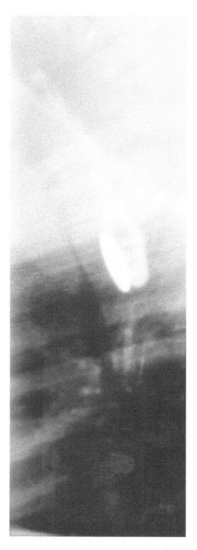

FIGURE 21.2 Pseudodiverticulum. Note that barium stints from top and outlines a small area in the proximal esophagus as the foreign body has migrated just anterior to the esophagus.

FOREIGN BODIES OF THE EAR

PRESENTATION

Otologic foreign bodies vary in presentation depending on the site within the ear, the duration present, and the nature of the object. Objects that are self-placed by a child may go undetected for extended periods because the child is hesitant to report such an action for fear of punishment. The parent may therefore be unaware of the situation until a complication has already occurred. Foreign bodies of the external canal are found most commonly among children between 2 and 4 years of age. They may be placed by a child or companion during play; curiosity, boredom, and imitation of others are thought to be causes. Insects may find their way into the external canal without any assistance. Das reviewed 233 cases of foreign bodies of the ear and nose and found the most consistent causative factor to be irritation or inflammation of these orifices.[8] Children with chronic itching, otitis externa, or otitis media are more likely to place objects in their ears.

Earrings may become embedded in the auricle when the site becomes infected and granulation forms. The use of spring-loaded guns to pierce ears has resulted in numerous such cases. More sites on the pinna are now being pierced, so it can be expected that this form of complication will increase in frequency. Also, when cartilaginous parts of the auricle such as the helix or tragus are pierced and infection ensues, chondritis or perichondritis may occur. This will necessitate removal of the ring or stud and antibiotic (frequently intravenous) coverage. Antiseptic technique when placing such piercings is of utmost importance to prevent such problems. It is also strongly advised that diabetics avoid piercing through cartilage.

Nonreactive substances such as plastic in the external ear canal that are not completely obstructing or touching the tympanic membrane may remain asymptomatic. Insects tend to incite local irritation, causing discomfort, erythema, and occasionally drainage. Vegetable matter can absorb moisture, swell, and cause increasing obstruction and inflammation. If complete obstruction occurs, a conductive hearing loss will occur. Very small objects may be difficult to visualize if lodged in the anterior sulcus or if the external canal is edematous. Filling the medial half of the canal with water to act as a concave lens may allow better visualization of this area.[9]

A relatively new type of foreign body, the alkaline button battery, bears special mention. Several reports have described the leakage of battery acid causing rapid onset local tissue destruction with pain, swelling, and drainage.[10–12] In addition to potentially serious injury to the external canal, tympanic membrane perforation has been reported to have occurred within 8 hours of entry.[10] Because this can lead to damage in the middle ear, removal must be immediate. Magnets may be helpful in removing these and other metallic objects.[13]

MANAGEMENT

Removal of most foreign bodies should be undertaken expeditiously but not emergently (except for the button batteries). Proper instrumentation should be at hand before beginning. The location and composition of the foreign body will help determine which instruments to use. First, an uncooperative child (and this includes most children in this situation) must be properly restrained in the parent's lap or a papoose. Excessive movement will lead to trauma of the ear with bleeding and decreased visibility.

An operating (open) otoscope or microscope should be available for best visualization. An alligator forceps, ear curette, right angle pick, and Frazier tip suction may be needed. Gentle irrigation may be used in certain instances, but should not be used with vegetable substances, which will swell. Irrigation should also be avoided when the tympanic membrane cannot be visualized because a perforation may already be present. Insects should be killed prior to removal by instilling mineral oil or 4% xylocaine into the external ear canal. Removal may then be accomplished with a suction or alligator forceps.

After removal of a foreign body, the external canal and tympanic membrane must be carefully examined. Aqueous-based acidic drops may be used for several days if the external canal appears injured or inflamed. The ear should be protected from water until resolution is complete.

COMPLICATIONS

Complications can be caused by the foreign body or by traumatic removal. Inflammation of external canal is usually not serious. It can be caused by an object that is mildly corrosive, reactive, or has been in the ear for a long time. Treatment includes water precautions and topical acidic drops. When a very corrosive object is involved, the complications may be serious. Necrosis and scarring of the soft tissue may develop. When circumferential, this can lead to canal stenosis. Debridement of the necrotic tissue, and packing or stenting of the external canal can prevent this outcome. If significant stenosis occurs, reconstructive surgery will be necessary. Necrosis of the tympanic membrane with permanent perforation, middle ear scarring, and conductive hearing loss can occur if a corrosive agent leaks deeper into the ear, as is the case with alkaline button batteries.

Lacerations of the external canal and tympanic membrane can occur due to impaction of sharp objects or traumatic removal. Balbani et al. reviewed 93 cases of ear foreign bodies and found that all 12 complications (11 canal lacerations and 1 tympanic membrane perforation) occurred in patients who had undergone previous attempts at removal.[14] Iatrogenic injuries can usually be avoided by using appropriate instruments, optimizing visualization, and employing proper restraint when necessary. An operating microscope is recommended when available and is imperative when the tympanic membrane cannot be seen. For lacerations of the canal wall, water precautions and acidic drops will likely prevent infection and further problems.

Tympanic membrane perforation requires careful examination with a microscope. If a flap of membrane has folded into the middle ear, it must be unfolded to encourage healing and to prevent cholesteatoma formation. When the tympanic membrane is not intact, the middle ear space may become contaminated and otitis media can develop. If the perforation does not heal spontaneously, patching or tympanoplasty may be necessary.

In summary, foreign bodies of the ear should be removed expeditiously. Urgent removal should be undertaken for button batteries or when evidence indicates tympanic membrane injury. If the proper equipment and ability to restrain the child are unavailable, consultation with an otolaryngologist is mandatory. Examination and removal may necessitate general anesthesia.

FOREIGN BODIES OF THE NOSE

PRESENTATION

The predicaments that lead to foreign bodies in the nose are similar to those of the ear. Boredom, curiosity, and acts of imitation are frequent factors; Das found chronic rhinitis to be the most common factor.[8] Foreign objects occasionally enter the nose accidentally while the child is sniffing or smelling. The overall incidence increases when toy sales increase, such as at Christmas and in summer.[15]

Children will typically not confess to having placed a foreign object in the nose. The most common finding is unilateral purulent, often foul smelling discharge. In fact, unilateral rhinorrhea in a young child should be considered evidence of a foreign body until proved otherwise. Less often, epistaxis may be the presenting symptom.[16] When an alkaline disc battery is lodged in the nose, symptoms and signs of acute inflammation may be present. Tissue damage may occur rapidly, as in the ear, due to electrical burn, liquefaction necrosis, and pressure necrosis.[17] These findings may go unnoticed until secondary complications have developed.

Diagnosis is made upon careful inspection of the nasal cavities. This will require powerful illumination, a nasal speculum, suction, possibly a nasal endoscope, and always cooperation or proper restraint. X-rays may be helpful if the object is radiopaque or has become calcified. An incidental finding of a nasal foreign body on a routine dental roentgenogram has been reported.[18] U.S. toy manufacturers are required by law to make toy parts radiopaque; however, toys and parts manufactured outside the U.S. need not conform to this regulation. In their review of children with nasal foreign bodies, Tong et al. found that 28 of 71 (31%) radiographs demonstrated a foreign object.[15]

MANAGEMENT

Nasal foreign bodies should be removed as quickly as possible to prevent local inflammation, tissue damage, and aspiration. Topical application of a decongestant and anesthetic will help visualization and cooperation. When cooperation is not forthcoming and restraint is inadequate, general anesthesia is advisable. Nasal secretions should be suctioned and the foreign body removed with a forceps. One of the authors finds a Hartmann forceps to be the most useful. Following removal, both nasal cavities should be inspected — optimally, with an endoscope — to look for other foreign bodies or a residual fragment of the removed object. A foreign substance that has been allowed to remain in the nose for an extended period of time may become calcified and form what is known as a rhinolith. Removing rhinoliths is often difficult and bloody.

Several alternative methods of removing nasal foreign bodies have been described that can be attempted in the office. Placing pepper in the nose to induce a sneeze or blowing in the child's mouth while occluding the contralateral nostril have been described; however, the authors do not recommend them. In a more controlled fashion, nebulized adrenaline together with nose blowing has yielded success.[19] Finkelstein reported success with oral ambu-bag insufflation while placing the patient in Trendelenberg position.[20] Removal with a Fogarty or small Foley catheter has been described; the catheter is passed through the nose beyond the foreign body and then inflated with 2 to 3 cc of saline. It is then pulled forward, expelling the foreign body.[7,21] Of course, there is a risk of pushing the object distally in the nose and possibly the nasopharynx, which can lead to aspiration.

Soft, friable objects can be removed with a Frazier tip suction. Firm objects that are flat or have a thin edge can be removed with a Hartmann or alligator forceps. A wire loop or ear curette may be passed beyond the foreign body and pulled forward to expel a firm or spherical object. After the foreign body is removed, local inflammation may manifest as purulent or bloody discharge or crusting. Saline drops or antibiotic ointment may then be instilled for several days. If the foreign body was an alkaline battery, sterile water should be used instead of saline.

COMPLICATIONS

As with the ear, problems can occur due to the foreign body or because of its removal. Complications include epistaxis, local infection, inflammation, and irritation. Scarring can occur between the nasal septum and turbinate if raw surfaces are near each other; this is called a synechia. One can prevent this by placing a stent of nonreactive material such as silastic or absorbable Gelfilm between raw surfaces. Nasal septal perforation has been reported in the literature and has recently been seen by one of the authors in a 7-year-old boy as a result of a disc battery that had been lodged in the anterior nasal cavity for almost 2 years.[15] It was discovered when the child was brought in for evaluation of a collapsing nasal dorsum and saddling of the nose.

Sinusitis can occur if the foreign body or the surrounding inflammation obstruct the middle meatus and the sinus ostia. This will present with pain and tenderness over the involved sinus or opacification on a radiograph. Treatment includes antibiotics, nasal decongestant spray, and possibly, nasal steroid spray. The most feared complication of a nasal foreign body or its attempted removal is aspiration. This can happen when the object is accidentally pushed backward into the nasopharynx. It is therefore imperative that an object lodged in the posterior nasal cavity, particularly a smooth, spherical object, be removed as soon as possible. The child must be restrained appropriately with proper lighting and instrumentation available. When the foreign object is difficult to grasp or the patient cannot be restrained adequately, extraction should take place in the operating room using general anesthesia and endotracheal intubation.

CONCLUSIONS

Foreign bodies of the esophagus, ear, and nose tend to occur in smaller children who will often not report the incident. The symptoms and signs of this problem vary widely, depending on the location, nature, and duration of the foreign object. Radiography may aid in the diagnosis. Removal is best performed by skilled personnel in a controlled environment with a full array of equipment. Regardless of their location, alkaline disc batteries must be removed emergently. Complications can result from the foreign body or its removal.

REFERENCES

1. *Injury Facts*, National Safety Council, Chicago, 1999.
2. Witt, W.J. The role of rigid endoscopy in foreign body management. *Ear Nose Throat J.,* 1985, 64, 70.
3. Turtz, M.G. and Stool, S.E. Foreign bodies of the pharynx and esophagus. In Bluestone, C.D. and Stool, S.E., Eds. *Ped. Otolaryngol.*, 2nd ed., Philadelphia: W.B. Saunders, 1990.
4. Singh, B. et al. Complications associated with 327 foreign bodies of the pharynx, larynx, and esophagus. *Ann. Otol. Rhinol. Laryngol.,* 1997, 106, 301.
5. Giordano, A. et al. Current management of esophageal foreign bodies. *Arch. Otol.,* 1981, 107, 249.
6. Derkay, C.S. et al. Retrieving foreign bodies from upper aerodigestive tracts of children. *AORN J.* 1994, 60, 53.
7. Henry, L.N. and Chamberlain, J.W. Removal of foreign bodies from the esophagus and nose with the with the use of a Foley catheter. *Surgery,* 1972, 71, 918.
8. Das, S.K. Etiological evaluation of foreign bodies in the ear and nose. *J. Laryngol. Otol.,* 1984, 98, 989.
9. Peltola, T.J. and Scarent, R. Water used to visualize and remove hidden foreign bodies from the external ear canal. *J. Laryngol. Otol.,* 1992, 106, 157.
10. Capo, J.M. and Lucente, F.E. Alkaline foreign bodies of the ear and nose. *J. Laryngol. Otol.,* 1986, 98, 989.
11. Rachlin, L.S. Assault with battery [letter]. *N. Engl. J. Med.,* 1984, 311, 921.
12. Skinner, D.W. and Chiu, P. The hazards of "button-sized" batteries as foreign bodies in the nose and ear. *J. Laryngol. Otol.,* 1986, 100, 1315.
13. Landry, G.L. and Edmanson, M.B. Attractive method for battery removal [letter]. *JAMA,* 1986, 256, 3351.
14. Balbani, A.P. et al. Ear and nose foreign body removal in children. *Int. J. Pediatr. Otorhinolaryngol.,* 1998, 46, 37.
15. Tong, M.C. et al. Nasal foreign bodies in children. *Int. J. Pediatr. Otorhinolaryngol.,* 1996, 35, 207.
16. Yanigasawa, E. and Citardi, M.J. Endoscopic view of a foreign body in the nose. *Ear Nose Throat J.,* 1995, 74, 8.
17. Alvi, A. et al. Miniature disc battery in the nose: a dangerous foreign body. *Clin. Pediatr.,* 1997, 36, 427.
18. Kittle, P.E. et al. Incidental finding of an intranasal foreign body discovered on routine dental examination. *Pediatr. Dent.,* 1991, 13, 49.
19. Douglas, A.R. Use of nebulized adrenaline to aid expulsion of intranasal foreign bodiesin children. *J. Laryngol. Otol.,* 1996, 110, 559.
20. Finkelstein, J.A. Oral ambu-bag insufflation to remove unilateral nasal foreign bodies. *Am. J. Emerg. Med.,* 1996, 14, 57.
21. Nandapalan, V. and McIlwain, J.C. Removal of nasal foreign bodies with a Fogarty biliary balloon catheter. *J. Laryngol. Otol.,* 1992, 106, 157.

Section VI

Airway and Endoscopy

22 Extubation Problems in Infants and Children

Ellen S. Deutsch and George H. Zalzal

The more prepared you are for problems, the less likely they are to occur.

William C. Gray, M.D.

CONTENTS

AWARENESS

Intubation is an important and beneficial component of modern medical care. It entails many serious risks and medical practitioners devote a great deal of thought and effort toward organizing and accomplishing this task safely. Extubation also entails many serious risks, but it may not always receive the same attention. For example, many clinicians are surprised to learn that potentially serious complications, such as desaturation and laryngospasm, are more common immediately after tracheal extubation than during induction in patients undergoing elective general anesthesia.[1]

Postextubation problems may result from the extubation, or the extubation may unmask or reveal abnormalities that were previously obscured while the patient was intubated. Some problems may have developed during the intubation or during the period in which intubation was maintained, or they may be related to the underlying condition that necessitated the intubation. Some problems become obvious at the time of extubation; others manifest weeks to months later.

EXTUBATION RISK FACTORS

Anatomic and mechanical factors, as well as co-morbid conditions, may contribute to postintubation airway complications. Sorting out their relative impact, particularly for acquired lesions with delayed manifestations, can be difficult. Skilled and attentive medical and nursing care is essential to minimize potential intubation complications. Intensive care physicians responsible for many aspects of the care of intubated patients need to be aware always of the incidence of late complications.[2]

ANATOMY AND DEVELOPMENT

Several factors make the infant's subglottis, containing the cricoid cartilage, particularly vulnerable to injury. In contrast to adults, for whom the vocal fold region makes up the narrowest portion of the airway, the subglottis is the narrowest portion of the upper conductive airway in infants and young children.[3,4] In a healthy, full-term newborn, the diameter of the normal subglottic region is approximately 4.5 mm.[2] In addition, unlike the thyroid and tracheal cartilages, the cricoid cartilage comprises a rigid and complete ring, so swelling must impinge on the lumen, at the expense of the airway.[2,4] Because airflow resistance is inversely related to the fourth power of the radius, even 1 mm of circumferential edema can significantly impair airflow and gas exchange; subglottic edema that would be asymptomatic in an adult could be life threatening in an infant.[4]

Many additional anatomic differences distinguish infants' airway physiology from adults'. Infants have a larger tongue and relative retrognathia.[3] The infant's larynx is more cephalad, usually between the second and fourth cervical vertebrae; it reaches the adult level of C-5 or C-6 by about 4 years of age. The anterior attachment of the vocal folds is lower or more caudal, and the trachea is directed somewhat posteriorly.[3] The 5.7-cm average tracheal length predisposes infants to accidental extubation or endobronchial intubation with movement of the endotracheal tube tip that occurs with changes in head position.[3]

PULMONARY PHYSIOLOGY

Although the work of breathing is the same in a term infant and adult (about 1 to 2% of minute oxygen consumption), minute oxygen consumption is approximately twice as high in infants as in adults because of a higher metabolic rate.[3] Adults use approximately 2 to 4% of total resting oxygen consumption for quiet breathing; premature infants use approximately 6%. In disease states, an infant's total oxygen consumption may increase to 30% or more; if prolonged, this extreme work of breathing can result in exhaustion and ventilatory failure.[5]

Preterm infants and term infants in the first weeks of life have an immature central respiratory drive and may respond to hypoxia with paradoxical respiratory depression; hypothermia also decreases ventilatory drive.[3] The immature respiratory musculature and soft, compliant cartilaginous thoracic wall can retract or collapse when faced with increased pulmonary resistive forces.[3] The more horizontal rib position decreases the contribution of the intercostal muscles to ventilation and makes gas exchange primarily reliant on the diaphragm, whose movement can be impeded by the relatively large abdominal cavity, particularly if it becomes distended.[3]

MECHANICS AND PHYSICAL PROPERTIES

Duration of Intubation and the Physical Characteristics of the Tube

Duration of intubation and the physical characteristics of the tube, particularly its size and unfavorable shape, are considered the two most important factors predisposing to injury.[2] There are no "rules" for the optimum duration of intubation. In general, endoscopic assessment is indicated in most adults after 5 to 7 days of intubation, in children after 1 to 2 weeks, and in infants when attempted extubation has been unsuccessful.[2] Intubation can be relatively safely continued, possibly with an endotracheal tube of smaller diameter, when the changes seen include edema in the vocal folds, edematous protrusion of the ventricles, surface mucosal ulceration, generalized erythema, and minor granulation tissue at the vocal process. Of particular importance is the absence of deep ulceration indicating perichondritis.[2] The size of the endotracheal tube relative to the child is important.[6] Many, but not all, authors recommend that an uncuffed endotracheal tube should be small enough to allow an inspiratory leak in conjunction with a positive pressure breath at approximately 20 cm H_2O pressure.[2,5]

Traumatic Intubation, Repeated Intubation, and Tube Movement

Traumatic intubation, repeated intubation, and tube movement may result in laryngeal injury. The risk increases with urgent intubation attempts, with an inexperienced operator, if the introducer (stylette) is used improperly, or if the child has an underlying anatomic abnormality.[2,5,6] Laryngeal injury produced during intubation in a patient requiring long-term intubation may be the nidus for a significant long-term laryngeal complication.[7] To decrease the need for reintubation, incidents of premature extubation or occlusion of the endotracheal tube should be minimized. Care needs to be taken to minimize endotracheal tubes' occlusion by kinking or by mucus obstruction, particularly in young infants with small diameter endotracheal tubes.[8] Motion of the child or motion of tube relative to the child, such as from bucking, coughing, head motion, transmitted ventilator movements, and manipulation of the tube or the child during procedures, should be minimized. Sedation may be indicated.[2,5,6]

Cuff Injuries

Cuff injuries are now seldom seen because large-volume, low-pressure cuffs have been designed to prevent tracheal damage; however, even these cuffs can be converted into injurious high-pressure cuffs by overinflation.[2,5,7,9] In the past, tracheal stenoses were more common and were caused primarily by pressure necrosis from the traditional high-pressure endotracheal tube cuffs.[9]

Prolonged Positioning

Prolonged positioning such as prone or Trendelenburg positioning may also predispose to laryngeal injury in intubated patients.[5]

Endotracheal Tube Composition

Endotracheal tube composition has been suggested as a risk factor for injury. Endotracheal tubes made of inexpensive polyvinylchloride contain numerous chemical additives that may leach into surrounding tissues; silicone tubes are less reactive and have reduced bacterial adherence.[10]

Nasogastric Tubes

Nasogastric tubes also increase the risk of reflux. They can cause postcricoid ulceration and necrosis and, rarely, acquired tracheoesophageal fistulae. If necessary, soft small tubes should be selected.[2,10]

CO-MORBID CONDITIONS

Extraesophageal Gastric Reflux

Extraesophageal gastric reflux contributes to granuloma formation, exacerbation of subglottic stenosis, and other laryngeal injuries.[10–12] After extubation, patients with reflux may have stridor, laryngospasm, chronic cough, and obstructive apnea.[11] Vigorous treatment of reflux,[2,10] including head elevation and, possibly, promotility agents, H_2 blocking agents, or proton pump inhibitors, should be considered.

Underlying Anatomic or Metabolic Conditions

Underlying anatomic or metabolic conditions may predispose to laryngotracheal injury or contribute to respiratory difficulty after extubation. Intrinsic laryngeal or tracheal cartilage abnormalities or extrinsic cartilage compression may contribute to respiratory difficulty after extubation. The risk of injury is increased with a history of croup, external laryngeal trauma, current or recent upper respiratory tract infection, acute laryngotracheitis, or impaired mucociliary clearance.[2,5,6] Medical conditions associated with subglottic stenosis include cleft lip and palate, Crouzon's disease, and Down syndrome.[5] Acromegaly and Wegener's granulomatosis are associated with laryngeal stenosis.[5] The risk of complications is increased in patients who have undergone surgical procedures in the head and neck, with nutritional deficits, such as those from burns, and with acute or chronic disease states such as anemia; hypoxia; hypotension; chronic infection; superinfection; significant heart, kidney, or liver disease; or other systemic illness.[2,5,12]

MECHANISM OF INJURY

An endotracheal tube will always lie in and exert pressure on the posterior larynx affecting three possible sites of major damage: the medial surfaces of the arytenoid cartilages, cricoarytenoid joints, and vocal processes; the posterior glottis and interarytenoid region; and the subglottis involving the inner surface of the cricoid cartilage, usually the posterior lamina.[2,7] When this pressure is greater than mucosal capillary pressure, ischemia occurs, first with irritation and then with congestion, edema, and eventually, ulceration. Injury can also be caused by frictional erosion.[13]

Progressive ulceration causes perichondritis, chondritis, and finally, necrosis: a "laryngeal bedsore."[2] Glottic edema and mucosal ulceration are common and may occur within hours of endotracheal tube intubation, while epithelial loss may occur after only 3 hours of endotracheal intubation.[4,12,14,15] Granulation tissue proliferates at the margins of the injured area and persistent granulation tissue becomes a localized intubation granuloma. New collagen matures to fibrous, firm scar tissue with progressive narrowing of the airway as the scar slowly contracts. Although the incidence of tracheal injury has decreased with the use of low-pressure cuffs, no corresponding decrease has been seen in the incidence of laryngeal injuries.[2]

EXTUBATION

PREPARATION

It is necessary to evaluate whether the condition initially resulting in intubation has been resolved or adequately improved and to ascertain whether any other congenital, acquired, or developmental lesions may directly or indirectly interfere with successful extubation. Potential upper airway sources of obstruction include nasal or choanal lesions, enlarged tonsils and adenoids, macroglossia, retrognathia, and temporomandibular joint ankylosis, as well as foreign bodies such as throat packs or blood clots.[16] Central airway lesions may include vocal fold paralysis; laryngeal, tracheal, or bronchial stenosis or malacia; or tracheomegaly (Figure 22.1).[6,9] Adverse pulmonary conditions include bronchopulmonary dysplasia, reactive airway disease, infections, and thoracic cavity abnormalities such as those from Lejeune's disease, camptomelic dysplasia, and diaphragmatic hernia. Fluid restriction or diuresis may be indicated.[5]

It is necessary to evaluate whether potential extubation difficulties from complications or management during intubation have been appropriately addressed. Aggressive positive pressure ventilation can result in barotrauma injuries.[3] Atelectasis from endotracheal tube advancement or mucus plugs may have occurred. Nasally intubated infants weighing less than 1500 g are at increased risk of postextubation atelectasis.[17] Musculoskeletal and neurologic conditions may interfere with airway maintenance and protection. Residual effects from neuromuscular blocking medications, narcotics, and sedatives can also be problematic.[3]

Preparation for extubation generally includes titration of any sedation and the prophylactic administration of large doses of steroids, although conclusive evidence of efficacy is lacking.[6,7] The equipment and personnel necessary for reintubation should be available. Most extubations are accomplished in the intensive care unit, but extubation in the operating room may be more

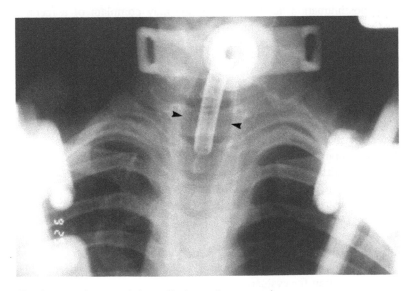

FIGURE 22.1 Tracheomegaly around the cuff of a tracheotomy tube.

appropriate, based on the likelihood and potential difficulty of reintubation as well as the resources in each location. During extubation, difficulty in removing an endotracheal tube is rare, but can be caused by an undeflated or excessively large cuff catching on the vocal folds; adhesion of the tube to the tracheal wall because of an absence of lubricant; or transfixion by a suture or wire to an adjacent structure, particularly following neck or chest surgery.[16]

PERIEXTUBATION EXAMINATION

A flexible fiberoptic examination with the endotracheal tube *in situ* in the intensive care unit without general anesthesia is generally not helpful. Removing the endotracheal tube allows an unimpeded assessment of the posterior glottis and the subglottis. Rigid postextubation endoscopy is generally performed under a general anesthestic. However, with small, relatively flaccid infants in an neonatal intensive care unit (NICU) or pediatric intensive care unit (PICU) setting and neonatologist or intensivist at bedside, extubation with rigid endoscopic visualization may be safely considered in selected circumstances.

POSTEXTUBATION ASSESSMENT

Delayed manifestations of airway problems can present from hours to months or even years after extubation.[12,15,18] Pain, dyspnea, stridor, and persistent sore throat should alert the physician to a possible airway injury. A patient who develops symptoms of airway obstruction and who has been intubated and ventilated in the recent past should be considered to have an organic lesion until the case is proved otherwise.

One can observe for increased work of breathing, with nasal flaring, chest retractions and stridor; cervical auscultation is also useful.[7] Hoarseness is common early after extubation but usually resolves rapidly.[15] Postextubation edema is evidenced by a barking or brassy cough, hoarseness, inspiratory stridor, and chest wall retractions.[5] Manifestations of laryngeal injury range from a mild change in vocal quality to severe stridor, hoarseness, and dyspnea.[15]

Radiologic studies may be helpful in evaluating postextubation airway lesions, but airway endoscopy provides the most useful information. Sedation or general anesthesia with sustained spontaneous ventilation facilitates the endoscopic evaluation of dynamic, as well as anatomic, lesions such as vocal fold paralysis or tracheomalacia and decreases the risk of airway collapse. Use of general anesthesia with paralysis will allow nondynamic evaluation of anatomic lesions.[15]

Patients with postintubation laryngeal granuloma may complain of a feeling of fullness or foreign body in the throat.[12] Instead of improving gradually over weeks, patients with severe glottic, subglottic, or tracheal injury show persistence or worsening of their symptoms as granulomas form and scar tissue contracts.[2,15] Symptoms of subglottic or tracheal stenosis may include exertional or progressive dyspnea, stridor, wheezing that progresses to stridor, trouble clearing secretions, discomfort in the chest and throat, and chronic cough.[15,18] In contrast, sedentary patients can tolerate surprising degrees of airway constriction.[12,18] Diagnosis can be delayed because the symptoms are often mistakenly attributed to pathologic pulmonary processes.[15]

Simple diagnostic radiologic studies, such as postero-anterior and lateral soft tissue neck and chest x-rays, easily demonstrate many airway lesions.[18] For selected lesions, tracheobronchography adds information about airflow dynamics in the distal airway, as well as a unified, rather than planar slice, view of the airway.[19] Helical thin section high-resolution computed tomography (CT) with three-dimensional reconstruction can provide helpful information, particularly for tracheal injuries. Magnetic resonance (MR) imaging is useful, but adds little diagnostic information over plain radiography, despite its added expense.[15] The new application of "virtual endoscopy," using three-dimensional image projection from digitized CT or MR imaging may prove to be very useful.[20] Diagnostic pulmonary function testing with flow volume curves may be of interest, but offers limited practical information for evaluating severe stenosis.[18]

MANAGEMENT OF POSTEXTUBATION PATHOLOGY

GENERAL PRINCIPLES

Immediate postextubation management (see Chapter 6) may include supplemental oxygen, cool humidification, systemic steroids, racemic epinephrine or racemic epinephrine with nebulized dexamethasone[3,5], and use of helium–oxygen mixtures ("heliox").[5,7,21] Additional interventions may include the application of continuous positive airway pressure (CPAP), particularly in infants; placement of a nasopharyngeal airway; and placing the patient in a high Fowler's position or the patient's position of comfort.[5] Mitomycin-C, an antineoplastic antibiotic that inhibits fibroblast proliferation, is currently being investigated as an adjunctive agent to prevent restenosis after treatment and may have applicability in managing acute injuries.[25-27]

SPECIFIC LESIONS

Glottic or Subglottic Edema

Glottic or subglottic edema typically maximizes within 4 hours after extubation; symptoms include inspiratory stridor, croupy cough, and possibly, respiratory distress (Figure 22.2A–C).[2,5,6] When not accompanied by ulceration or perichondritis, edema is usually reversible and symptoms typically resolve within 24 hours.[2,5] Diffuse swelling of the mucosa of the laryngeal ventricles is common and is described as "protrusion of edematous mucosa of the ventricle," which quickly subsides once the endotracheal tube is removed.[2] The decrease in airway caliber, however, causes an exponential increase in airway resistance that may precipitate respiratory failure necessitating reintubation.[2,5] Persistent vocal fold edema occasionally manifests as chronic Reinke's edema with a permanently husky voice.[2]

Ulceration

Superficial ulceration heals when the endotracheal tube is removed, but deep ulceration into perichondrium or cartilage may progress to form scar tissue and eventual stenosis. Benjamin describes a classic injury of an "ulcerated trough" as an obvious, wide, deep area of erosion and round ulceration of the medial aspect of the arytenoid and cricoid cartilages. Weeks or months after extubation, healing and fibrosis lead to a contracted linear "healed furrow" associated with chronic dysfunction or even fixation of the cricoarytenoid joint.[2] Severe injuries with deep ulceration into the cartilage of the arytenoid, cricoid, or cricoarytenoid joint indicate the need for extubation or tracheotomy as soon as possible so that the endotracheal tube can be removed.[2]

Granulation Tissue

Granulation tissue may form at the site of irritation and ulceration caused by tube pressure (Figure 22.3).[2] Large, flap-like "tongues of granulation tissue" begin to arise within 48 hours of intubation. They can cause severe valve-like obstruction almost immediately after extubation, but usually resolve completely. Occasionally, unilateral removal is necessary; microbiology culture for antibiotic coverage may be helpful. If persistent, granulation tissue can cause partial airway obstruction, as well as a husky, weak voice when vocal fold apposition is impaired.[2]

Granulomas

Granulomas may result from ulcerations within the larynx or, less frequently, trachea (Figure 22.4). Some resolve spontaneously and others can present with a husky voice many weeks after extubation.[2,12] Pedunculated granulomas can be removed with a biopsy forceps or laser; sessile lesions

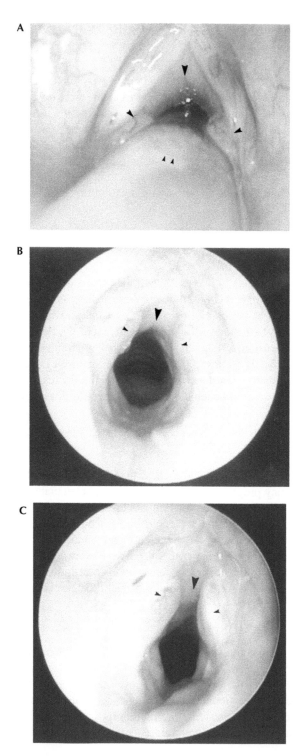

FIGURE 22.2 Demonstration of progression of edema and airway obstruction following extubation of an 8-week-old premature gestation triplet: A. view of larynx while intubated; B. lumen of airway immediately after extubation; C. lumen of the airway several minutes after extubation. Without the airway stenting effect of the endotracheal tube, the edematous tissue expands, narrowing the airway. Small arrows: granulation tissue; larger arrow: subglottic edema; double arrows: endotracheal tube.

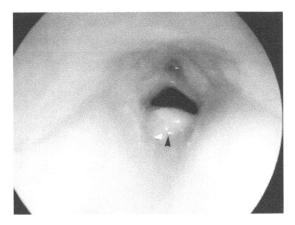

FIGURE 22.3 Premature, 11-week-old gestation infant. Removal of posterior glottic granulation tissue (arrow) enabled successful extubation.

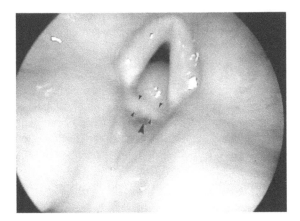

FIGURE 22.4 Posterior glottic synechiae in a 10-year-old boy intubated for 2 weeks following a motor vehicle crash, who presented with a hoarse voice and exercise intolerance. The granuloma and the central portion of the synechiae (small arrows) were resected. Note the small opening between synechiae and posterior glottis (large arrow) that distinguishes this from posterior glottic stenosis.

may require careful resection to avoid injuring the perichondrium. After removal, antibiotics and systemic corticosteroids are helpful.[15]

Laryngeal Webs

Laryngeal webs in the anterior commissure can be treated endoscopically using laser therapy under suspension microlaryngoscopy. Repair of a thick, fibrotic web may require reinforced stents fixed in place endoscopically with translaryngeal sutures to prevent restenosis after treatment.

Interarytenoid Synechia

Interarytenoid synechia from ulceration involving the vocal processes of the arytenoids can lead to granulation tissue, which may fuse and then fibrose into a firm, fibrous band that pulls the arytenoid cartilages together, thus limiting vocal fold abduction (Figure 22.5).[2,14] The lesion is frequently hidden on nasoendoscopic view, and the anterior opening may be mistaken for the glottis,

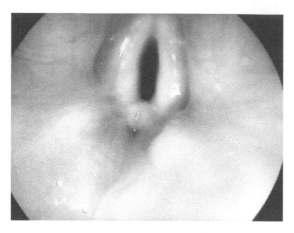

FIGURE 22.5 Ulceration progressed over 4 weeks to an interarytenoid synechiae in a 4.5-month-old boy intubated for respiratory illness. Note the small opening posterior to synechiae.

leading to an erroneous diagnosis of bilateral adbuctor paralysis. Scar division or excision with laser or microsurgical instruments provides dramatic improvement.[2,14]

Vocal Fold Paralysis

Vocal fold paralysis is thought to result from compression of the anterior branches of the recurrent laryngeal nerve between the arytenoid and the laryngeal cartilages by the endotracheal tube cuff.[2,10,15] Spontaneous recovery from this neuropraxia usually occurs within 6 months.[2,10] Because this lesion is extremely rare, mechanical posterior laryngeal disorders should be considered. Laryngeal electromyography may be useful in confirming normal innervation.[14,22]

Artenoid Dislocation or Subluxation/Cricoarytenoid Fixation or Ankylosis

Arytenoid dislocation or subluxation from intubation may result in cricoarytenoid fixation or ankylosis, a condition often misdiagnosed or poorly assessed.[2,8] Mucosal ulceration over the arytenoid cartilage may invade the cricoarytenoid joint, causing an active arthritis with ultimate fusion of the cricoarytenoid joint.[10] Patients can present with persistent hoarseness and odynophagia.[2,10] If the cricoarytenoid joints are ankylosed with the vocal cords in the adducted position, inspiratory airway obstruction may be present with a nearly normal voice.[2]

Mobility of the arytenoid on the articular facet of the cricoid can be seen and "felt" during direct laryngoscopy. Using a rigid instrument to exert gentle pressure on the medial aspect of the arytenoid cartilage allows assessment of lateral movement; similar pressure on the lateral aspect allows assessment of medial movement.[2] Cricoarytenoid joint abnormalities may be difficult to demonstrate, but should be considered if surrounding changes such as posterior glottic stenosis, a healed furrow, or a healed fibrous nodule are also present.[2]

If dislocation of the cricoarytenoid joint is detected during the acute phase, repositioning should be attempted, although there is little evidence that this can be effectively achieved.[2] When arytenoids and the interarytenoid space have been eroded, steroid injection into the submucosa of the interarytenoid and immediate cricoarytenoid regions may be helpful.[10] However, most cases of cricoaryntenoid joint ankylosis present late, with limited movement or fixation in the joint; attempts to manipulate the cartilage into position using endoscopic or open surgical approaches are difficult and unlikely to be successful.[2,10,15] Other management options include arytenoidectomy, which can be accomplished using a laser; however, this is potentially associated with worsening of the voice or subsequent aspiration-induced pneumonia.[15]

Posterior Glottic Stenosis

Posterior glottic stenosis may result from deep annular ulceration in the posterior glottis with secondary fibrosis and scar formation. Its presence indicates the need for extubation or tracheotomy in order to allow removal of the endotracheal tube.[2] The transverse fibrotic scar may be a thin and crescentic web, but is usually firm and thick.[2] Vertical incision of the interarytenoid web of scar tissue from the subglottic region to the interarytenoid region, with extension into the muscle when necessary, temporarily releases the stenosis, but restenosis is likely and may require repeated division.[2,15] Laryngofissure allows access to excise the web-like scar for placement of a free or pedicled mucosal graft to cover the denuded area; this may be spot welded in place using the CO_2 laser or arytenoidectomy, vocal cord lateralization, or cartilage graft.[2,15] Severe scarring of the posterior commissure is relatively difficult to treat, and the results of endoscopic or open surgical approaches are often poor.[15]

Acquired Subglottic Stenosis

Acquired subglottic stenosis is the most common serious long-term consequence of neonatal intubation (Figure 22.6A and B).[23] Nonsurgical management options include expectant management, removal of granulation tissue, and the use of systemic steroids. Dilation or laser procedures are used only in limited circumstances and can contribute to increased trauma and fibrosis, as well as near-total or total obliteration of the lumen.[2] Open surgical management options include tracheotomy; cricoid split; laryngotracheal reconstruction or laryngotracheoplasty, with or without placement of a stent; and cricotracheal resection.

Subglottic Cysts

Incidences of subglottic cysts appear to be increasing in frequency with the increased utilization of prolonged intubation (Figure 22.7). They most likely represent mucoceles that occur following trauma to the ducts of the abundant mucus glands within the subglottic mucosa.[23] The cysts enlarge gradually but may cause significant airway obstruction; patients often present months after extubation.[2] The cysts may be marsupialized or removed with laser vaporization or laryngeal microinstumentation.[2,23]

Tracheal Stenosis

Tracheal stenosis is almost always the result of pressure necrosis from an endotracheal tube cuff.[15] In an acute emergency situation, dilatation under general anesthesia provides temporary relief, but excessive pressure may rupture the membranous wall of the trachea rather than pass through the stenosis.[9,15] Full-thickness destruction of the tracheal wall rarely responds to conservative measures, and prolonged stenting, repeated dilatations, local or systemic use of steroids, and destruction of scar tissue by biopsy forceps, electrocoagulation, cryosurgery, or laser generally provide only temporary relief.[9]

Although rare, thin tracheal webs and areas of granulation may be permanently cured with laser therapy. Application of laser therapy, however, has not achieved long-term success in most patients with postintubation tracheal stenosis and may ultimately cause more scarring and stricturing.[9,15,18,24] Most tracheal stenoses are best treated by resection and reconstruction using a neck and/or upper sternotomy approach.[9,15,24] Tracheostomy is only instituted if correction of the stenosis must be delayed. If the lesion is accessible through the neck, a tracheotomy should be made through the damaged trachea at the level of the stenosis.[9] Alternatively, a tracheal T-tube can be used for patients with a functional glottis who are not surgical candidates.[15]

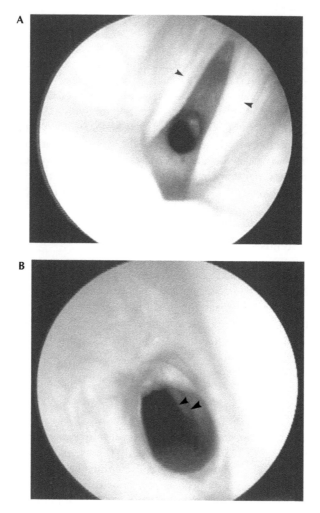

FIGURE 22.6 Neonatally acquired subglottic stenosis in an 11-year-old boy: (A) view from above the vocal folds (arrows); (B) close-up; tracheal rings can be seen beyond the stenosis (arrows).

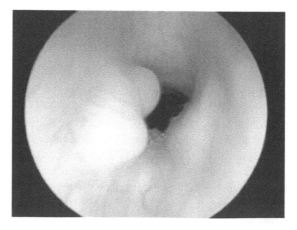

FIGURE 22.7 Multiple subglottic cysts.

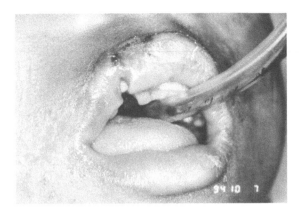

FIGURE 22.8 Tooth displaced and lip eroded in a child intubated, sedated, and chemically paralyzed following laryngotracheal reconstruction.

Incidental Injuries

Incidental injuries can occur in a variety of ways in intubated patients. Patients intubated orally may sustain tongue paresis, paralysis, or necrosis; palatal necrosis, clefting, grooving, or asymmetry; alveolar and lip ulceration; primary tooth dilaceration; cross-bite; poor speech intelligibility; and enamel hypoplasia (Figure 22.8).[8,11,17,28,29]

SURGICAL INTERVENTION

GENERAL CONSIDERATIONS

If surgical intervention is indicated, procedures that can be accomplished in adults and even larger children may not be feasible in small children because of limitations related to airway and instrument size. Pediatric-trained support staff, anesthesiologists, and intensivists are an essential consideration. Appropriate instrumentation for newborns and children must be available. The surgeon must be experienced with laser procedures as well as with the complicated head and neck airway procedures indicated for newborns and young children. When in doubt, continued intubation with transport to a facility with greater resources for definitive diagnosis and management is an appropriate consideration.

CRICOID SPLIT

The cricoid split operation, i.e., anterior cricoid decompression, is designed to alleviate subglottic stenosis without resorting to a tracheotomy.[30] In contrast to laryngotracheal reconstruction, it is generally performed in smaller patients with fresh, rather than mature, subglottic injury. Generally, candidates have subglottic edema or stenosis but are otherwise ready for extubation and weigh at least 1500 g.

The cricoid split is performed on an intubated child under general anesthesia. The cricoid cartilage is exposed in the manner of performing a tracheotomy. A vertical midline incision is made in the anterior lamina of the cricoid and the first two tracheal rings, allowing the edges of the cricoid cartilage to "spring" open.[30] The incision may also be extended superiorly into the lower portion of the thyroid cartilage. Some surgeons will use endoscopic guidance to direct their cartilage incision to minimize potential injury to the anterior commissure. Dividing the posterior lamina or making lateral cuts in the cricoid ring may also be performed depending on the identified pathology.

The cartilagenous middle third of the (infant) hyoid can be harvested as a graft and then shaped and sutured into the anterior incision. Similarly, a portion of the superior thyroid lamina cartilage may be used. The patient is then reintubated on the operating table with a larger endotracheal tube. A passive drain is placed to allow any air escaping from the cricotracheal incision egress through the skin. The patient remains intubated for up to 7 to 10 days; sedation, paralysis, mechanical ventilation, and supportive care are used. Intravenous steroids are given for the final 24 hours and then extubation is attempted.[31]

The cricoid split has been described as a "simple" surgical procedure involving potentially complicated and problematic postoperative care.[32] Potential complications from prolonged paralysis and sedation must be adequately assessed and addressed prior to extubation. The potential for unsuccessful extubation from continued or progressive airway pathology must be acknowledged when informed surgical consent is obtained from the family, with the understanding that additional surgical procedures may be required.

CONCLUSION

Intubation is a life-saving medical intervention for many infants and children, but serious complications may occur. Constant vigilance is required to decrease the incidence of laryngeal and tracheal injury in intubated patients, who often cannot protect themselves because of underlying conditions or pharmacologic intervention. An understanding of the pathophysiology of injury will improve strategies for prevention. Knowledge and awareness of the subtle distinctions between various airway lesions is essential to helping select appropriate management. The techniques of surgical resection and reconstruction of subglottic and tracheal stenoses have been refined over the last three decades and can be applied safely and successfully in most circumstances. Glottic injuries remain a more challenging problem.

REFERENCES

1. Asai, T., Koga, K., and Vaughan, R.S. Respiratory complications associated with tracheal intubation and extubation. *Br. J. Anaesth.*, 1998, 80, 767–775.
2. Benjamin, B. Prolonged intubation injuries of the larynx: endoscopic diagnosis, classification, and treatment. *Ann. Otol., Rhinol., Laryngol.*, 1993 (Suppl.), 160, 1–15.
3. Suresh. S., Birmingham, P.K., and Ravindranath, T.M. Ventilatory support for infants in emergency and in the intensive care unit. *Indian J. Pediatr.*, 1995, 62, 395–419.
4. da Silva, O.P. Factors influencing acquired upper airway obstruction in newborn infants receiving assisted ventilation because of respiratory failure: an overview. *J. Perinatol.*, 1996, 16, 272–275.
5. Marley, R.A. Postextubation laryngeal edema: a review with consideration for home discharge. *J. Perianesth. Nursing*, 1998, 13(1), 39–53.
6. Maze, A. and Bloch, E. Stridor in pediatric patients. *Anesthesiology*, 1979, 50(2), 132–145.
7. McCulloch, T.M. and Bishop, M.J. Complications of translaryngeal intubation. *Clin. Chest Med.*, 1991, 12(3), 507–521.
8. Page, N.E., Giehl, M., and Luke, S. Intubation complications in the critically ill child. *AACN Clin. Issues*, 1998, 9(1), 25–35.
9. Grillo, H.C. and Donahue, D.M. Post intubation tracheal stenosis. *Semin. Thoracic Cardiovasc. Surg.*, 1996, 8(4), 370–380.
10. Weymuller, E.A., Jr. Prevention and management of intubation injury of the larynx and trachea. *Am. J. Otolaryngol.*, 1992, 13(3), 139–144.
11. Burton, D.M., Pransky, S.M., Katz, R.M., Kearns, D.B., and Seid, A.B. Pediatric airway manifestations of gastroesophageal reflux. *Ann. Otol., Rhinol., Laryngol.*, 1992, 101(9), 742–749.
12. Balestrieri, F. and Watson, C.B. Intubation granuloma. *Otolaryngol. Clin. North Am.*, 1982, 15(3), 567–579.
13. Bishop, M.J., Weymuller, E.A., Jr., and Fink, B.R. Laryngeal effects of prolonged intubation. *Anesth. Analg.*, 1984, 63, 335–342.

14. Carrat, X., Verhulst, J., Duroux, S., Pescio, P., Devars, F., and Traissac, L. Postintubation interarytenoid adhesion. *Ann. Otol. Rhinol. Laryngol.*, 2000, 109, 736–740.

15. Streitz, J.M., Jr. and Shapshay, S.M. Airway injury after tracheotomy and endotracheal intubation. *Surgical Clin. North Am.*, 1991, 71(6), 1211–1230.

16. Hartley, M. and Vaughan, R.S. Problems associated with tracheal extubation. *Br. J. Anaesth.*, 1993, 71, 561–568.

17. Spence, K. and Barr, P. Nasal vs. oral intubation for mechanical ventilation of newborn infants (*Cochrane Rev.*). *Cochrane Lib.*, Issue 4, 2000. Oxford: Update Software.

18. Grillo, H.C. and Donahue, D.M. Postintubation tracheal stenosis. *Chest Surg. Clin. North Am.*, 1996, 6(4), 725–731.

19. Deutsch, E.S., Smergel, E., Crisci, K., and Panitch, H. Tracheobronchography in children. *Laryngoscope*, 1996, 106(10), 1248–1254.

20. Hartwick, C.J., Chung, S., Emery, K.H., and Myer, C.M., III. Imaging case study of the month: pediatric virtual bronchoscopy. *Ann. Otol. Rhinol. Laryngol.*, 2002, 111, 281–283.

21. Smith, S.W. and Biros, M. Relief of imminent respiratory failure from upper airway obstruction by use of helium–oxygen: a case series and brief review. *Acad. Emerg. Med.*, 1999, 6(9), 953–956.

22. Wohl, D.L., Kilpatrick, J.K., Leshner, R.T., and Shaia, W.T. Intraoperative pediatric laryngeal electromyography: experience and caveats with monopolar electrodes. *Ann. Otol., Rhinol., Laryngol.*, 2001, 110, 524–531.

23. Tierney, P.A., Francis, I., and Morrison, G.A.J. Acquired subglottic cysts in the low birth weight, preterm infant. *J. Laryngol. Otol.*, 1997, 111, 478–481.

24. Wood, D.E. and Mathisen, D.J. Late complications of tracheotomy. *Clin. Chest Med.*, 1991, 12(3), 597–609.

25. Rahbar, R., Shapshay, S.M., and Healy, G.B. Mitomycin: effects on laryngeal and tracheal stenosis, benefits, and complications. *Ann. Otol. Rhinol. Laryngol.*, 2001, 110, 1–6.

26. Rahbar, R., Valdez, T.A., and Shapshay, S.M. Preliminary results of intraoperative mitomycin-C in the treatment and prevention of glottic and subglottic stenosis. *J. Voice*, 2000, 14(2), 282–286.

27. Ward, R.F. and April, M.M. Mitomycin-C in the treatment of tracheal cicatrix after tracheal reconstruction. *Int. J. Pediatr. Otorhinolaryngol.*, 1998, 44, 221–226.

28. Angelos, G.M., Smith, D.R., Jorgenson, R., and Sweeney, E.A. Oral complications associated with neonatal oral tracheal intubation: a critical review. *Pediatri. Dentistry*, 1989, 11(2), 133–140.

29. Macey-Dare, L.V., Moles, D.R., Evans, R.D., and Nixon, F. Long-term effect of neonatal endotracheal intubation on palatal form and symmetry in 8- to 11-year-old children. *Eur. J. Orthodontics*, 1999, 21, 703–710.

30. Cotton, R.T. and Seid, A.B. Management of the extubation problem in the premature child anterior cricoid split as an alternative to tracheotomy. *Ann. Otol.*, 1980, 89, 508–511.

31. Morrissey, M.S.C. and Bailey, C.M. Diagnosis and management of subglottic stenosis after neonatal ventilation. *Arch. Dis. Childhood*, 1990, 65(10), 1103–1104.

32. Grundfast, K.M., Coffman, A.C., and Milmoe, G. Anterior cricoid split: a "simple" surgical procedure and a potentially complicated care problem. *Ann. Otol., Rhinol., Laryngol.*, 1985, 94(5), 445–449.

23 Aerodigestive Endoscopy

Eric A. Mair, Jon Robitschek, and Joseph Haddad, Jr.

Educate the eye and the fingers.

Chevalier Jackson, M.D.

CONTENTS

INTRODUCTION

Pediatric aerodigestive tract endoscopy can be arguably considered one of a core of clinical arenas that have enabled pediatric otolaryngology to develop into a distinct subspecialty within the comprehensive surgical specialty of otolaryngology — head and neck surgery. All such surgery residents are now required to receive training in the technical specifics and subtleties of aerodigestive tract endoscopy in children and adults. In many training programs and clinical practices, however, increasingly fewer cases require pediatric endoscopy when compared with adult numbers. Nonetheless, the need for well-developed technical skill, instrumentation knowledge, and clinical acumen is no less critical for these procedures when caring for children.

Adult patients present their own set of potential clinical issues, such as severe major organ disease. However, in children, the margin of anatomic and physiologic airway reserve, often the determining factor between the safe execution of endoscopy and disaster, is more likely to be critically smaller than in their older counterparts. The objective of this chapter is to help the reader identify and prevent potential problems that can occur with rigid and flexible endoscopy of the upper aerodigestive tract in children.

GUIDING PRINCIPLES

The endoscopist's level of experience with the operative technique and his or her knowledge of underlying pathology must be recognized as definitive indicators for assuring accurate diagnosis and safe, effective therapeutic intervention.

BACKGROUND

Technological advancements in flexible and rigid instrumentation have enabled the endoscopist to better evaluate the upper aerodigestive tract in children. Flexible fiberoptic endoscopes now allow relatively easy access to the upper airway passages in infants and young children in an office setting; they provide a great deal of information on breathing and swallowing anatomy and physiology. When general anesthesia is necessary and appropriate for endoscopic aerodigestive tract procedures, their safety and success will depend not only on preparation and ready availability of instrumentation but also on clear communication among the endoscopist, nursing staff, and anesthesia team. Unfortunately, even with appropriate attention to detail, complications may still occur.

HOW OLD IS THE PATIENT?

Key maturational distinctions in age-related anatomy and physiology must be recognized.

Infants

- Obligate nasal breathers until 9 to 12 weeks of age
- Larynx located at the fourth cervical vertebrae, distensible, apt to laryngospasm, and a third the size of the adult with a shortened cricothyroid membrane
- Arytenoids with vocal processes equaling roughly the same length as the membranous vocal folds
- Narrowest area is subglottic lumen, more often compromised due to soft tissue edema, warranting extreme caution during intubation and endoscopic instrumentation[1]
- Poor lung compliance with relatively narrow lower airway, absence of collateral ventilation, and elevated oxygen consumption contributing to poor reserve capacity and increased risk of hypoxemia

Children

- Larynx reaches adult size at age 12 to 14 and is located at the seventh cervical vertebrae.
- Arytenoids with vocal processes approach the adult cartilaginous:membranous vocal fold ratio.
- Narrowest area gradually becomes the glottic aperture as larynx matures; mucosa is still more prone to inflammatory edema than in adults.
- Adenoid and tonsils approach maximum size at age 5 to 7, contributing to airway symptomatology.[1]

WHERE IS THE PROPER LOCALE?

Do not attempt a procedure in a setting in which you are unlikely to be able to extricate safely from an adverse occurrence.

Office or Out-Patient Clinic

- Primary setting for flexible laryngoscopy without sedation/anesthesia
- Topical anesthesia acceptable, usually applied intranasally; beware potential to decrease laryngeal sensory reflexes if applied in excess
- Limited capacity to monitor the child's cardiorespiratory status adequately, address airway emergencies, or provide sedation/anesthesia

Intensive Care Unit

- Available monitoring of cardiorespiratory status
- Access to readily available emergency airway equipment
- Intravenous access (usually) already established
- Sedation protocols and clinical support from pediatric anesthesia or intensive care unit medical staff

Operating Room

- Ideal setting for the vast majority of endoscopic procedures due to availability of comprehensive monitoring equipment, anesthesia, and airway support resources
- Full array of instrumentation readily available for complicated cases and for managing acute airway emergencies

WHAT ARE THE CLINICAL OBJECTIVES?

Diagnosis

- Following a thorough history and general otolaryngologic office examination, including assessment of voice/cry and cervical auscultation, a fiberoptic laryngoscopy (generally without laryngeal topicalization for infants or young children) may be considered to assess for laryngmalacia, vocal fold mobility, supraglottic and glottic lesions, and laryngopharyngeal reflux changes within the hypopharynx and laryngopharynx. On occasion, subglottic pathology may also be identified.
- Despite an adequate history and thorough office examination, an endoscopic examination under general anesthesia is often required to establish a definitive diagnosis, particularly with subglottic and tracheobronchial pathology.
- The need to evaluate dynamic airway anatomy and function determines which anesthetic technique to use in the operating room theater — whether spontaneous breathing vs. jet or apneic with intermittent positive pressure ventilation.
- The differential diagnosis determines what part, or all, of the upper aerodigestive tract is evaluated.
- The diagnosis and clinical impact determine the relative timing and mode of therapeutic intervention.

Therapeutic Intervention

- Definitive management can follow diagnostic endoscopy; obtain consent in advance when deemed reasonable for patient and family.
- Establish best combination of anticipated postoperative airway patency and physiologic function with a planned minimum of tissue instrumentation and ablation.

- Preparation, parent/child understanding, and continued endoscopic diagnostic reevaluation, with possible continued therapeutic intervention, contribute to safe and successful outcomes.
- Potential for in-patient status postoperatively should be discussed in advance.

EARLY RECOGNITION AND TIMELY INTERVENTION

The majority of airway complications during aerodigestive tract endoscopy are preventable with adequate oxygenation, ventilation, close respiratory monitoring, and adequate anesthesia of the larynx.

BASIC ANESTHESIA PRINCIPLES

- Acknowledge that a team approach to sharing the airway with anesthesia is mandatory, with emphasis on planned continuous communication between anesthesia and the endoscopist throughout the procedure.
- General anesthesia is required for rigid bronchoscopy and rigid esophagoscopy and is commonly used for accompanying direct laryngoscopy.
- Sedation is considered for selected cases of flexible fiberoptic bronchoscopy and flexible fiberoptic esophagoscopy.
- Assure education of the child and family on sedation and anesthetic techniques; elective preoperative anesthesia consult is appropriate in most "airway" cases.
- Assure knowledge of importance of NPO status prior to the procedure, preferably with multiple reminders including the day before or when hospital day-of-surgery arrival times are (usually) provided.
- Assure that appropriate preoperative medical work-up is up to date; this is particularly relevant in patients with
  - Continued oxygen requirements
  - Potential cervical spine pathology (such as c1-c2 subluxation seen in some children with trisomy 21)
  - Known major organ disease (cardiac, renal, hepatic pathology), seizure history, or intracranial or neuromuscular disorders
  - Family history (or prior surgical history) of anesthetic complications
- Establish timing and planned location of IV access prior to entering the OR/procedure room in nonemergency cases.
- Assure appropriate pediatric equipment for pulse oximetry, CO_2 monitoring, electrocardiogram leads, and blood pressure monitoring before bringing the child into the operating room.
- Assure availability of continued postoperative monitoring as patient recovers from general anesthesia, sedation, and narcotic analgesia.

THINGS TO WATCH FOR

Progressively serious potential sequelae that may occur during aerodigestive tract endoscopy include hypoxemia, laryngospasm, bronchospasm, bradycardia, and aspiration (see Chapter 5 and Chapter 6).

- Oral trauma is a potentially common occurrence with aerodigestive tract endoscopy (see Chapter 5 and Chapter 6).
- Dental injuries may result from the use of rigid laryngoscopes, suspension laryngoscopy, bronchoscopes, or esophagoscopes as a result of excessive pressure to the alveolar tissue and teeth, particularly the maxillary central incisors.

- Three variations of dental trauma include fracture, displacement, and avulsion. This can be prevented by careful intubation/extubation technique, protecting the teeth with a mouth guard, and examining the teeth/gingiva before and after the procedure.
- With deciduous teeth trauma, the tooth may be removed manually or allowed to displace with time.
- Permanent tooth trauma is classified according to involvement of enamel, enamel and dentin, or extension completely to the central pulp. With enamel chipping, it is appropriate to consider a dental evaluation adding a composite material to the tooth with reshaping as needed. With enamel and dentin fracture — associated with pain, temperature sensitivity, or mobility, and diagnosed with oral radiographs — a dental evaluation is required for possible surgical therapy. If the central pulp is involved in the dental injury, with a presentation similar to enamel and dentin fracture, a thorough dental evaluation is required for optimal therapy.
- Tooth displacement can often be managed with gentle replacement of the tooth into position; however, a dental evaluation to consider splinting for proper stabilization is recommended.
- An avulsed tooth needs to be located with abdominal and chest radiographs obtained to rule out aspiration if the tooth is not identified with a thorough intraoral and pharyngeal examination. If able to be retrieved, acutely, the permanent tooth should be replaced into the socket with an immediate dental evaluation for stabilization.[2]

LARYNGOSCOPY

Flexible and direct (rigid) laryngoscopies are complementary tools for evaluating the supraglottic and glottic area. The flexible fiberoptic laryngoscope provides optimal visualization of the unsedated larynx to examine dynamic vocal fold mobility and function. The critical subglottic space is more safely evaluated under general anesthesia with direct laryngoscopy and rigid telescopic or microscopic visualization due to the flexible fiberoptic laryngoscope's lack of airway control, limited visibility, and parabolic image provided. Direct (rigid) laryngoscopy will also provide space for microsurgical instrumentation.

FLEXIBLE LARYNGOSCOPY

Indications

Flexible laryngoscopy is a minimally invasive diagnostic tool employed in the clinic and operative setting that provides excellent dynamic visualization for complete examination of the nasal passage, pharynx, and larynx. Indications are broad and include assistance for intubation and extubation. This method can also be used for diagnostic evaluation of supraglottic, glottic, and (potentially) subglottic pathology such as laryngomalacia, hypopharyngeal foreign body, vocal fold paralysis, dysphonia, laryngotracheal stenosis, hemangioma, papilloma, and laryngopharyngeal reflux (see Table 23.1).

Anatomic Hurdles

- Potential anatomic hurdles to flexible fiberoptic endoscope advancement include deviated nasal septum, polyps, and nasal/choanal stenosis.
- A clear understanding of *normal* glottic function is imperative in the diagnostic evaluation of functional stability.
- Almost 20% of diagnosed cases of larynogomalacia may have other associated airway abnormalities.[3]

TABLE 23.1
Comparison of Rigid and Flexible Endoscopic Techniques

	Flexible laryngoscopy	Direct laryngoscopy	Rigid bronchoscopy	Flexible bronchoscopy	Rigid esophagoscopy	Flexible esophagoscopy
Ideal location	Clinic – OR – ICU	ICU – OR	OR	ICU – OR	OR	OR – ICU
Anatomical approach	Primarily nasal; oral (pacifier) as alternative in infants	Oral	Oral	Primarily nasal; oral as alternative	Oral	Oral
Anesthesia	Topical airway anesthetic	General via laryngoscope	General via ventilatory bronchoscope	IV sedation or general via ETT or LMA	General via ETT	IV sedation or general via ETT
Ventilation	Spontaneous respirations	Primarily spontaneous; also apneic w/IPPV for microsurgery	Primarily spontaneous, also apneic w/IPPV	Spontaneous respirations	Spontaneous respirations	Spontaneous respirations
Risk assessment	Low	Low	Medium–high; foreign body[a]	Low–medium	Medium–high; foreign body[a]	Low
Areas best examined	Supraglottic and glottic structures	Supraglottic, glottic, and subglottic structures	Subglottic, primary tracheobronchial tree	Tracheobronchial tree with subsegmental bronchi	Proximal esophagus (above the aortic knob)	Distal esophagus (below the aortic knob)
Visual capabilities	Good	Excellent	Excellent	Fair	Excellent	Good
Scope durability	Medium	High	High	Low	High	Medium
Major complications	Epistaxis; laryngospasm; loss of airway	Oral trauma; laryngospasm; loss of airway	Laryngospasm; loss of airway; tracheal trauma; aspiration pneumonia	Laryngospasm; loss of airway; aspiration pneumonia	Muscoal trauma; perforation; aspiration pneumonia; hemorrhage	Muscosal trauma; perforation; aspiration pneumonia; hemorrhage

Notes: ETT = endotracheal tube; LMA = laryngeal mask airway; OR = operating room; ICU = intensive care unit; IPPV = intermittent positive pressure ventilation.

[a] Presence of foreign body puts the child at greater risk for perforation, poor oxygenation, and loss of airway.

- Superior subglottic visualization is attained in up to 75% of cases, although hampered by secretions, overhang of the epiglottis, and vocal fold paralysis.[4]
- If the endoscope cannot be passed through the nose, attempt the other nostril. In the case of infants, attempt a ped-endo pacifer, which permits oral passage of a 4-mm flexible endoscope through a pacifier. Alternatively, a small flexible endoscope (<2 mm diameter) may be used, especially if nasal anomalies are also suspected.
- Compliance with office fiberoptic endoscopy may be a factor in young children; infants are easily restrained with a parental hug and older children can generally be talked through the procedure.
- Use of various topical anesthetic agents, whether by spray, ointment, or lubricant, is helpful; however, beware of potential overdose and desensitization of the glottis if they are overused.

Complications

Epistaxis

- Secondary to trauma, epistaxis is prevented by prudent, unforced advancement; adequate visualization; and proper application of lubrication and topical nasal decongestant. Alternatively, a smaller scope can be attempted.
- Treat epistaxis with direct pressure by pinching the nose. If applying pressure fails, consider spot cautery or nasal packing and reassess for persistent hemorrhage.

Laryngospasm

- Avoiding contact with the larynx is the first step toward preventing laryngospasm.
- Do not pass the flexible laryngoscope through the vocal folds without prior sedation and topical laryngeal anesthesia — and without emergency resuscitation equipment on hand.
- Treatment of severe laryngospasm in the out-patient office setting may present a life-threatening emergency, again emphasizing the need to assess the locale and available tools.

DIRECT LARYNGOSCOPY

Indications

Direct laryngoscopy is a diagnostic and therapeutic tool utilized to obtain direct visualization of the pharyngeal, supraglottic, glottic, and subglottic anatomy. Clinical indications include a need for critical evaluation of airway anomalies or lesions with possible biopsy. Its therapeutic potential is enhanced considerably with suspension microlaryngoscopy, allowing the use of a rigid telescope or a microscope for bimanual laryngeal microsurgery (see Table 23.1).

Anesthesia and Ventilation

Pediatric patients usually undergo general anesthesia through intravenous and/or inhalational routes, generally using one of three techniques (see the chapter on anesthesia).

Spontaneous Ventilation

- Anesthetic gases are delivered via a metal cannula placed within the oral cavity or located on the side of the laryngoscope or through a flexible tube placed transnasally into the nasopharynx.

- Alternatively, intravenous anesthesia may be used, although it may be associated with a longer recovery.
- Advantages:
  - Improved visualization of laryngeal structures; no intervening foreign body, i.e., endotracheal tube
  - Reduced risk of barotrauma and endotracheal tube trauma
- Risks:
  - Apnea if the level of anesthesia becomes too deep
  - Laryngospasm if the level of anesthesia is too light (balance achieved through constant communication with pediatric anesthesiologist)
  - Difficult to perform in children > 12 years of age due to entrainment of room air; may combine with intravenous anesthesia (see the chapter on anesthesia)
  - No anesthetic gas scavenging system typically employed

Jet Ventilation

- Requires continuous neuromuscular blockade with rapid high-pressure ventilation via the laryngoscope (supraglottic) or a flexible midtracheal tube (Ben Jet or Hunsaker tube)[5]
- Advantages:
  - Good laryngeal visualization; minimal foreign body obstruction
  - Safe technique with experienced anesthesiologist or if spontaneous ventilations are unsuccessful
- Risks:
  - Laryngeal edema/dessication
  - Barotrauma: mediastinal emphysema and/or pneumothorax; must always visualize open glottis prior to jetting; requires "real time" communication with anesthesiologist or via on-screen imaging

Apneic with Intermittent Positive Pressure Ventilation

- This is often used in cases of microsurgery when an immobile larynx is desired.
- A small-diameter endotracheal tube may be placed anterior or posterior to pathology to afford direct visualization of the appropriate glottic structures.
- Advantage:
  - Classical technique familiar to many anesthesiologists
- Risks:
  - Intermittent endotracheal intubation and oxygenation with secondary hypoxemia, loss of airway, and potential for mucosal irritation

Patient Positioning

Infant

- The infant should be supine, with head extended with flexion of the neck into the sniffing position.
- Place a rolled towel or small shoulder roll under the shoulders in an effort to approximate the infant's relatively large head with the chest and neck.

Child

- Supine, sniffing position

Adolescent

- Supine, sniffing position
- Towel beneath the occiput

Choice of Laryngoscope

Intubating/Diagnostic Laryngoscopes

- These are smaller laryngoscopes that have a right-sided opening or removable slider for ease of intubating; the older generation had "bottom-sliders."
- Such laryngoscopes are useful for providing anatomic access for diagnostic telescopic bronchoscopy, or for introducing ventilating bronchoscope or endotracheal tube.
- They offer multiple options with specific uses, such as "anterior commisure laryngo-scope"; the endoscopist should have a representative array immediately available for use.
- Curved anesthesia blades (e.g., MacIntosh) are not preferred due to the blade's bulky size; the potential for trauma is greater and maneuverability is limited within the pediatric oropharynx.

Operating/Laser Laryngoscopes

- These scopes offer a considerably larger field in which to operate with no intubation port.
- They provide more room to maneuver a laser beam, mircodebrider, or controlled micro-instrumentation therapeutically.
- Multiple choices are available, with specific uses such as a (pediatric and neonatal) "subglottiscope"; the endoscopist should have a representative array immediately available for use.
- These are always used with suspension, with appropriate precautions and care employed to avoid intraoral trauma (discussed earlier).

Length of Laryngoscope

- Choose an appropriate length; if too short, the proximal end will be within oral cavity and if too long, the distal working end may be proportionally larger than appropriate.
- *Rule of thumb:* the distance from the base of the palm to the tip of the middle phalanx approximates the length of the child's airway from the upper incisors to the larynx. Alternatively, relative age/size charts are available.

Anatomic Hurdles

- Positioning the tongue to the left, the laryngoscope is inserted and advanced along the right side of the oral cavity using the left hand, being careful not to entrap the lips, leverage against the superior alveolar surface, or ensnare the palatine tonsil tissue.
- The right hand can gently extend the head without excessive rotation.
- The laryngoscope is elevated along a vector of motion perpendicular to the blade of the laryngoscope with the tip of the blade placed in the vallecula to avoid glottic trauma.[6]
- If one is unable to visualize the larynx,
  - Apply anterior pressure to the cricoid in an attempt to improve visualization.

- Apply suction in the event of copious secretion.
- Reposition the child assuring a midline approach.
- Because of infants' elevated larynx (C-4), deep placement of the laryngoscope is a common problem; reposition accordingly. Consider angling the head to the left, thereby shortening the distance to the larynx as the laryngoscope is advanced along the right pharyngeal gutter.
- Consider specialty intubating laryngoscopes (e.g., an anterior commisure laryngoscope) in children with craniofacial abnormalities.
- Consider flexible laryngoscopy through a facemask or laryngeal mask airway.[7]
- Consider suspension laryngoscopy for bimanual airway manipulation.
  - Remain aware of superior alveolar pressure, lip entrapment, and intraoral trauma; beware torquing injury from increased suspension energy translated to vulnerable mucosal and endolaryngeal pressure points.
  - The suspension should be stabilized to the operating table and not the child's chest.
  - Ensuring proper oxygenation and delivery of anesthesia should be continually reassessed throughout the procedure — a responsibility shared with anesthesia — reinforcing the importance of communication and the team approach.

Complications

Loss of the Airway

- Laryngospasm, hemorrhage, and subglottic edema are secondary to traumatic intubation or aggressive instrumentation.
- Assuring oxygenation, adequate visualization, suctioning, and topical anesthesia are the initial management principles.

Dental Trauma

- Upward displacement of teeth into the maxilla is a well-recognized complication.
- Prevention, inspection, and immediate treatment are called for. For older children with permanent teeth, consider using a molded plastic dental guard.

Barotrauma

- This is a risk with positive pressure ventilation, but especially with midtracheal jet ventilation in a nonparalyzed child with a closed glottis.
- Diagnosis is based on clinical suspicion (observed trauma, oxygen desaturation, asymmetric or abnormal lung auscultation, tachycardia) and chest radiograph.
- Treatment varies depending on clinical and radiographic findings.
- Conservative management includes analgesia and supplemental oxygen. Cases of pneumothorax and pneumomediastinum are treated accordingly.[1,8]

BRONCHOSCOPY

Flexible as well as rigid bronchoscopy is a powerful diagnostic and also a (potential) therapeutic tool in pediatrics. Each has distinct advantages and complements the other exceedingly well. Both modalities should be part of the endoscopist's armamentarium.

Rigid Bronchoscopy

Indications

Major clinical indications for rigid bronchoscopy include diagnostic evaluation for a variety of congenital or acquired airway disorders in infants and children (Table 23.1), foreign body removal, and urgent airway control in cases of obstructing airway masses or massive hemoptysis. A ventilating bronchoscope may also serve as a conduit for laser (via fiber or coherent beam), electrocautery, cryotherapy, stent placement, balloon dilation, and microinstrumentation.

Absolute contraindications for rigid bronchoscopy include hemodynamic instability, cervical spine instability, and severe chronic lung disease with refractory hypoxemia arising from airway instability.[9] Relative contraindications include cervical ankylosis, kyphoscoliosis, baseline hypoxemia, and coagulapathy/bleeding disorder.

Anesthesia and Ventilation

The majority of children undergo rigid bronchoscopy under general anesthesia, following the principles outlined for direct laryngoscopy with a few additional guidelines regarding rigid bronchoscopy.

Topical Anesthesia

- Prior application of topical lidocaine to the larynx can help prevent the potential for laryngospasm as the bronchoscope is manipulated with leverage placed upon the endolaryngeal structures; absorption rate through laryngeal mucosa varies.
- Intermittent endobronchial application of topical anesthetic can help reduce the potential for bronchospasm as the brochi and mucosa are manipulated; 100% absorption rates through tracheobronchial mucosa should be anticipated and maximum allowable amounts should be calculated beforehand.
- Dosing lasts 20 to 30 min with onset occurring within 3 to 4 min; dose limit is 5 mg/kg; dosing interval times (approximately 30 min) should be kept in mind.[10]

Spontaneous Ventilation

- This technique is ideal for shorter procedures, younger patients, foreign body removal, and laser therapy.
- It is possible to convert to apneic with intermittent positive pressure ventilation (IPPV) or spontaneous-assisted ventilation (SAV); however, an airway must be secured prior to ceasing spontaneous ventilation.
- Prior application of topical anesthesia to the larynx can help prevent the potential for laryngospasm as the bronchoscope is manipulated with leverage placed upon the endolaryngeal anatomy.
- Intermittent endobronchial application of topical anesthetic can help reduce the potential for bronchospasm if the brochi mucosa is manipulated; 100% absorption rates should be anticipated and maximum allowable amounts should be known beforehand.

Jet Ventilation

- This method is more suitable for the older pediatric patient (age > 12) and prolonged procedures.
- Intermittent negative pressure ventilation (INPV) and external high-frequency oscillation (EHFO) have been studied with varied applications.[11]

Apneic with Intermittent Positive Pressure Ventilation

- Today, this technique is not as common as the two previous approaches.
- A neuromuscular blocker is administered with 100% oxygen via face mask.
- Telescopic bronchoscopy should be performed with intermittent mask ventilation or intubation to prevent hypoxemia.
- Disadvantages:
  - Risk of hypoxemia, hypercapnea, and tachycardia
  - Frequent intubations with subsequent repetitive trauma to the airway (e.g., distal advancement of recurrent respiratory papillomatosis)

Choice of Bronchoscopes

- Select an appropriate length and diameter bronchoscope for the task.
  - Use the smallest diameter that still allows easy inflow of oxygen and anesthetic vapors but not so narrow as to restrict outflow of carbon dioxide and dead space vapors; see the chapter on anesthesia for information on bronchoscope–telescope compatibility.
  - Select length adequate for anticipated procedure; lengths are generally set at 20 or 30 cm, with overlap for only a limited number of inner diameters.
  - Rule of thumb: the size of distal interphalangeal joint on the fifth digit approximates the normal tracheal diameter in a child; alternatively, relative age/size charts are available.

Anatomical Hurdles

There is no substitute for knowledge of anatomy and for experience.

Technique Pearls

- The long side of the beveled end of the rigid bronchoscope is anteriorly oriented and can be used to lift the epiglottis.
- With the arytenoid complex accurately identified, the bronchoscope is gently advanced with 90° of rotation to provide direct visualization of the vocal folds.
- One full vocal fold should be identified in the field of vision to assure that the long end of bevel is oriented vertically between the two vocal folds. The bronchoscope should be gently advanced into the trachea — gently rotating another 90°, if necessary, to allow advancement through glottis and subglottis.

In general, three basic techniques can be used to insert a rigid bronchoscope.

Direct Intubation

- The rigid bronchoscope, preferably with telescopic visualization, is introduced into the oropharynx and advanced with appropriate angulation through the larynx into the trachea.
- Direct intubation is the most difficult of the three techniques, with increased risk of direct trauma to the pharynx, esophagus, and larynx.
- This approach is not recommended for patients with poorly defined anatomy or suspected difficult intubation.

Endotracheal-Assisted Intubation

- This technique is performed in patients who are already intubated.

- The bronchoscope is advanced under direct visualization, preferably with telescopic visualization, until vocal folds are in clear view.
- The endotracheal tube is removed and the bronchoscope is advanced under direct vision into the trachea.
- Beware of entrapped tracheal secretions obscuring glottis upon extraction; assure adequate suctioning of the endotracheal tube prior to removal.
- This is a useful technique, particularly in infants and patients who are difficult to intubate, by theoretically reducing risk because the bronchoscope is already positioned at the laryngeal introitus prior to extubation.
- Accidental extubation while positioning the bronchoscope should be avoided.

Laryngoscopic Intubation

- Laryngoscopic intubation begins with direct visualization of the vocal folds using a laryngoscope with a side slide or an open side slot; alternatively, the laryngoscope can be placed in the vallecula and lifted anteriorly to expose the laryngeal introitus. Once the scope is positioned, the side slide should be removed without shifting laryngoscope position.
- The rigid bronchoscope is introduced and advanced past the vocal folds into the proximal trachea, preferably under telescopic visualization. The laryngoscope is then removed.
- In comparison with direct intubation, laryngoscopic intubation provides optimum visualization of the larynx with reduced risk of direct trauma to arytenoid complexes, vocal folds, and subglottis.
- This is the preferred approach in the majority of children because of its safety and reduced level of risk.

Complications

Potential injuries related to passage and placement of a rigid bronchoscope through the oral cavity, oropharnx, hypopharynx, and larynx are presented in laryngoscopy section.

Direct Trauma to the Airway

- Avoidance
  - Direct visualization affords early recognition.
  - Appropriate bronchoscope size should be selected and the bronchoscope advanced cautiously, with clear visualization of anatomical landmarks (see Table 23.2).
- Recognition
  - Intraoperative findings may include visualized mucosal disruption, tracheobronchial bleeding, and clinical findings consistent with pneumothorax.
  - Postoperative findings may include hemoptysis or subcutaneous emphysema with progressive airway obstruction.
- Management
  - Excessive mucosal trauma may necessitate an extended sedated intubation period (overnight to several days) or even a controlled tracheotomy in severe cases of laryngeal trauma.
  - Repair of mucosal tears should initially be considered to provide coverage of exposed cartilage.
  - Persistent subcutaneous emphysema may require external drainage or an endoscopic or external approach to repair the airway laceration.
  - Clinically significant and/or progressive pneumomediastinum or pneumothorax will most likely require a chest tube.

TABLE 23.2
Approximate Age to Size Correlation for Rigid and Flexible Endoscopes

	Flexible laryngoscopy (Olympus w/o suction port) O.D. (mm)	Direct laryngoscopy (Karl Storz) blade length (cm)	Rigid bronchoscopy (Karl Storz)	Flexible bronchoscopy (Olympus w/suction port) O.D. (mm)	Rigid esophagoscopy (Karl Storz)	Flexible esophagoscopy (Olympus) O.D. (mm)
Infant	1.8	8	3	2.8	4–5	4.8
Child: 1–4 years	1.8	10.5	3.5–4	2.8	6	5.3
Child: 4–10 years	4.0	12	5	3.6	7	6.0
>10 years	4.0	16	6	4.8	8	6.0

- Intravenous steroids are generally administered in an effort to diminish the acute inflammatory response but are not recommended for a prolonged course.
- Uncontrolled bleeding (rare) may require emergent transfusion and thoracotomy to control the source of hemorrhage.

FLEXIBLE FIBEROPTIC BRONCHOSCOPY

Indications

Employing a pediatric flexible bronchoscope, instead of a nasopharyngolaryngeal endoscope, allows full visualization down to the subsegmental bronchi. This is primarily a diagnostic tool with limited therapeutic capabilities. Major clinical indications include evaluation of persistent noisy breathing such as stridor, wheezing, hoarseness, or unexplained cough (see Table 23.1).

- Inspiratory stridor is the most common indication for flexible bronchoscopy. Associated with glottic and subglottic pathology in 14% of cases, this necessitates complete lower airway evaluation per flexible bronchoscopy in all patients with unexplained persistent stridor.[12]
- Suspected airway obstruction is secondary to foreign body, mucus plug, neoplasm, infections, granulation formation, or congenital anomaly.
- Miscellaneous indications include pulmonary toilet or cultures for persistent pneumonia, atelectasis, hypoxia, hemoptysis, immunocompromised related pulmonary disease, and assistance in percutaneous tracheotomy or endotracheal tube placement.

Relative Contraindications

Relative contraindications include uncontrolled hemoptysis, baseline hypoxemia, and coagulapathy/bleeding disorder.

Anesthesia and Ventilation

Children generally undergo fiberoptic bronchoscopy under intravenous sedation in an effort to reduce airway obstruction risks, improve diagnostic yield, and enhance patient comfort. The child undergoing flexible fiberoptic bronchoscopy, as opposed to rigid bronchoscopy, may spontaneously ventilate around the flexible bronchoscope rather than through the rigid bronchoscope. If the child is sedated, supplemental oxygen can be provided through a face mask, inserting the fiberoptic bronchoscope through the inlet port on the mask. If the child is intubated, the fiberoptic bronchoscope can be threaded through the endotracheal tube via an L-adaptor ("double-swivel").

Laryngeal Mask Airway

The use of a laryngeal mask airway (LMA) has become a useful adjunctive technique with demonstrated efficacy in children with moderate to severe hypoxemia or with a difficult airway.[7]

- Advantages of the LMA over intubation include
  - Minimal hemodynamic response secondary to reduced laryngeal stimulation
  - Lower level of anesthesia with improved oxygenation secondary to greater diameter tube
- Disadvantages of the LMA over intubation include
  - Insertion is blind, but direct visualization via flexible laryngoscopy can confirm the position.
  - Experience with this fairly new technique varies among endoscopists.
  - There is a potential for oro-hypopharyngeal injury from cuff inflation following prolonged placement.[13]
  - There is a greater risk of aspiration with the LMA when compared with the endotracheal tube.

Anatomical Hurdles

General

Suctioning the nostrils and administering a topical vasoconstrictor prior to introducing the bronchoscscope afford improved visualization and minimize resistance. Sequential topicalization of the larynx and trachea through the suction channel reduces reflex coughing and the potential for laryngospasm and bronchospasm.

Nasal Advancement

- This occurs between middle and inferior turbinate — usually the widest opening of the nasal airway — and is the preferred recommended approach.
- The nasal floor is parallel to the inferior turbinate. Beware limited maneuverability distally secondary to acute angle with respect to the nasopharyngeal inlet.
- Beware of intranasal asymmetry, most commonly from a deviated nasal septum; if significantly increased resistance is encountered, attempt advancement through the contralateral side.
- Alternatively, if nasal advancement cannot be adequately achieved, the fiberoptic endoscope may be passed orally, although direct oropharyngeal trauma is a recognized risk.

Pharyngeal Hypotonia

Whether from an underlying neurological disease or from oversedation, pharyngeal hypotonia may result in collapsed mucosal planes obscuring the location of the larynx.

- Attempt a jaw thrust maneuver initially for laryngeal exposure.
- Alternatively, administer oxygen through the suction channel or through a separate catheter introduced through the opposite nares.
- Consider placement of an orogastric tube to address gastric distension and the potential accompanying diminished respiratory capacity.
- In the event of continued poor visualization, consider employing a rigid laryngoscope for direct visualization or consider flexible bronchoscopy under general anesthesia through an endotracheal tube.

Copious Secretions or Mucus Plug

If secretions are inadequately disposed of with the 1.2-mm suction channel, consider

- Administering normal saline lavage with applied suction
- Introducing a rigid bronchoscope for enhanced suction and instrumentation or requiring general anesthesia in a child
- Using limited volumes of *N*-acetylcysteine in an attempt to dissolve the plug

Suboptimal Visualization

- Visualizing the anterior glottis is improved with the transnasal flexible route while potentially sacrificing adequate posterior views and vice versa when compared with rigid bronchoscopy (a consideration in cases of suspected tracheoesophageal fistulas or laryngeal cleft that may benefit from the rigid scope's posterior range and instrumentation for palpation).
- Vocal fold movement evaluation is optimized in patients with minimal to no sedation, employing an office flexible fiberoptic endoscope. Subsequent rigid laryngoscopy under anesthesia permits direct palpation to rule out cricoarytenoid joint fixation.[14]

Complications

Pneumothorax

Pneumothorax is a rare occurrence secondary to airway barotrauma that usually arises from over-aggressive ventilation with positive pressure through supporting airway apparatus. Mechanical injury may result in loss of mucosal integrity with potential for air escape. Avoid wedging the end of bronchoscope into an airway segment for any protracted period of time. Avoid using flexible transluminal instrumentation for biopsy or other therapy without sustained adequate visualization of the operative field. The treatment of a pneumothorax varies depending on the patient's respiratory status and ranges from observation to chest tube placement.

Postprocedure Stridor

Laryngeal or tracheal swelling may occur from the procedure, and this potential should be discussed beforehand with the patient and family. Postprocedural stridor is usually minor and transient. Acutely, humidified air or a racemic epinephrine treatment may be considered. A single dose of intravenous steroids, such as dexamethsone, may be helpful, although supportive studies are limited.

Pneumomediastinum

Although it is very rare for a mucosal tear with violation of the major airways to occur, this may result from forced advancement, instrumentation, or a deep transbronchial biopsy. Treatment varies, depending on clinical significance and progression of symptoms, and ranges from observation to mediastinal tube placement.

Bronchoalveolar Lavage

A useful adjunctive procedure with fiberoptic bronchoscopy is bronchoalveolar lavage (BAL) to obtain cytology (e.g., for lipid-laden macrophages) or culture samples as well as to remove mucus secretions or plugs from the airway. Try to avoid in children with persistent hypercapnia or hypoxemia (unable to correct to $PaO2 \geq 75$ mmgHg).[5] Potential specific complications from BAL include aspiration and sample contamination. Aspiration is prevented by securely wedging the bronchoscope into the airway segment to be lavaged so as to avoid proximal distribution; however, the tip should not be wedged for a protracted period of time because atelectasis or progressive air-trapping may ensue. Minimize the potential for sample contamination from oral and nasal secretions by keeping the suction channel clean until the specimen is collected and by using sterile normal saline for the lavage. With BAL, beware of the potential bacteriostatic effect of lidocaine and avoiding topicalization to the lower airway if possible.

ESOPHAGOSCOPY

INDICATIONS

Pediatric esophagoscopy is a useful procedure for cases of foreign body or caustic substance ingestion, failure to thrive, difficulty feeding, suspected gastroesophageal reflux, or suspected congenital abnormality of the esophagus. Flexible and rigid esophagoscopy are complementary, with each having distinct advantages in specific clinical scenarios (see Table 23.1).[15]

ANATOMICAL HURDLES

General Considerations

The esophagus lacks a surrounding serosa layer; combined with a thin buccopharyngeal fascia plane, it is susceptible to perforation, with limited ability to wall off the perforated site and isolate a potential infection.

Narrowing Points

Three narrowing points are described. Technique accommodations should be anticipated as routine when advancing through these regions.

- Cricopharyngeus — when in appropriate location and orientation, gradually dilate with slow steady pressure, under direct visualization with rigid esophagoscope.
- Aortic knob — appreciate surrounding cardiac pulsations and advance gently unless significant resistance is encountered.
- Esophagogastric junction — similar to the cricopharyngeal region, slow steady pressure in the appropriate location and orientation will permit passage of the esophagoscopy into the stomach.

Anatomical Variances

Be aware of known diverticula(e), fistula(e), extreme curvature of the spine, and stricture(s) to reduce potential for complications. Radiologic evaluation with a plain radiograph, gastrograffin swallow, computed tomography, or fluoroscopy should be considered in patients with suspected anatomic variance, foreign body, or perforation.

RIGID ESOPHAGOSCOPY

Indications

"Open tube" rigid esophagoscopy is ideal for evaluating the hypopharynx, cricopharyngeus, and proximal esophagus (above the aortic knob). Its capabilities for foreign body extraction and instrumentation parallel that of rigid bronchoscopy and exceed its fiberoptic complementary counterpart.

Anesthesia and Ventilation

Children should have rigid esophagoscopy performed under general anesthesia. Endotracheal intubation is almost always employed prior to esophageal cannulation to secure the airway and prevent aspiration, although the occasional exception for a "brief" cricopharygeal foreign body removal has been made.

Esophagoscope Advancement

A rigid laryngoscope may be used to assist with location of the cricopharygeal inlet prior to introduction of the esophagoscope. An endoscopic telescope provides improved visualization of the hypopharynx, cricopharyngeus, and proximal esophagus; it should remain proximal to the esophagoscope distal end. The esophageal lumen is visualized at all times throughout advancement, with care taken to keep the lumen in the center of the field as best as possible. Steady, gentle pressure with excellent visualization of the central lumen is the key to successful esophageal advancement.

Positioning and Technique Pearls

- The rigid esophagoscope is lubricated with (lidocaine) jelly at the distal end of the tube prior to placement to aid smooth advancement. Care is taken to avoid lubricating the telescope because this will blur the image.
- The esophagoscope is stabilized by the left hand at the level of the dentition or hard palate and carefully advanced by the right hand at the proximal end.
- The long side of the smooth beveled end of the rigid esophagoscope is anteriorly oriented and can be used to lift the larynx to visualize the esophageal opening. Alternatively, an intubating laryngoscope may be used to elevate the larynx and expose the cricopharyngeus for esophagoscope placement.
- The telescope is positioned within the esophagoscope just proximal to the tip of the esophagoscope. Such positioning allows full visualization of the esophageal lumen as the normally collapsed lumen is dilated by the preceding open tube. Protruding the telescope distal to the esophagoscope tip does not permit optimal visualization of the lumen.
- Because the distended esophagus is of greater diameter than the trachea, the rigid esophagoscope diameter is usually greater than that of the rigid bronchoscope. However, large-diameter rigid esophagoscopes (especially if anteriorly displaced) may compromise the tracheal airway distal to the tip of the endotracheal tube.
- Rigid bronchoscopes should not be used as rigid esophagoscopes. Rigid bronchoscopes may cause mucosal damage to the esophagus due to sharper edges and extra holes along the side of the tube.
- Copious gastroesophageal secretions are commonly encountered in rigid esophagoscopy. Suctioning within the esophagus is optimally accomplished with a small-diameter, atraumatic, flexible suction under telescopic visualization.
- An assistant elevating the patient's shoulder may help passage of the rigid esophagoscope distally.

FLEXIBLE FIBEROPTIC ESOPHAGOSCOPY

Indications

Evaluation of the mid and distal esophagus, including the esophagogastric junction, is best achieved with the flexible esophagoscope due to the insufflation capabilities. A thorough examination of the hypopharynx and proximal esophagus remains a technical challenge with the flexible esophagoscope. However, foreign body removal from the mid and distal esophagus is safe and usually effective. The relatively wider diameter of the flexible esophagoscope permits better visualization when compared with the thinner flexible bronchoscope (see Table 23.2). Forceps for foreign body removal are smaller (much like flexible bronchoscopy). If the foreign body is unusual or large, rigid esophagoscopy is preferred.

Anesthesia and Ventilation

Children usually undergo IV sedation or general anesthesia with endotracheal intubation. General anesthesia with intubation is recommended in children with difficult airways or in foreign body cases.

Esophagoscope Advancement

Great care must be taken in passing the flexible esophagoscope through the cricopharyngeus because this is a relatively blind portion of the procedure with little control. Once the esophagoscope is beyond the cricopharyngeus, insufflation permits esophageal distension and excellent visibility of the mid and distal esophagus (and stomach).

COMPLICATIONS

Esophageal Perforation

Esophageal perforation is a rare, though life-threatening (mortality as high as 30%), complication occurring more frequently with rigid esophagoscopy than with flexible fiberoptic esophagoscopy.

Pathogenesis

Risk factors for perforation include inflammation, infection, and mucosal ulceration (foreign body). Mucosal tears offer a nidus for infection with abscess formation or the development of an intramural hematoma. Supprative infection involving areodigestive flora (staphylococcus, bacteroides, pseudomonas) can ensue within 8 to 12 h. Anatomically, the thoracic esophageal perforation is at greatest risk for developing mediastinitis. Cervical perforations may tract down caudally, leading to mediastinitis, although the more likely finding is abscess formation.

Two principal mechanisms of injury include

- Puncture — the narrowing at the cricopharyngeus and presence of diverticulum represent the biggest pitfall, especially with a rigid scope. Prudent advancement, proper orientation, and optimal visualization of the entire lumen are the critical preventive measures.
- Dilation — contributing the greatest number of instrument perforations, dilation in the context of strictures must be performed cautiously. While balloon is favored over bougienage in an effort to reduce an axial force, it is difficult to avoid mucosal-limited tears. Because complete perforation occurs proximal to the stricture, close inspection is warranted. Assisted fluoroscopic guidance of contrast-enhanced balloon dilation of esophageal strictures adds to endoscopic safety in difficult cases.

Clinical Presentation

Localized pain to the neck or chest is the most common complaint. Other symptoms and signs include fever, tachycardia, tachypnea, cervical/mediastinal emphysema, and dyspnea secondary to pleural effusion.

Diagnosis

A high index of suspicion on the part of the endoscopist is critical for making a timely and accurate diagnosis. It is not uncommon to perforate the thin mucosal wall unknowingly. Physical examination is helpful with 60% sensitivity for cervical emphysema and 30% for mediastinal.[16]

- Perform a complete head and neck examination.
- A plain radiograph of the chest and abdomen (supine and upright) should be performed. (Note: Timing of the radiograph must be recognized as a diagnostic factor, given that emphysematous change and effusion may take several hours before being evidenced on film.)
- A gastrograffin swallow study should be performed. If the results are negative, consider a more sensitive study with barium. Consider performing the swallow study in the upright and lateral decubitus position to detect cervical perforation.

- CT is useful as an adjunctive study to evaluate for abscess, mediastinal air, or fistula formation.
- Avoid rescoping the patient to make the diagnosis. (Note: All endoscopic procedures should be videotaped if the technology is available so that they may be reviewed for a source and location of perforation.[17])

Prevention

- Visualization
- Knowing the underlying esophageal pathology
- Clinical experience — in the awake patient, swallowing aids in scope advancement into and through the cervical esophagus. Always avoid forced advancement, especially in a blinded setting.
- Fluoroscopy — a useful adjunct to address anatomical complexities, particularly with strictures

Management
Esophageal perforation represents a life-threatening emergency and a thoracic trained surgeon should be consulted immediately. Treatment includes surgical and nonsurgical options. Surgery is considered the mainstay of treatment unless the child is deemed unfit for surgery, in which case medical management represents a reasonable alternative.

- Initial management:
  - Care begins with broad-spectrum intravenous antibiotics, NPO status, and esophageal suction via oral or nasal route.
- Surgical management:
  - Two possible approaches are drainage by itself and drainage with exploration and esophageal repair.
  - Cervical perforation can often be addressed with open drainage of the neck.
  - Thoracic perforations require open surgery with direct repair of defect or ligation and subsequent revision.
- Medical management:
  - This is limited to poor surgical candidates and involves parenteral nutrition, close monitoring, antibiotic therapy, and continuous esophageal suction.
  - Worsening of the child's condition demands reevaluation with CT scan to evaluate for the presence of abscess and consideration of emergent surgery.

SPECIFIC PATHOLOGY

FOREIGN BODY IN THE AIRWAY

General Considerations

Peak Incidence
Foreign body in the airway is found in children under 3 years of age, with foreign body aspiration representing a source of considerable pediatric morbidity and mortality.[18]

Diagnostic Dilemma
Presenting symptoms can be transient, ranging from choking, cyanosis, and hemoptysis to voice changes, chronic cough, and drooling. Given the spectrum of presentations and time course of

diagnosis, treatment is variable. In conjunction with radiologic evaluation, the primary therapeutic and diagnostic tool is rigid bronchoscopy.[19]

When to Employ Rigid Bronchoscopy

This approach is used for cases of diagnostic uncertainty in the context of suggestive symptoms, history, or radiologic findings.

Perioperative Steroids

Equivocal data offer some evidence for increased risk of postoperative atelectasis and pneumonia. The strongest indication occurs in cases of chronically aspirated foreign bodies with granulation and mucosal erosion.

Predictive Factors for Complications

Type of Foreign Body

- Organic
  - Antigenic substances including nuts, seeds, and vegetables are apt to induce bronchial swelling and an inflammatory reaction of the bronchial mucosa.
  - Extraction is complicated by risk of fragmentation, poor visualization secondary to bronchial secretions, and hemorrhage from inflamed mucosa.
- Inorganic
  - Sharp objects, particularly needles, safety pins, and nails, cause direct trauma to the bronchial mucosa and represent a technical challenge for extraction.
  - Ensuring a secure grasp of the object without mucosal traction to avoid laceration injury is key to minimizing operative risk.
  - Trouble areas include grasping object, bronchial branch points, and glottis.

Timing and Duration of the Procedure

The longer the foreign body has been in place, the more the chance for mucosal damage, granulation formation, and erosion is increased. Prolonged cases are at increased risk for laryngeal edema and compromised airway (demonstrated in cases > 30 min).[20]

Instrumentation

- Preparation is paramount to ensure age-appropriate instrumentation is on hand. Practicing extraction using an identical foreign body is recommended.
  - Bronchoscopic sheaths ranging from 3.5 to 6 mm (see Table 23.2)
  - 0 and 30° telescopes of appropriate lengths and diameters
  - Wide range of grasping optical forceps including dual and single action
  - Functional balloon catheter that may facilitate dislodging of deeply impacted foreign body
  - Appropriate suction catheters of adequate length

Anesthesia and Ventilation

As previously mentioned, there are several accepted methods for administering general anesthesia in rigid bronchoscopy. Employing IV anesthesia, spontaneous ventilation with 100% oxygen is recommended with Venturi jet ventilation as needed, thus offering an acceptable adjunct (noted risk of barotrauma).

Complications

Loss of Airway

Persistent hypoxia is the leading contributor to mortality. Etiologies include laryngeal edema, pneumothorax, hemorrhage, and degassing (foreign body is aspirated into another bronchus during attempted extraction).

- Airway management: key issues
  - The topical anesthetic should be applied to the larynx prior to intubation with the rigid bronchoscope.
  - Direct mucosal trauma should be avoided, especially in the subglottic space, with close observation for hemorrhage, ventilatory status, and adequate oxygenation.
  - Pneumonia is the most common postoperative complication; use perioperative antibiotics with low threshold.

Unsuccessful Extraction

After extraction has been attempted once, a second attempt in 2 to 4 days should be considered, depending on the endoscopist's experience level, location of the foreign body, equipment and facilities available, and the child's condition. Reasons for unsuccessful extraction include

- Poor visualization (especially with infants using a 2.5-mm rigid bronchoscope) — attempt to administer suction and irrigation.
- Foreign body larger than bronchoscope lumen — grasp the foreign body outside the bronchoscope lumen and extract the bronchoscope with the attached foreign body as one unit.
- Fragmentation (not uncommon with organic material) — avoid this by using a prudent extraction technique. Extract what fragments are grasped followed by continued extraction for fragmented pieces. Consider BAL with suction to obtain distal fragments.[21]

Alternative Approaches

Thoracotomy

Thoracotomy with external removal of the foreign body should be considered for trapped, sharp foreign bodies when extraction has a high degree of potential to result in tissue disruption.

Use of Flexible Bronchoscopy

This has been documented in cases with minimal potential risk; however, routine use for foreign body removal varies among endoscopists. A combination approach of rigid and flexible bronchoscopy is recommended in some cases (flexible scope through secure rigid bronchoscope), especially in cases of distal lower airway involvement.

- Argument for:
  - Useful when removing distal airway foreign bodies
  - IV sedation used without general anesthesia
- Argument against:
  - Obstructs airway while failing to offer ventilatory support
  - Inability to grasp and stabilize foreign bodies due to small instrument size[22]

Foreign Body in the Esophagus

General Considerations

Esophageal foreign bodies remain a considerable source of pediatric morbidity and mortality. Time of diagnosis is variable as is the clinical presentation, which ranges from hematemesis to fever to airway obstruction.

Critical Management Issues

Identity and Location of the Foreign Body

Coins are the most common smooth objects and often pass on their own; however, sharp bodies are prone to cause mucosal laceration. In particular, batteries require emergent treatment secondary to increased risk of perforation. Whether the object is lodged at the level of the cricopharyngeal muscle (most common) or in the middle (carina/aortic knob) or distal esophagus, position is a major factor in presentation and determining treatment approach.

Duration of Time Following Ingestion

The risk of esophageal perforation secondary to a prolonged inflammatory response must be realized and should motivate the physician toward definitive and expeditious treatment.

Age and Condition of the Child

Issues of airway compromise, hemodynamic stability, and co-morbidities (strictures, previous surgeries, respiratory/GI disease) must be addressed in an effort to afford the patient optimum treatment.

Studied Risk Factors for Complication

A total white count > 11,000 and impaction > 24 h have been demonstrated to increase risk (between 5 to 10 times) for a major complication (aortaesophageal fistula, retropharyngeal abscess, perforation, mediastinitus).[23]

Management

Primarily rigid or flexible esophagoscopy or conservative medical management is called for.[24]

- Rigid and flexible esophagoscopy are safe and efficacious (morbidity < 1%), emphasizing the anatomical advantages garnered with rigid (above the aorta) as opposed to flexible (below the aortic knob).
- Given the cost difference, general anesthesia risk, and comparable success rates between the two approaches, it is not unreasonable to attempt flexible esophagoscopy initially with rigid esophagoscopy reserved in refractory cases.[25]
- Alternatives include balloon catheter and conservative management.

When to Employ Flexible Esophagoscopy

- This procedure is performed under sedation, the airway is NOT secured and must be factored in when assessing the safety of the procedure in the individual child.
- Flexible esophagoscopy with suction and forceps is ideal for smooth objects (coins, food, plastic).
- Limited grasping ability, poor visualization of the proximal esophagus, and maneuverability may prevent extraction of jagged or pointed objects.
- Do NOT hesitate to employ a rigid scope if the flexible is not getting the job done.

When to Employ Rigid Esophagoscopy

- This is performed under general anesthesia; the airway is secured.
- Patient positioning, scope advancement, and adequate visualization are paramount.
- Greater range of forceps and fine movements on the part of the surgeon make rigid esophagoscopy ideal in the instance of pointed- or sharp-body extraction.

Alternatives

- Dilators, nasogastric tubes, or esophageal bougienage are prone to mucosal trauma and subsequent perforation.
- Foley balloon catheter under fluoroscopic guidance is employed in cases of proximal objects; however, the risk of dislodging the foreign body with aspiration may be considerable. When this is used, appropriate back-up resources should be immediately available.
- The use of papain is discouraged secondary to the associated risk of esophageal perforation.[26]

Technique Pearls

- An esophageal foreign body in most cases is NOT an acute emergency. Careful preparation of the child for foreign body removal by an experienced endoscopist under proper conditions maximizes safety and minimizes trauma. Hasty, ill-prepared decisions with improper instrumentation or anesthetic expertise may do more harm than good. Of course, treatment for an esophageal perforation or ingestion of a battery cannot be delayed.
- Instruments and forceps are selected and tested using a duplicate foreign body before surgery. Optical forceps are preferred when appropriate. Several different forceps are chosen anticipating unforeseen circumstances, including delicate, "light-touch," non-crushing forceps and firm-grasping forceps.
- Radiographs are critically reviewed for foreign body location and consistency.
- The foreign body should not be grabbed as soon as it is visualized, but rather studied to ascertain its shape, size, and potential for unforeseen parts (e.g., sharp points buried deep to the visualized area). The esophagoscope tip or selected forceps may be used to modify the foreign body position as necessary.
- Suction is generally used to remove secretions from around the foreign body — not to attempt removal.
- The forceps should be advanced until they lightly touch the foreign body. Next, the rigid esophagoscope is rotated and retracted slightly to allow the blades of the forceps to be opened. Under telescopic guidance, the opened forceps blades are advanced so that they are beyond the center of mass of the foreign body. Care is taken not to push the foreign body distally.
- Once the foreign body is grasped, the forceps and esophagoscope are removed as one unit. The foreign body is rotated to the largest lumen diameter (coronally in the esophagus). Care is taken to ensure that the endotracheal tube remains secure upon removal of the esophageal foreign body.
- Alternatively, the flexible esophagoscope may be used for foreign bodies in the mid and distal esophagus. Irregularly shaped or impacted foreign bodies are usually easier and safer to remove with a rigid esophagoscope and a secured airway.
- A Fogarty embolectomy catheter may be gently placed behind the foreign body, inflated, and pulled forward to dislodge a smooth foreign body that is difficult to remove. The

airway should be protected with an endotracheal tube to prevent inadvertent aspiration of the foreign body.

- Complete esophageal inspection is mandatory. Multiple foreign bodies may be present. Mucosal tears or strictures in the esophagus are examined.

Complications

Mucosal Trauma and Perforation

- Most common complication of foreign body extraction
- Greatest risk at the cricopharyngeal muscle with advancement of the rigid scope
- Other risk factors: esophageal erosions and insufflation per the flexible scope
- Presenting symptoms: fever, tachycardia, and hematemesis
- Initial diagnostic study should include gastrograffin swallow study
- Reference preceding section on perforation management

Specific Esophageal Pathology

Open Safety Pin

Open safety pins are a rare occurrence (declining incidence secondary to disposable diapers); nevertheless, they pose a challenge to safe extraction without significant hemorrhage or perforation.

- Risk of perforation is high and warrants immediate removal with a rigid scope.
- The orientation of the safety pin dictates the approach and again emphasizes the need for radiologic evaluation.
- Pointing caudally, the safety pin can be pulled within the sheath of the scope and extracted without further trauma. When open ends point cephalad, the extraction becomes a technical challenge and especially prone to complication. The suggested approach is to advance the open pin into the stomach and reverse its direction with subsequent extraction.[27]
- Alternatives include attempted extraction within the rigid sheath and gastrotomy in extremely difficult cases. Insufflation may improve visualization of the open tip; however, caution should be exercised, recognizing edema, inflammation, and delayed treatment as risk factors for perforation.[28,29]

Battery

- Swallowed batteries pose a high risk of perforation secondary to chemical erosion.
- Immediate endoscopic removal is indicated.
- Noted caveats include a battery in the stomach that, depending on clinical context, may be observed with serial radiographs.

Caustic Ingestion

- Flexible esophagoscopy and direct laryngoscopy are indicated in the assessment of injury extent.
- The greatest risk lies with alkali substances; burns are best identified 24 to 48 h after ingestion with direct inspection of the oro-hypopharynx and the esophagus.
- There is less risk with acid substances — "coagulation necrosis."

- Contraindications include severe burns with associated laryngeal edema or a patient on high-dose steroids.
- Follow-up radiographic studies should be performed to assess for stricture (more common with circumferential burns as opposed to longitudinal).[30]

CONCLUSIONS

Pediatric aerodigestive tract endoscopy is a practiced technique requiring continued application to maintain one's skills. Given the relative size and labile mucosal physiology, the critical margin of reserve in children may be exceptionally small; even a slight misjudgment may have clinically significant impact on the patient's well-being.

REFERENCES

1. Benjamin, B. Anethesia for the pediatric airway endoscopy. *Otolaryngol. Clin. North Am.*, 2000, 33, 29–46.
2. Rosenburg, M.B. Anesthesia-induced injury. *Int. Anesthesiol. Clin.*, 1989, 27, 120–125.
3. Mancuso, R.F. et al. Laryngomalacia. The search for the second lesion. *Arch. Otolaryngol. Head Neck Surg.*, 1996, 122, 1417–1418.
4. Hawkins, D.B. and Clark, R.W. Flexible laryngoscopy in neonates, infants, and young children. *Ann. Otolaryngoolgy.*, 1987, 96, 81–85.
5. Hilbert, G. et al. Bronchoscopy with bronchoalveolar lavage via the LMA in high-risk immunosuppressed patients. *Crit. Care Med.*, 2001, 29, 1848–1849.
6. Holinger, L.D. *Pediatric Laryngology and Bronchoesophagology*. New York: Lippincott–Raven, 1997.
7. Tunkel, D.E. and Fisher, Q.A. Pediatric flexible fiberoptic bronchoscopy through the laryngeal mask airway. *Arch. Otolaryngol. Head Neck Surg.*, 1996, 122, 1364–1367.
8. Bunting, H.E. and Allen, R.W. Barotrauma during jet ventilation for microlaryngeal surgery. *Anethesia*, 1995, 50, 374–375.
9. Ayers, M.L. and Beamis, J.F. Rigid bronchoscopy in the 21st century. *Clin. Chest Med.*, 2001, 22, 355–364.
10. Amitai, Y. et al. Serum lidocaine concentration in children during bronchoscopy with topical anesthesia. *Chest*, 1990, 98, 1370–1373.
11. Natalini, G. et al. Negative pressure ventilation vs external high frequency oscillation during rigid bronchoscopy. *Chest*, 2000, 118, 18–23.
12. Torres, I.D. and Noviski, N. Flexible fiberoptic bronchoscopy. *Mt. Sinai J. Med.*, 1995, 62, 36–40.
13. Brietzke, S.E. and Mair, E.A. Laryngeal mask versus endotracheal tube in a ferret model. *Ann. Otol., Rhinol., Laryngol.*, 2001, 110, 827–833.
14. Wood, R.E. Pitfalls in the use of the flexible bronchoscope in pediatric patient. *Chest*, 1990, 97, 199–203.
15. Eisen, G.M. et al. Modifications in endoscopic practice for pediatric patients. *Gastrointest. Endosc.*, 2000, 52, 838–842.
16. Sarr, M.G. et al. Management of instrumental perforations of the esophagus. *J. Thoracic Surg.*, 1983, 17, 311–318.
17. Panka, J. et al. Endoscopic perforations of the upper digestive tract: a review of their pathogenesis, prevention, and management. *Gastronenterology*, 1994, 106, 787–802.
18. Lima, J.A. and Fischer, G.B. Foreign body aspiration in children. *Paediatr. Respir. Rev.*, 2002, 3, 303–307.
19. Reilly, J.S. et al. Prevention and management of aerodigestive foreign body injuries in childhood. *Pediatr. Clin. North Am.*, 1996, 43, 1403–1411.
20. Zaytoun, G.M. et al. Endoscopic management of foreign bodies in the tracheobronchial tree: predictive factors for complication. *Otolaryngol. Head Neck Surg.*, 2000, 123, 311–316.

21. Banerjee, A. et al. Larnyngo-tracheo-bronchial foreign bodies in children. *J. Laryngol. Otol.*, 1988, 102, 1029–1032.

22. McGuirt, W.F. et al. Tracheobronchial foreign bodies. *Laryngoscope*, 1988, 98, 615–618.

23. Loh, K.S. et al. Complications of foreign bodies in the esophagus. *Otolaryngol. Neck Surg.*, 2000, 123, 613–616.

24. McGahren, E.D. Esophageal foreign bodies. *Pediatr. Rev.*, 1999, 20, 129–133.

25. Berggreen, P.J. et al. Techniques and complications of esophageal foreign body extraction in children and adults. *Gatrointestinal Endoscopy*, 1992, 39, 626–630.

26. Holsinger, J.W. et al. Esophageal perforation following meat impaction and papain ingestion. *JAMA*, 1968, 204, 188–189.

27. Salley, L.H., Jr. and Wohl, D.L. Nasal foreign body: removal of an open safety pin from the left nostril. *Ear Nose Throat J.*, 2000, 79(2), 118–119.

28. Marsh, B.R. The problem of the open safety pin. *Ann. Otol. Rhinol. Laryngol.*, 1975, 84, 624–626.

29. Bizakis, J.G. et al. The challenge of esophagoscopy in infants with open safety pin in the esophagus: report of two cases. *Am. J. Otolaryngol.*, 2000, 21, 255–258.

30. Holinger, L.D. *Pediatric Laryngology and Bronchoesophagology.* 1997, New York, Lippincott–Raven.

24 Pediatric Tracheotomy

Ian N. Jacobs and George H. Zalzal

To be prepared against surprise is to be trained. To be prepared for surprise is to be educated.

James P. Carse, *Finite and Infinite Games*

CONTENTS

INTRODUCTION

Although the tracheotomy may be a life-sustaining vehicle for many critically ill children, it carries many significant risks and burdens. Mucous plugging or tracheotomy tube dislodgment may lead to cardiopulmonary arrest, anoxic brain injury, and even death. There are also significant delays in speech and language development. In addition, when a tracheotomy is performed in an infant, one can anticipate that it will remain in place for several years. Optimal home care and support will minimize the morbidity and mortality associated with pediatric tracheotomy. Newer technologies, including customized tracheotomies and alternatives to tracheotomy and traditional modes of ventilation, may be helpful in the future.

INDICATIONS

There are three main indications for tracheotomy in infants and children. These include airway obstruction, long-term ventilation, and pulmonary toilet. Infants with congenital or acquired upper airway obstruction may require a tracheotomy at an early age because of extubation failure. Severe cases of congenital laryngeal stenosis may require a tracheotomy immediately after delivery. However, most cases of laryngeal stenosis occur in premature infants requiring long-term ventilation. Bilateral vocal cord paralysis usually results in severe airway obstruction when the vocals cords remain in the paramedian position. A tracheotomy is required in over 50% of cases.[1,2] Neonates may sustain long periods of intubation and ventilation with an endotracheal tube; however, long-term ventilation for bronchopulmonary dysplasia (BPD) will require a tracheotomy. Many premature children with BPD are managed at home with tracheotomies, ventilators, and supportive equipment. In addition, many children with neurological problems and/or loss of brain stem function may require a tracheotomy for pulmonary toilet.

PROCEDURE AND TECHNIQUE

Any child who is candidate for a tracheotomy should undergo a comprehensive examination of the airway prior to the tracheotomy. This is essential to make sure that there are no severe anomalies in the distal airway, such as vascular compression or long-segment tracheal stenosis, prior to performing a tracheotomy. There are special considerations when a tracheotomy is performed in an infant or small child. First, the anatomical landmarks make it more difficult to localize the trachea in these patients than in adults. The major landmarks, including the cricoid and the thyroid cartilage, are not prominent. The trachea is smaller and not as superficial, as well as quite mobile and easy to push over to the side. Furthermore, the rapid placement of a tracheotomy in the cricothyroid membrane ("slash trach") should be avoided in infants and small children.

Routine tracheotomy for infants and small children requires careful dissection with an established airway such as an orotracheal tube. If an artificial airway is not in place, the child undergoes bronchoscopy or intubation prior to the tracheotomy. Occasionally, a tracheotomy may be performed under local anesthesia in older children or adolescents, but this should be avoided, if possible, in small children. In certain cases, the airway may be managed by face mask ventilation or a laryngeal mask airway; however, an endotracheal tube is always preferred.

Once the airway is established, the child is positioned for tracheotomy (Figure 24.1). All indwelling tubes, such as nasogastric tubes, should be removed. A shoulder roll is used for hyperextension. The patient's head is near the anesthesiologist, who has immediate access to the airway at all times. The landmarks, including the cricoid cartilage and the midline sternum, are marked out. A transverse incision is made with the scalpel and deepened through the subcutaneous tissue of the pretracheal fascia. The strap muscles are identified, separated, and used to localize the midline. The upper tracheal rings are identified. In rare instances, the isthmus of the thyroid gland must be divided to expose the upper tracheal ring, unless there is subglottic pathology requiring lower placement.

The tracheotomy tube is usually placed between the second and third tracheal ring. Two stay sutures are placed on either side of the tracheotomy incision and a vertical incision is made through the two tracheal rings (Figure 24.2). The surgeon inserts the tube and ventilation is established. The assistant holds the tube as the surgeon secures the tracheotomy tube with the tracheotomy ties. The authors use the tracheotomy ties with foam wrap to protect the skin and hydrosorb for the

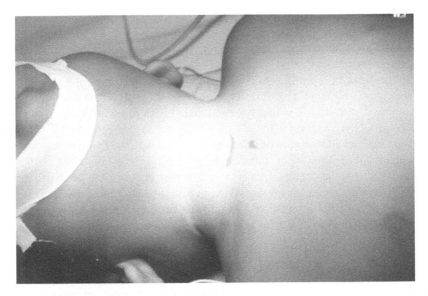

FIGURE 24.1 The patient in the hyperextended position for tracheotomy. The cutaneous surgical landmarks for tracheotomy including the cricoid cartilage, midline sternal notch, and the hyoid bone.

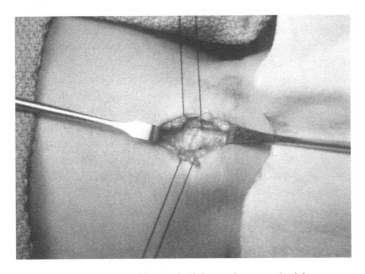

FIGURE 24.2 Two stay sutures placed on either end of the tracheotomy incision.

undersurface of the tracheotomy and almost never suture the tracheotomy to the skin. Occasionally, the edges of the trachea may be sutured to the skin edge, but this will often lead to a persistent tracheal-cutaneous fistula.

TRACHEOTOMY TUBE TYPES

A very important issue is the selection of the tracheotomy tube. Newer manufacturing technologies have increased the number of options. Tracheotomy tubes come in varying lengths, diameters, and materials; they can be cuffed or uncuffed. The age, size, and medical condition of the patient help to determine the tube type. Tracheotomy tubes have three dimensions: inner diameter (ID), outer diameter (OD), and length. The size of the tube is based upon the patient's age and the size of the airway. The dimensions of the tracheotomy tube should roughly correspond to the endotracheal tube that is in place. Table inserts in many of the tracheotomy tube boxes compare the dimensions of the three most commonly used tracheotomy tubes: Shiley®, Bivona®, and Portex®. Shiley tubes are made of polyvinyl chloride, which is rigid. Bivona tracheotomy tubes are made of silicone, which is softer, but can be reinforced with wire. The selection is based upon needs and preference.

Tracheotomies may also come with a cuff. A cuffed tracheotomy tube may be needed for a child requiring higher ventilatory pressures. The three types of cuffs are: high-volume, low-pressure; foam; and tight to shaft (TTS). The first two are inflated with air, while the last requires saline. It is imperative to avoid overinflation with the cuff, which may lead to problems with tracheal erosion and stenosis. On interval endoscopies, it is important to visualize the tracheotomy with cuff inflated with the usual amount of air or saline and then deflate the cuff to examine the surrounding trachea for signs of erosion. If some degree of erosion occurs, then it is imperative to use less pressure or change tracheotomy tube types. Mucosal erosion can lead to pressure necrosis and eventual stenosis of the distal airway. In certain situations, customized tracheotomies may be needed. A specific dimension may be required to overcome a problem such as tracheal granulation tissue.

ROUTINE TRACHEOTOMY CARE

Because many tracheotomy-related complications take place at home, an optimal home-care environment is necessary. The caregivers must have the necessary resources, education, and motivation to provide safe care for the child and should be trained in all aspects of routine and emergent tracheotomy care. They should be prepared for all potential disasters and should be able to perform tracheotomy tube changes easily and quickly. In the event that the tracheotomy becomes plugged or dislodged, the caregiver should be prepared to replace the tracheotomy quickly. He or she should also be trained in CPR.

Adequate tracheotomy equipment, including spare tracheotomies, smaller size tracheotomies, tracheotomy ties, dressing, suction equipment, manual resuscitation bag, humidity devices, and monitors, should be available for home and travel (Figure 24.3). Pulse oximeters are often used although no standard for telemetry exists. Because parents cannot provide 24 hours of home care, home nursing care is usually needed as well. All home care nurses or health-care providers should be trained and competent in all aspects of tracheotomy care. The amount of home nursing care depends on the individual needs of the patient and family; generally, a family should be expected to provide 8 hours of care and require 16 hours of assistance each day. Again, this depends on needs, resources, and capabilities.[3]

- Correct size tracheotomy and obturator
- Tracheotomy — size smaller
- Pipe cleaners
- Container for sterile water
- Sterile water
- Gauze
- Portable suction machine
- Long flexible suction catheters
- Humidity valves
- Gauze tracheotomy dressing
- Oxygen
- Tracheotomy collar

FIGURE 24.3 Equipment needed for tracheotomy tube care.

- Correct size tracheotomy and obturator
- Blanket roll
- Lubricant
- Tracheotomy ties
- Scissors
- Clean wet and dry gauze
- Stethoscope
- Tracheotomy — size smaller
- Resuscitation bag with mask
- Oxygen source

FIGURE 24.4 Equipment needed for tracheotomy tube change.

TRACHEOTOMY TUBE CHANGES

Routinely changing tracheotomy tube is an essential aspect of home care. Most families will perform a weekly tracheotomy tube change, although there are no set standards. All caretakers should learn routine tracheotomy care prior to the patient's discharge from the hospital. Preparation is always essential and problems should be anticipated; it is imperative to have proper equipment available for tracheotomy tube changes (see Figure 24.4). Proper lighting and position are important as well.

Two skilled caregivers are needed to perform a routine tracheotomy tube change. One person is the primary tracheotomy "changer" and the other is the "partner." The steps of a routine change should be followed in order:

1. Hyperoxygenate the child for 10 to 15 minutes.
2. Assemble all supplies and emergency equipment.
3. Determine the partner and position the child.
4. Hyperextend the child on a shoulder roll with the neck well exposed.
5. Be prepared for a difficult cannulation as well as significant bradycardia or desaturation.
6. Have all supplies readily available.
7. The person inserting the tracheotomy takes charge. On his count, the partner removes the tracheotomy and the clean tracheotomy is placed at a right angle into the stoma and advanced into the lumen.
8. The partner reattaches the ventilator and listens for breath sounds.
9. Clean the stoma and apply new gauze.
10. Place, secure, and check tracheotomy ties for correct tension. Only one finger should fit under the tie.
11. Always be prepared for the worst and stay calm.

COMPLICATIONS

Tracheotomy-related complications are classified as immediate, early, and delayed. Some complications, such as hemorrhage or pneumediastinum/pneumothorax, may occur in the perioperative period. Others, such as tracheal granulation tissue, occur late. In addition, certain complications, such as accidental dislodgment or mucous plugging of the tracheotomy tube, may occur anytime. In the past, the mortality rate in children with tracheotomies has been reported to be as high as 24%.[4] Most recent reports indicate mortality rates ranging from 0.5 to 5%.[5–7] Many of these deaths may be preventable with improvements in home care.

Operative Hemorrhage

Excessive bleeding, which is the most common operative complication during tracheotomy, is usually related to technique. Meticulous attention to detail is important. One must be careful with thyroid tissue overlying the trachea. In many cases in the infant or neonatal tracheotomy, the isthmus of the thyroid gland may be avoided; however, if it must be divided, suture ligation is essential. One should stay in the midline and avoid dissecting off laterally because only midline exposure is needed. Coagulation defects should be detected and corrected prior to surgery. Hemostasis should be adequate at the end of the procedure. In situations when excessive oozing is encountered, packing the wound with Surgicel (Johnson & Johnson) may be helpful.

Pneumothorax

Because the apical pleura are higher in infants and small children, injury to the pleura and lung is more likely in these patients than in adults. However, this complication is uncommon and easily avoided by minimizing dissection into the inferior portion of the neck. The authors routinely obtain a chest x-ray (CXR) in the operating room or intensive care unit after the tube is in place. However, some clinicians have reported that the routine use of CXR may not be necessary after pediatric tracheotomy.[6] The best way to avoid this complication is to dissect meticulously and stay in the midline during the dissection. If pleural tissue seems to bulge into the dissection site, that site is best avoided. Sometimes, however, air may track down into the mediastinum. In most cases, this resolves spontaneously; however, in rare circumstances, chest tube placement is needed.

Accidental Decannulation

Obviously, in the early postoperative period, accidental decannulation may be quite hazardous. Because the tracheotomy stoma is not healed, it may suddenly close up and be difficult to reinsert. One may also get into a false passage during the emergent placement of the tracheotomy tube. Accidental decannulation is best avoided by proper adjustment of tracheotomy ties so that only one finger may be placed under the ties. The nursing staff should avoid changing the tracheotomy strings or dressing until the first tracheotomy tube change at 1 week postoperative. In addition, the authors routinely place stay sutures on each side of the trachea near the tracheotomy incision. These stay sutures, which are marked "left" and "right," are necessary in the event that the tracheotomy tube falls out and cannot be reinserted. In the event of an accidental decannulation, it may also be necessary to intubate the patient if laryngeal stenosis is not significant. It is also imperative to keep a smaller size tracheotomy tube by the bedside.

False Passage

During tracheotomy insertion, a false passage will be entered and the patient will not be ventilated. This usually takes place in the operating room during the initial surgery or in the first several days in case of accidental decannulation. This complication is avoided by placing two sutures on both sides of the tracheotomy incision and making a large enough incision into the trachea. It also helps to avoid forcing the tracheotomy into the site. If one enters a false passage, it is prudent to pull up on the tracheotomy ties and try to find the correct passage. At the bedside, a flexible suction catheter can sometimes localize the correct passage and the tracheotomy tube can be inserted over the catheter. In the operating room, a rigid bronchoscope passed into the tracheostome site may be helpful.

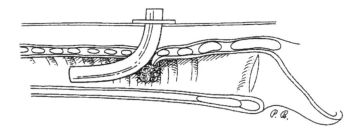

FIGURE 24.5 One surgeon excises the suprastomal granulation polyp through the stoma as the assistant surgeon examines the airway with a rigid ventilating bronchoscope. (From Gray, R.F., Todd, N.W., and Jacobs, I.N., *Laryngoscope*, 1998, 108, 10; Figure 1. With permission.)

EARLY COMPLICATIONS

Local Infection/Skin Breakdown

The peristomal skin may break down because of pressure from the tracheotomy tube. Skin breakdown may take weeks to heal by secondary intention. It is best to avoid this complication with meticulous wound care. Protective dressings such as hydrosorb may protect the skin from breakdown. It is important to secure the tracheotomy with tracheotomy ties that are not excessively tight. It should be possible to insert one finger beneath the tracheotomy ties.

LATE COMPLICATIONS

Tracheal Granulation Tissue

The tracheotomy tube, which is a foreign body, may produce granulation tissue at different sites. Most commonly, many children develop suprastomal granulation tissue above the tube.[8] Routine excision of granulation tissue is not recommended because granulation tissue will usually recur.[9] However, totally obstructive suprastomal granulation tissue puts the child at greater risk for sudden death if the tracheotomy tube plugs or falls out. A sphenoid punch or single skin hook is used to excise the granulation tissue under bronchoscopic visualization (Figure 24.5). Granulation tissue may be peristomal as well and make tracheotomy tube changes more difficult. Generally, silver nitrate is used to shrink such tissue on the exterior surface.

Distal tracheal granulation tissue may be a difficult problem related to aggressive suctioning and improper size and position of the tracheotomy tube. Prevention is the best treatment. Distal obstructive granulation may be removed with the laser (CO_2 or KTP), treated with corticosteroids, or bypassed with a longer tracheotomy tube, but one is limited by the carina.

Suprastomal Collapse (Tracheomalacia)

Suprastomal collapse results from pressure of the tracheotomy tube and local infection and chondritis. Severe suprastomal collapse may prevent decannulation.[8] This complication is minimized by use of appropriately sized tracheotomy tubes and meticulous tracheotomy/stomal care. However, this complication may not always be avoided; in many cases, surgical correction of the collapse may be necessary. In most cases, this can be performed endoscopically by passing an absorbable suture between the suprastomal cartilage and the stomal skin (Figure 24.6). In severe cases, it may be necessary to perform an open tracheoplasty with cartilage grafting in a single-stage fashion.

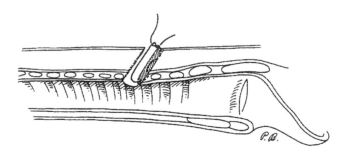

FIGURE 24.6 Repair of suprastomal collapse through the stoma as the assistant observes through the ventilating bronchoscope. (From Gray, R.F., Todd, N.W., and Jacobs, I.N., *Laryngoscope*, 1998, 108, 10; Figure 2. With permission.)

Tracheal or Subglottic Stenosis

Stenosis may develop at, above, or distal to the tracheotomy tube. It is not uncommon to have some degree of mild tracheal stenosis just at or above the level of the tracheotomy tube. The tracheotomy tube may cause granulation tissue formation and chondritis of the suprastomal cartilage, which can limit decannulation. It may be necessary to perform a single-stage laryngotracheoplasty to augment the trachea at that site. An improperly placed high tracheotomy may also contribute to high tracheal or subglottic stenosis. It is essential to place the pediatric tracheotomy below the first tracheal ring and maintain clean, meticulous care.

Tracheal stenosis may also occur distal to the end of the tracheotomy tube. This may be caused by an oversized tracheotomy tube, excessive motion, cuff erosion, or excessive suctioning. Tracheoscopy in the office or at the bedside may elucidate the problem. The tracheotomy tube cuff should be kept deflated as tolerated. The proper size of tracheotomy tube should be used.

Tracheal-Cutaneous Fistula

A persistent tracheal-cutaneous fistula has been reported to occur in 19%[5] and 42%[10] of patients who have had a tracheotomy for more than 1 year. The tracheotomy fistula may be a potential route for external contaminants to spread to the trachea and bronchi. Treatment is by complete surgical excision of the tract and skin closure. Potential complications include pneumomediastinum and pneumothorax. This is avoided by performing primary closure over a rubber band drain and a short period of intubation. The tract could also be excised and then a small tracheotomy tube placed overnight. The tube is removed the following morning and the tract closes by secondary intention. The first method may lead to a better cosmetic result.[11]

Innominate Artery Erosion

This feared complication may occur because the innominate artery crosses in front of the trachea. This artery may ride high and be predisposed to this complication, which is caused by erosion of the tracheotomy or cuff into the anterior tracheal wall. It may present with a sentinel bleed and may become quickly fatal unless it is diagnosed immediately. Diagnosis requires a high index of suspicion. Arteriography may be necessary to define the bleeding vessel. Treatment involves the surgical ligation of the innominate artery by the cardiothoracic team.

Dysphagia

Many children with tracheotomies have severe swallowing and feeding issues because the tracheotomy contributes to an increased tendency to aspirate. The tracheotomy may fix the larynx and prevent elevation. In addition, diminished laryngeal closure and subglottic pressure will be present with a tracheotomy in place[12] and concomitant airway-related pathology, such as vocal cord paralysis or tracheal-esophogeal fistula (TEF), may increase the risk of aspiration. Furthermore, children tracheotomized for neurological reasons may have global neurological impairment with delayed pharyngeal and esophageal motility. Children with tracheotomy also cannot smell and thus cannot taste their food; the airway problem may limit normal airflow to the nasal cavity. Other associated problems, such as gastroesophogeal reflux (GER), may contribute to decreased laryngeal sensitivity.[13]

The Passy–Muir speech valve, which redirects airflow through the glottis, may enhance deglutition for multiple reasons. The valve should be considered in children who demonstrate an adequate airway. In addition, children with tracheotomies should undergo a formal feeding evaluation if any problems with a modified barium swallow or an endoscopic feeding evaluation are identified. The flexible endoscopic evaluation of swallowing (FEES) can be easily performed on infants and children of all ages in the ambulatory setting. The FEES study can address the airway and feeding issues at the same time. It is important to address the feeding problems early, especially if reconstructive airway surgery is required.[14]

Speech and Language Delays

Profound delays in speech and language acquisition are common in tracheotomized children. This may be related to a critical airway with the inability to move air around the tracheotomy tube. The tracheotomy tube may block the flow of air. In many cases, the problem is alleviated when the airway problem is corrected and the tracheotomy is removed. In children with an adequate airway above the tracheotomy tube, who can move sufficient air around the tube, a Passy–Muir speech valve may help with speech production. This valve will act as a one-way valve and allow tracheotomized children to phonate. It is essential to know the airway situation before recommending a valve and to use the valve under close supervision. The valve should be removed during sleep and upper respiratory infections.

DECANNULATION

GENERAL CONSIDERATIONS

A standard approach to decannulation should be followed to ensure the safe and expeditious removal of the tube as soon as it is feasible to do so. In order to achieve decannulation, three conditions must be met[8]:

- The original condition requiring the tracheotomy should be resolved or improved.
- The airway needs to be adequate for the respiratory needs of the individual patient.
- The child should be able to protect the airway and should not need the tracheotomy for pulmonary toilet reasons.

In addition, there should be no other reason to maintain the tracheotomy — for example, an upcoming surgery that affects the airway such as cleft palate or craniofacial surgery.

If the child meets the criteria for decannulation, he or she should undergo a comprehensive endoscopic evaluation of the airway and correction of any obstructive problems prior to decannulation. This will ensure that the airway is indeed adequate for everyday function. It is necessary to evaluate the dynamics of the larynx, making sure that vocal cord mobility is normal and no evidence of supraglottic collapse or stenosis is present. In addition, it is important to make sure that the nasopharyngeal airway is patent. If large adenoids and tonsils are obstructive, they should be removed prior to decannulation. It is also important to examine the subglottic and tracheal airway with the rigid ventilating bronchoscope or telescope to ensure that no stenosis or distal tracheobronchomalacia exists here.

Suprastomal collapse and granulation polyps must be corrected prior to decannulation. In many cases there is a significant degree of collapse of the suprastomal airway. This can be repaired endoscopically by placing a suture through the collapsing cartilage and peristomal epithelium to "pexy" up this collapsing cartilage. An assistant surgeon holds the ventilating bronchoscope as the primary surgeon works at the stoma and visualizes the repair on a monitor. Granulation polyps can be excised with a forceps, Kerrison, optical forceps, or CO_2 laser (Figure 24.5).

DECANNULATION METHODS

The final process of decannulation varies from institution to institution, but close telemetry in the initial decannulation period is essential. Some prefer to downsize and cap off the tracheotomy. The smallest possible tracheotomy is placed and a tracheotomy cap is placed on the end of the tracheotomy. The patient then respires around this. A short period of observation (overnight) is followed and, if successful, the tracheotomy is removed. Other clinicians simply remove the tracheotomy when the airway is deemed adequate. Whatever method is chosen, it is important to observe the patient closely for problems and to individualize the approach.

ALTERNATIVE MODES OF VENTILATION (NONINVASIVE VENTILATION)

Innovations in pulmonary medicine and critical care have led to the development of noninvasive modes of ventilation and oxygenation. These techniques may obviate the need to maintain a tracheotomy. The commonly employed mode of noninvasive ventilation is nasal mask ventilation. A face mask (bilevel positive airway pressure) can be used to administer positive pressure during the inspiratory and expiratory phases of ventilation. The levels of pressure can be adjusted and a polysomnography study can confirm whether the nasal mask ventilation is providing adequate ventilation. Patients who still require supplemental oxygen can be decannulated; oxygen dependency is no reason to remain cannulated. Supplemental oxygen may be administered by nasal canula. In certain situations, a patient with continuous oxygen requirement may receive transtracheal oxygen delivery. An oxygen canula can be left in the old tracheostome site after decannulation.[15,16]

SUMMARY

Tracheotomy, which carries significant risks, should never be taken lightly. A number of severe life-threatening risks can be minimized. By adherence to meticulous surgical technique and very careful postoperative care, one can avoid these severe problems. Standard protocols for routine and emergent tracheotomy care need to be followed. Adherence to these detailed protocols will be helpful for optimizing safe tracheotomy care in the home and in the community.

REFERENCES

1. Rosin, D.F., Handler, S.D., Potsic, W.P. et al. Vocal cord paralysis in children. *Laryngoscope,* 1990, 100, 1174–1179.
2. Dedo, D.D. Pediatric vocal cord paralysis. *Laryngoscope,* 1979, 89, 1378–1384.
3. Panitch, H.B., Downs, J.J., Kennedy, J.S., Kolb, S.M., Parra, M.M., Peacock, J., and Thompson, M.C. Guidelines for home care of children with chronic respiratory insufficiency. *Pediatr. Pulmonol.,* 1996, 21, 52–56.
4. Fearon, B. and Cotton, R.T. Subglottic stenosis in infants and children: the clinical problem and experimental surgical correction. *Can. J. Otolaryngol.,* 1972, 1, 281–289.
5. Wetmore, R.F., Handler, S.D., and Potsic, W.P. Pediatric tracheostomy: experience during the past decade. *Ann. Otol. Laryngol.,* 1982, 91, 628–632.

6. Wetmore, R.F., Marsh, R.R., Thompson, M.E., and Tom, L.W.C. Pediatric tracheostomy: a changing procedure? *Ann. Otol. Rhinol. Laryngol.,* 1999, 108(7), 695–699.
7. Darden, D., Towbin, R., and Dohar, J. Pediatric tracheostomy. Is postoperative chest x-ray necessary? *Ann. Otol. Rhinol. Laryngol.,* 110(4), 345–348, 2001.
8. Gray, R.F., Todd, N.W., and Jacobs, I.N. Tracheostomy decannulation in children: approaches and techniques. *Laryngoscope,* 1998, 108, 8–12.
9. Rosenfeld, R.M. and Stool, S.E. Should granulomas be excised in children with long-term tracheotomy? *Arch. Otol. Head Neck Surg.,* 1992, 118, 1323–1327.
10. Joseph, H.T., Jani, P., Preece, J.M. et al. Pediatric tracheostomy: persistent tracheal-cutaneous fistula following decannulation. *Int. J. Pediatr. Otorhinolaryngol.,* 1991, 22, 231–236.
11. Stern, Y., Cosenza, M., Walner, D.L. et al. Management of persistent tracheocutaneous fistula in the pediatric age group. *Laryngoscope,* 1999, 108(9), 880–883.
12. Cameron, J., Reynolds, J., and Zuidema, G. Aspiration in patients with tracheotomies. *Surg. Gynecol. Obstetr.,* 1973, 136, 68–70.
13. Thompson, L.D., Rudolph, C.D., and Willging, J.P. Swallowing disorders in children. *Curr. Op. Otolaryngol.,* 1999, 7, 313–319.
14. Willging, J.P. Benefit of feeding assessment before pediatric airway reconstruction. *Laryngoscope,* 2000, 210, 825–833.
15. Preciado, D.A., Thatcher, G., Panitch, H.B., and Rimell, F.L. Transtracheal oxygen catheters in a pediatric population. *Otol. Rhinol. Laryngol.,* 2002, 111(4), 310–314.
16. Hoffman, L.A., Johnson, J.T., Wesmiller, S.W. et al. Transtracheal delivery of oxygen: efficacy and safety for long-term continuous therapy. *Ann. Otol. Rhinol. Laryngol.,* 1991, 100, 108–115.

25 Laryngotracheal Reconstruction

Gregory F. Hulka and Daniel L. Wohl

The feasibility of an operation is not the best indication for its performance.

Henry, Lord Cohen of Birkenhead

CONTENTS

INTRODUCTION

Following the introduction of prolonged endotracheal intubation for infants with premature lungs in the mid-1960s, the incidence of laryngotracheal stenosis began to rise. Advances in the surgical management of these infants and children have steadily progressed since that time,[1] paradoxically corresponding with a current decrease in overall incidence as better awareness and medical advances have significantly reduced the number of children requiring prolonged intubation. It is incumbent, therefore, for physicians who choose to care for these children to remain aware of ongoing advancements while also continuing to develop and maintain their skills.

Airway management, in general, is a team concept. Although the otolaryngologist–head and neck surgeon may take a primary role in the diagnosis and management of these children, their care almost always involves a competent cadre of specialists, including intensivists, anesthesiologists, and pulmonologists, as well as gastroenterologists, pediatric surgeons, and emergency physicians. Additionally, the team will include participation by hospital and home nurses, respiratory therapists, and possibly nurse practitioners and nurse anesthetists. The primary care physician is usually intimately involved. Perhaps the most demanding role, however, is provided by the parents and family, or their legal equivalent, because these individuals must attend to the ongoing daily needs of these children during and after their "technology-dependent" years.

AVOIDANCE OF COMPLICATIONS

PREPARATION AND PLANNING

Major pediatric airway surgical procedures depend upon much more than a skilled surgeon. Careful planning of operative and postoperative care will minimize the likelihood of related complications. Success requires a knowledgeable team, including anesthesia, operating room personnel, respiratory therapy, intensive care unit staffing, nursing personnel, and home health personnel.

Open communication — before, during, and after the event — and an understanding among all involved increase the opportunity for a successful outcome. Preoperative planning is an opportunity for the medical team to get to know the patient. It also offers a chance for the patient and family to get to know and begin the relationship with the health care team — in addition to beginning to understand the underlying pathology of the child patient's airway pathology. Planning continues with the intraoperative endoscopic assessment of the airway, which may also serve to introduce the patient to the operating room personnel as well as to other members of the team.

PREOPERATIVE ASSESSMENT

It is important to keep in mind that there is rarely only one choice in taking care of an airway problem in a child. The surgeon should begin outlining the general options during the initial office or bedside assessment. Only after a firm diagnosis has been ascertained and described to the family should a detailed discussion proceed as to more specific options for therapy, along with their inherent risks and benefits.

Today, more families perform reviews of the literature and often read about options for therapy. Maintaining an open mind when considering family concerns, beliefs, and suggestions is fundamental in the care of these children. It is important to remember the overlap in appropriate indications and treatment of subglottic and tracheal stenosis. Furthermore, two physicians may differ as to which form of therapy would be best, based on the individual surgeon's experience with certain techniques. Subsequently, the family should understand the risks and benefits of all options. In some instances, not only would a tracheostomy be an alternative, but it might also be the best option compared with reconstruction.

Sometimes families are unsure or uncomfortable choosing what may seem to them to be a more radical procedure than they had considered. A general rule may be to discuss the most conservative form of therapy initially. No procedures are risk free or 100% successful. Complications or failure arising from a procedure that a surgeon has too enthusiastically encouraged a reluctant family to choose can leave everyone involved with second thoughts as to whether they made the right choice.

PREOPERATIVE MEDICAL AND SURGICAL HISTORY

The vast majority of patients considered for laryngotracheal reconstruction have other medical problems, and many of these patients also have other forms of airway disease, including upper or lower airway compromise.

Sequelae of prematurity. Very frequently, patients requiring airway reconstruction have been born prematurely. Bronchopulmonary disease and cardiac disease are common in this group and appropriate, but prolonged, intubation may result in airway pathology. Congenital cardiovascular anomalies may place the left recurrent laryngeal nerve at risk during cardiac surgery or may result in a degree of extrinsic tracheal compression. One must understand the degree of the pathology and acute tolerance of transient as well as long-term hypoxia and intubation, in addition to postsurgical sequelae such as increased tracheal bloody secretions, in these infants with other reasons for cardiopulmonary compromise.

Generally, direct communication with the pulmonologist, cardiologist, and other specialists is important to determine whether these patients are realistic candidates for surgical procedures that involve transient airway compromise, long operative times, and postoperative care that includes intensive care unit management. Are other surgical procedures being considered? If the child presently has a tracheostomy tube in place, it may be best simply to postpone any surgical management of the airway until after the other surgical procedures are performed. This will minimize postrepair trauma to the reconstructed airway from intubation for other surgical procedures.

Steroid use. Medical problems requiring the use of steroids also must be identified. Not only forms of pulmonary disease may require steroid use, but also autoimmune disorders, inflammatory disease processes, and the patient's status after bone marrow or solid organ transplant. The use of corticosteriods is associated with graft failure, which should be considered when surgical correction may involve grafting techniques in patients using such medications. Subsequently, other procedures including cricotracheal resection with reanastomosis may still be an alternative, but the effects of corticosteroids on wound healing must be considered.

Gastroesophageal reflux. The effects of application of gastric acid to the airway of an animal model have clearly demonstrated exacerbation of subglottic narrowing[2] that is improved with reflux medication. Although for humans this seems to be a reasonable conclusion, it is debatable.

In some patients, reflux can clearly be identified as a contributing factor to fixed subglottic narrowing. Whether it is worthwhile to perform a complete gastrointestinal evaluation on all asymptomatic patients is arguable. The utility of esophagoscopy with biopsy, barium swallow, and pH probe testing, as well as other forms of diagnostic testing, is reviewed in Chapter 19. However, if one does choose to obtain a pH probe study, it is important that it be a two-channel pH probe. A child with multiple episodes of reflux into the distal esophagus, without a single event occurring in the hypopharyngeal region, is at much less risk for exacerbation of subglottic disease than the child with only a handful of episodes of reflux over 4 hours, but with each episode a full column (including hypopharyngeal) regurgitation.

With the role of reflux disease not entirely clear cut, it is certainly worthwhile to consider empiric therapy,[3] even in asymptomatic patients. The relative toxicity of anti-reflux medications given perioperatively is low enough that they may offer more to be gained than lost by avoiding their potential risks. In some cases, airway reconstruction is not indicated because the underlying pathology has been identified — not as fixed subglottic narrowing, but rather submucosal edema, which may be associated with gastroesophageal reflux or other inflammatory (and reversive) processes.

Age of patient. As knowledge and experience in laryngotracheal reconstruction have progressed, various restrictions in age and weight have been replaced by a reasoned consideration of all clinical factors. In some children, a "cricoid split" in the extended neonatal period may be accompanied by rigid tissue interposition, including rib cartilage, thyroid cartilage, or hyoid bone. These procedures are more appropriately considered as a larygotracheal reconstruction.

ENDOSCOPIC DIAGNOSIS

A comprehensive evaluation of the child's upper and lower conductive airway by an experienced endoscopist is critical to ascertaining an accurate diagnosis. Concomitant airway compromise needs to be determined to decide if the patient is actually a candidate for eventual decannulation. Knowing that subglottic or tracheal stenosis exists does not rule out the existence of other etiologies of airway compromise.

Midfacial and mandibular anomalies need to be considered. Glossoptosis, laryngomalacia, vocal cord paralysis, or any other concomitant laryngeal pathology needs to be identified. Laryngeal clefting, tracheoesophageal fistula, and tracheomalacia need to be looked for as well. The presence of any of these pathologies may preclude the possibility of immediate repair and decannulation and the option of tracheostomy may be favorable. Similarly, adenotonsillar hypertrophy can develop in these patients, just as in the general pediatric population, and needs to be assessed at an appropriate time prior to decannulation.

One should accurately define the site's pathology. A mature scar with normal mucosal covering is a much better candidate for possible repair than edema, hyperemia, and granulation tissue, which may indicate an active, undiagnosed underlying reactive mucosal process. Differentiation between subglottic cysts and extrinsic and intrinsic masses within the airway vs. subglottic narrowing seems obvious, but these can occasionally be confused and not recognized until the airway is open. Even with a very thorough and complete intraoperative evaluation of the airway, the preoperative discussion with the family must leave open the door for change in plan once the airway has been intraoperatively evaluated. For example, what is identified as a thin web at the time of the endoscopic evaluation of the airway may turn out to be much thicker than originally realized, and other pathology may become apparent.

Four characteristics of laryngotracheal stenosis that should be determined are

- Where: define the region(s) of anatomy involved.
- Lumen size: calibrate the smallest diameter.
- Maturity: assess for the firmness and relative thickness of the fibrosis.
- Length: calibrate the length of the scar band.

TECHNIQUE

A wide variety of techniques are used to repair airway compromise related to subglottic and tracheal stenosis, and impressions of which procedure is best applied to identical types of pathology vary as well. Rather than discuss the indications for different forms of stenosis,[4] we will describe different categories of techniques and discuss potential complications of which to be aware within each category.

SINGLE-STAGE VS. TWO-STAGE PROCEDURES

Generally, single-stage procedures are used in patients with less severe narrowing of the airway; by definition, they do not leave the "safety valve" of a tracheostomy tube in place.[5–7] Immediate postextubation/poststent removal risks include collapse of the airway secondary to slippage of the graft. This is not necessarily a technical complication. Rather, it could be related to the loss of cartilage graft integrity subsequent to necrosis at the suture sites.

Granulation tissue[8] and restenosis with two-stage procedures are more likely to occur than in single-stage procedures and may form at the upper or the lower margins of the stent. At the site of the previous tracheostomy tube, there may be an area of weakening of the trachea, anteriorly; this may secondarily result in unrecognized collapse. Failure to achieve extubation may also be due to a dynamic airway lesion previously disguised by the now repaired dominant lesion.[9]

CRICOTRACHEAL RESECTION VS. GRAFTING

Cricotracheal resection and grafting may be reasonable techniques to address the same form of pathology, and success may prove to be similar between them. Cricotracheal resection is more likely to put the recurrent laryngeal nerves at risk simply because dissection takes place in the pathway of this nerve. However, this is an infrequent complication, and there is no reason to think of this as a more significant risk than recurrent laryngeal nerve injury with thyroid surgery. With cricotracheal resection, the level of pathology must be well enough below the level of the glottis so that, at the time of reanastomosis, there is enough room to place sutures without suturing the vocal folds. Generally, a minimum 5 mm of distance below the undersurface of the vocal folds is necessary in order to have adequate margins for reanastomosis. With cricotracheal resection, if care is not taken in placing sutures extramucosally when bringing the two halves of the airway together, their presence intralumenally may increase the likelihood of granulation tissue and postoperative restenosis can occur. With cricotracheal resection, immediate or late airway obstruction may present secondary to arytenoid prolapse; treatment of symptomatic patients can be successfully managed with endoscopic partial arytenoidectomy.[10–12]

GRAFTING MATERIAL

The material used for grafting to the stenotic section of airway may vary, depending on the surgeon. The most often used and best described is the costal cartilage of rib graft.[13] Other potential grafts include hyoid bone interposition, conchal cartilage,[14] thyroid ala cartilage, and hydroxyapatite, as well as other materials.[15] Each of these has advantages, ranging from their rigidity to availability to lack of need for donor site. The use of biodegradable external stents is being investigated. They may prove effective but their application remains experimental.[16] When cartilage is taken from a separate incision, complications must be considered at the site of donation.

The risk of greatest concern with rib grafts is pneumothorax. One should check for a leak at the time of closing the wound and a chest x-ray postoperatively is also worthwhile; pneumothorax can arise from obtaining the rib graft or possible injury to a high apical segment of the lung, which may have been injured at the surgical site. With conchal cartilage, some surgeons place pressure dressings much as they place for treatment of auricular hematoma.

TYPE OF STENT

It is generally accepted that rigid stents are superior to soft stents. The orthopedic literature has described well that important aspects of wound healing for bone and structural cartilage are stability and immobility. Without these, nonunion is more likely to occur. Similarly, it is generally accepted that the material of which a stent is made should be nonreactive. Whether to use a Teflon stent, a laryngeal stent formed in the shape of the airway, or a segment of an endotracheal tube is argued by many; each has its benefits and risks. The duration of stenting or post single-stage intubation should be determined based on the assessment of reconstruction stability.[1,17] In general, combined anterior and posterior grafting results in less stability and will require a longer period of intubation.

USE OF MITOMYCIN

The use of topically applied mitomycin to minimize the potential of postoperative subglottic narrowing is advocated by some surgeons. Because it is a known carcinogen, this drug should be used cautiously; long-term data regarding its application to the airway are not yet available.[18]

NEUROMUSCULAR BLOCKADE AND PROLONGED SEDATION

Some professionals advocate complete avoidance of neuromuscular blockade, while others strongly feel that it is essential to minimize the motion of an internal stent. A period of immobility is strongly favored, particularly with the use of an endotracheal tube in patients who have had a cricotracheal resection or single-stage procedure.[19]

RECOGNITION AND MANAGEMENT OF COMPLICATIONS

Even with the best planning, techniques, and medical care, complications will occur.[20] Anticipating and preparing for their possibility are important to ensure that when they occur, the impact on patients is minimized. Some cases require a quick response; others simply require an application of appropriate management while keeping in mind a long-term plan.

INTRAOPERATIVE COMPLICATIONS

Intraoperative complications are frequently related to mechanical ventilation. Many of these patients have underlying pulmonary disease, and leaks around the endotracheal tube during the time of surgery can lead to the decreased capacity to provide ample positive pressure for ventilation. Understanding the need for positive pressure is the key to minimizing these problems; packing with pledgets in an open airway will help minimize these leaks. Similarly, minimizing the amount of blood that runs into the trachea is important. Subsequent bronchospasm from blood or other fluid leaking into the lungs can have transient as well as long-term, devastating consequences, so minimizing this risk is important.

Another classic time to develop a very avoidable complication occurs at the time of changing the tube used for ventilation over to another endotracheal tube or stent and tracheostomy tube combination. Very often, during the switch-over, the child is taken off pressure or rate control ventilation and hand bagged for several breaths. Unless one is careful, the enthusiasm to bag can be such that enough pressure is generated to rupture blebs within the lungs of once premature patients. This can happen even with an experienced anesthesiologist; however, communication to avoid such potential problems is generally all that is required.

IMMEDIATE POSTOPERATIVE COMPLICATIONS

One hopes to prevent pneumothorax; however, awareness of its possibility and identifying it early are most important. Most surgeons recommend obtaining a chest x-ray in the immediate postoperative period to identify a pneumothorax, even if bilateral breath sounds are appreciated.

Esophageal injuries can also occur. Generally, these are more common when a posterior graft is used. Often, an esophageal tear will be identified at the time of grafting, but sometimes it is only identified when subcutaneous air is palpated, or worse when mediastinitis subsequently develops. Awareness of its possibility is important, and intraoperative esophagoscopy may be performed if it is suspected that the esophagus has been injured. Endotracheal tube plugging can develop in single-stage procedures or with a cricotracheal resection. Mucus and blood clot plugging of the endotracheal tube may be so severe that it cannot be suctioned clear. Often, this requires the premature removal of the tube. As this decision is usually made so quickly that a member of the otolaryngology team may not be present, it is important to evaluate the airway as soon as safely possible.

Tracheostomy tube plugging in a two-staged procedure can also occur. When the tracheostomy tube is a part of the stent, an inner cannula can generally be quickly removed. When the tracheostomy tube is in place inferior to a stent, it may be necessary simply to remove it and place a new, clean tracheostomy tube. If a single-chamber pediatric or neonatal tracheotomy tube is used and attached to a stent, it may be urgently necessary to cut any attachments to an internal stent in order to place a new tube.

Recurrent laryngeal nerve injury, particularly if associated with cricotracheal resection, may be the result of a transient paresis and not from permanent injury. Patience is beneficial here, allowing an opportunity for spontaneous resolution. Electromyography (EMG) testing may be considered to assess for the presence of motor unit action potentials (MUAP). The finding of intact MUAP, however, is only indicative of neuromuscular synapse integrity and does not provide useful information regarding partial denervation or early muscle fatigue.

Pneumonia is one of the most common immediate complications associated with larygnotracheal reconstruction. Insufficient pulmonary toilet in the ICU may result in segmental areas of atelectasis, which result in trapped secretions or blood that has passed into the trachea. Iatrogenic infections obtained from a prolonged stay in an ICU must also be guarded against and quickly treated once identified.

Premature extubation may occur during transportation of the patient or in the ICU. Usually, during transportation the patient is sedated and paralyzed, minimizing the chance of accidental extubation from voluntary motion of the patient. Assiduous attention to ICU airway protection protocols should also reduce the possibility of accidental extubation as the patient is being moved about in the bed or during times when inadvertent voluntary movement is possible.

EXTENDED POSTOPERATIVE COMPLICATIONS

Granulation tissue may occur at the end of stents, sometimes related to motion of the stent. Excessive amounts need to be removed, but modest accumulation usually resolves following stent removal. Slipped and broken stents can occur. Stents can settle into a position within the trachea where they are hard to remove. Broken stents can occur, usually from direct neck trauma, and should be replaced.

Superficial wound infections are often identified but should respond to wound care and topical and/or intravenous antibiotics. Cutaneous ulceration at the site of the tracheostomy tube flange can occur. Use of skin protective material, such as Duoderm, can minimize the friction and pressure trauma from extended contact.

Other ICU complications include narcotic withdrawal, weakness from long-term neuromuscular blockade, and RSV infections. Weakness from neuromuscular blockade and narcotic withdrawal can occur; the best way of preventing this is to be aware of the possibility and minimize the amount and length of usage of these drugs. These clinical matters are usually best managed by the intensivists involved in the care of these patients.

LONG-TERM COMPLICATIONS

The well-prepared surgeon will have assessed potential long-term concerns when planning an airway reconstructive procedure. Family preparedness, including emotional readiness for major surgery and the possibility of extended postoperative care and monitoring, is an important consideration. Furthermore, the family that lives in an extremely rural environment far from the local emergency room requires special consideration with regard to postoperative care.

Home monitoring, nursing care, and supplies are concerns to be addressed. The amount of nursing care and monitoring will vary depending on the kind of procedure and the capabilities of the family. As a general rule, it is better to provide too much for the family with limited medical resources than to begin without enough care and run into catastrophe. Training in infant and child CPR is necessary for all families and should be verified. Training in tracheostomy tube care is usually already established but should be verified. If a tracheostomy tube becomes dislodged, it is better if more than one family member has been instructed in how to replace it.

Availability of appropriate medical care may be limited for some families. A surgeon may choose a more conservative approach toward airway management when families are not able to access health care readily. Availability of 911 service means that for patients who live in more rural communities, the presence of a telephone within the home (or readily accessible nearby) and an established route for EMS to the family should be dealt with prior to discharge.

The surgical team contact person should expect multiple phone calls. It is practical to have a designated person on staff who can provide knowledgeable responses in a timely manner. An emergency contact number should also be provided so that families know how to contact the team for urgent issues.

REVISION LARYNGOTRACHEAL RECONSTRUCTION

When revision is necessary, the most important aspect in the evaluation of the patient is to try to determine why the initial procedure failed. The child's medical history and prior airway interventions should be completely evaluated, and previous surgical procedures and postoperative management should be reviewed. An updated endoscopic evaluation, checking for dynamic and static findings, is essential. Often, something can be identified, but sometimes failure is for an unknown or unpredictable reason.[21]

A change of technique, whether it is the surgeon's own failed laryngotracheal reconstruction (LTR) or a referral from another surgeon, is worth considering. In a patient who previously had a grafting technique, cricotracheal resection may be a better alternative for revision if the failure was because of resorption or displacement of the graft for unknown causes.

CONTINUING EDUCATION ISSUES

Unless a surgeon benefits from a steady inflow of new patients (whether from within his own institution or referred into his practice), laryngotracheal reconstruction in children should be cautiously considered. The success of these procedures depends on the level of skill and experience of many resources and is not limited to the skill and experience of the surgeon alone. It is important to remain current by reading journals and attending relevant meetings. An honest self-assessment is one of the most useful continuing education tools in existence. Reviewing one's successes and failures and trying to improve one's techniques for evaluation, management, and understanding of airway disease processes in children is a constant check ensuring continued improvement of patient care.

CONCLUSIONS

Although the incidence of infants and children requiring major airway reconstructive procedures should continue to decrease, surgical and nonsurgical innovations in technique and improvements in technology will continue to be developed and applied. The involved surgical team should become familiar with the advantages and disadvantages of these potential advancements in management and remain aware of the following key nontechnical points in determining long-term success in laryngotracheal reconstruction:

- Make an accurate diagnosis of the airway pathology.
- Apply knowledgeable decision making to determine the procedures to perform.
- Determine who is an appropriate candidate.
- Ongoing education is critical to assure an informed family.
- Assure availability of appropriate and necessary postoperative care.

REFERENCES

1. Myer, C.M., III and Hartley, B.E.J. Pediatric laryngotracheal surgery, *Laryngoscope*, 2000, 110, 1875–1883.
2. Carron, J.D., Greinwald, J.H., Oberman, J.P., Werner, A.L., and Derkay, C.S. Simulated reflux and laryngotracheal reconstruction: a rabbit model. *Arch. Otolaryngol. Head Neck Surg.*, 2001, 127(5), 576–580.
3. Ludemann, J.P., Hughes, C.A., Noah, Z., and Holinger, L.D. Complications of pediatric laryngotracheal reconstruction: prevention strategies. *Ann. Otol. Rhinol. Laryngol.*, 1999, 108 (11 Pt. 1), 1019–1026.

4. Backer, C.L., Mavroudis, C., Gerber, M.E., and Hollinger, L.D. Tracheal surgery in children: an 18-year review of four techniques. *Eur. J. Cardio-Thoracic Surg.*, 2001, 19(6), 777–784.

5. Gustafson, L.M., Hartley, B.E., Liu, D.T., Chadwell, J., Koebbe, C., Meyer, C.M., and Cotton, R.T. Single-stage laryngotracheal reconstruction in children: a review of 200 cases (review; 11 refs). *Otolaryngol. Head Neck Surg.*, 2000, 123(4), 430–434.

6. Saunders, M.W., Thirlwall, A., Jacob, A., and Albert, D.M. Single- or two-stage laryngotracheal reconstruction; comparison of outcomes. *Int. J. Pediatr. Otorhinolaryngol.*, 1999, 50(1), 51–54.

7. Rhee, J.S. and Toohill, R.J. Single-stage adult laryngotracheal reconstruction without stenting. *Laryngoscope*, 2001, 111(5), 765–768.

8. Jewett, B.S., Cook, R.D., Johnson, K.L., Logan, T.C., and Shockley, W.W. Effect of stenting after laryngotracheal reconstruction in a subglottic stenosis model. *Otolaryngol. Head Neck Surg.*, 2000, 122(4), 488–494.

9. Rutter, M.J., Link, D.T., Liu, J.H., and Cotton, RT. Laryngotracheal reconstruction and the hidden airway lesion. *Laryngoscope*, 2000, 110, 1871.

10. Cicero, P.J., Martin, R., Ramirez, M.S., and Navarro, F. Laryngotracheal reconstruction in subglottic stenosis: an ancient problem still present. *Otolaryngol. Head Neck Surg.*, 2001, 125(4), 397–400.

11. Wolf, M., Shapira, Y., Talmi, Y.P., Novikov, Il, Kronenberg, J., and Yellin, A. Laryngotracheal anastomosis: primary and revised procedures. *Laryngoscope*, 2001, 111(4 Pt. 1), 622–627.

12. Rutter, M.J., Link, D.T., Hartley, B.E.J., and Cotton, R.T. Arytenoid prolapse as a consequence of cricotracheal resection in children. *Ann. Otol. Rhinol. Laryngol.*, 2001, 110, 210.

13. Kaschke, O., Otze, H., and Sandmann, J. Use of cartilage grafts in the treatment of laryngotracheal stenosis and defects in children. *Eur. J. Pediatr. Surg.*, 2001, 11(3), 147–153.

14. Silva, A.B., Lusk, R.P., and Muntz, H.R. Update on the use of auricular cartilage in laryngotracheal reconstruction. *Ann. Otol. Rhinol. Laryngol.*, 2002, 109(4), 343–347.

15. Long, C.M., Conley, S.F., Kajdacsy–Balla, A., and Kerschner, J.E. Laryngotracheal reconstruction in canies: fixation of autologouscostochondral grafts using polylactic and polyglycolic acid miniplates. *Arch. Otolaryngol. Head Neck Surg.*, 2001, 127(5), 570–575.

16. Robey, T.C., Eiselt, P.M., Murphy, H.S., Mooney, D.J., and Weatherly, R.A. Biodegradable external tracheal stents and their use in a rabbit tracheal reconstruction model. *Laryngoscope*, 2000, 110, 1936.

17. Gustafson, L.M., Liu, J.H., Hartnick, C.J., and Cotton, R.T. Duration of stenting in single-stage laryngotracheal reconstruction with anterior costal cartilage grafts. *Ann. Otol. Rhinol. Laryngol.*, 2001, 110, 413.

18. Hartnick, C.J., Hartley, B.E., Lacy, P.D., Liu, J., Bean, J.A., Willging, J.P., Meyer, C.M., and Cotton, R.T. Topical mitomycin application after laryngotracheal reconstruction: a randomized double-blind, placebo-controlled trial. *Arch. Otolaryngol. Head Neck Surg.*, 2001, 127(10), 1260–1264.

19. Jacobs, B.R., Salman, B.A., Cotton, R.T., Lyons, K., and Brilli, R.J. Postoperative management of children after single-stage laryngotracheal reconstruction. *Crit. Care Med.*, 2001, 29(1), 164–168.

20. Ludemann, J.P., Hughes, C.A., Noah, Z., and Hollinger, L.D. Complications of pediatric laryngotracheal reconstruction: prevention strategies. *Ann. Otol. Rhinol. Laryngol.*, 1999, 108, 1019.

21. Choi, S.S. and Zalzal, G.H. Pitfalls in laryngotracheal reconstruction. *Arch. Otolaryngol. Head Neck Surg.*, 1999, 25(6), 650–653.

Section VII

Rhinology

26 Rhinosinusitis

Ellis M. Arjmand and Rodney P. Lusk

The art of healing comes from nature, not from the physician. Therefore the physician must start from nature, with an open mind.

Paracelsus

CONTENTS

INTRODUCTION

Sinusitis is a common childhood illness whose incidence is difficult to define due to ambiguity regarding diagnostic criteria. Viral rhinitis, allergic rhinitis, adenoiditis, and adenoid hypertrophy may all be misdiagnosed as sinusitis. The potential for misdiagnosis, overtreatment, and undertreatment is great, and additional difficulties arise from the lack of well-defined treatment protocols. Few antibiotics are formally indicated for treatment of pediatric sinusitis; thus, dose and duration of treatment are not well established.

Antibiotic therapy is based, to a large extent, on parallels to otitis media. CT scan has become something of a "gold standard" for the diagnosis of chronic pediatric sinusitis.[1,2] Plain radiographs or CT scans are generally not required for the diagnosis of acute sinusitis. The high incidence of radiographically apparent sinus abnormalities in asymptomatic children has led to increased awareness that the CT scan must be interpreted in the context of patient history and physical examination.[3–6]

Bacteriology, radiographic imaging, and relevant anatomy will be reviewed in this chapter. Complications of medical treatment of sinusitis and complications of sinus disease will be presented and discussed. The importance of accurate diagnosis and direct treatment will be emphasized. Related information can be found in discussions of diagnostic imaging, allergy and immunology, and endoscopy.

BACKGROUND

A common misconception among parents and some primary care physicians is that the paranasal sinuses are not present in infants and young children. However, complications of maxillary or ethmoid sinus disease can occur at any age. The frontal sinus develops later, although complications of frontal sinusitis (e.g., osteomyelitis or cerebritis) may be seen in children in the first decade of life. Because of the erroneous belief that the sinuses are not present, undertreatment of sinusitis in children may lead to the development of complications of sinusitis; however, supporting data are difficult to obtain.

Conversely, the diagnosis of sinusitis may be made erroneously, for example, in cases of nasal foreign body or choanal atresia. The treating or consulting physician must be aware of the possibility of other diagnoses, particularly if the expected response to treatment is not seen. Other instances in which the anticipated response to treatment might not be seen are ciliary dyskinesia, cystic fibrosis, and immune deficiency.

OBTAINING AN ACCURATE DIAGNOSIS

The distinction between acute sinusitis and viral upper respiratory infection (URI)/rhinitis is often unclear.[7] The primary determinants are duration of illness and presence of purulent rhinorrhea. Symptom complex (fever, rhinorrhea, facial pain, cough, postnasal drainage) of greater than 7 days' duration and the presence of purulent rhinorrhea are suggestive of acute sinusitis, rather than viral URI. Sinus opacification, air–fluid level, or mucoperiostial thickening may be seen with acute sinusitis or viral URI.

The presence of purulent secretions in the middle meatus is strongly suggestive of sinusitis. Examination is facilitated by topical decongestion (e.g., aerosolized oxymetazoline) and anterior rhinoscopy. The distinction is important. Overtreatment (use of antibiotics to treat viral URI) unnecessarily exposes the child to the risk of complications of treatment (e.g., pseudomemembranous colitis, drug allergy, diarrhea) and increases the risk of drug-resistant bacteria evolving. Undertreatment (non-use of antibiotics when bacterial sinusitis is present) poses the risk of increased incidence of regional complications, asthma exacerbation, and prolonged illness. Although many cases of acute sinusitis are self-limited, the duration of the illness is likely to be less if antibiotics are used.

Chronic sinusitis may be diagnosed on the basis of duration of illness (ranging from 3 weeks to 3 months) or persistence of infection following antibiotic therapy. The diagnostic criteria are poorly established and extremely variable. Some authors have reported that the symptom complex of chronic sinusitis differs from that of acute sinusitis in that children with chronic sinusitis more frequently have headache, postnasal drainage, and cough and less often have fever and anterior rhinorrhea.[8]

BACTERIOLOGY

Knowledge of bacteriology guides antibiotic selection. Because sinonasal cultures are traditionally thought to correlate poorly with cultures obtained by direct sinus aspirate, much of the treatment of sinusitis is empiric. Although some recent studies have challenged this long-held notion, the use of nasal culture to guide antibiotic selection is not widely accepted.

The pathogens causing most cases of acute sinusitis in children are well known, and parallels to the bacteriology of acute otitis media are close. *Streptococcus pneumoniae*, *Haemophilus influenzae*, and *Moraxella catarrhalis* are most commonly seen; much less often, *Streptococcus pyogenes* and *Staphylococcus aureus* are also identified on culture.[7]

In contrast, the bacteriology of chronic sinusitis is less well characterized. It appears that *Streptococcus pneumoniae*, *Haemophilus influenzae*, and *Moraxella catarrhalis* are far less common with chronic sinusitis, and *Staphylococcus aureus* is considerably more common. Anaerobic bacteria are seen on culture in some reports, as are fungal species, occasionally. The results vary from study to study[9,10] and the true role of anaerobes is unclear (i.e., pathogen or colonizer). Mixed infections are relatively common. However, in a substantial percentage of cases, the cultures show no growth, although typically the cultures are taken intraoperatively after treatment with antibiotics.

MEDICAL COMPLICATIONS

Children with sinusitis are often treated with multiple medications. Many over-the-counter medications — frequently administered by parents without physician guidance — contain various combinations of mucolytics, decongestants, antihistamines, analgesics, and cough suppressants. Each active ingredient carries with it the potential for side effects, adverse effects, and unexpected effects. The recent withdrawal of phenylpropanolamine from the market illustrates the risk of serious adverse reactions, even with drugs that appear to have been safely used for many years. The introduction and subsequent withdrawal from the market of numerous antihistamines over the past decades (e.g., Hismanal, Seldane) illustrates the risks of drug interactions, even with medications extensively tested prior to FDA approval.

The treatment of chronic sinusitis generally includes a 3-week course of a broad-spectrum antibiotic, although drug selection, dosing, and duration of treatment have evolved more by common practice than by systematic study. Complications of antibiotic therapy (e.g., allergic reactions, diarrhea, pseudomembraneous colitis) are probably more likely with prolonged use of broad-spectrum antibiotics.

Some investigators have reported encouraging results using home IV antibiotics to treat children with chronic sinusitis.[11] The additional risks posed by this method of treatment include the risks of general anesthesia (for placement of long-term venous access) and the risks of indwelling venous catheter at home (e.g., thrombophlebitis and line sepsis). Long-term outcomes of this method of treatment are not available.

The treating physician must be specific and goal directed in selecting medications and constantly aware of the potential for atypical reactions. Specifically, antibiotic selection should be guided whenever possible by knowledge of past response, local resistant rates, and empiric knowledge of bacteriology. Care must be taken to comply with dosing and administration guidelines. Overly long as well as improperly short duration of treatment is to be avoided; unfortunately, the available literature on optimum duration of treatment is relatively sparse. Mucolytics and topical decongestants have few attendant risks; however, parents must be informed of the risks of rhinitis medicomentosa with the prolonged use of oxymetazoline or neosynephrine. Pseudoephedrine is widely available in various pediatric preparations, and it appears to be very safe, although the recent experience with phenylpropanolamine is cautionary.

Nasal (topical) steroids, some of which are now approved for use in children as young as 2 years of age, have potential risks ranging from nasal drying and epistaxis to growth disturbance. Guidelines for prolonged nasal steroid use are still evolving.

Antihistamines have little place in the treatment of sinusitis, although they have a valuable preventive role in patients with allergies. Complications of antihistamine use (drying effect, thickening of secretions, decreased mucociliary clearance, and drug interactions) can be limited by avoiding their use. However, doing so requires careful parental education to prevent the use of the widely available over-the-counter cold-and-allergy or sinus medications, which contain combinations of antihistamines and decongestants.

The otolaryngologist has a unique role in establishing the diagnosis through the use of nasal and nasopharyngeal endoscopy. The distinction between sinusitis and other conditions with somewhat similar presentation (e.g., adenoiditis or nasal foreign body) can be made by careful examination and history taking. The potential for complications that result from well-intentioned treatment based on an inaccurate diagnosis can thus be reduced.

COMPLICATIONS OF ACUTE SINUSITIS

Several regional complications can develop from acute sinusitis.[12–14] The orbital complications typically present with obvious physical findings. Central nervous system (CNS) complications may be more difficult to diagnosis due to nonspecificity of symptoms. Surgical intervention and the use of parenteral antibiotics are often required. The high rate of loss of vision or death from these complications in the preantibiotic era illustrates their severity and the need for aggressive management.

ORBITAL COMPLICATIONS

Complications of acute sinusitis develop by spread along venous channels or through bony dehiscences, e.g., in the lamina papyracea. Orbital complications of sinusitis were classified by Hubert in 1937[15] and a widely used modification of the classification presented in 1970[16] follows:

- Inflammatory edema (preseptal cellulitis)
- Orbital cellulitis without abscess
- Orbital cellulitis with subperiostial abscess
- Orbital cellulitis with orbital abscess
- Cavernous sinus thrombosis

Preseptal cellulitis (also referred to as periorbital cellulitis) causes edema of the preseptal soft tissues, sometimes to a pronounced degree, without proptosis or ophthalmoplegia. Sinogenic preseptal cellulitis must be differentiated, on the basis of history and physical examination, from the relatively more common periorbital cellulitis caused by haemophilus influenza. Treatment of preceptal cellulitis, in the absence of abscess, includes broad-spectrum oral antibiotics for coverage of pathogens that cause acute sinusitis, topical and systemic decongestants, and warm compresses to the eye.

Orbital cellulitis, subperiostial abscess, and orbital abscess present with similar physical findings. The distinction between them may in some cases be difficult; nevertheless, the treatment varies and the diagnosis must be made promptly and accurately.[17–19]

Proptotis may be present at each stage (II–V), and acute loss of vision can develop as a consequence of increased intraocular pressure, decreased ophthalmic artery flow, and traction on the optic nerve. Orbital cellulitis characteristically causes axial (frontally directed) proptosis, whereas subperiostial abscess (SPA) typically leads to eccentric (nonaxial) proptosis, away from the site of the abscess. Because most SPAs are in the medial orbit lateral to the lamina papyraea, the globe is usually displaced laterally. When an abscess is present within the orbital fat (stage IV, orbital cellulitis with abscess), the proptosis is usually severe and axial; opthalmoplegia is severe.

Cavernous sinus thrombosis is a rare complication of sinusitis. When present, it leads to proptosis on the side that is initially affected, followed by extension to bilateral findings of orbital edema.

Evaluation of visual acuity is of critical importance whenever proptosis is present. An ophthalmology consult should be obtained. If visual acuity is normal and the proptosis is axial, orbital cellulitis is the most likely diagnosis. Treatment with intravenous antibiotics and decongestants is begun. The eye examination must be followed closely; if disease progresses or fails to improve in 24 to 48 hours, a CT scan must be obtained to rule out abscess formation. Surgery (endoscopic or external ethmoidectomy, with or without maxillary antrostomy) is indicated for orbital cellulitis with lack of response to intravenous antibiotics.

A CT scan is obtained immediately if SPA or orbital abscess is suspected on the basis of physical examination findings; presence of an abscess is an indication for surgery. A SPA may be drained by external approach or endoscopically. Studies demonstrate a more rapid recovery if the endoscopic approach is used,[17,18] and external incision can be avoided if the abscess is drained endoscopically along with endoscopic ethmoidectomy. However, the sinus disease can be treated with an open or endoscopic surgical approach.

A few studies involving small numbers of patients have demonstrated effective treatment of SPA without surgery.[20,21] However, due to the possibility of rapid extension of the abscess (it increases in size by direct extension from the sinus, rather than by a process of suppuration), the risk of loss of vision, and the difficulty in assessing visual acuity in a child with orbital inflammation, nonsurgical treatment of SPA is not recommended.

Orbital abscesses also require surgical drainage. The risk of loss of vision is higher with intraconal abscess than with superiostal abscess. The sinus disease may be treated endoscopically, but an external approach is preferred for definitive abscess drainage. In most cases, the endoscopic approach does not offer adequate exposure for drainage of an abscess located within the orbital fat. Ophthalmology consultation and close follow-up are required. Intravenous antibiotics and nasal decongestants are administered, as they are for orbital cellulitis and SPA.

Cavernous sinus thrombosis is a rare complication of acute sinusitis. Management includes prompt surgical treatment of the sinus disease, ophthalmology consultation, intravenous antibiotics, and nasal decongestants. The use of anticoagulants is controversial.

REGIONAL AND INTRACRANIAL COMPLICATIONS

Acute sinusitis may also lead to intracranial complications or to osteomyelitis of the anterior wall of the frontal sinus.[12,13] The intracranial complications include meningitis, epidural abscess, subdural abscess, cerebritis, and brain abscess. Intracranial complications develop most often from frontal and sphenoid sinusitis.

Meningitis presents as an acute process, with characteristic findings of fever, lethargy, nucchal rigidity, and diffuse headache. In contrast, the presenting signs and symptoms of abscess or cerebritis are variable because acute as well as chronic conditions may be seen. Signs and symptoms include those of increased intracranial pressure (e.g., nausea, vomiting, lethargy, papilledema), fever, headache, seizure, behavioral change, and focal neurological signs. Patients with epidural abscess generally complain of a continuous dull headache; those with a subdural abscess usually have severe headache, focal neurologic changes, and papilledema.

Lumbar puncture (LP) is required when intracranial complications are present or suspected. Brain imaging should be performed prior to LP to determine whether mass effect (and risks of brain herniation) is present. CT scan has traditionally been the test of choice for initial evaluation, although MRI appears to be superior for detecting small epidural or subdural abscesses and for delineating the extent of brain inflammation.

Treatment depends on the location and extent of disease. Medical therapy involves the use of antibiotics that cross the blood–brain barrier and are directed toward the pathogens that cause acute sinusitis. Activity against *Staphylococcus aureus* and anaerobic bacteria is also needed. Duration of treatment is individualized and an infectious disease consultation should be obtained.

Steroid treatment is controversial and is generally not recommended when an intracranial abscess is present. Surgical treatment is determined on the basis of disease location and extent. Early neurosurgical consultation should be obtained. The sinus disease can often be treated endoscopically. An external approach is needed in some cases of direct spread of disease from the sinuses to the cranial fosse.

Osteomyelitis of the anterior wall of the frontal sinus (Pott's puffy tumor) develops by spread of infection through the valveless diploic veins. Similarly, posterior spread of infection may lead to a frontal subdural empyema. Presenting signs and symptoms of frontal osteomyelitis include frontal pain, tenderness, and swelling. In unusual cases, the presentation may be subacute, with frontal swelling but no tenderness or erythema.

CT is recommended to access the location and extent of the infection. Parental antibiotics with activity against *Staphylococcus aureus*, nonenterococcal streptococcal, and oral anaerobes are used. Surgical treatment includes abscess drainage (if present) and removal of devitalized bone. Frontal sinus obliteration is rarely indicated.

COMPLICATIONS OF CHRONIC SINUSITIS

Chronic sinusitis may lead to a range of nonspecific and poorly localized symptoms, some of which can be quite debilitating. Headaches and chronic cough are frequently seen and poor appetite, behavioral change, and irritability have been reported. In young or developmentally delayed children, head banging and hair pulling may be seen. The otolaryngologist must be aware that physical findings such as fever and rhinorrhea may not be evident in children with chronic sinusitis; he or she must be alert to the possibility of chronic sinusitis in the child with relatively nonspecific symptoms. Suppurative complications may arise from chronic sinusitis, e.g., frontal osteomyelitis. However, these complications (particularly orbital complications) are thought to develop from acute sinusitis in the great majority of cases.

CONCLUSIONS

Acute sinusitis is a common childhood illness; suppurative orbital and intracranial complications are possible. Complications may develop from no treatment or undertreatment of the primary infection, but the issue is complicated by the fact that treatment guidelines for pediatric sinusitis are relatively poorly defined. Indications for surgical intervention are fairly clear when suppurative complications are present, but they are much less clear in other situations.

The otolaryngologist plays a key role in differentiating acute sinusitis from other disease processes with a similar symptom complex. With accurate diagnosis, complications of inappropriate treatment can often be avoided and secondary complications of the disease are less likely to arise. The otolaryngologist must also be aware of the early signs and symptoms of orbital and intracranial complications, when prompt evaluation (often including radiographic imaging) is needed.

BIBLIOGRAPHY

Arjmand, E.M. and Lusk, R.P. Management of recurrent and chronic sinusitis in children. *Am. J. Otolaryngol.*, 1995, 16, 367–382.

Lusk, R.P. Surgical management of sinusitis. In Lusk, R.P., Ed. *Pediatric Sinusitis*. New York: Raven Press, 1992.

REFERENCES

1. McAllister, W.H., Lusk, R.P., and Muntz, H.R. Comparison of plain radiographs and coronal CT scans in infants and children with recurrent sinusitis. *Am. J. Roentgenol.*, 1989, 153, 1259–1264.
2. Lazar, R.H., Younis, R.T., and Parvey, L.S. Comparison of plain radiographs, coronal CT, and intraoperative findings in children with chronic sinusitis. *Otolaryngol. Head Neck Surg.*, 1992, 17, 29–34.
3. Diament, M.J., Senac, M.O., Gilsanz, V. et al. Prevalence of incidental paranasal sinuses opacification in pediatric patients: a CT study. *J. CT*, 1987, 11, 426–431.
4. Lesserson, J.A., Kieserman, S.P., and Finn, D.G. The radiographic incidence of chronic sinus disease in the pediatric population. *Laryngoscope*, 1994, 104, 159–166.
5. Calhoun, K.H., Waggenspack, G.A., Simpson, C.B. et al. CT evaluation of the paranasal sinuses in symptomatic and asymptomatic populations. *Otolaryngol. Head Neck Surg.*, 1991, 104, 480–483.

6. Glasier, C.M., Mallory, G.B., and Steele, R.W. Significance of opacification of the maxillary and ethmoid sinuses in infants. *J. Pediatr.*, 1989, 114, 45–50.

7. Wald, E.R. Diagnosis and management of acute sinusitis. *Pediatr. Ann.*, 1988, 17, 629–638.

8. Parsons, D.S. and Phillips, S.E. Functional endoscopic surgery in children: a retrospective analysis of results. *Laryngoscope*, 1993, 103, 899–903.

9. Muntz, H.R. and Lusk, R.P. Endoscopic sinus surgery in children with chronic sinusitis — a pilot study. *Laryngoscope*, 1990, 100, 654–658.

10. Brook, I. Bacteriologic features of chronic sinusitis in children. *JAMA*, 1981, 246, 967–969.

11. Buchman, C.A., Yellon, R.F., and Bluestone, C.D. Alternative to endoscopic sinus surgery in the management of pediatric chronic rhinosinusitis refractory to oral antimicrobial therapy. *Otolaryngol. Head Neck Surg.*, 1999, 120, 219–224.

12. Lusk, R.P., Tychsen, L., and Park, T.S. Complications of sinusitis. *Pediatr. Sinusitis*, 1992, 11, 127–146.

13. Hengerer, A.S. and Yanofsky, S.D. Complications of nasal and sinus infections. In Bluestone, C.D., Stool, S.E. et al., Eds. *Pediatric Otolaryngology,* 3rd ed. Philadelphia: W.B. Saunders, 43, 866–873.

14. Schramm, V.L., Jr., Carter, H.D., and Kennerdell, J.S. Evaluation of orbital cellulitis and results of treatment. *Laryngoscope*, 1982, 92, 732–738.

15. Hubert, L. Orbital infections due to nasal sinusitis. *NY State J. Med.*, 1937, 37, 1559–1563.

16. Chandler, J.R., Langenbrunner, D.J., and Stevens, E.R. The pathogenesis of orbital complications in acute sinusitis. *Laryngoscope*, 1970, 80, 1414–1428.

17. Arjmand, E.M., Lusk, R.P., and Muntz, H.R. Pediatric sinusitis and subperiosteal orbital abscess formation: diagnosis and treatment. *Otolaryngol. Head Neck Surg.*, 1993, 109, 886–894.

18. Manning, S.C. Endoscopic management of medial subperiosteal orbital abscess. *Arch. Otolaryngol. Head Neck Surg.*, 1993, 119, 789–791.

19. Patt, B.S. and Manning, S.C. Blindness resulting from orbital complications of sinusitis. *Otolaryngol. Head Neck Surg.*, 1991, 104, 789–195.

20. Souliere, C.R., Antoine, G.A., Martin, M.P. et al. Selective nonsurgical management of subperiosteal abscess of the orbit: computerized tomography and clinical course as indication for surgical drainage. *Int. J. Pediatr. Otorhinolaryngol.*, 1990, 19, 109–119.

21. Rubin, S.E., Rubin, L.G., Zito, J. et al. Medical management of orbital subperiosteal abscess in children. *J. Pediatr. Ophthalmol. Strabis.*, 1989, 26, 21–27.

27 Pediatric Endoscopic Sinonasal Surgery

Gary D. Josephson, Jordan S. Josephson, and Charles W. Gross

Ethmoidectomy ... one of the easiest operations with which to kill a patient

Harris P. Mosher

CONTENTS

INTRODUCTION

Sinonasal surgery has experienced some of its greatest changes and advances during the last decade. With the advances in endoscopic technology and instrumentation over the last two decades came renewed interest in and considerable study of sinus disease by the otolaryngology community worldwide. As a result, functional endoscopic sinus surgery (FESS) has developed. FESS has greatly enhanced surgical technique in the operating room; more importantly, the nasal endoscope has afforded the otolaryngologist other advantages including

- A more accurate way to diagnose sinus disease in the office
- A more comprehensive approach to treating chronic sinus disease
- A way to provide accurate and meticulous postoperative care

Thus, FESS should be considered as a comprehensive treatment plan by first making an accurate diagnosis and then targeting the treatment plan first to treat the patient medically. The advantages gained in the operating room are a plus for patients who are not improving medically to a satisfactory extent and need surgery to relieve obstruction of the sinus passageways. Surgery should be considered as an adjunct to the medical treatment of chronic sinusitis. This is almost always the case because chronic sinusitis is mostly a chronic disease that usually requires long-term medical therapy. For the purposes of this chapter, we shall consider FESS a total sinus approach to treating patients.

The endoscope is responsible for affording the surgeon the instrumentation to improve the quality of care to the patient greatly; unfortunately, it can also provide the novice or less proficient surgeon with a false sense of security in the operating room. Even in the best hands, FESS still remains a considerable challenge and is fraught with the same potentially significant risks and complications associated with traditional sinus surgery. More recent refinements in instrumentation, the development of powered tools, and the introduction of navigation systems have subsequently improved the safety and efficacy of treating sinonasal disease, although each of these also has added risks.

Approximately 15 years ago, otolaryngologists were performing traditional sinus surgery to treat patients with sinus disease. It is only since then that most of the surgical community has learned about and converted to FESS from the former traditional techniques. It is apparent that many are more familiar and comfortable with traditional techniques, which still have their place in the treatment of sinus disease. However, with time, fewer surgeons will need to resort to traditional techniques.

As with many surgical procedures, pediatric applications often lag behind those in the adult population. Safety issues are usually more heavily scrutinized in the pediatric population. Because of the smaller anatomy, the developing facial skeleton, and a developing immune system, one might say that FESS in the pediatric population is more difficult and at an increased risk for complications in comparison with those associated with the adult population. Although it continues to be defined, the role of endoscopic sinus surgery in the pediatric population has grown and developed into a safe and effective approach for treating sinonasal diseases in children.[1] With a strong knowledge of the nasal anatomy and sinus development in the growing child, the otolaryngologist can become skilled in the surgical management of pediatric sinonasal disease while avoiding potential complication.

In properly trained hands, the FESS approach is safe and effective. It is important, however, for the skilled surgeon to be well versed in treatment of the potential complications resulting from the disease or the surgery.

HISTORY

Certainly the novice, as well as the experienced surgeon, is discouraged when he or she reads in the first paragraph of a published manuscript that a surgical procedure is the "blindest and most dangerous (operation) in all surgery" or "one of the easiest operations with which to kill a patient." These quotes were reported to come from the admonitions of the early 20th century surgeon, Harris P. Mosher,[2,3] in his discussion of intranasal ethmoidectomy. The risk of surgical complications and poor outcomes has been significantly reduced over the past two decades because of

- The advent of high-resolution nasal endoscopes
- Better lighting and more advanced grasping, cutting, and powered instrumentation to perform intranasal and sinus surgery
- Better resident teaching
- Comprehensive instruction courses and conferences

HISTORY OF ENDOSCOPIC SINUS SURGERY

Endoscopic evaluation of the nasal cavity, middle meatus, and antrum was performed as early as 1903 by Hirschman.[4] The 4.0-mm endoscope he used is probably the true precursor to the nasal endoscope used today. However, it was not until the 1950s that von Riccabona's and Nehls' work in Europe led to the revitalization of nasal endoscopy. The improved resolution, large field of vision, and accurate color provided by the endoscopes developed by H.R. Hopkins led to enhanced diagnostic capabilities.[5,6] Work by Stammberger, Messerklinger, and others in the 1970s renewed interest in the use of these endoscopes for nasal, paranasal, and upper airway diagnosis and management.[7] Kennedy is credited for the true transmigration of endoscopic sinus surgery from Europe to the United States in 1985.[8,9]

Today, the indications to use endoscopic surgical techniques in the sinonasal cavity have expanded well beyond their original descriptions for sinus disease. Publications as early as 1989 have described the technique of endoscopic sinus surgery in children as a safe and effective treatment tool for chronic rhinosinusitis.[1]

COMPLICATIONS

The word *complication* in today's society is often misunderstood; in no way should it be considered synonymous with the word *malpractice*. Unfortunately and incorrectly, it is often misconstrued as such by the legal community. Complications do occur even in the best of hands and it is to be understood that complications of the procedure and complications of the disease process exist. For instance, meningitis is a well-known complication of sinus infection. It may occur before or after surgery as a result of the infection spreading to the intracranial cavity. If it occurs after surgery, one must not jump to the conclusion that it is a complication of the surgery because it may, in fact, be a complication of the disease process.

The method used by the surgeon to deal with complications can be broken down into three general principles: (1) avoidance, (2) recognition, and (3) management. To avoid complications, the surgeon should be well studied in surgical anatomy and principles recognizing danger areas and potential hazards. Furthermore, accurate patient selection, detailed preoperative preparation, and diligent postoperative care should occur.[10] If the surgeon is unfortunate enough to experience a complication, it is important for the clinician to identify the problem early so that treatment can be instituted early to avoid worsening of the complication. Also, every physician should have in his or her armamentarium the acumen to manage the possible surgical complications of the procedures performed. One should never hesitate to obtain assistance or to ask for consultation from other medical and surgical specialists.

This chapter will focus on complications of FESS and their management. Complications will be divided into major and minor categories and further subdivided by the type of complication and its management. An otolaryngology surgical atlas should be consulted for anatomy, general principles, and surgical technique because these are beyond the scope of this chapter.

MINOR COMPLICATIONS

Periorbital Hematoma

Entrance into the orbit through the lamina papyracea may result in periorbital hematoma or periorbital ecchymosis. It may also result from inadvertent injury to the anterior or posterior ethmoid artery with or without retraction. If lid edema occurs, the patient may complain of visual loss from the lid swelling. With isolated ecchymosis, discoloration without visual symptoms is the most common complaint. The patient may also complain about periorbital pain.

Once the injury is recognized, close observation is necessary to be sure that it is limited to the periorbita. Ice packs to the affected eye for the first 24 to 48 hours are recommended to stop the bleeding and to decrease lid swelling. Visual checks every 2 to 4 hours should be performed immediately following the appearance of the hematoma, and the physician should be alerted of any changes to visual acuity. Reassuring the parents may be all that is necessary. The ecchymosis usually resolves within 1 to 2 weeks without any long-term sequelae. Warm compresses are recommended after 48 hours and will usually hasten the resolution of the hematoma and discoloration.

Subcutaneous Orbital Emphysema

If the lamina papyracea is violated, the communication with the orbit offers a route for air to enter into the subcutaneous tissues. However, it is worth mentioning that this can also occur in the absence of anatomical violation to the lamina papyracea as the surgeon operates in close proximity to the lamina papyracea. If the patient blows his nose hard enough, an emphysema can occur. This may be further exacerbated if the patient cries, sneezes, coughs, or strains. Periorbital swelling and crepitus are identified during examination. Ecchymosis may accompany the emphysema.

The physician should first perform a visual check to be sure that the injury does not involve the affected eye. Light pressure and warm compresses for 24 to 48 hours are recommended. The patient and family should be instructed to limit straining and nose blowing for at least 1 week, thus allowing the fracture in the lamina papyracea to heal and prevent additional air entry. The air will usually reabsorb within 1 week. Reassuring the family is important.

Periorbital Cellulitis (Preseptal)

Infection that enters the preseptal space by direct extension through the lamina papyracea will cause erythema, edema, pain, and possibly, fever. This is a complication of the sinus infection and often occurs prior to surgical intervention. This may also be a delayed complication recognized days to weeks after endoscopic sinus surgery. Postoperative periorbital cellulitis may be caused by obstruction of the middle meatus with dried blood or crusts. Thus, it is important to provide proper postoperative follow-up cleaning and debridements. Uncooperative children in the office may require a second-look procedure under general anesthesia so that an adequate postoperative cleaning can be performed. Lateral wall osteitis from chronic infection or a resistant organism to the selection of the postoperative antibiotics may also be the inciting factor. Early recognition and treatment are important in order to avoid continued spread of infection into the orbit.

A good ophthalmologic evaluation is important to be sure that the infection and swelling are limited to the preseptal space and to assist in the management. If this is the case, nasal toilet and topical decongestants should be used. Directed antibiotic therapy based on culture results found at surgery should be instituted. If the physician wishes, oral antibiotics may be tried first, as long as close follow-up can be performed within the first 24 hours after initiation of therapy. If no improvement is noted or if symptoms worsen, broad-spectrum intravenous antibiotics should be started. Warm compresses to the affected eye may assist in the treatment of the lid edema.

Orbital Abscess

Orbital abscess, which can occur after endoscopic sinus surgery, is usually due to the underlying infection. Chapter 26 discusses orbital abscess in detail.

Epiphora

The nasolacrimal duct, covered by hard bone, courses in the lateral nasal wall, lateral to the anterior tip of the middle turbinate inferiorly and lateral to the agger nasi cell superiorly. The duct may be injured during antrostomy, especially if the surgeon removes the bone anterior to the natural maxillary ostium. Even if the duct is injured, epiphora is usually temporary and the duct will recanalize into the nasal cavity. If scarring, stenosis, or infection to the duct occurs, long-standing epiphora can result and be quite bothersome for the child and parents. In the case of osteitis or infection, dacrocystitis and purulent drainage from the puncta in the medial corner of the affected eye may occur.

Most cases of epiphora will resolve by themselves as the injured duct recanalizes into the nasal cavity, and therefore, no treatment is required. However, persistent cases may require ophthalmology consultation for nasolacrimal duct probing or stenting, with severe cases requiring dacrocystorhinostomy. Antibiotic-steroid eye cream and or oral antibiotics may be required in patients with evidence of infection. Warm compresses, nasal saline spray, and topical decongestants can help.

Synechiae

Synechiae have been reported as the most common postoperative complication of FESS. The role of debriding (cleaning) the cavity in uncooperative children, whether in the office or during a second-look procedure, cannot be overemphasized. Adhesions often occur in areas of narrowing or when two adjacent mucosal surfaces have been denuded or abraded. This further supports the concept of directed sinus surgery toward areas of disease, cutting tissue with through-cut instrumentation or shavers, and avoidance of tearing tissue. Adhesions commonly occur between the middle turbinate and lateral nasal wall or in narrow areas such as the frontal recess, the middle meatal antrostomy, and sphenoid ostium. If synechiae or scarring occurs, occlusion of the surgical antrostomy or osteomeatal complex may cause recurrent disease and return of the patient's presenting symptoms. Scarring in the olfactory cleft may lead to anosmia or hyposmia.

Avoiding the occurrence of synechia and scarring is the best treatment. Multiple approaches to this end have been tried with varying successes. First and foremost, delicate dissection and cutting tissue directed toward the diseased areas while avoiding mucosal abrasion and tearing is essential. Once the dissection is complete, placing Merogel® between the middle turbinate and lateral nasal wall may help healing while avoiding lateralization and scarring of the middle turbinate. Application of mitomyacin-C has also been reported to decrease the incidence of scarring and ostium closure.

Various other products and devices have been used to prevent synechiae; their prevention of scarring is controversial. No matter how skilled the surgeon and/or how meticulous the dissection is, or regardless of the packing or other devices used, some degree of scarring may occur. Therefore, the postoperative care using saline lavage and intranasal steroid sprays and potentially long-term postoperative debridement of the surgical cavity in the office or in the operative suite are paramount. Close follow up in the postoperative period until all denuded surfaces are re-epithelialized is the most successful method of preventing significant synechiae. Persistent synechiae, with resultant recurrence of symptoms and disease, may necessitate revision endoscopic sinus surgical procedures.

Natural Ostia Closure

Middle meatal antrostomy closure or synechia formation closing off the natural ostium or separating the natural ostium from the antrostomy even if the surgical antrostomy remains open may lead to the recirculation of mucus. This can result in the recurrence of maxillary sinus disease with its associated symptoms. Avoidance is the best treatment and can best be accomplished by making sure that the antrostomy is connected to the natural ostium. Even a large antrostomy does not assure patency. As with synechiae, good postoperative debridement is paramount in making sure that the surgical site does not scar. Revision endoscopic surgical antrostomy may be necessary if scarring becomes too difficult to treat with office postsurgical debridement.

Diplopia

Diplopia is most often related to direct injury of the medial rectus muscle or its neurovascular supply. Edema of the medial rectus will cause a transient diplopia that will resolve in time. Persistent diplopia requires ophthalmologic consultation and, possibly, surgical correction.

Facial Growth

Altered facial growth as a result of chronic sinusitis and after endoscopic sinus surgery in children has been debated.[11,12] Recent investigation with quantitative anthropometric evaluation and qualitative assessment of facial growth in young children has revealed no evidence that facial growth alteration is clinically significant 10 years after endoscopic sinus surgery in children.[13]

MAJOR COMPLICATIONS

Hemorrhage

Before any surgical procedure, a medical and family history should be obtained to identify any obvious potential coagulopathies. Evaluation and management of the coagulopathic child are detailed further in Chapter 13.

Hemostasis during endoscopic sinus surgery is extremely important because bleeding may make the surgical dissection more difficult by tarnishing the lens and obscuring the surgeon's view. Before starting the surgical procedure, decongestion with topical vasoconstrictors on nasal pledgets, followed by good infiltration with 1% lidocaine with epinephrine, is essential. Failure to wait at least 7 to 10 minutes for the injection to take effect is a common mistake. Good injections and allowing the appropriate time for adequate vasoconstriction can mean the difference of a bloodless dissection.

Bleeding can occur and can become problematic for several reasons. If tissue is torn rather than meticulously cut, generalized oozing may occur. More aggressive bleeding may occur if the anterior or posterior ethmoid artery or sphenopalatine artery has been violated. Finally, in the region of the sphenoid sinus, the carotid artery courses laterally in the sphenoid sinus encased by its bony covering. In a small percentage of patients, the artery may be dehiscent. The cavernous sinus may also be violated during the dissection in this area.

Generalized oozing from tissue trauma usually resolves on its own. The surgeon may need to apply a topical vasoconstrictive pledget in the sinus cavity to achieve hemostasis. Other times, uncontrolled bleeding may require the use of electrocautery or nasal packing. Packing one side of the nose while proceeding with surgery on the other may allow surgery to proceed safely. Certainly, if bleeding obscures the ability to proceed safely with proper surgical dissection, the procedure should be aborted and hemostasis controlled.

Injury to the ethmoid vessels should alert the surgeon to the close proximity of the eye and the skull base. Retraction of the vessel into the eye can result in orbital hematoma and visual loss. The sphenopalatine vessel can inadvertently be injured as it crosses the face of the rostrum.

Cavernous sinus bleeding usually results in brisk bleeding that can be controlled with light packing. If this occurs, the patient must undergo a CT scan or MRI to assure intracranial integrity and lack of intracranial bleeding. Close monitoring is extremely important. Finally, injury to the carotid artery is possible because it runs laterally in the sphenoid sinus and may be dehiscent. Violation of the carotid artery could result in disastrous bleeding, stroke, and death. Pressure over the injured vessel may afford additional time until the bleeding vessel is controlled and neurosurgical assistance is obtained.

Cerebral Spinal Fluid Leak

The roof of the ethmoid sinus and floor of the cranial cavity have significant variability. Therefore, it is important to study the CT scan and have it in the operating suite during the surgical dissection. The roof may vary from being almost vertical to being almost horizontal. The difference in height between the cribriform plate and the roof may vary from 4 to 16 mm.[14] Entrance into the intracranial cavity can occur anywhere along the skull base, but most commonly takes place at the roof of the ethmoid sinus immediately posterior to the ethmoid dome and in the area of the posterior ethmoid superior to the sphenoid sinus.[15]

Identifying and following landmarks during the surgical dissection can decrease the incidence of cerebral spinal fluid (CSF) leak. The middle turbinate should be the lateral landmark of the dissection to prevent violation of the cribriform plate. The anterior and posterior ethmoidal neurovascular bundles serve as the superior limit of the ethmoid cavity. If bleeding occurs during the dissection of the ethmoidal dome, it should be assumed that the skull base has been reached. The operative field is further demarcated by the dome of the ethmoid, the frontal recess, the sphenoid rostrum, and the medial orbital wall (the anatomic approach to endoscopic intransal ethmoidectomy is well described by Schaefer[16]).

Occasionally, the last ethmoid cell is anterior to the sphenoid sinus. The surgeon should not assume that this is because, posteriorly, the last ethmoid cell is usually lateral to the sphenoid sinus and is in close proximity to the optic nerve. If this is the case, then entering the sphenoid by continuing the dissection through the most posterior ethmoid cell may cause optic nerve damage and/or intracranial entrance. Therefore, when sphenoidotomy is necessary, the authors recommend the method of entering the sphenoid by identifying the natural ostium medial to the middle turbinate, rather than entering the sphenoid sinus through the dissection of the posterior ethmoid sinus. Admittedly, other excellent surgeons advocate entering via the posterior ethmoid.

The possibility of microfracture or even dehiscence of the skull base can occur even in the best of hands when the surgeon removes the bone of the cells at the skull base or when turbinate or septal surgery is performed. Most of these injuries probably occur without injury to the dura. Therefore, CSF leak is not detectable immediately and can worsen later. The surgeon must always be cognizant of this and must be alert to any symptoms such as unusual postoperative headaches.

Intraoperative Identification

If, during the surgical dissection, the physician believes he has violated the dura and entered into the cranial cavity, immediate identification of the defect will enable surgical correction. Using a blunt metal probe to mark the point of injury and performing a lateral skull film will confirm the suspicion. If the defect is small, most likely it will heal spontaneously; however, obvious leaks noted endoscopically should be repaired. A patch of mucosa, temporalis fascia, or a flap of tissue from the septum or middle turbinate may be used to close the defect. Tissue glue may be helpful in securing graft placement. Light packing to buttress the graft in place may be necessary.

Consultation with a neurosurgical colleague is always useful, even if the surgeon believes the defect is small and has been corrected with a tissue flap. A CT scan should be performed to assure absence of intracranial injury, bleed, or pneumocephalus. Postoperatively, the patient should be placed on bed rest, with minimal activity that may increase intracranial pressure, including but not limited to nose blowing, straining, and coughing. Neurosurgical monitoring should also be performed to further allow for early identification of any delayed intracranial injury. The use of prophylactic antibiotics is controversial.

Postoperative Identification

CSF leaks may be identified in the postoperative patient who complains of persistent clear rhinorrhea and/or headaches, or they may present with meningitis that may or may not be recurrent. Occasionally, in the case of a microfracture or dehiscence without a dural tear, the patient may have a CSF leak pneumoencephally or meningitis at a later date by blowing the nose, straining, or coughing. The physician is obligated to secure the diagnosis so that treatment can begin as early as possible.

Diagnosis can be confirmed by several tests. First, the physician can have the child lean his or her head forward and then observe the clear rhinorrhea as it drips onto a gauze. The presence of a halo on the white gauze should increase suspicion, although this does not confirm CSF. Maintaining the head in this position will allow the clinician to obtain a sample for further analysis. Index of suspicion can be further increased by testing the specimen for glucose. A quantitative measure is preferred because commercially available sticks can pick up trace levels of glucose that can be present in mucus secretions. Simultaneous blood glucose levels need to be drawn because CSF levels of glucose are 40 to 60% those of blood levels. The remainder of the sample should be sent to the laboratory and tested for beta 2 transferrin. This will definitively confirm the presence of CSF rhinorrhea.

Once the diagnosis is suspected, the child should be placed on bed rest and avoid any activity that can increase intracranial pressure. Most cases will resolve on their own within a 1-week period. In the presence of meningitis, the inflammation of the meningis with subsequent fibrosis in the dehiscent area may result in cure. If the leak persists despite these conservative methods, the physician may wish to supplement bed rest by inserting a spinal drain to further decrease intracranial pressure while allowing the leak to heal.

Surgical therapy is considered for cases refractory to conservative measures. In these cases, in order for the leak to be repaired successfully, localization of the dehiscent site is paramount. This can be done with endoscopic visualization. Those difficult to identify may require a metrizamide scan or intrathecal injection of flouroscein to further localize the area. The physician must realize that injection of localization dyes into the cerebral spinal fluid space carries a remote possibility of morbidity.

Once the leak is localized, endoscopic repair can be performed as described earlier in the section on intraoperative identification. When the dehiscence is large and multiple endoscopic attempts have been unsuccessful, neurosurgical consultation for craniotomy and intracranial repair may need to take place.

Blindness and Visual Disturbance

Two major catastrophic events can lead to visual disturbance or blindness from endoscopic sinus surgery. One is transection of the optic nerve, and the other is retrobulbar hemorrhage. Each will be discussed individually.

The surgeon should take all precautions and be cognizant during surgery because early recognition of an orbital complication can prevent a poor outcome. This is best done by reviewing the anatomy on the CT scan prior to surgery and having the scan on the view box in the operating suite for easy reference. The authors prefer to have the patient's eyes uncovered during the procedure for easy access and to allow for visualization of the pupil and availability for palpation during the procedure. Lacrilube can be placed in the eyes to prevent dryness and corneal ulceration. Tape is placed gently over the lateral aspect of the lid to keep the lid gently closed but allow easy access.

Excellent local intranasal injection is paramount in preventing significant bleeding during the procedure. This is important because bleeding can impair visualization of important landmarks during the surgical dissection. The authors prefer a step-wise approach to surgery in children. They first identify the natural maxillary sinus ostia and sometimes perform the maxillary middle meatal antrosomy before proceeding with ethmoidectomy in children. This landmark is used to demarcate the lateral limit of the dissection, delineates the line of the lamina papyracea, and prevents inadvertent entrance into the orbit. Ethmoidectomy can then be safely undertaken by staying medial to this landmark. Care is also taken when making the infundibulotomy incision because inadvertent entrance into the orbit can occur during this part of the dissection.

Optic Nerve Transection

Injury to the optic nerve can occur during ethmoidectomy. The nerve may be dehiscent secondary to congenital absence of the bony covering, an overly large air cell posteriorly over the nerve, or chronic infection. Such an isolated injury would be extremely rare but can occur. The hallmark findings indicating this injury are that the afferent pupillary reflex is absent and light will not stimulate the pupil to constrict. The direct and consensual pupillary reflexes are affected. Pupillary reflexes may also be affected but should not be absent by deep general anesthesia. These should return to normal as the child is aroused. Topical decongestion that accidentally leaks onto the eye during surgery may also alter pupillary responses. Unfortunately, transection of the optic nerve is untreatable and permanent.

Orbital Hematoma

The vascular supply to the nose, paranasal sinuses, and orbit involves connecting arteries and localized veins that can be interrupted during surgery.[17] Two types of orbital hematoma can occur. The arterial type is caused by injury to the anterior or posterior ethmoidal artery, and the venous type results from penetration of the lamina papyracea and disruption of the orbital veins.

If disruption of the anterior or posterior ethmoid artery occurs at the junction where the artery emerges from the orbit into the nose, the artery may retract into the orbit, causing an immediate orbital hematoma. This can result in marked proptosis, pupillary dilatation, lid edema, chemosis, vision loss, and immediate high-orbital pressures.[18] Venous injury causes hematoma and symptoms more slowly. The superior and inferior ophthalmic veins and their branches provide the main venous supply to the eye and optic nerve. This bleeding occurs from direct trauma to the vessels by inadvertent penetration through the lamina papyracea. Because of the low-pressure system of these vessels, bleeding usually is self-limited. However, in some cases, a continual bleed into the subperiosteal or postseptal space can lead to gradual pressure build-up, thus compromising the vascular supply to the optic nerve and leading to blindness. This can occur over several hours to days.

Whether the hematoma is caused by an arterial or venous injury, the resulting visual disturbance or blindness is caused by a compromise to the venous supply of the optic nerve. This causes decreased perfusion and drainage, leading to increased ocular pressures. Therefore, all treatments are aimed at reducing intraocular pressure while improving venous drainage. This allows the optic nerve continued perfusion and drainage.

As described earlier, the two causes of orbital hematoma are arterial and venous. Because of the immediate pressure caused by an arterial hemorrhage as opposed to the slow build-up over time in a venous bleed, it is believed that the danger to the optic nerve is greater with an arterial bleed. Two protocols borrowed from Stankiewicz[18] are suggested: arterial bleed (Figure 27.1) and venous bleed (Figure 27.2). Ophthalmology consultation is essential in managing these problems.

Medical Therapies for Orbital Hematoma

Eye massage. Eye massage directly reduces eye pressure by redistributing intraocular and extraocular pressure. This is performed by keeping the hand open and the fingers together. Gentle massage

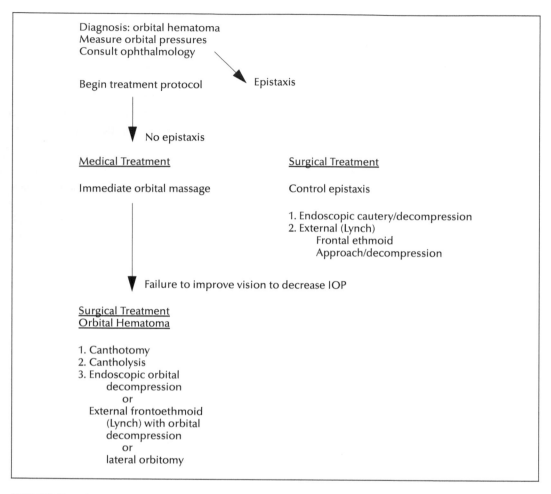

Diagnosis: orbital hematoma
Measure orbital pressures
Consult ophthalmology

Begin treatment protocol　　　Epistaxis

No epistaxis

Medical Treatment　　　　　　　　Surgical Treatment

Immediate orbital massage　　　Control epistaxis

　　　　　　　　　　　　　　1. Endoscopic cautery/decompression
　　　　　　　　　　　　　　2. External (Lynch)
　　　　　　　　　　　　　　　　Frontal ethmoid
　　　　　　　　　　　　　　　　Approach/decompression

Failure to improve vision to decrease IOP

Surgical Treatment
Orbital Hematoma

1. Canthotomy
2. Cantholysis
3. Endoscopic orbital
　　decompression
　　　　or
　External frontoethmoid
　　(Lynch) with orbital
　　decompression
　　　　or
　　lateral orbitomy

FIGURE 27.1 Protocol for treatment of arterial hematoma. (From Stankiewicz, J.A. and Chow, J.M. *Oto-laryngol. Head Neck Surg.*, 1999, 120, 841–847. With permission.)

can be repeated while waiting for other therapies such as diuretics to work. Orbital massage is contraindicated in patients who have had previous eye surgery, including glaucoma-filtering surgery, corneal transplant, retinal detachment surgery, or cataract surgery.[17]

Diuretics. Mannitol given intravenously reduces intraocular pressure maximally in 30 to 60 minutes. It works hyperosmotically to dehydrate the vitreous humor and the orbital tissue. A dose of 1 to 2 g/kg is infused as a 20% infusion over 30 to 60 minutes.[19] Electrolytes must be monitored because massive diuresis occurs. Acetazolamide is a second choice to mannitol, but also may be used at an initial dose of 500 mg intravenously, repeated in 2 to 4 hours. It acts by lowering intraocular pressure by decreasing the production of aqueous humor.[17]

Miotics (pilocarpine, carbachol, and epinephrine). Miotic eye drops can effectively reduce intraocular pressure. These drops may be considered after ophthalmic consultation and should only be used under direct supervison of an ophthalmologist. These medications do interfere with pupillary response and can cloud clinical progress.

Steroids. Although high-dose intravenous steroid administration has been used to decrease edema from surgical and infectious insults, no good literature is available to indicate if it is useful in the treatment of retrobulbar hemorrhage.

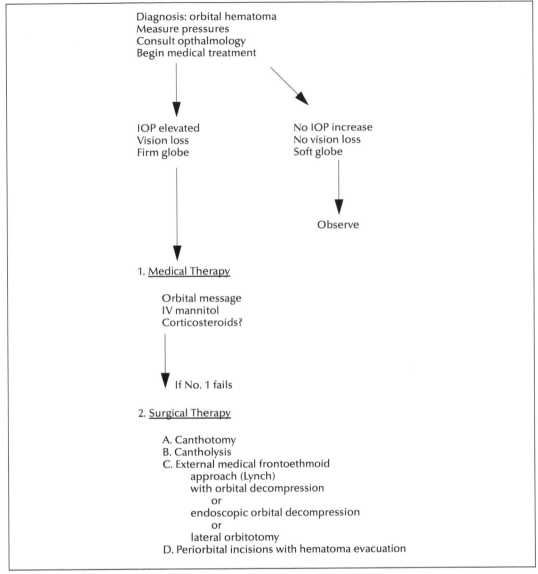

FIGURE 27.2 Protocol for treatment of venous hematoma. (From Stankiewicz, J.A. and Chow, J.M. *Otolaryngol. Head Neck Surg.*, 1999, 120, 841–847. With permission.)

SURGICAL THERAPIES

Lateral Canthotomy and Cantholysis

Lateral canthotomy and cantholysis produces instant pressure reduction by expanding orbital volume. A scissors or scalpel is used to make a lateral incision that allows the intraorbital contents to expand and release the intraorbital pressure.

Medial Orbital Decompression and Optic Nerve Decompression

After lateral decompression, orbital pressure should be monitored closely with a tonometer. If sufficient pressure is not reduced, medial orbital decompression with optic nerve decompression is the final surgical option in the treatment of blindness secondary to retrobulbar hemorrhage. This technique is beyond the scope of this chapter. The periorbita should be incised for additional drainage.

Following successful control of vision loss and proptosis, the child should be admitted to the intensive care unit for bed rest and sedation. Frequent eye evaluations for proptosis, vision or pupillary changes, or increasing eye pain must be performed, and ophthalmology consultation should be obtained. Decision making regarding continuing diuretics or miotics should be made with the help of the consulting ophthalmologist.

Pneumocephalus

Pneumatoencephaloceles are a result of entrance into the cranial vault through a dural tear that allows air entry without cerebral spinal fluid leak. This one-way ball valve effect causes a mass effect as the pocket of air enlarges, especially during increased intranasal pressure such as during nose blowing, sneezing, or coughing. Depending on the volume and rapidity of air entry, the resultant intracranial shift will determine symptoms and urgency of treatment. If pneumocephalus is suspected, CT scan of the head will confirm the diagnosis. Intensive care unit observation and neurosurgical consultation are required and surgical intervention may be necessary. The technique is essentially the same as that for sealing CSF rhinorrhea.

Meningitis and Brain Abscess

Introduction of pathogens into the intracranial cavity may result in meningitis or develop into a brain abscess. Approximately 15% of patients with an inadequately controlled CSF leak will develop meningitis.[20] The child may develop headaches, fever, and meningeal signs. Lumbar puncture and CT scanning help in obtaining the diagnosis.

Early diagnosis and appropriate treatment of sinus disease, especially in the frontal and sphenoid sinus will help prevent intracranial spread of infection. Meticulous dissection during surgery while respecting surgical landmarks will help prevent CSF leaks. Again, prophylactic antibiotic therapy for CSF leak is controversial. Some surgeons feel it is important, but others feel that it will mask potential meningitis. If the patient is diagnosed with meningitis, encephalitis, or intracranial abscess, intravenous antibiotic therapy should be instituted immediately. Neurosurgical and infectious disease consultations are important in determining appropriate antibiotic coverage as well as the need for surgical intervention.

Image-Guided System

The close proximity of the sinuses to the orbit and cranium leaves even the experienced surgeon vulnerable to complications. In the pediatric patient, the sinonasal cavity may be small and undeveloped, so the risks are increased compared with the risks in the adult population. This is more complicated in the face of revision surgery or extensive disease.

Image-guidance systems to assist in safely performing sinus surgery are becoming more popular among otolaryngologists. However, the physician should not substitute image guidance for his or her basic knowledge of nasal surgical anatomy and important landmarks that outline surgical dissection. Anatomic relationships, as well as didactic and laboratory workshops should continue to be the primary source by which the otolaryngologist gains experience and learns to perform FESS.

Image-guided surgery requires the surgeon to learn how to use the equipment. The set-up time in the operating room will increase the time of the surgical procedure, especially for the novice. In addition, the surgeon must remember that the image-guided systems (Instatrak, Visualization Technology Inc. and Stealthstation systems, Sofamor Danek) are reported to be accurate to within 2 mm. Although this may be reassuring to the surgeon, it also may offer a false sense of security. This technology is no substitute for knowledge and proficiency in using anatomic landmarks to direct surgical dissection.[21]

CHOANAL ATRESIA REPAIR

Choanal atresia can be unilateral or bilateral. Unilateral atresia usually presents as unilateral nasal drainage and does not require immediate repair as opposed to bilateral atresia, which presents as airway distress and requires treatment urgently. Several methods can be used to repair the atresia surgically; the most common is transpalatal or transnasal endoscopic. The pearls and pitfalls of the transnasal endoscopic repair will be discussed because this is the preferred method in the hands of the experienced endoscopist.

RESTENOSIS

One of the most common and frustrating complications or sequelae from choanal atresia repair is restenosis of the surgical site. It is believed that this occurs for several reasons, including excessive tissue trauma during the surgical dissection, inadequate removal of the lateral bony wall, and inadequate removal of the bony septum.[22]

With powered instrumentation (shavers and drills) and direct visualization with endoscopes, surgical dissection can carefully be performed with minimal trauma to surrounding tissue. In addition, stenting is controversial; when it is used, the stent should be placed for as short a time as possible. The authors are using stenting for unilateral atresia repairs less frequently. The length of time to use stenting still remains controversial.

Adequate removal of the lateral boney wall and the posterior nasal septum creates a large neochoanae decreasing the likelihood of restenosis. One should be cognizant that the optic nerve is housed in bone in this lateral wall. The CT scan should be available in the room during the procedure to help identify surgical landmarks and prevent complications.

Mitomycin, an aminoglycoside antibiotic, has been used as an antineoplastic agent to inhibit DNA synthesis and break DNA strands and chromosomes.[23] Topical application has found it to have properties that inhibit figroblast growth and migration.[24] In the surgical site after choanal atresia repair, topical application has shown promise in increasing patency rates after surgical therapy to create a neochoanae.[25] As with endoscopic sinus procedures, endoscopic choanal atresia repair can lead to intracranial and intraorbital complications, which should be handled as discussed previously.

PALATAL FISTULA

The authors advocate placing a nasopharyngeal sponge by way of the oral cavity before beginning the dissection. This displaces the palate inferiorly as well as serves as a guide for the surgeon when the nasopharynx is entered. If the surgeon is not posterior enough in the formation of the neochoanae, a palatal fistula could possibly be created. If this is recognized early and a small opening is created, primary closure of the defect through the oral cavity should be performed. In the case of a large defect, closure as performed for cleft palate by creating advancement flaps of the palatal mucosa may need to be performed at a later date. Image guidance systems may also be used during this procedure to decrease the incidence of complications.

SEPTOPLASTY

Complications from septoplasty in children, facial plastics, and reconstructive surgery are covered in Chapter 33. Nevertheless, it deserves mention in this chapter as well because of the concerns of nasal surgery on craniofacial growth. Several authors have debated whether septoplasty should be performed in children because midfacial growth has been proposed to be disrupted at injury of the growth plates in the septum.[26–28] However, trauma alone causing significant septal deviation may be enough to effect facial growth. Others have recommended "conservative" septoplasty on children to be safe and necessary in children with severe septal deviations causing nasal airway obstruction.[29,30] Other complications of septoplasty may include failure to correct the deviation, septal perforation, CSF leak, and over-resection causing saddle nose deformity.

CONCLUSIONS

Endoscopic sinonasal surgery is a safe and effective method to treat nasal disease in children. With the introduction of FESS, otolaryngologists worldwide have found renewed interest in the treatment of sinus disease. This has caused a plethora of courses, conferences, research, and literature, which ultimately allow the otolaryngologist to provide a better and safer quality of care to the patient.

A thorough knowledge of the anatomy is paramount; cadaveric dissections are recommended prior to performing FESS in the operating room. A comprehensive history and physical examination must be performed, including an endoscopic nasal exam when possible. Accurate diagnosis should precede comprehensive medical therapy. Medical therapy should always be the first line of therapy and surgery should be considered an adjunct to it. Surgery is reserved for patients who fail to respond to medical therapy and/or for those who have an anatomic problem causing symptoms. A CT scan should be studied preoperatively and in the operating room during the procedure. When indicated, image guidance may be helpful.

The surgeon should recognize his or her limitations and should abort surgery in the case of excessive bleeding or if the dissection is more complex than initially thought preoperatively. The surgeon can always come back another day to finish the surgery if he or she feels the need to abort the procedure. Surgeons who are better versed in traditional sinus surgery than in FESS may feel it necessary to rely on some of these traditional techniques to avoid complication. As with any procedure, as more otolaryngologists have become familiar with FESS, the complication rate has decreased. For difficult cases, the surgeon should obtain consultation from more experienced colleagues who often perform revision surgery. This is particularly appropriate for the pediatric patient.

In conclusion, the endoscopic nasal approach offers the surgeon a superior approach to treating sinus disease in the pediatric patient. As a result, pediatric patients can now be offered the highest quality of care with a decreased complication rate in treating nasal disease.

REFERENCES

1. Gross, C.W., Guruchiari, M.J., Lazar, R.H., and Long, T.E. Functional endonasal sinus surgery (FESS) in the pediatric age group. *Laryngoscope*, 1989, 99, 272–275.
2. Mosher, H.P. The applied anatomy and intranasal surgery of the ethmoid labyrinth. *Trans. Am. Laryng. Assoc.*, 1912, 94, 25–39.
3. Mosher, H.P. The surgical anatomy of the ethmoid labyrinth. *Ann. Otolaryngol.*, 1929, 38, 869–901.
4. Draf, W. *Endoscopy of the Paranasal Sinuses.* New York: Springer–Verlag, 1983.
5. Von Riccabona, A. Erfahrungen mit der Kieferhohlenendoskopie. *Arch. Ohr-Nas-Kehlk-Heilk*, 167, 359, 1955.
6. Nehls, G. Antroskopopieerfahrung Eine Beitrag Zur Nasennebenhohllendiagnostik. *HNO* (Berlin), 5, 158, 1955.
7. Stammberger, H. *Functional Endoscopic Sinus Surgery. The Messerklinger Technique.* Philadelphia: B.C. Decker, 1991.
8. Stammberger, H. The evolution of functional endoscopic sinus surgery. *Ears Nose Throat J.*, 1994, 73, 451–455.
9. Vining, E. and Kennedy, D. The transmigration of endoscopic sinus surgery from Europe to the United States. *Ear Nose Throat J.*, 1994, 73, 456–460.
10. Josephson, J.S. and Linden, B.E. The importance of post-operative care in the adult and pediatric patient treated with functional endoscopic sinus surgery. *Operative Tech. Otolaryngol. Head Neck Surg.*, 1990, 2, 112–116.

11. Carpenter, K.M., Graham, S.M., and Smith, R.J. Facial skeletal growth after endoscopic sinus surgery in the piglet model. *Am. J. Rhinol.*, 1997, 11, 211–217.
12. Medina, J., Hernandez, H., Tom, L.W. et al. Development of the paranasal sinuses in children. *Am. J. Rhinol.*, 1997, 11, 203–209.
13. Bothwell, M.R., Piccirillo, J.F., Lusk, R.P., and Rodenour, B.D. Long-term outcome of facial growth after functional endoscopic sinus surgery. *Otolaryngol. Head Neck Surg.*, 2002, 126, 628–634.
14. Keros, P. Uber Die Praktische Beteundung der Niveau-Unterschiede der Lamina criosa des ethmoids (1962). Cited in Naumann, H.H., Ed., *Head and Neck Surgery: Face and Facial Skull*. Vol 1. Philadelphia: W.B. Saunders, 1980.
15. Josephson, J.S., Rice, D., and Josephson, G.D. Functional endoscopic sinus surgery. In Krespi, Y. and Ossoff, R., Eds. *Complications in Head and Neck Surgery*. W.B. Saunders Co. 1993, 131–142.
16. Schaefer, S.D. An anatomic approach to endoscopic intranasal ethmoidectomy. *Laryngoscope*, 1998, 108, 1628–1634.
17. Stankiewicz, J.A. Blindness and intranasal ethmoidectomy: prevention and management. *Otolaryngol. Head Neck Surg.*, 1989, 101, 322–329.
18. Stankiewicz, J.A. and Chow, J.M. Two faces of orbital hematoma in intranasal (endoscopic) sinus surgery. *Otolaryngol. Head Neck Surg.*, 1999, 120, 841–847.
19. Josephson, J.S., Balwally, A.N., and Josephson, G.D. Complications of functional endoscopic sinus surgery. *Insights Otolaryngol.*, 7(4), 1992, 1–8.
20. Ommaya, A.K. Spinal fluid fistulae. *Clin. Neurosurg.*, 1976, 23, 363.
21. Metson, R., Gliklich, R.E., and Cosenza, M. A comparison of image guidance systems for sinus surgery. *Laryngoscope*, 1998, 1164–1170.
22. Josephson, G.D., Vickery, C.L., Giles, W.C., and Gross, C.W. Transnasal endoscopic repair of congenital choanal atresia. *Arch. Otolaryngol. Head Neck Surg.*, 1998, 124, 537–540.
23. Jassir, D., Buchman, C.A., and Gomez–Marin, O. Safety and efficacy of topical mitomycin c in myringotomy patency. *Otolaryngol. Head Neck Surg.*, 2001, 124, 368–373.
24. Daniels, J.T., Occleston, N.L., Crowston, J.G., and Khaw, P.T. Effects of antimetabolite induced cellular growth arrest on fibroblast–fibroblast interactions. *Exp. Eye Res.*, 1999, 69, 117–127.
25. Prasad, M., Ward, R.F., April, M.M., Bent, J.P., and Froehlich, P. Topical mitomycin as an adjunct to choanal atresia repair. *Arch. Otolaryngol. Head Neck Surg.*, 2002, 128, 398–400.
26. Sarnat, B.G. Differential effect of surgical trauma to the nasal bones and septum upon rabbit snout growth. In Sanvenero–Rosselli, G. and Boggio–Robutti, G., Eds. *Transactions of the Fourth International Congress of Plastic Surgery*. Rome, Amsterdam: Excerpta Medica, 1967.
27. Meeuwis, C.A., Verwoerd–Verhoef, H.L., van der Heul, R.O., and Verwoerd, C.D.A. Morphological changes of the cartilaginous nasal septum after partial resection in young rabbits. *Clin. Otolaryngol.*, 1985, 10, 231–232.
28. Loosen, J.V., Verwoerd-Verhoef, H.L., and Verwoerd, C.D.A. The nasal septal cartilage in the newborn. *Rhinology*, 1988, 26, 161–165.
29. Josephson, G.D., Levine, J., and Cutting, C.B. Septoplasty for obstructive sleep apnea in infants after cleft palate repair. *Cleft Palate Craniofacial J.*, 1996, 33(6), 473–476.
30. Healy, G. An approach to the nasal septum in children. *Laryngoscope*, 1986, 96, 1239–1242.

Section VIII

Otology

28 Otitis Media

David H. Darrow and Craig S. Derkay

The fact that your patient gets well does not prove that your diagnosis was correct.

Samuel J. Meltzer

CONTENTS

INTRODUCTION

Complications of otitis media include infectious and inflammatory processes that result from spread of infection beyond the middle ear space, as well as long-term effects of middle ear disease on tympanic structures and language development. The incidence of otitis media in the United States is rising. This is due, in large part, to the rapid spread of upper respiratory illness facilitated by daycare facilities that are increasingly attended by younger children and infants who, anatomically and immunologically, are most susceptible to developing otitis media. Middle ear disease of long-standing duration may result in delays in development of language, social, or motor skills. Inappropriate use of antimicrobial therapy has resulted in increased antibiotic resistance increasing the risk for local, regional, and systemic complications.

In childhood, otitis media is most commonly associated with eustachian tube dysfunction, requiring surgical middle ear ventilation with tympanostomy tubes that may alter the tympanic membrane resulting in long-term hearing loss. Furthermore, although otogenic complications have become relatively rare since the advent of modern antibiotic therapy, intratemporal and extracranial complications of otitis media may still occur and remain a major health concern. In addition, the effectiveness of modern therapy in lowering the incidence of complications, however beneficial, may have secondarily resulted in precipitating a relative lack of familiarity among treating clinicians with the manifestations of these serious, potentially life-threatening disorders.

OTITIS MEDIA — A BRIEF REVIEW

BACKGROUND, DEFINITION, INCIDENCE, AND ETIOLOGY

Otitis media (OM) is a major health issue, costing the U.S. health system more than $5 billion per year. American children suffer an estimated 28 million cases of acute otitis media per year.[1] More than 25% of the 120 million prescriptions for antibiotics and 40% of all antibiotic prescriptions for children under the age of 10 are written for OM, and indirect costs for treatment of OM probably exceed the direct costs.[2] Myringotomy with insertion of tubes is the most common surgical procedure in children. In 1996, about 1 of every 110 children had tubes inserted.[3]

OM is, by definition, inflammation of the middle ear without reference to its etiology or pathogenesis. Acute otitis media (AOM) is associated with the rapid onset of symptoms and signs of acute infection in the middle ear space, including fever, otalgia, and purulent middle ear effusion. Otitis media with effusion (OME) refers to inflammation of the middle ear associated with serous, mucoid, or mucopurulent fluid. The effusion in OME can be the result of AOM or eustachian tube dysfunction; it may be acute in origin or chronic in nature. In contrast, chronic otitis media (COM) represents progressive and long-standing tympanic disease characterized by clinically significant tympanic membrane retraction and atelectasis, perforation, otorrhea, cholesteatoma, and chronic suppurative disease; this is discussed in Chapter 29.

OM is primarily a disease of infancy and early childhood with the peak age-specific attack rate occurring between 6 and 18 months of age. Children who have had little or no OM by 3 years of age are unlikely to have subsequent severe recurrent disease. Risk factors for OM have been established by numerous investigators[4–8] and include

- Attendance at group daycare
- Sibling history of recurrent OM
- Early occurrence of initial OM
- Lack of breastfeeding
- Male gender
- Allergy
- Possibly, exposure to smoke in the household

OM is also more common among Native Americans and Eskimos and, in these groups, is frequently complicated by perforation of the tympanic membrane and persistent suppurative drainage. Factors beyond genetics that may predispose these children to otitis include crowded living conditions, poor sanitation, and inadequate medical care.[8]

The pathogenesis of OM is multifactorial, including infection, impaired eustachian tube function, immune status, and allergy. In most cases, OM begins with a viral infection of the upper respiratory tract that causes congestion of the eustachian tube and impairment of normal tubal function, including middle ear ventilation, ciliary clearance, and drainage. As a result, pathogens colonizing the nasopharynx may gain access to the middle ear space and multiply due to impairment of the normal protective mechanisms. Immune responses, with or without antimicrobial therapy, will normally eradicate the infection; however, effusion may persist until normal tubal function returns. Effusion may also occur in the absence of infection, typically in ears in which severely impaired eustachian tube function results in transudation of fluid into the middle ear. Such cases are frequently associated with atelectasis and retraction of the tympanic membrane.

BACTERIOLOGY AND ANTIBIOTIC RESISTANCE

Most bacteriological studies of AOM demonstrate the importance of *Streptococcus pneumoniae* and *Haemophilus influenzae* and a minor role for *Moraxella catarrhalis*.[9] Children with OME also have these bacterial pathogens present, suggesting that bacteria play a role in the development and persistence of the effusion. Respiratory viruses, alone and in combination with bacterial pathogens, have been identified in as many as one third of middle ear effusions.[10] The rising incidence of pathogen resistance in otitis media to antimicrobial agents has become a significant issue. Although regional differences are undoubtedly present, recent data from Children's Hospital of Pittsburgh indicate that up to 40% of AOM episodes are due to *S. pneumoniae,* with more than 40% of these penicillin resistant; 25% are due to *H. influenzae* with about 25% penicillin resistance; 12% are due to *M. catarrhalis* with 100% penicillin resistance; and about 23% are due to other pathogens.[11]

The risk factors postulated for development of antimicrobial resistance are low dose and prolonged treatment with beta-lactam antibiotics, recent exposure to antibiotics, attendance in large child daycare environment, young otitis-prone infants, and winter season.[8,12] Unfortunately, these bacterial strains are also highly resistant to other beta-lactam antibiotics, as well as trimethaprim-sulfa and macrolides. Poole and colleagues[13] have reported rates of drug-resistant *Streptococcus pneumoniae* as high as 90% in some communities and macrolide resistances exceeding those of beta-lactams in some populations. Sutton and colleagues[12] found penicillin resistance in 38% of *S. pneumoniae* cultures, and beta-lactamase production in 65% of *Haemophilus influenzae* and 100% of *Moraxella catarrhalis* cultures, in effusions from children undergoing tympanostomy tube surgery.

Over the past decade, penicillin resistance to *Streptococcus pneumoniae* has become a world-wide problem. Not only has this made medical management more problematic, but resistant bacteria have also been associated with the potential for a higher incidence of infectious complications with otitis media.[14] Inappropriate prescribing of antibiotics in the treatment of pediatric infections has been implicated as the key component in the development of drug-resistant OM, and a significant effort has been made to educate the medical profession and public. The indiscriminate treatment of upper respiratory infections and uncomplicated middle ear effusion with antibiotics has now been strongly discouraged.[15] In addition, the wisdom of long-term use of low-dose, daily antibiotics to manage recurrent AOM prophylactically has been questioned because this method has demonstrated minimal efficacy, if any, and would seem to place ideal evolutionary pressure on the development of resistant strains of bacteria.[16]

DIAGNOSTIC VARIABILITY

The accurate diagnosis of otitis media is a key principle in determining appropriate management. Usually, a parent or primary caregiver initially provides a child's history of otitis media. In general, he or she has a strong emotional investment in the outcome of the office visit, and however well intentioned, the ability to differentiate between the various potential causes of fever and generalized pain — key criteria in the diagnosis of OM — is often limited. It is the responsibility of the clinician, therefore, to determine, as accurately as possible, the true symptoms, periodicity, and clinical impact of a child with suspected otitis media.

Furthermore, there may be wide latitude in physical examination acumen between clinicians within a primary care group and within a specialty practice. An inflamed tympanic membrane does not necessarily mean that middle ear effusion is present. The presence of a middle ear effusion does not necessarily mean that the child has AOM. The use of the term "ear infection" is widely abused in today's society, fomented in large part by the popular media. In children, the use of pneumatic otoscopy is considered the most optimal examination method, but it is not universally used within all clinical specialties.[17] Availability of quality pediatric audiology services may be limited. Office tympanometry can be helpful but is still subject to the interpretation and findings of the examining clinician. Improvement and refinement in the teaching of primary care resident physicians regarding the diagnosis of otitis media and its clinical variations, accompanied by sustained interspecialty dialogue throughout their careers, will help reduce this potential and perceived gap in diagnostic accuracy.

MEDICAL MANAGEMENT

Although over 70% of episodes of AOM are likely to clear without antibiotic therapy, treatment appears to resolve symptoms more rapidly and reduces the risk of complication.[18] Antimicrobial agents should show efficacy against the three major bacterial pathogens. The selection of a particular drug is based upon clinical and microbiological efficacy, acceptability of the preparation, absence of side effects and toxicity, convenience of dosing schedule, and cost. In most cases, amoxicillin is appropriate first-line therapy, using high doses for children considered at risk for resistant pneumococcus. Second-line therapy should be guided by the likelihood of untreated drug-resistant organisms.[9,19] Duration of antibiotic therapy is typically up to 10 days, depending on the oral antimicrobial agent used, although a shorter duration of therapy may be appropriate in older children or in less severe cases.[20]

The typical clinical course of a child who receives an appropriate antimicrobial agent includes significant resolution of acute signs within 48 to 72 hours; a change of antibiotic coverage should be considered if acute signs persist beyond that time. Children with severe otalgia, sepsis, immune compromise, or suppurative complications of OM may benefit from tympanocentesis to identify the causative organism or tympanostomy tube placement to facilitate drainage and improve ventilation.[19] As discussed earlier, prolonged antimicrobial therapy for prophylaxis against recurrent AOM is not recommended.[21]

Persistent noninfected middle ear effusion does not need to be managed with repeat antibiotic courses. In most cases, the middle ear effusion is self-limiting; resolution can be anticipated in up to 60% of children by 1 month, 80% by 2 months, and 90% by 3 months.[6] Persistent effusion following antibiotic treatment for AOM is more likely if there is[2]

- An episode of OM within the preceding month
- Daycare attendance with greater than 10 other children
- Bilateral disease
- Age less than 2
- Age of less than 6 months at first otitis
- More than three acute episodes of otitis in the preceding 6 months
- The presence of passive smoke exposure
- The occurrence of otitis during the winter months
- A family history of ear disease

Medical therapies such as systemic or topical decongestants, antihistamines, and homeopathic remedies have not demonstrated efficacy in the management in OM,[22,23] and the effects of allergic immunotherapy in OM have not been well studied. Trials of corticosteroid therapy for persistent OME have yielded mixed results.[24] Interventions such as eustachian tube inflation and chiropractic manipulation do not improve outcomes.[25,26] Early trials of the protein-conjugated heptavalent pneumococcal vaccine (Prevnar®), developed to reduce invasive pneumococcal disease in infants, have demonstrated efficacy against vaccine-specific serotypes of S. pneumoniae, but only a modest reduction in urgent visits for middle ear disease has been seen.[27,28]

SURGICAL MANAGEMENT

Insertion of tympanostomy tubes is often recommended to improve middle ear ventilation in children with recurrent AOM and persistent OME. First introduced by Armstrong in 1954, tympanostomy tube insertion is now the most common surgical procedure performed in children under general anesthesia. Multiple studies have demonstrated a reduced frequency of infection in children with a history of recurrent AOM, and tubes are generally recommended for children who have experienced four episodes in a 6-month period or six episodes in a 12-month period.[29]

In studies of children with persistent OME, ventilation tubes have achieved longer disease-free intervals and improved hearing than has medical management alone.[30] Tube insertion recommendations are usually considered when bilateral effusions associated with (conductive) hearing loss for 3 months or a unilateral effusion persistent for 6 months is identified. Other factors, such as potential impact of recurrent AOM or persistent OME on speech acquisition language development and patient or parent quality of life, antibiotic intolerance, and allergies or complications may play a role in the consideration for ventilation tube placement.

Adjunctive adenoidectomy has been advocated for otitis media management and clinically validated over time.[31,32] This position is not universally accepted, however, because of disagreement on the timing or potential utility for removing the adenoids.[33] Most otolaryngologists understand the rationale and acknowledge the potential long-term benefits of adenoidectomy, particularly in a child with renewed, persistent OME following ventilation tube extrusion or with a strongly supportive history of coexisting upper airway obstruction or chronic rhinosinusitis. The decision to perform adjunctive adenoidectomy, however, may be influenced by the emotions of the parents, the referring physicians, or the consulted specialist. This negotiation is ideally best achieved with open and honest dialogue between an empathetic otolaryngologist and a knowledgeable parent or care giver who has been educated and empowered to provide consent on behalf of the child for whom they are all responsible.

DEVELOPMENTAL COMPLICATIONS

Children with middle ear effusion typically suffer a temporary loss of ipsilateral hearing that improves when the status of the middle ear returns to normal. In most cases, the hearing loss is conductive with pure tone and speech awareness thresholds elevated by 20 to 30 decibels (dB), but thresholds may vary from 0 to 50 dB. Hearing loss may be asymmetrical, even when both ears are involved. Far more common in the preantibiotic age, some clinicians believe that sensorineural hearing loss may still occur in a small percentage of cases as a result of bacterial toxins that cross the round window membrane.[34]

Compromise of auditory function is, at best, a short-term complication for children in a critical period of speech acquisition and language development and for those struggling with academic performance. It is less clear whether fluctuating or long-standing conductive hearing loss causes more significant developmental delays. Although some investigators have observed a delay in acquisition of speech and language skills that improves rapidly after clearance of middle ear disease, others suggest that such effects are small and that intervention may not be necessary.[35] A more detailed discussion of these issues is found in Chapter 9.

SOCIAL AND ECONOMIC COMPLICATIONS

The true cost of managing OM cannot be calculated strictly on the basis of the cost of the prescription and the initial office visit. The typical child with otitis will have an initial visit and at least one to two subsequent ear checks. At each visit, there are expenses for time lost for the working parent, transportation costs to and from the physician's office, babysitting cost for the children who remain at home, and an educational cost from time lost at daycare, preschool, or elementary school. For the child with severe or recurrent disease, costs expand to include visits to specialists, such as otolaryngologists, audiologists, speech and language therapists, and the fees for the tests and therapy provided by these professionals.

Lifestyle costs are also related to this disease. Many parents inappropriately limit the water exposure of their children with OM under the misguided notion that the swimming pool water may penetrate through an intact eardrum. Even in the presence of a tympanostomy tube, it appears genuinely safe for children to participate in water sports as long as they do not swim more than 6 feet below the surface, jump or dive off the diving board, or expose their ears to water mixed with soap or shampoo.[36] Some parents will alter travel plans if they are concerned about otalgia due to barotitis in children with OM or eustachian tube dysfunction who fly in airplanes.

Rosenfeld and colleagues developed a tool to quantify the quality of life of children with OM and then used it in a prospective observational trial of children undergoing tympanostomy tubes for otitis media. Parents rated their children's physical suffering (ear pain, ear discomfort, and high fevers); emotional distress (irritability, frustration, restlessness, and poor appetite); and their own concerns (worry, concern, or inconvenience because of the child's ear infections or fluid) as the most significant negative aspects of their children's otitis on their quality of life. Large improvements in quality of life were found in 56% of children with physical symptoms; caregiver concerns, emotional distress, and hearing loss improved most and significant changes were also measured for improvement in activity limitations and speech impairment.[37]

COMPLICATIONS OF MYRINGOTOMY AND VENTILATION TUBE PLACEMENT

TECHNIQUE

Intraoperative complications of performing myringotomy and placing a ventilating tube are few. Although dislocating the incudostapedial joint, severing the facial nerve, and puncturing an exposed jugular bulb are dreaded complications, they are described only in rare case reports. More likely, minor external canal trauma may result from difficult cerumen evacuation or inadvertent suction catheter or myringotomy knife shaft (or blade) pressure on canal skin; secondary overenlargement of the myringotomy incision may occur because of the necessarily more aggressive suctioning used for the more difficult to remove desiccated effusions.

In children with extremely small external auditory canals, placement and follow-up of ventilation tubes can be a challenge. This is especially an issue in children with Down syndrome and craniofacial disorders. Smaller diameter speculae with longer shafts may be required. Following myringotomy, tubes found to be larger than the lumen of the speculum can be placed in the ear canal prior to the speculum and manipulated into the myringotomy site using otologic picks. The small external auditory canal may also influence the surgeon to choose a smaller grommet style tube, such as a Tiny-Tef® tube, although these have the disadvantage of staying in the eardrum for a shorter period of time.

Children with chronic eustachian tube dysfunction may require repeated insertion of ventilation tubes. This may result in an atelectatic tympanic membrane, which poses a surgical challenge for the reinsertion of the tube. Under these circumstances, the tube can often be inserted high in the anterior quadrant. If the tympanic membrane is excessively flaccid, a reparative tympanoplasty may need to be considered and discussed (see Chapter 29).

ANESTHESIA

One of the major concerns that parents have when tympanostomy tube insertion is considered is the safety of the general anesthetic. Hoffmann and colleagues[38] evaluated 4000 consecutive children who had had tubes placed for possible complications of the general anesthesia and found no serious complications or deaths. Far fewer than 1% had airway obstruction that required intervention with muscle relaxants or insertion of an endotracheal tube. They concluded that myringotomy with ventilation tube placement is an extremely safe procedure.

OTORRHEA

The most common immediate postoperative complication of tympanostomy tube insertion is otorrhea through the lumen of the tube. Following tube insertion, otorrhea occurs in approximately 10% of cases, most commonly when a mucoid or purulent effusion is aspirated at the time of myringotomy; this typically will clear with ototopical therapy. Delayed otorrhea that occurs after the initial postoperative period usually results from nasopharyngeal secretion reflux into the middle ear, an upper respiratory infection, tube-associated granulation tissue, or contamination within the external canal. Most children with tympanostomy tubes will have at least one episode of otorrhea per year that the tubes stay in place.[36,39]

Ototopical antibiotics alone have shown great efficacy in resolving otorrhea from most causes; the addition of oral systemic antibiotics may be helpful in the presence of a severe upper respiratory infection (URI) with nasopharyngitis or when cellulitis complicates the external otitis. Granulation tissue surrounding the tube is best treated initially using steroid-containing preparations. Ofloxacin and ciprofloxacin/hydrocortisone — fluoroquinolone antibiotic preparations with no known oto- toxicity — are the newest generation of ototopical agents available for use in patients with draining ears and tympanic membrane perforations. These appear to be at least as efficacious as neomy- cin/polymyxin B/hydrocortisone in the prevention of postoperative otorrhea after placement of ventilation tubes.[40] Neomycin/polymyxin B/hydrocortisone and ophthalmic preparations used off- label carry the theoretical risk of ototoxicity, although it is estimated such cases occur in fewer than 1 in 10,000 people treated.

Comprehensive reviews of clinical and animal research studies conclude that ototoxicity is very uncommon or poorly recognized.[41] Some investigators suggest that tubes impregnated with silver oxide may reduce the incidence of postoperative otorrhea.[42] Alternatively, tubes manufactured with an ion-balanced method reportedly have theoretical advantage from less biofilm accumulation tendency, with presumed decrease in the incidence of postoperative otorrhea.[43] Postoperative tube obstruction may be reduced by the use of topical phenylephrine at the time of tube placement.[44]

Oberman and Derkay recently reviewed management of pediatric tympanostomy tube otorrhea and came to several conclusions based upon a review of the medical literature.[45] Ear canal preparation prior to tympanostomy tube placement *does not* reduce the incidence of early post-tympanostomy tube otorrhea. The presence of an active middle ear infection as manifested by mucoid, mucopuru- lent, or purulent middle ear effusion *does* increase the risk of early otorrhea. Perioperative ototopical drops probably decrease the incidence of early post-tympanostomy tube otorrhea. The use of systemic antibiotics with activity against the common middle ear pathogens may reduce the risk of early otorrhea, but this has not yet been confirmed with randomized placebo-controlled clinical trials.

The overall risk of otorrhea and the bacterial pathogens may demonstrate seasonal variation. Patient age and gender do not appear to be a risk factor in the development of early otorrhea. Rarely, tympanostomy tubes incite a chronic infectious or inflammatory reaction that fails to respond to routine office management and requires removal of the ventilation tube. More rarely still, the presence of an unrecognized retained tympanostomy tube in the middle ear cleft may be the etiology of a chronic infectious or inflammatory middle ear process. Water precautions for surface swimming in children with tympanostomy tubes are now considered unnecessary for most children, with postactivity otorrhea rates comparable with or without dry ear precautions.[36] Diving, head dunking, and water type are independent variables that may warrant precautions. Furthermore, some children appear to be "otorrhea prone"; in such cases, more aggressive intervention and stricter adherence to water precautions are warranted.

DURATION AND EXTRUSION

The average grommet style tube stays in the tympanic membrane for about 1 year and rarely requires surgical removal. Ventilation tube duration and extrusion rates do not appear to be related to site of placement.[46] The vast majority of children exhibit normal tube extrusion parameters requiring, perhaps, office management for crusting and debris build-up or for an extruded tube still resting within the external canal. Based on the length of time within the tympanic membrane, tube type, secondary tympanic membrane features, age of child, and otorrhea history, a significantly retained tube will occasionally require removal under general anesthesia.

Sequelae related to tympanostomy tube insertion include scarring of the tympanic membrane (tympanoslerosis or as myringoslerosis) and tympanic membrane atrophy, which may be localized or diffuse and may or may not be associated with retraction pockets or secondary conductive hearing loss. Tympanosclerosis may occur in up to 50% of tympanic membranes that have had a ventilation tube in them by the time the tube has extruded, but the tympanosclerosis is rarely identified within the middle ear and the hearing is not usually affected.[39] Atrophy and atelectasis result from the loss of the middle fibrous layer of the healed tympanic membrane after tube extrusion. Continued eustachian tube dysfunction causes retraction of the tympanic membrane with a predilection for these sites, increasing the risk of cholesteatoma formation within a retraction pocket. Less commonly, a perforation may remain at the insertion site following extrusion of the tube. Rates of perforation vary depending upon the type of tube, ranging from 0 to 4% for grommet style tubes to 12 to 25% for unmodified Goode T-tubes.[39] Rare complications include the development of cholesteatoma at the site of the tube insertion due to ingrowth of squamous epithelium at the edge of the tympanostomy and intrusion of the tube into the middle ear cavity.[39,47]

IMPACT OF MANAGED CARE

Many otolaryngologists feel that managed care has resulted in delayed diagnosis of otitis media as well as over- and undertreatment of some children. This becomes an especially contentious issue with regard to the follow-up of children with tympanostomy tubes by the surgeon who performed the operation. In a survey study initiated by the Pediatric Otolaryngology Committee of the American Academy of Otolaryngology–Head and Neck Surgery, 1200 general and pediatric otolaryngologists responsible for the placement of 75,000 myringotomy and tube insertions in children per year were asked to comment on their current practice for tympanostomy tube follow-up.

There was a strong consensus to see the children back within the first month by 96% of respondents and at least every 6 months until extrusion by 94% of respondents. The respondents estimated an incidence of 17 out of every 100 children experiencing at least a minor complication of their underlying eustachian tube dysfunction or of the procedure — usually sustained otorrhea. They reported that approximately 1 of every 20 children in their practice had experienced a complication or sequelae of their underlying ear disease as a direct result of a delayed referral to see the otolaryngologist. Practice guidelines for primary care physicians were presented, including an ear, nose, and throat follow-up within the first month and then at regular intervals until the tubes are out and the eustachian tube function has normalized. The Committee concluded that referral to an otolaryngologist should be made when[47]

- A tube is occluded or cannot be visualized.
- Otorrhea or granulation tissue fails to resolve after an appropriate course of therapy.
- Hearing loss or speech or language delays occur in children with ventilation tubes.
- There is evidence of structural ear disease, such as atelectasis, retraction pockets, or squamous debris.

The American Academy of Pediatrics has recently adopted these recommendations into published guidelines for its members.[48]

INTRATYMPANIC COMPLICATIONS

Intratympanic complications of OM may result from acute or chronic middle ear disease. This includes tympanic membrane atrophy, retraction pockets or perforations, adhesive OM, acquired cholesteatoma, and tympanosclerosis. Such complications are best avoided by maintaining a high level of vigilance and a low threshold for ventilation and surgical intervention in susceptible ears.

TYMPANIC MEMBRANE ATROPHY, RETRACTION POCKETS, AND ADHESIVE OTITIS MEDIA

Weakening of the tympanic membrane due to recurrent perforation and chronic eustachian tube dysfunction may result in tympanic membrane atrophy, retraction pockets, and adhesive OM. Over time, the inherent stiffness of the tympanic membrane is lost from progressive disruption disorganization of the middle fibrous layers, thus resulting in attenuation and flacidity, with progressive retraction and potential atelectasis. Ongoing negative middle ear pressure results in the formation of retraction pockets within the tympanic membrane, most commonly at previous perforation or tympanostomy sites. When retractions become sufficiently deep, they may retain squamous debris and pose the risk of cholesteatoma.

Ventilation of the middle ear with a tympanostomy tube will often arrest tympanic membrane retraction progression. Placement of a cartilage graft underneath the flaccid segment may be useful once better ventilation has been established. Occasionally, when progressive retraction is not addressed promptly, a fibrous adhesion may develop between the tympanic membrane and the ossicles and/or the medial wall of the middle ear. This "adhesive otitis" is typically associated, initially, with a mild conductive hearing loss, which may progress if the ossicles, particularly the long process of the incus, become eroded. Tympanoplasty with or without mastoidectomy is indicated when hearing loss is moderate to severe or when significant risk of cholesteatoma is present, as discussed in Chapter 29.

ACUTE PERFORATION

When pressure from pus accumulating in the middle ear space with AOM increases, an acute perforation of the tympanic membrane may occur. Many clinicians consider such perforations a part of the disease process rather than a complication, especially because the vast majority heal uneventfully within 1 to 2 weeks. The inner connective tissue layer of the tympanic membrane, however, is often lost during the healing process and perforation is more likely to occur in ears with repeat episodes of AOM that already have attenuated tympanic membranes.

When drainage and exfoliated skin accumulate significantly, debridement of the external canal will assist with resolution of secondary otitis externa. Obtaining a culture of the drainage following debridement of the canal may be useful in guiding medical therapy. Combined oral and topical antibiotic therapy is usually appropriate in these circumstances when middle ear and outer ear pathology is present. A chronic perforation may result when the outer squamous layer of the tympanic membrane fuses with the epithelium of the middle ear on its undersurface. Patients with chronic perforations must be periodically monitored for hearing loss and development of cholesteatoma.

ACQUIRED CHOLESTEATOMA

Keratinizing squamous epithelium may accumulate within the tympanic membrane or the middle ear space from the formation of deep retraction pockets that accumulate desquamated epithelium from the surface of the eardrum or from chronic tympanic membrane perforations in which the squamous layer has gained access to the middle ear space. These acquired cholesteatomas may increase in size; bone resorption may result from direct pressure or due to collagenase production within the lesion, ultimately resulting in hearing loss. In advanced cases, the process may erode bone covering other vital middle ear structures and cause labyrinthine fistula, facial nerve paralysis, or intracranial complications. Treatment of acquired cholesteatomas is surgical and, in advanced cases, may require two stages: one to eradicate the disease and make the ear "safe" and the second to reconstruct the hearing mechanism, as discussed in Chapter 29.

TYMPANOSCLEROSIS

The formation of calcified plaques within the tympanic membrane or middle ear mucosa is called tympanosclerosis. When only the tympanic membrane is involved, it is more accurately called myringosclerosis. This process occurs secondary to degeneration of collagenous fibrous tissue, which then becomes interlaced with deposits of calcium and phosphate crystals. The plaques typically appear in regions of the tympanic membrane adjacent to prior injury, such as perforation or tympanostomy tube insertion; they may also occur, with less frequency, in tympanic membranes with a history limited to recurrent infections. If limited to the tympanic membrane, tympanosclerosis is usually of little clinical consequence unless extensive enough be associated with marked conductive hearing loss from loss of vibratory elasticity. Conductive hearing loss may also occur if the ossicular chain is affected by tympanosclerosis involving the ossicular tendons and ligaments, the oval window, or the epitympanum, where the ossicular heads are housed. There is no known preventative treatment. Tympanoplasty is indicated in cases with moderate to severe conductive hearing loss.

PROGRESSION AND EXTENSION OF OTITIS MEDIA

An unfortunate consequence of the development of effective antibiotics and the precipitous decline of otogenic complications has been decreased recognition of impending complications of OM outside the middle ear. Fever and other signs and symptoms that once heralded the progression of otitic disease are now frequently suppressed by medical therapy. Furthermore, the effectiveness of modern therapy and the low incidence of complications have resulted in a degree of complacency in the treatment of infections of the middle ear as well as a lack of familiarity with the manifestations of complications. The clinician must bear in mind that complications of OM, even in their mildest form, will compromise quality of life; left untreated, they may rapidly progress with potentially life-threatening consequences.

FACTORS IN THE SPREAD OF OTITIC INFECTION

Most reports published during the antibiotic era suggest that intratemporal and intracranial otogenic complications more commonly result from AOM in the pediatric age group, while complications from chronic middle ear disease are more common among older patients.[49–51] Spread of infection occurs when acute or chronic processes in the middle ear spread through intact bone via small venules or preformed pathways, or due to the slow erosion of bone by cholesteatoma. Such spread may involve adjacent sites within the temporal bone, the posterior or middle cranial fossae, the extratemporal soft tissues, or more distal sites reached by hematogenous spread (Figure 28.1).

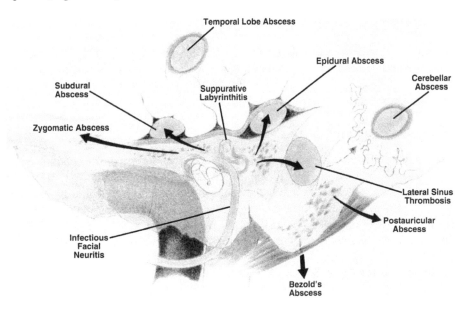

FIGURE 28.1 Common pathways in the spread of otitis media.

Species and Virulence of the Organism

Streptococcus pneumoniae (15 to 40%) and *Streptococcus pyogenes* (10 to 20%) are the most frequent offenders in acute mastoiditis. Aerobic bacteria may be cultured from approximately 70% of middle ears with chronic suppurative OM (CSOM), and *Proteus* and *Pseudomonas aeruginosa* are the most common offending organisms.[52] Anaerobes are present in nearly equal frequency, most notably *Bacteroides* sp., *Peptococcus/Peptostreptococcus* sp., and *Propionibacterium acnes*. Mixed infections are present in over 50% of these cases. It should be noted, though, that many organisms cultured from chronic suppurative effusions may represent colonization of the ear, and their preponderance may mask the presence of more virulent organisms.

Host Conditions

The host tissue responds to the release of toxic substances from the infecting organisms by mounting an inflammatory reaction. Cells involved in the inflammatory response assist in the removal of the bacteria. Several conditions associated with immune compromise, such as infancy, old age, diabetes, malnutrition, malignancy, AIDS, and immunodeficiency, are likely to diminish the effectiveness of this response and may, therefore, increase the likelihood of spread and the risk of complications. Under conditions of relative immune compromise, opportunistic organisms may predominate among the spectrum of flora, and those already colonizing the upper respiratory tract may become more virulent.

Prior Therapy

Inappropriate use of antibiotic therapy in the management of AOM and OME has resulted in increasing rates of infection by multidrug-resistant organisms. Recent studies demonstrate conflicting results regarding the risk of otogenic complications in such infections.[14,53,54] In CSOM, prior therapy and resistance appear to be less significant factors, although some organisms have demonstrated resistance. In CSOM, timely surgical intervention aimed at debridement of the middle ear and mastoid spaces, establishment of adequate ventilation and drainage, and reconstruction of defects in the tympanic membrane remain the cornerstone of therapy in the prevention of otogenic complications.

PATHWAYS IN THE SPREAD OF OTITIC INFECTION

When the mucosal defense system is unable to deter the progression of disease, the integrity of the bone of the middle ear becomes critical because most complications of OM occur outside the bony confines of the ear. Spread of infection through the osseous barrier may occur in one or more of the ways described in the following subsections.

Direct Extension as a Result of Disease

Direct extension by erosion through bone demineralized by cholesteatoma or chronic inflammation extension is the route most commonly implicated in complications due to CSOM. Extradural abscesses, subperiosteal abscesses, and lateral sinus thrombosis usually occur by this mechanism. Patients will commonly present with a prodrome of partial or intermittent impairment of structures affected by the advancing infection, most notably pain, abducens nerve palsy, or facial paralysis due to involvement of the cranial nerves and vertigo due to involvement of the labyrinth.

Direct Extension through Anatomic Pathways

Extension of disease through normal anatomic pathways may result in otogenic complications. Such pathways include the oval and round windows, cochlear and vestibular aqueducts, and bony dehiscences and fissures such as the temporal bone suture lines, neural cannaliculi, and fallopian canal. Spread through small fissures is common in acute infections and in acute exacerbations of chronic infection and may lead to complications such as labyrinthitis.

Direct Extension through Traumatic Defects

Head trauma or prior surgery of the middle ear or mastoid may result in defects or fractures of the temporal bone, representing potential routes through which future infections may directly extend.

Thrombophlebitis

Thrombophlebitic spread can occur through small veins and Haversian canals to the surrounding dural sinuses. Spread through small veins during AOM is the most common etiology of otogenic meningitis, while brain abscess usually results from thrombophlebitis of cerebral veins.

CLASSIFICATION

Complications of otitis media are generally grouped into two main categories:

- Complications within the temporal bone and extratemporal soft tissues:
  - Acute mastoiditis
  - Subperiosteal and Bezold's abscesses
  - Facial paralysis
  - Labyrinthitis
  - Petrous apicitis
- Complications within the cranial cavity:
  - Extradural abscess
  - Lateral sinus thrombosis
  - Brain abscess
  - Meningitis
  - Subdural infection
  - Otitic hydrocephalus

Intratemporal complications are more common than intracranial complications, with acute mastoiditis accounting for the majority. Facial paralysis and subperiosteal abscess are the most common second-stage complications.[55,56] Among the intracranial complications, meningitis is probably the most frequently encountered,[50,57–59] although some authors report more cases of brain abscess[60,61] and epidural abscess[54,58] in their series. Brain abscess is generally considered to have the highest rate of mortality.[49,58] In 25 to 50% of cases, two or more otogenic complications are present concomitantly,[59,61,62] usually reflecting the path of least resistance chosen by the spreading infection. During an exploration for lateral sinus thrombosis, for example, it is not uncommon also to find a perisinus abscess from which it may have originated or a brain abscess to which it may have progressed.

SYMPTOMS AND SIGNS OF IMPENDING COMPLICATION

Complications of AOM are most often heralded by symptoms of the middle ear infection. Fever, hearing loss, and severe otalgia are seen in most cases; children are often inconsolable and cannot sleep. However, in cases of "masked" mastoiditis and aditus block, the presentation may be somewhat more subtle, thereby complicating the diagnosis early in the progression of the disease. Progression of AOM to facial paralysis, meningitis, serous labyrinthitis, or subdural abscess may often occur in the absence of any additional signs or symptoms. In contrast, most patients first develop acute coalescent mastoiditis when extradural abscess, sigmoid sinus thrombosis, brain abscess, or otitic hydrocephalus secondarily complicates AOM. This intermediate stage is characterized by mastoid erythema, tenderness, and swelling associated with anterior displacement of the auricle. Postauricular fluctuance is associated with subperiosteal abscess and confirms the presence of coalescence within the mastoid cavity.

The presentation of complicated CSOM is well described.[51,63,64] Early signs and symptoms include fetid otorrhea, deep pain, and headache. The development of malodorous, purulent discharge from the ear is highly suggestive of bone destruction; it is postulated that the longer the period of drainage is, the greater the amount of bone destruction present.[63] Pain is a symptom generally not associated with chronic OM, but may arise in exacerbation of the disease or with progressive destruction of bone or obstruction of drainage of purulent material from the mastoid space via the aditus. Exacerbations are usually associated with more transient pain, whereas pain due to bone erosion or obstructed drainage is commonly deep and constant; the latter may suggest a developing complication. Fever, nausea, and altered mental status may be present at the time of diagnosis, but generally occur later in the course of the infection. More rare findings at presentation include dysequilibrium, hearing loss, subperiosteal abscess, cranial neuropathies, nuchal rigidity, and seizures, all of which imply that a complication is imminent or has occurred.

INITIAL MANAGEMENT

General Considerations

A thorough history and physical should be performed on all patients suspected of having a complication of OM, including microscopic assessment of the ear. Symptoms of headache, neck pain, and visual changes suggest intracranial involvement; patients with signs of papilledema, impaired extraocular movement, nuchal rigidity, or hemiparesis demand immediate neurosurgical evaluation. When intracranial extension is uncertain, lumbar puncture may be helpful in arriving at a diagnosis after imaging studies have ruled out increased intracranial pressure with risk of herniation. All patients suspected of having intracranial disease should be observed by neurosurgical personnel.

Diagnostic Imaging

Computerized axial tomography (CT) scanning with intravenous contrast is the imaging modality of choice in screening for complications of OM. Although magnetic resonance imaging (MRI) and angiography are useful in the definitive diagnosis of certain of these complications, CT is positive in the vast majority of cases of intracranial extension; in all cases, it gives the most accurate assessment of bone involvement. CT scanning should be considered an indispensable part of the evaluation of all patients suspected of having otogenic complications.

Antimicrobial Therapy

Intravenous antibiotic therapy should be started as soon possible, preferably directed by tympanocentesis or myringotomy in AOM or by culture of otorrhea through the tympanic membrane perforation in CSOM. Empiric therapy in complications of AOM should include coverage of *S. pneumoniae*, *H. influenzae*, *S. pyogenes*, *S. aureus*, and anaerobes at doses appropriate to treat resistant organisms. High-dose ampicillin/sulbactam provides good single-agent coverage in such cases; however, cefotaxime and ceftriaxone should also be considered if meningitis is suspected. Polymicrobial infection is common with CSOM and its complications; broad-spectrum coverage is indicated. Multiple drug therapy may occasionally be necessary to accomplish this goal. Ticarcillin/clavulanic acid is excellent coverage for *Pseudomonas aeruginosa*, *Proteus* sp., anaerobes, and the other organisms most frequently implicated in these infections and achieves reasonable cerebrospinal fluid (CSF) levels in the presence of meningeal inflammation.[65]

Surgical Considerations

In most cases, it is desirable to delay surgical treatment of the infected ear until the patient is neurologically and systemically stable. However, clinical deterioration and progression of infection despite the effective delivery of initial therapy are indications for earlier intervention. In general, the goals of therapy are to prevent further disease progression by evacuating the purulent material and to facilitate the resolution of the precipitating infection through judicious and careful re-establishment of middle ear and mastoid ventilation.

COMPLICATIONS OF OTITIS MEDIA

INTRATEMPORAL COMPLICATIONS

Acute Mastoiditis

Pathophysiology
The middle ear space and mastoid air cell system are freely connected via the "valveless" aditus ad antrum. Once inflammation or infection is present in the middle ear, it rapidly involves the mastoid as well. Both spaces typically develop inflamed mucosa and can accumulate purulent debris. Resolution of the middle ear disease by drainage through the eustachian tube, or through a perforation of the tympanic membrane, normally leads to resolution of the disease in the mastoid. However, when inflamed mucosa or granulation tissue causes obstruction of the aditus or posterior epitympanum, disease may remain "backed up" within the mastoid. Failure of the blockage to resolve on antibiotic therapy and middle ear aeration may result in spread of the inflammatory process through the mucosa to the periosteum, producing physical findings of postauricular pain, erythema, and swelling.

Treated promptly, acute mastoiditis (AM) with periosteitis will usually respond to aggressive antibiotic coverage, and progression to coalescent mastoiditis should not occur. In contrast, pus under pressure in the mastoid air cells more commonly causes necrosis and demineralization of the bony septae resulting in acute coalescent mastoiditis, a disease that must be treated surgically.

Nearly all children who develop AM are under age 10. The disorder has been diagnosed with increasing frequency in infants, owing to the aggressive use of antibiotics in older children or to the difficulty in diagnosing AM in younger children.[66–68] Prior treatment with antibiotics can also result in "masked" or partially treated mastoiditis, further complicating the diagnosis.[69,70] The treatment suppresses the otologic and systemic symptoms of the infection, but may be insufficient to treat isolated osteitis or purulent material in the mastoid.

Most patients who develop AM are previously healthy and have no prior history of OM. Although OM is more common in patients infected with the human immunodeficiency virus (HIV),[71,72] there are no data regarding the incidence of AM in HIV-infected children. Subacute mastoiditis is more common among patients with diabetes.[69,70] The association of AM with other types of immunocompromised patients is not well established, but physicians caring for such individuals should be aware of the risk.

The organisms isolated in AM are, in order of frequency, *Streptococcus pneumoniae*, *Streptococcus pyogenes*, *Staphylococcus aureus*, and *Haemophilus influenzae*.[73] Anaerobes and Gram-negative bacilli account for less than 15% of isolates. Although this distribution does not reflect that of AOM, it may reflect the relative virulence of the pathogens in AOM and their propensity for bony invasion.

Diagnosis
Acute mastoiditis classically presents with postauricular pain, erythema, tenderness, and swelling causing anterior displacement of the pinna; however, any combination of these findings may be present. Signs of AM may be present 1 to 2 weeks prior to the presentation of physical examination

features, and a history of prior OM cannot always be elicited. Otoscopy will typically demonstrate a purulent middle ear effusion with or without perforation of the tympanic membrane. Visualization of the tympanic membrane may be hindered to some extent by edema of the posterior canal wall. In cases of aditus block, the tympanic membrane and middle ear space may look relatively normal. The tissues surrounding the mastoid tip should be examined for the development of subperiosteal fluctuance or Bezold's abscess within the sternocleidomastoid muscle. On occasion, moderate to severe acute otitis externa may mimic some of the signs and symptoms of AM with canal inflammation and drainage and postauricular erythema from posterior inflammatory extension; a tender tragal cartilage is a key distinguishing physical finding not routinely encountered in AM.

The development of coalescent mastoiditis is best assessed by computerized tomography (CT) of the temporal bone. This study, used with contrast, is also useful in determining whether the infection has spread outside the confines of the temporal bone. In coalescent AM, the normal bony trabeculae are lost and the mastoid cortex is thinned. Sclerosis of the bone may be present in cases of long-standing disease. CT may also help to distinguish other causes of swelling in this area, including rhabdomyosarcoma, eosinophilic granuloma, branchial cleft anomalies, or severe otitis externa.

Management

Treatment of acute mastoiditis begins with aggressive antimicrobial therapy as previously discussed. Except in cases of subacute AM or AM with periosteitis, the threshold for myringotomy with tube insertion should be quite low because this will provide material for culture and immediately establish drainage of the infection and ventilation of the middle ear. Results achieved by myringotomy with or without tube insertion are similar to those achieved by mastoidectomy.[74] Cortical mastoidectomy should therefore be reserved for refractory cases of noncoalescent mastoiditis, but may be considered early in the management of coalescent AM, particularly if other complications are present.

Subperiosteal Abscess

Pathophysiology

In the antibiotic era, subperiosteal abscess has become a relatively uncommon sequela of OM. It is usually associated with the development of acute mastoiditis following an episode of AOM. Far less commonly, except in some third-world nations,[75] subperiosteal abscess may complicate CSOM.

In their 1908 text,[76] Bezold and Siebenmann describe the primary extracranial routes of spread of mastoid infection. The most common of these is extension through the lateral surface of the mastoid cortex, resulting in a subperiosteal abscess. Progression of the abscess detaches periosteum superiorly and posteriorly but is limited inferiorly by muscle attachments. When infection breaks through the large, thin-walled cells internal to the digastric groove at the mastoid tip, an abscess may form beneath the sternocleidomastoid muscle, presenting as a tender, fluctuant mass in the neck. This abscess, known as Bezold's abscess, may progress along fascial planes to the larynx, the mediastinum, or the retropharyngeal space.

A third route of spread described by the authors is through the root of the zygoma. This region may occasionally be pneumatized, and involvement of these cells with mastoiditis may cause elevation of the periosteum under the temporalis muscle. The offending organisms in subperiosteal abscess usually reflect those of the preceding mastoiditis. *Streptococcus* sp. and *Staphylococcus* sp. are common in acute infections, whereas *Proteus* and *Pseudomonas* are more common in cases due to chronic otitis media.

Diagnosis

Patients with subperiosteal abscesses most commonly present with a history of acute otitis media that progressed to include postauricular pain and swelling. In infants, by virtue of their having only an aerated antrum, fluctuance will present in a more superior orientation in this region. Less commonly, but associated with a similar history, pain and swelling may occur in the area of the zygomatic arch. A protuberant upper half of the auricle, raised away from the skull by a fluctuant mass, is a defining feature in most cases of subperiosteal abscesses. To establish the diagnosis of subperiosteal abscess in cases in which no fluctuances present, CT scanning with contrast enhancement can be useful in localizing small lesions or a Bezold's abscess in the neck.

Management

Treatment of subperiosteal abscesses is surgical and consists of incision and drainage of the abscess, accompanied by a mastoidectomy. The minimal operation should be a complete simple (cortical) mastoidectomy; however, more extensive procedures should be performed as indicated in order to establish drainage and aeration of the affected air cells. Inspection of the posterior and middle cranial fossae to rule out epidural abscess[64] may be warranted based on the presenting signs and symptoms. Treatment of a Bezold's abscess should include a neck exploration as well. Broad-spectrum antibiotic coverage started preoperatively should be continued after surgery and altered when culture results become available. Several days of intravenous therapy in the hospital should be considered prior to discharge on oral antibiotics. When a diagnosis of osteomyelitis is made, intravenous therapy should be continued for approximately 6 weeks.

Facial Paralysis

Facial Paralysis from Acute Otitis Media

Facial paralysis may occur as a complication of acute otitis media and chronic otitis media. In the acute setting, the nerve is usually affected through a dehiscence of the fallopian canal, which may be present in over 50% of patients.[77] The nerve becomes inflamed and edematous, and a neuropraxia results. A direct neurotoxic effect may also contribute to the disorder, but this has not been experimentally confirmed.[51] Conservative treatment with systemic antibiotics and myringotomy, with or without tube placement, is usually sufficient to eliminate the infection; the prognosis for full return of facial function is excellent although patients with complete paralysis may have a prolonged recovery.[78] Operative decompression of the facial nerve is not indicated unless progressive degeneration of the nerve is suggested by evoked electromyography or electroneuronography.

Facial Paralysis from Chronic Otitis Media

Facial paralysis due to prolonged AOM (longer than 2 weeks) or to COM usually results from erosion of the bony canal by infection or cholesteatoma. The infectious process eventually compresses the nerve, causing invagination of the nodes of Ranvier and segmental demyelination in the compressed region.[51] This process reduces the resistance of the axonal membrane to stretch and may ultimately result in nerve degeneration. Onset of symptoms is slow and progressive, and symptoms may be partial and intermittent. Lacrimal function remains intact unless a concomitant proximal lesion is present. Rarely, facial paralysis may be due to a suppurative labyrinthitis in which a bony sequestrum remains or to chronic osteomyelitis of the petrous pyramid.[50]

The etiology is determined by thorough microscopic examination of the ear. CT scanning should also be performed in order to localize cholesteatoma and assess its size. In long-standing facial paralysis, nerve excitability testing, maximal stimulation testing, and electroneuronography may help determine the prognosis for recovery of the nerve.[79]

Immediate exploration of the middle ear is indicated in all cases of facial paralysis due to chronic otitis media. Mastoidectomy is performed and all diseased bone and cholesteatoma are removed. The facial nerve is exposed by removing cholesteatoma matrix, leaving attached granulation tissue to avoid further injury to the nerve. Healthy bone above and below the disease is "eggshelled" and removed with a Rosen needle to allow the nerve room to swell. Some authors advocate exploration of the fallopian canal from the geniculate ganglion to the stylomastoid foramen.[51] In areas where epineurium is violated, the sheath is opened and dehiscences may be repaired by appropriate grafting procedures. Intraoperative cultures are taken to determine appropriate postoperative antibiotic therapy.

Postoperatively, intravenous antibiotics are administered for approximately 1 week. Broad-spectrum antibiotic coverage is indicated pending culture results. Additional care should include protection and moisturization of the eye. The prognosis for recovery is good if axonal degeneration has not occurred preoperatively.

Petrositis

Pathophysiology

Acute otitis media and chronic suppurative otitis media may affect pneumatized spaces anywhere within the petrous temporal bone. When drainage of these air cells is inadequate, the disease process may affect the surrounding structures causing petrositis, associated with cranial neuropathies, and in some cases, extension into the middle cranial fossa. The pathogenesis of chronic petrositis is similar to that of chronic mastoiditis.

Organisms may gain access to the petrous apex from the middle ear and mastoid through five separate cell tracts.[80] The posteromedial and posterosuperior tracts pass superomedially around the labyrinth and may extend to the anterior cells of the apex. The subarcuate tract, which passes through the arch of the superior semicircular canal, may also reach anteriorly to the apex. The peritubal tract travels a very short distance to the petrous apex in an anteromedial direction around the carotid artery. The cells of this tract are bordered inferiorly by the carotid canal and superiorly by Meckel's cave and are therefore the least accessible. Finally, the perilabyrinthine tract extends from the epitympanum to the posterior cells of the labyrinthine region. The presence of the bony labyrinth impairs drainage from this area and increases the risk of intracranial extension of disease. Furthermore, the presence of air cells immediately adjacent to bone marrow in nonpneumatized areas of the apex increases the risk of osteomyelitis.

Cadaveric dissection has also demonstrated venules coursing through the anterior petrous apex from the cavernous sinus to the inferior petrosal sinus or jugular bulb, suggesting another possible pathway for the spread of infection.[81] Offending bacteria include *Pseudomonas* sp. and *Proteus* sp., but mixed infection is common.

Diagnosis

In 1904, Gradenigo described the triad of abducens nerve palsy, severe pain around the eye in the trigeminal distribution, and persistent otorrhea and recognized its association with infection of the petrous apex.[82] Subsequently, petrositis was identified as a frequent, potentially lethal complication of otitis media requiring aggressive treatment. In fact, radical mastoidectomy with labyrinthectomy was the early procedure of choice for treatment of this disorder.

In the antibiotic era, it has become quite rare for patients with petrositis to present with pure "Gradenigo's syndrome." The two most constant symptoms are deep boring pain and persistent otorrhea following simple mastoidectomy. Occipital, parietal, or temporal pain suggests involvement of the posterior cells, whereas frontal or orbital pain suggests more anterior involvement. Diplopia may be present as a result of sixth nerve palsy due to involvement of the abducens as it passes through Dorello's canal beneath the petroclinoid ligament. Patients may also present with low-grade fever, transient facial paralysis, and mild vertigo.

CT scanning with contrast enhancement is often helpful in confirming the diagnosis. The study may reveal coalescence or bone destruction in the area of the petrous pyramid or, less commonly, an epidural abscess at the apex. Gallium and technetium bone scanning may be useful when CT scanning is inconclusive.

Management

Most cases of acute coalescent petrositis may be treated with aggressive intravenous antibiotic therapy in combination with mastoidectomy. However, petrositis due to CSOM often involves low-grade osteomyelitis of the petrous pyramid and may be resistant to conservative therapy. Exploration of the petrous apex is indicated when, despite mastoidectomy, pain remains intractable or symptoms of diplopia, facial weakness, or vertigo are present. In such cases, broad-spectrum intravenous antibiotics are continued postoperatively, with osteomyelitis of the petrous pyramid requiring 6 weeks of therapy with periodic reassessment bone scanning.

Surgery is directed at removal of existing disease, establishment of adequate ventilation, and preservation of the facial nerve, carotid artery, and labyrinth. The approach to the air cells of the petrous apex is curettage of fistulous tracts extending anteriorly from the mastoid antrum. Bone softened due to osteitis is simply removed and the path of infected cells is followed adjacent to the labyrinthine capsule. There is surgical risk, especially in long-standing infections, of inadvertent entry into a semicircular canal, which will usually result in complete loss of hearing in the affected ear. When osteitic involvement of the labyrinth is severe, a labyrinthectomy may be considered to facilitate access to the apical cells. Osteitis of the fallopian canal may also place the facial nerve at risk.

In cases in which fistulous tracts and osteitic bone are not apparent, an exploration of the pneumatized tracts to the apex may be necessary. Numerous approaches have been described,[83–87] and it is incumbent upon the operating surgeon to be familiar with all of these because pneumatization of air cell tracts is not always predictable by preoperative imaging.

Labyrinthitis

Pathophysiology

Labyrinthine complications of otitis media arise as a result of the spread of infection from the middle ear to the cochlea and vestibule. Commonly, bacteria and inflammatory mediators gain access to the labyrinth through the round window or oval window or through acquired bony defects. In other cases, the perilymphatic space may be violated by advancing cholesteatoma or contaminated by CSF from pre-existing meningitis.

Schuknecht[88] has classified the labyrinthine complications into four types based on the offending noxious agent:

- Acute serous (toxic) labyrinthitis due to bacterial toxins or other mediators of inflammation
- Acute suppurative labyrinthitis due to invasion by bacteria
- Chronic labyrinthitis due to ingrowth of granulation tissue or cholesteatoma into the labyrinth
- Labyrinthine sclerosis due to replacement of normal labyrinthine structures by fibrous tissue and bone

Ludman[62] has observed that the distinction between serous and suppurative labyrinthitis is one made in retrospect after auditory and vestibular function have returned and, therefore, minimizes its clinical significance. Nevertheless, this classification is illustrative of the correlation of pathogenesis with clinical outcome.

Serous labyrinthitis is believed to be the most common complication of otitis media and may be associated with AOM or CSOM. This complication develops as an extension of the inflammatory process from the middle ear via preformed pathways or from the passage of infected CSF through the internal auditory meatus, cochlear aqueduct, or vestibular aqueduct. It is common in cases of labyrinthine fistula, but may occur in the presence of any perilabyrinthine infection. Characteristically, a dilation of the labyrinthine blood vessels is followed by the movement of inflammatory cells across the round window membrane and into the perilymph. A serofibrinous exudate then accumulates in the perilymphatic compartment around the portal of entry and may spread throughout the entire labyrinth. Over time, the exudate resorbs and is, in most cases, replaced by fibrosis in the perilymphatic space.

Acute suppurative labyrinthitis occurs less commonly than acute serous labyrinthitis. The incidence of suppurative labyrinthitis of meningogenic origin is uncertain, but tympanogenic suppurative labyrinthitis in the antibiotic era is estimated at less than 1%.[89] The spread of bacterial infection through the labyrinth is similar to that in serous labyrinthitis, but the destruction of tissue is permanent and more severe. The penetration of the basilar membrane by bacteria and inflammatory cells places the organ of Corti at significant risk. In contrast, the resistance of Reissner's membrane to cellular penetration creates an osmotic pressure differential between endolymph and perilymph resulting in endolymphatic hydrops. Spread of infection to the meninges from the labyrinth is unusual, but quite morbid when it occurs.

Chronic labyrinthitis most often occurs in association with osteitic or cholesteatomatous fistulas through which soft tissue has grown into the labyrinth. The incidence of chronic labyrinthitis is unknown, but cholesteatomatous fistulas are thought to occur in 10% of cases of chronic mastoiditis;[88,90] 75% of cases involve the horizontal semicircular canal.[51] These fistulas are often clinically silent and are discovered unexpectedly at operation. In most cases, they remain covered by cholesteatoma matrix, which prevents inflammatory and suppurative processes from affecting the labyrinth. Loss of this protection due to progression of the fistula permits bacterial invasion and ingrowth of granulation tissue, ultimately with loss of labyrinthine function. The replacement of labyrinthine structures by fibrous or osseous tissue constitutes labyrinthine sclerosis.

Diagnosis

In general, symptoms of suppurative labyrinthitis occur more suddenly and are more severe than those of serous labyrinthitis, and recovery is far less common. Symptoms of chronic labyrinthitis are usually slowly progressive. Vestibular and cochlear symptoms in labyrinthitis often occur together, but vestibular symptoms may appear first in cases of cholesteatomatous fistula involving a semicircular canal. Spontaneous nystagmus begins as an irritative-jerk nystagmus beating toward the infected ear, but becomes a paralytic-jerk nystagmus beating toward the opposite ear. Vertigo, ataxia, and past pointing accompany the ocular symptoms. Hearing loss is usually of the high-frequency, sensorineural type. Onset is usually sudden and severe in suppurative labyrinthitis, but may be progressive or fluctuating in serous or chronic labyrinthitis. Diplacusis and distortion of sound may also present.

Patients in whom labyrinthitis is suspected should undergo neurologic evaluation to rule out meningeal involvement prior to otologic testing. Caloric testing, if possible, will usually demonstrate some residual function in serous labyrinthitis, but loss of function is common in more advanced stages of the disease. Detection and localization of labyrinthine fistulas have been discussed in detail by McCabe.[91] Positive and negative pressures are applied to the ear canal through a pneumatic otoscope; a positive fistula test causes transient vertigo. Conjugate deviation of the eyes and nystagmus toward the opposite ear are seen when positive pressure is introduced. High-resolution CT scanning may be useful in preoperative detection of labyrinthine erosion by cholesteatoma.

Management

Treatment of labyrinthitis due to otitis media begins with culture of the purulent material and establishment of drainage. In acute infections, myringotomy and insertion of a tympanostomy tube are useful for these purposes. In chronic suppurative otitis media, mastoidectomy is indicated, although some authors advocate delaying surgery until acute symptoms have subsided in order to avoid the risk of spreading infection.[62] Appropriate antibiotic therapy is administered, and the patient is placed on strict bed rest with minimal head movement. Antiemetics are given to control vomiting, and intravenous hydration is ordered to replace losses due to emesis. If hearing loss becomes total and vertigo is intractable, meningitis is considered imminent. Lumbar puncture should be performed and antibiotic therapy modified to achieve adequate CSF levels.

Conservative management of labyrinthine fistulas is critical to the preservation of auditory and vestibular function. Fistulas involving the vestibule and cochlea place the inner ear at high risk, and it has been suggested that the disease within these lesions be left undisturbed and exteriorized.[51] Similarly, attempts to clear large or deep fistulas carry significant risk.[92] On the other hand, most surgeons believe that it is safe to leave cholesteatoma matrix over the fistula in an open cavity procedure as long as there is no infected granulation tissue deep to it. Growth of new bone will close the defect over time. In cases in which the nature of the underlying tissue is uncertain, McCabe has advocated biopsy and frozen section examination.[91] In these cases, cholesteatoma is removed with careful preservation of the endosteum. If cholesteatoma matrix is left in an intact canal wall procedure, re-exploration in 6 to 12 months is indicated to remove the remaining epithelial pearl.[93]

In the antibiotic era, indications for opening the labyrinth for drainage are exceedingly few. Labyrinthectomy should be considered only when the disease process has caused a total loss of function or when meningitis develops despite aggressive antibiotic therapy.

INTRACRANIAL COMPLICATIONS

Extradural Abscess

Pathophysiology

Cholesteatoma and granulation tissue frequently complicate chronic suppurative otitis media and have a propensity to erode adjacent bony structures. When these processes reach the periphery of the mastoid space, erosion often proceeds until dura is exposed, but is then impeded by this relatively resistant structure. The result is an inflammation of the dura known as pachymeningitis, which is often followed by the production of granulations along the dura. The accumulation of purulent material results in a collection of pus between dura and the bony wall known as an extradural or epidural abscess.[94]

Commonly, resorption of bone will occur in the region of the tegmen, resulting in an extradural abscess of the middle cranial fossa. The infectious process in such cases begins lateral to the attachment of the dura at the arcuate eminence, which serves to limit the extent of the abscess. An abscess developing medial to the eminence may abut the petrous apex, involving the fifth and sixth cranial nerves and resulting in facial pain and diplopia (Gradenigo's syndrome). In the middle fossa, lateral to the arcuate eminence, the dura is loosely attached and large abscesses may develop accompanied by neurologic signs of mass effect. Lateral erosion through the cranium produces the subperiosteal abscess known as Pott's puffy tumor. Posterior fossa extradural abscesses usually result from the erosion of bone in Trautmann's triangle or over the lateral sinus. The latter, known as a perisinus abscess, is frequently associated with the development of lateral sinus thrombosis. Untreated posterior fossa abscesses may also extend to the neck via the jugular foramen.

Diagnosis

Symptoms of extradural abscess may include temporal headache, ear pain, or low-grade fever; however, often physician and patient become aware of its presence only after exposure during elective mastoidectomy. Extradural abscesses of long standing are an exception to this rule and are often accompanied by mild nuchal rigidity and signs of meningismus (Kernig's and Brudzinski's signs). Characteristically, symptoms that are present are suddenly relieved during periods of spontaneous drainage into the mastoid. Exacerbation of the aural discharge on compression of the ipsilateral jugular vein is also highly suggestive. Lumbar puncture may reveal an increased white cell count, but usually with lymphocyte predominance. Glucose levels are normal and no organisms are seen. When extradural abscess is suspected prior to surgery, CT scanning is preferred for confirmation of the diagnosis.

Management

Surgical intervention is indicated whenever examination or CT scan is suggestive of extradural abscess; antimicrobial therapy will not effectively penetrate the walls of the abscess. Mastoidectomy is performed and the tegmen and sinus plates are removed. Loose granulation tissue is removed and a border of normal dura is exposed peripherally around the affected site. Manipulation of adherent granulations is to be avoided so that the dura is not inadvertently violated and the subdural space remains protected. Cholesteatoma matrix covering a dural exposure may be left behind if well exteriorized. Removal of cholesteatoma is otherwise completed, and a Penrose drain is placed into the cavity at the end of the procedure. Postoperative antibiotics, systemic and topical, are useful in preventing the spread of residual organisms through the remaining granulations and should be determined based on the results of intraoperative cultures. A 6-week course of antibiotic therapy is generally recommended in cases in which a diagnosis of osteomyelitis is made.

Lateral Sinus Thrombosis

Pathophysiology

Extension of the inflammatory process in the mastoid cavity to the adjacent venous sinuses may occur directly from progression of the erosive process through the dura or by spread along mastoid or middle emissary veins. The transverse sinus, which begins at the internal occipital protuberance, exits the tentorium as the sigmoid sinus. Before leaving the cranium as the internal jugular vein, the sigmoid is joined by the superior and inferior sinuses. The segment of the transverse-sigmoid complex immediately beneath the mastoid air cells is known as the lateral sinus and is the region most susceptible to thrombosis or thrombophlebitis due to mastoid disease. However, otogenic involvement of other dural sinuses has been reported.[95]

Thrombosis of the dural sinuses usually begins as a result of damage to the tunica intima by an adjacent inflammatory process, most commonly an extradural perisinus abscess. Fibrin formation and platelet aggregation are initiated by the damage to the vessel wall and may be enhanced by the thrombogenic capacity of the neighboring bacteria, creating a mural thrombus.[96] Classically, the thrombus becomes infected by penetration of the abscess through the dura and wall of the vessel. However, it has also been suggested that seeding occurs primarily due to thrombophlebitic spread from the pneumatized spaces and that dural inflammation and fibrosis due to perisinus abscess actually serve to improve resistance to direct spread of infection.[64] Thrombus may then propagate along vessel walls causing local invasion, or it may produce bacteremia, septicemia, or septic embolization. Involvement of the cerebrum, meninges, and cerebellum has been reported in 45% of patients with lateral sinus thrombosis.[97]

Recent publications indicate an evolving microbiology in this disorder. Once dominated by the beta-hemolytic streptococcus and pneumococcus, cultures now reflect the flora of chronic otitis media, revealing multiple pathogens including Proteus, *Staphylococcus aureus*, Bacteroides, and *Escherichia coli* as well as aerobic and anaerobic streptococci.[62,95,98] Such results support a higher incidence of dural sinus thrombosis in chronic ear disease,[62,95,98,99] although in one recent series acute ear disease was the more common etiology.[57]

Diagnosis

The use of aggressive antibiotic therapy has altered the once dramatic presentation of this disease to one of a less acute nature. The classical high-spiking "picket fence" fever and rigor are seen rarely. Cervical or orbital extension of the clot often resulted in paralysis of cranial nerves or proptosis of the eye, which are now unusual findings. Commonly, patients present after about 2 weeks of symptoms with headache, which is usually lateral in location.[62,95] The headache is frequently preceded by ear pain and/or discharge on the ipsilateral side and may be accompanied by nausea and vomiting. Visual changes, nuchal rigidity, and dysequilibrium are rare complaints.

Physical examination will almost universally reveal purulent drainage from a perforated tympanic membrane. Pitting edema and tenderness over the postauricular area due to involvement of the mastoid emissary vein (Griesinger's sign) may be noted. Fever remains a prominent feature in the vast majority of patients, and papilledema due to increased intracranial pressure is present in over 50%.[62,95] Less commonly, the clinician may note palsy of the abducens nerve, believed to result from compression of the nerve by a distended inferior petrosal sinus within the closed space of Dorello's canal (Gradenigo's syndrome).[95] Nuchal rigidity and nystagmus are less common findings.

Routine blood work will usually reveal an elevated white cell count with a shift to the left, as well as an elevated erythrocyte sedimentation rate. Blood cultures, except in the presence of extreme fever due to bacteremia, are usually negative. Lumbar puncture should be performed unless uncal herniation is likely to result from the procedure. Commonly, an elevated CSF pressure is noted, due probably to impaired reabsorption through the arachnoid granulations. CSF chemistry and cell counts are usually unremarkable. A positive Queckenstedt's or Tobey–Ayer test, once considered pathognomonic of the disorder, has been found to be unreliable and to elevate intracranial pressure to dangerous levels.[62] The test is considered positive when compression of the internal jugular vein on the side of the thrombosis fails to raise CSF pressure, but compression of the contralateral vein results in a rapid and marked increase in pressure.

Definitive diagnosis of dural venous thrombosis is now based primarily on imaging studies. Although the gold standard study has been cerebral angiography,[100] magnetic resonance imaging (MRI) with magnetic resonance angiography (MRA) has emerged as a highly accurate and less invasive modality.[100–102] The thrombosis is determined by the absence of flow-induced signal loss.[100] CT scanning is also highly sensitive and is an excellent adjunctive study in screening for concomitant otogenic complications.[103]

Management

Modern day treatment of lateral sinus thrombosis is based on control of infection by minimal surgical debridement and intensive antibiotic therapy. When thrombosis of the sinus is suggested by physical examination and initial laboratory studies, intravenous antibiotics should be started to minimize hematogenous spread. It has been suggested that coverage should include some combination of two or more of the following: ampicillin, chloramphenicol, a cephalosporin, and an aminoglycoside.[99] Surgical intervention is directed by imaging studies. Mastoidectomy is performed with wide exposure of the sigmoid sinus. Bone is removed until normal dura is exposed peripherally around the region of suspected thrombosis. Dural granulations are carefully removed and the sinus wall is inspected.

A normal-appearing, compressible sinus wall requires no further surgical treatment. On the other hand, if the sinus wall is inflamed or immobile on palpation, evaluation of the sinus lumen is indicated. A small-gauge needle may be used to aspirate the sinus; if bleeding is encountered, no further surgical treatment is necessary. Failure to obtain blood on aspiration suggests thrombosis, and aspiration of pus indicates infection of the thrombus. The discovery of pus upon aspiration requires the accepted treatment for all abscesses, which is to drain the collection. Under these circumstances, evacuation of the infected clot should be performed. Control is gained distally proximally within the mastoid cavity by extraluminal compression using absorbable sponges between the sinus wall and the overlying bone. An incision is then made in the lateral sinus wall in the direction of the vessel. If blood is obtained, the incision may be simply covered with absorbable sponge or temporalis muscle. If infected thrombus is noted, it is removed until only healthy clot remains.

The patient is maintained on intravenous antibiotics. Ligation of the internal jugular vein, once popular in the management of lateral sinus thrombosis, is now reserved only for cases that are unresponsive to initial surgical and antibiotic therapy, and in those in which septic emboli are developing.[58,104] Anticoagulation is still used by many clinicians to prevent extension of the thrombus and to reduce the risk of thrombosis of the cavernous sinus.[105] Use of anticoagulant therapy, however, incurs the risks of septic embolization and hemorrhage due to breakdown.[58] More controversial is the dry tap of the sinus, which may be managed conservatively by aggressive antibiotic therapy or by opening the sinus and evacuating the clot.

Brain Abscess

Pathophysiology

For many years, brain abscess was most frequently associated with otitic infection, and its management lay primarily with the otologist. However, the development of antibiotics during the early part of the 20th century, combined with improved neurosurgical management of early intracranial complications, has seen a dramatic decline in the incidence of otogenic brain abscess. Recent data suggest an association with otitis media in 15 to 25% of all brain abscesses.[106,107]

Despite the effect of antibiotic therapy on the incidence of otogenic brain abscess, the disorder remains the deadliest complication of otitis media. Death rates reported in the literature of the last 30 years range from 4 to 47%,[58,106,107] although otogenic brain abscess seems to have a better prognosis than brain abscess from other sources.[107] It is therefore essential that the otologist consider the possibility of brain abscess when treating any otogenic complication.

Retrograde venous thrombophlebitis, often in association with extradural abscess, is the mechanism most commonly implicated in the development of a brain abscess. Temporal lobe abscesses, which usually result from spread through the tegmen tympani,[94] occur twice as frequently as cerebellar abscesses, which are more commonly associated with suppurative labyrinthitis and/or lateral sinus thrombosis.[64] Local pachymeningitis induces thrombophlebitic or periarteriolar spread to the cortex of the temporal lobe or the cerebellum. Edema and encephalitis subsequently develop within the white matter, causing softening of this layer. A collagen capsule, formed by response of fibroblasts to the inflammation, serves to localize the process over a period of approximately 2 weeks, while liquefaction and infection of entrapped brain tissue progresses. In rare cases, a well-encapsulated abscess will enter a latent period, only to be reactivated months or even years later.

Expansion of the abscess generally proceeds in the direction of the ventricle and produces an increase in intracranial pressure, as well as localizing symptoms and signs. Cerebellar abscesses occur within the restricted space of the posterior fossa adjacent to the brain stem and, therefore, generally produce earlier symptoms and more lethal sequelae than their temporal counterparts. Respiratory arrest may result from herniation of the cerebellar tonsils through the foramen magnum. Left untreated, temporal abscess will ultimately rupture into the ventricular or subarachnoid spaces, resulting in fatal meningitis. Occasionally, rupture onto the surface of the brain may result in the formation of a fistulous tract between the abscess cavity and the ear.

Numerous pathogens have been implicated in the formation of otogenic brain abscesses, but the flora of such an abscess does not necessarily reflect that of the otitic infection from which it arose. Multiple organisms are isolated in one third to one half of cases.[64,108] Recent data suggest that anaerobic Gram-positive cocci, such as *Peptococcus, Peptostreptococcus,* and unspecified anaerobic streptococci, are most commonly involved.[106,109] However, aerobic Gram-positive cocci and Gram-negative bacilli may also be isolated, with *Streptococcus, Staphylococcus,* and *Proteus* most common among the organisms in this group.

Diagnosis

Signs and symptoms of brain abscess progress through four stages.[51] The first stage corresponds to the initial encephalitis that results from the invasion of brain tissue. The symptoms of this stage are largely constitutional and mild, consisting of general malaise, headache, fever, chills, nausea, and vomiting. During the second or "latent" stage, the abscess localizes and the symptoms abate or disappear. The third stage is characterized by signs and symptoms of increased intracranial pressure and irritation and compression of specific locations in the brain secondary to abscess enlargement. As a rule, the general features of mass effect are more constant and present earlier than those of a more focal nature. Severe headache is present in 70 to 90% of patients and nausea and vomiting, often projectile in this stage, occur in 25 to 50% of cases.[110] Seizures, menigismus, and papilledema are each seen in 20 to 50% of patients.[110,111] Fever is usually low grade to subnormal.[112] Visual changes may result from ocular paralysis. Pressure on the vagus center may cause a slowing of the pulse, and arrhythmic breathing may result from compression of the respiratory center.

Temporal lobe lesions may be associated with visual field defects, usually quadrantic homonymous hemianopias. Other symptoms associated primarily with temporal lobe abscess include hemiparesis and nominal aphasia. Motor exam will confirm weakness of the contralateral side.

Patients with cerebellar abscess may present with intention tremor or ataxia, with a tendency to fall toward the affected side. Patients with abscess will demonstrate ipsilateral dysmetria and dysdiadochokinesia and spontaneous nystagmus, which increases on gaze to the side of the lesion. Later symptoms may include drowsiness and stupor. The final stage is that in which the abscess ruptures into the ventricle or the subarachnoid space. This event usually results in a rapid clinical decline and, ultimately, death.

Routine laboratory testing adds little to the diagnosis of brain abscess. The white cell count may be elevated, but is normal or mildly elevated in 40% of cases.[111] The results of lumbar puncture are usually abnormal but nonspecific, and transtentorial herniation has been reported in up to one third of cases in which the procedure was performed.[110]

CT and MRI scanning are the standard of care in the diagnosis of brain abscess. On contrast-enhanced scans, the pyogenic material appears as an area of decreased density and is surrounded by a high-density ring representing the smooth, thin collagenous wall. In turn, the abscess is encircled by an area of low density representing edema in the surrounding brain tissue. The findings of gas within the lesion and ventricular or meningeal enhancement are also common.

MRI is equally diagnostic and offers some advantages over CT. First, better contrast between the area of peripheral edema and the surrounding brain is noted on MRI and may suggest the diagnosis of brain abscess at a very early stage. In addition, MRI gives more accurate assessment of extraparenchymal spread as demonstrated by intraventricular hyperdensity and periventricular enhancement.[113] However, because bone destruction due to concomitant complications is quite common in the presence of brain abscess, CT scanning should be considered in most cases.

Management

Initial management of a brain abscess is dictated by the clinical condition of the patient. Although they may inhibit host defenses against the spreading infection, corticosteroids may effectively lower the intracranial pressure in cases of coma or rapid deterioration. Mannitol may also be useful for this purpose. Antibiotic therapy should be started as soon as the diagnosis of brain abscess is made. Most authors favor the initial use of cefotaxime and/or high-dose nafcillin or penicillin, at least until culture results are available. When chronic otitis media is the suspected etiology, an anti-pseudomonal penicillin or an aminoglycoside should be added, along with metronidazole for anaerobic coverage.

Numerous reports advocating medical management of brain abscess have been summarized by Haines et al.,[110] who found medical therapy to be successful in 37 of 50 cases (74%) with a mortality of only 4%. However, these authors and others[111] conclude that medical therapy should be reserved for cases of multiple brain abscesses, after a causative organism has been identified by aspiration, and for control of cerebritis present in the early stages of the disease or following spillage of abscess contents during drainage. In general, surgery remains the therapy of choice in order to confirm the diagnosis, identify the causative organism, and decompress the mass lesion. In addition, operative intervention will usually reduce the course of adjunctive antibiotics and shorten the hospital stay.

The primary surgical modalities in the treatment of brain abscess are aspiration with or without irrigation and excision. Excision is generally reserved for encapsulated lesions and should not be performed on those in the cerebritis stage. In general, residual neurological deficits appear to be more profound with excision than with aspiration because surrounding white matter is often removed with the lesion. However, recurrence appears to be lower for excised lesions than for aspirated ones.[110,111] In addition, mortality rates have been shown to be similar for aspiration, aspiration followed by excision, and primary excision.[110] Excision may therefore be considered the procedure of choice for superficial and solitary abscesses. Aspiration may be more feasible for lesions located in deep or critical areas of the brain, for patients who are too ill for general anesthesia, and for cases involving multiple abscesses.

Antibiotic therapy is continued for several weeks, and the patient is followed closely through serial imaging studies. Recurrences require reoperation and have been known to occur even years after the initial procedure. Management of the offending ear involves wide-field, complete mastoidectomy with drainage as soon as the patient's neurological condition permits.

Otitic Meningitis

Pathophysiology

Otitic meningitis is a generalized bacterial infection of the pia and arachnoid, with organisms identifiable in the CSF. In adults, meningitis is more likely to result from chronic infection of the middle ear than from AOM. In contrast, AOM is a more frequent cause of meningitis in the pediatric age group.[57]

Generalized meningitis in chronic otitis media most commonly begins as a localized meningitis or pachymeningitis in association with an extradural abscess or some other infectious otogenic focus. Bacteria gain access to the CSF and meninges primarily by direct extension through the dura and arachnoid. In suppurative labyrinthitis, infection may spread through the internal acoustic meatus and the aqueducts of the cochlea and vestibule. The CSF is an excellent culture medium with low concentrations of immunoglobulins, and bacteria multiply relatively freely consuming CSF glucose. Phagocytic cells are impaired by the low opsonic activity of the CSF, and some organisms possess a polysaccharide capsule, which further hinders the activity of these cells.

As a result of the infection, vessel permeability increases and allows an influx of proteins and leukocytes. Transport of fluid out of the CSF is impaired, causing a rise in intracranial pressure. Lactic acid accumulation causes a fall in pH and glucose metabolism is impaired. Accumulation of pyogenic exudate in the basal cisterns occludes the ventricular foramina, causing noncommunicating hydrocephalus, and obstructs the flow of subarachnoid CSF, causing communicating hydrocephalus.

Diagnosis

Patients typically present with high fever, severe generalized headache, photophobia, confusion, and stiff neck. Nausea, vomiting, and anorexia are also common. Back pain and myalgia may be severe, with the patient exhibiting a preference for the fetal position. On examination, temperatures over 39°C are the rule, often accompanied by a rapid pulse. A depressed level of consciousness may be noted. The patient is unable to extend the leg with the thigh flexed (Kernig's sign) and may exhibit flexion of the hip and knee when the head is bent (Brudzinski's sign). Cranial nerves are affected in 10% of patients.[114] Palsies of the abducens nerve generally resolve with treatment. In contrast, involvement of the eighth nerve may cause partial or complete heating loss, which is usually irreversible.[115] Papilledema is rare except when mass lesions are present simultaneously. Complications include cerebral edema, seizures, subdural effusion, and shock. Delirium may ensue in the late stages, followed by Cheyne–Stokes breathing, coma, and death.

The diagnosis may be made on examination of CSF alone. However, the examining physician must be alert for signs of other complications and should consider some form of brain imaging if other diagnoses are entertained. Opening CSF pressure will be high, and analysis will reveal an elevated white cell count with a predominance of leukocytes, as well as an elevated protein concentration. A depressed glucose concentration confirms the diagnosis because no other complication has this effect on the CSF. The offending organism is culturable in 85% of cases, as long as antibiotic therapy has not been started prior to lumbar puncture.

Management

The management of otitic meningitis consists primarily of high-dose antibiotics capable of CSF penetration. When CSOM is the cause, coverage for Gram-negative organisms is essential. Current recommendations for first-line agents are ceftriaxone or cefotaxime in combination with vancomycin, ampicillin, or penicillin G. These regimens provide excellent coverage for Gram-negative organisms, including *Haemophilus influenzae* and enterobacteria, as well as Gram-positive bacteria such as pneumococcus. When *Pseudomonas* meningitis is suspected due to CSOM, ceftazidime and antipseudomonal penicillins are also appropriate choices for systemic therapy. Intrathecal administration of gentamicin may be considered for resistant cases, but has been noted to induce seizures. Maintenance therapy is adjusted in accordance with CSF cultures. Duration of treatment is 7 to 21 days, with the longer antibiotic courses directed at negative and anaerobic infections.[65] Patients require repeated lumbar puncture to monitor their response to therapy. CSF cultures should be negative after 2 to 3 days of therapy, but cell counts and chemistries may be abnormal for several days longer.

Adjunctive therapy is helpful in reducing the morbidity of meningitis. When intracranial pressure is elevated, lumbar puncture may permit decompression and prevent neurologic sequelae. Dexamethasone, which may also be effective for this purpose, has been shown to deter sensorineural hearing loss and death in children with meningitis.[116] Debridement of the ear is useful in treating the focus of the infection, and mastoidectomy is indicated when the patient is neurologically stable. Patients may be monitored for sensorineural hearing loss by otoacoustic emissions during the recovery period.[117]

Subdural Infection

Pathophysiology

Otogenic infection of the subdural space is rare, and usually occurs in infants as a result of thrombophlebitic spread in meningitis. Less commonly, CSOM may also cause an accumulation of infected fluid behind the dura and arachnoid as a result of thrombophlebitic spread through intact dura or direct extension through the dura by erosion. This fluid collection, termed a dural effusion, may progress to frank purulence if left untreated. A subdural empyema results when pus collects over a large surface area. Subdural abscess is the entrapment of pus by granulation tissue and fibrous tissue in response to the spreading infection. The local morbidity of subdural infections is associated with their propensity to cause cortical compression. However, they are also known to generate multiple small cerebral abscesses by thrombophlebitic spread and to interfere with the normal flow of CSF. As a result, the mortality rate of these infections remains 27 to 35%.[118]

Classically, infection of the subdural space reflects the flora of infection of the upper respiratory tract. Streptococcal infection has been the rule, and anaerobes are isolated in approximately 50% of these cases.[64] However, of the group of eight cases of subdural infection reported by Gower and McGuirt, all were nonsterile effusions with cultures positive for *H. influenzae* and *S. aureus*.[57] Gram-negative rods may also be isolated.

Diagnosis

Clinically, subdural infection is manifested as nonspecific central neurologic symptoms. Severe headache and drowsiness are the rule, occasionally leading to frank stupor or coma. Meningeal signs are usually present and may be accompanied by focal cortical signs such as hemiplegia and aphasia. Hemianopia and deviation of the eyes to the affected side may occur; focal seizures have been observed in some 60% of these cases.[118] As a rule, neurologic findings are more focal than would be found in meningitis and more rapid in onset than would be found in the presence of a brain abscess.

Routine laboratory studies will reveal an elevated white cell count and sedimentation rate. Lumbar puncture may be dangerous and rarely aids in the diagnosis. When performed, an increased CSF pressure is demonstrated, a mild pleocytosis is present, protein concentration is elevated, and glucose level is normal. Definitive diagnosis is made by CT or MRI scan with contrast enhancement, although occasionally these abscesses are quite small and barely detectable by imaging.[111]

Management

Subdural infection is managed in conjunction with a neurosurgeon. Surgical therapy consists of bur holes for diagnosis, drainage, and irrigation as necessary. Prodigious doses of the intravenous antibiotics previously mentioned are initially directed against the otitic focus and altered in accordance with culture results. When the patient is stable, mastoidectomy should be performed in order to treat the otologic source of the infection.

Otitic Hydrocephalus

Pathophysiology

The development of increased intracranial pressure in the absence of brain abscess has been observed in a subset of patients with acute or chronic otitis media. Termed otitic hydrocephalus by Symonds in 1931,[119] the disorder is actually identical to the entity known as pseudotumor cerebri, originally described by Quincke in 1893.[120] As a result, most authors presently consider the term "otitic hydrocephalus" to be synonymous with pseudotumor cerebri resulting from otitis media, with these cases accounting for some 25% of all cases of pseudotumor.[121] The pathophysiology of otitic hydrocephalus remains unclear, but increased production or decreased resorption of CSF is thought to be responsible.[64] Impaired function of the arachnoid villi due to thrombosis of the dural venous sinuses or localized meningitis has been suggested as a cause.[122] The condition typically arises in children and adolescents whose ears have been infected for several weeks.

Diagnosis

Patients usually present with protracted headache occasionally associated with diplopia and vomiting. The most reliable clinical findings are bilateral papilledema and paralysis of the sixth nerve on the affected side. Focal neurologic signs are absent. Lumbar puncture reveals increased opening pressure, usually greater than 300 mm of water, with no cells and normal concentrations of protein and glucose. Imaging studies are helpful to rule out the presence of mass lesion; in particular, MRI may be useful in detecting associated thrombosis of the dural venous sinuses.[123,124]

Management

Treatment of otitic hydrocephalus is directed at management of the elevated CSF pressure so as to prevent optic atrophy from persistent papilledema. Serial lumbar punctures or placement of a lumbar drain will effectively diminish CSF pressures over the several weeks usually required for the condition to run its course. In prolonged cases, ventricular or subtemporal decompression may be indicated. Diuretics, steroids, and hyperosmolar dehydrating agents have also been suggested as an adjunct to therapy.[62] Mastoidectomy should be performed in order to manage the chronically draining ear.

CONCLUSIONS

Otitis media is a common and significant disease of childhood. Although it has been and continues to be a well studied infectious process, consensus is limited concerning the comprehensive management of otitis media in children across the spectrum of medical specialties. Otitis media will remain unsettled in the mainstream consciousness of our popular culture for many physiologic, pharmacologic, environmental, social, economic, and emotional reasons. Nonetheless, despite what must be considered the best efforts of dedicated professionals and their well-intentioned efforts to improve upon understanding and successful management of otitis media in children, a significant number and range of complications still occur.

In mild forms, complications of otitis media may compromise quality of life. If left untreated, there may be rapid clinical advancement with the development of intratemporal or intracranial complications that may result in profoundly life-affecting changes or potentially life-threatening sequelae. Vigilance, diagnostic acumen, and prompt intervention are essential to minimize the clinical impact from potential complications of otitis media. Even with the best care, medical or surgical complications may arise from application of reasonable treatment algorithms such as antibiotics or ventilation tubes. Developmental delays from the impact of prolonged middle ear disease can arise and should be considered a valid concern; the long-term cost to society may be substantial — although not necessarily appreciated in the short-term economic and emotional equations of society's thought process. Unfortunately, in today's culture and climate of equal parts skepticism and experimentation, a substantial incidence of complications may arise from the extreme avoidance or overzealous application of new or old therapies for otitis media in children.

REFERENCES

1. Vital and Health Statistics: Ambulatory and inpatient procedures in the U.S., Hyattsville, MD: National Center for Health Statistics, 1996.
2. Rosenfeld, R.M. and Bluestone C.D., Eds. *Evidence Based Otitis Media*. Hamilton, Ontario: B.C. Decker, Inc., 1999.
3. Isaacson, G.I. and Rosenfeld, R.M. Care of the child with tympanostomy tubes. *Pediatr. Clin. North Am.*, 1996, 43, 1183–1193.
4. Wald, E.R., Dashefsky, B., Byers, C. et al. Frequency and severity of infections in day care. *J. Pediatr.*, 1988, 112, 540–546.
5. Etzel, R.A., Pattishall, E.N., Haley, N.J. et al. Passive smoking and middle ear effusion among children in daycare. *Pediatrics*, 1992, 90, 228–232.
6. Teele, D.W., Klein, J.O., and Rosner, B. Epidemiology of otitis media during the first 7 years of life in children in Greater Boston: a prospective, cohort study. *J. Infect. Dis.*, 1989, 160, 83–94.
7. Paradise, J.L., Rockette, H.E., Colborn, D.K. et al. Otitis media in 2253 Pittsburgh area infants: prevalence and risk factors during the first two years of life. *Pediatrics*, 1997, 99, 318–332.
8. Uhari, M., Mantysaari, K., and Niemela, M. A meta-analytic review of the risk factors for acute otitis media. *Clin. Infect. Dis.*, 1996, 22, 1079–1083.
9. Dowell, S.F., Butler, J.C., Giebink, G.S. et al. Acute otitis media: management and surveillance in an era of pneumococcal resistance — a report from the drug-resistant *Streptococcus pneumoniae* therapeutic working group. *Pediatr. Infect. Dis. J.*, 2001, 20(1), 1–5.
10. Chan L.S., Takata, G.S., Shekelle, P. et al. Evidence assessment of management of acute otitis media: 1. The role of antibiotics in treatment of uncomplicated acute otitis media. *Pediatrics*, 2001, 108, 239–247.
11. Bluestone, C.D., Stephenson, J.S., and Martin, L.M. Ten year review of otitis media pathogens. *Pediatr. Infect. Dis. J.*, 1992, 11, S7–S11.
12. Sutton, D.V., Derkay, C.S., Darrow, D.H. et al. Resistant bacteria in middle ear fluid at time of tympanostomy tube surgery. *Ann. Otol. Rhinol. Laryngol.*, 2000, 109, 24–29.
13. Poole, M.D. Declining antibiotic effectiveness in otitis media: a convergence of data. *Ear Nose Throat J.*, 1998, 77, 444–447.
14. Zapalac, J.S., Billings, K., and Roland, P.S. Suppurative complications of acute otitis media in the era of antibiotic resistance. Abstract presented at the 16th annual meeting of the American Society of Pediatric Otolaryngology, May 11, 2000, Scottsdale, AZ.
15. Dowell, S.F., Butler, J.C., Giebink, G.S. et al. Acute otitis media: management and surveillance in an era of pneumococcal resistance — a report from the drug-resistant *Streptococcus pneumoniae* therapeutic working group. *Pediatr. Infect. Dis. J.*, 1999, 18, 1–9.
16. Paradise, J.L. Managing otitis media: a time for change. *Pediatrics*, 1995, 96, 712–715.
17. Pelton, S.I. Otoscopy for the diagnosis of otitis media. *Pediatr. Infect. Dis. J.*, 1998, 17, 540–543.
18. Rosenfeld, R.M. Implications of the AHRQ evidence report on acute otitis media. *Otolaryngol. Head Neck Surg.*, 2001, 125, 440–448.
19. Block, S.L., Hedrick, J.A., Tyler, R.D., Smith, R.A., and Harrison, C.J. Microbiology of acute otitis media recently treated with aminopenicillins. *Pediatr. Infect. Dis. J.*, 2001, 20, 1017–1021.
20. Paradise, J.L. Short-course antimicrobial treatment of AOM: not best for young children. *JAMA*, 1997, 278, 1640–1642.
21. Block, S.L, Harrison, C.J., Hedrick, J., Tyler, R., Smith, A., and Hedrick, R. Restricted use of antibiotic prophylaxis for recurrent acute otitis media in the era of penicillin nonsusceptible *Streptococcus pneumoniae*. *Int. J. Pediatr. Otorhinolaryngol.*, 2001, 61(1), 47–60.
22. Flynn, C.A. et al. Decongestants and antihistamines for acute otitis media in children. *Cochrane Libr.*, 2002, 3, 1–25.
23. Jacobs, J. et al. Homeopathic treatment of acute otitis media in children: a preliminary randomized placebo-controlled trial. *Pediatr. Infect. Dis. J.*, 2001, 20, 177–183.

24. Rosenfeld, R.M. and Post, J.C. Meta-analysis of antibiotics for the treatment of otitis media with effusion. *Otolaryngol. Head Neck Surg.*, 1992, 106(4), 378–386.
25. Chan, K.H. and Bluestone, C.D. Lack of efficacy of middle ear inflation: treatment of otitis media with effusion in children. *Otolaryngol. Head Neck Surg.*, 1989, 100, 317–323.
26. Froehle, R.M. Ear infection: a retrospective study examining improvement from chiropractic care and analyzing for influencing factors. *J. Manipulative Physiol. Ther.*, 1996, Mar–Apr, 19(3), 169–177.
27. Eskola, J., Klipi, T., Palmu, A. et al. Efficacy of a pneumococcal conjugate vaccine against acute otitis media. *New Engl. J. Med.*, 2001, 344, 403–409.
28. Black, S., Shinefield, H., Fireman, B. et al. Efficacy, safety and immunogenicity of heptavalent pneumococcal conjugate vaccine in children. *Pediatr. Infect. Dis. J.*, 2000, 19, 187–195.
29. Casselbrant, M.L., Kaleida, P.H., Rockette, H.E. et al. Efficacy of antimicrobial prophylaxis and of tympanostomy tubes insertion for prevention of recurrent acute otitis media: results of a randomized clinical trial. *Pediatr. Infect. Dis. J.*, 1992, 11, 278–286.
30. Bluestone, C.D. and Klein, J.O. *Otitis Media in Infants and Children*, 2nd ed. Philadelphia: W.B. Saunders. 1995, 145–240.
31. Boston, M.B., McCook, J., Burke, B., and Derkay, C.S. Incidence of risk factors for additional tympathy tube insertion in children. *Arch. Otol. HHS*, 2003, 129, 293–296.
32. Coyte, P.C. et al. Role of adjuvant adenoidectomy and tonsillectomy in the outcomes of insertion of tympanostomy tubes. *New Engl. J. Med.*, 2001, 344, 1188–1195.
33. Paradise, J.L., Bluestone, C.D., Colborn, D.K. et al. Adenoidectomy and adenotonsillectomy for recurrent acute otitis media: parallel randomized clinical trials in children not previously treated with typmanostomy tubes. *JAMA*, 2000, 282, 945–953.
34. Paparella, M.M., Oda, M., Hiraida, F., and Brady, D. Pathology of sensorinueral hearing loss in otitis media. *Ann. Otol. Rhinol. Laryngol.*, 1972, 81, 632–647.
35. Paradise, J.L., Feldman, H.M., Campbell, T.F. et al. Effect of early or delayed insertion of tympanostomy tubes for persistent otitis media on developmental outcomes at age of 3 years. *New Engl. J. Med.*, 2001, 344(16), 1179–1187.
36. Salata, J.A. and Derkay, C.S. Water precautions in children with tympanostomy tubes. *Arch. Otolaryngol. Head Neck Surg.*, 1996, 122, 276–280.
37. Rosenfeld, R.M., Bhaya, M.H., Bower, C.M. et al. Impact of tympanostomy tubes on child quality of life. *Arch. Otolaryngol. Head Neck Surg.*, 2000, 126, 585–592.
38. Hoffmann, K., Derkay, C.S., Thompson, G.K. et al. Perioperative anesthetic complications of tympanostomy tube placement in children. *Arch. Otolaryngol. Head Neck Surg.*, 2002, 8, 1040–1043.
39. Kay, D.J. and Rosenfeld, R.M. Meta-analysis of tympanostomy tube sequelae. *Otolaryngol. Head Neck Surg.*, 2001, 124, 374–380.
40. Morpeth, J.F. et al. Comparison of oflaxicin and neomycin/polymixin B/hydrocortisone as prophylaxis against post-tympanostomy otorrhea. *Int. J. Pediatr. Otorhinolaryngol.*, 2001, 61, 99–104.
41. Pickett, B.P. Ear drop ototoxicity: reality or myth? *Am. J. Otol.*, 1997, 18, 782–791.
42. Gourin, C.G. and Hubbell, R.N. Otorrhea after insertion of silver oxide-impregnated silastic tympanostomy. *Arch. Otolaryngol. Head Neck Surg.*, 1999, 125, 446–450.
43. Berry, J.A., Biedlingmaier, J.F., and Whelan, P.J. *In vitro* resistance to bacterial biofilm on coated fluoroplastic tympanostomy tubes. *Otolaryngol. Head Neck Surg.*, 2000, 123(3), 246–251.
44. Altman, J.S., Haupert, M.S., Hamaker, R.A. et al. Phenylephrine and the prevention of postoperative tympanostomy tube obstruction. *Arch. Otolaryngol. Head Neck Surg.*, 1998, 124, 1233–1236.
45. Oberman, J.P. and Derkay, C.S. Posttympanostomy tube otorrhea. *Am. J. Otolaryngol.*, 2004, 25(2), 110–117.
46. Walker, P. Ventilation tube obstruction versus site of placement. *Aust. N.Z. J. Surg.*, 1997, 67, 52–57.
47. Derkay, C.S., Carron, J.D., Wiatrak, B.J. et al. Post-surgical follow-up of children with tympanostomy tubes: results of the AAO-HNS Pediatric Otolaryngology Committee national survey. *Otolaryngol. Head Neck Surg.*, 2000, 122, 313–318.
48. AAP section of otolaryngology and bronchoesophagology, Follow-up management of children with tympanostomy tubes. *Pediatrics*, 2002, 109(2), 328–329.
49. Ballenger, J.J. Complications of ear disease. In Ballenger, J.J., Ed. *Diseases of the Nose, Throat, Ear, Head, and Neck*, 13th ed. Philadelphia: Lea and Febiger, 1985, 1170–1196

50. Glasscock, M.E., III and Shambaugh, G.E., Jr. Intracranial complications of otitis media. In: Glasscock, M.E., III and Shambaugh, G.E., Jr., Eds. *Surgery of the Ear*, 4th ed. Philadelphia: W.B. Saunders, 1990, 249–275.
51. Neely, J.G. Complications of temporal bone infection. In: Cummings, C.W., Fredrickson, J.M., Harker, L.A., Krause, C.J., and Schuller, D.E., Eds. *Otolaryngology — Head and Neck Surgery*, 4th ed. St Louis: C.V. Mosby, 1986, 2988–3015.
52. Harker, L.A. and Koontz, F.P. The bacteriology of cholesteatoma. In McCabe, B.F., Sade, J., and Abramson, M., Eds. *Cholesteatoma*. First International Conference. Birmingham, AL: Aesculapius Publishing, 1977.
53. Ryan, M.W. and Antonelli, P.J. Pneumococcal antibiotic resistance and rates of meningitis in children. *Laryngoscope*, 2000, 110, 961–964.
54. Go, C., Bernstein, J.M., de Jong, A.L. et al. Intracranial complications of acute mastoiditis. *Int. J. Pediatr. Otorhinolaryngol.*, 2000, 52, 143–148.
55. Goldstein, N.A., Casselbrant, M.L., Bluestone, C.D. et al. Intratemporal complications of acute otitis media in infants and children. *Otolaryngol. Head Neck Surg.*, 1998, 119, 444–454.
56. Kangsanarak, J., Fooanant, S., Ruckphaopunt, K. et al. Extracranial and intracranial complications of suppurative otitis media. Report of 102 cases. *J. Laryngol. Otol.*, 1993, 107, 999–1004.
57. Gower, D. and McGuirt, W.F. Intracranial complications of acute and chronic infectious ear disease: a problem still with us. *Laryngoscope*, 1983, 93, 1028–1033.
58. Samuel, J., Fernandes, C.M.C., and Steinberg, J.L. Intracranial otogenic complications: a persisting problem. *Laryngoscope*, 1986, 96, 272–278.
59. Kraus, M. and Tovi, F. Central nervous system complications secondary to otorhinologic infections. An analysis of 39 pediatric cases. *Int. J. Pediatr. Otorhinolaryngol.*, 1992, 24, 217–226.
60. Lund, W.S. A review of 50 cases of intracranial complications from otogenic infection between 1961 and 1977. Quoted by Glasscock, M.E., III Shambaugh, G.E., Jr., Eds. *Surgery of the Ear,* 4th ed. Philadelphia: W.B. Saunders, 1990, 251.
61. Kangsanarak, J., Navacharoen, N., Fooanant, S. et al. Intracranial complications of suppurative otitis media: 13 years' experience. *Am. J. Otol.*, 1995, 16, 104–109.
62. Ludman, H. Complications of suppurative otitis media. In Kerr, A.G., Ed. *Scott-Brown's Otolaryngology*. 5th ed. London: Butterworths, 1987, 264–91.
63. Schwaber, M.K., Pensak, M.L., and Bartels, L.J. The early signs and symptoms of neurotologic complications of chronic suppurative otitis media. *Laryngoscope*, 1989, 99, 373–375.
64. Snow, J.B. Cranial and intracranial complications of otitis media. In English, G.M., Ed. *Otolaryngology*. Philadelphia: Lippincott, 1989.
65. Sanford, J.P. *Guide to Antimicrobial Therapy 2000*. West Bethesda, MD: Antimicrobial Therapy, Inc, 2000.
66. Ginsburg, C.M., Rudoy, R., and Nelson, J.D. Acute mastoiditis in infants and children. *Clin. Pediatr.*, 1980, 19, 549–553.
67. Hoppe, J.E., Koster, S., Bootz, F. et al. Acute mastoiditis — relevant once again. *Infection*, 1994, 22, 178–182.
68. Luntz, M., Geren, G., Nusem, S. et al. Acute mastoiditis — revisited. *Ear Nose Throat J.*, 1994, 73, 648–654.
69. Holt, G.R. and Gates, G.A. Masked mastoiditis. *Laryngoscope*, 1983, 93, 1034–1037.
70. Badrawy, R., Abou–Bieh, A., and Taha, A. Masked diabetic mastoiditis. *J. Otolaryngol. Otol.*, 1975, 89, 815–821.
71. Williams, M.A. Head and neck findings in pediatric acquired immune deficiency syndrome. *Laryngoscope*, 1987, 97, 713–716.
72. Barnett, E.D., Klein, J.O., Pelton, S.I. et al. Otitis media in children born to human immunodeficiency virus-infected mothers. *Pediatr. Infect. Dis. J.*, 1992, 11, 360–364.
73. Blevins, N.H. and Lalwani, A.K. Acute mastoiditis. In Lalwani, A.K. and Grundfast, K.M., Eds. *Pediatric Otology and Neurotology*. Philadelphia: Lippincott–Raven, 1998, 265–275.
74. Harley, E.H., Sdralis, T., and Berkowitz, R.G. Acute mastoiditis in children: a 12-year retrospective study. *Otolaryngol. Head Neck Surg.*, 1997, 116, 26–30.
75. Ibekwe, A.C. and Okoye, B.C. Subperiosteal mastoid abscesses in chronic suppurative otitis media. *Ann. Otol. Rhinol. Laryngol.*, 1988, 97, 373–375.

76. Bezold, F. and Siebenmann, F. *Textbook of Otology.* Translated by J. Holinger. Chicago: E.H. Cole-grove, 1908, 179–185.
77. Schuknecht, H.F. and Gulya, A.J. *Anatomy of the Temporal Bone with Surgical Implications.* Phila-delphia: Lea & Febiger. 1986, 161–184.
78. Elliott, C.A., Zalzal, G.H., and Gottlieb, W.R. Acute otitis media and facial paralysis in children. *Ann. Otol. Rhinol. Laryngol.,* 1996, 105, 58–62.
79. Schaitkin, B.M., May, M., and Klein, S.R. *Topognostic, Otovestibular, and Electrical Testing: Diag-nosis and Prognosis. The Facial Nerve,* 2nd ed. New York: Thieme Medical Publishers, 2000, 213–230.
80. Schuknecht, H.F. and Gulya, A.J. *Anatomy of the Temporal Bone with Surgical Implications.* Phila-delphia: Lea & Febiger. 1986, 111–128.
81. Gadre, A.K., Brodie, H.A., Fayad, J.N. et al. Venous channels of the petrous apex: their presence and clinical importance. *Otolaryngol. Head Neck Surg.,* 1997, 116, 168–174.
82. Gradenigo, C. Ueber Circumscripte Leptomeningitis mit spinalen Symptomen. *Arch. Ohrenheilk,* 1904, 51, 60–62.
83. Eagleton, W.E. Localized bulbar cisterna (pontine) meningitis, facial pain, and sixth nerve paralysis and the relation to caries of the petrous apex. *Arch. Surg.,* 1930, 20, 386–420.
84. Frenckner, P. Some remarks on the treatment of apicitis (petrocitis) with and without Gradenigo's syndrome. *Acta Otolaryngol.* (Stockh.), 1932, 17, 97–120.
85. Eagleton, W.E. Unlocking of the petrous pyramid for localized bulbar (pontile) meningitis secondary to suppuration of the petrous apex. Report of four cases with recovery in three. *Arch. Otolaryngol.,* 1931, 13, 386–422.
86. Ramadier, J. Les osteites petreuses profondes (petrosites). *Otorhinolaryngol. Int.,* 1933, 17, 816.
87. Lempert, J. Complete apicectomy (mastoidotympanoapicectomy). New technic for complete exenter-ation of carotid portion of petrous pyramid. *Arch. Otolaryngol.,* 1937, 25, 144–177.
88. Schuknecht, H.F. *Pathology of the Ear.* Cambridge, MA: Harvard University Press, 1974.
89. Paparella, M.M. and Sugiura, S. The pathology of suppurative labyrinthitis. *Ann. Otol. Rhinol. Laryngol.,* 1967, 76, 554–586.
90. Bates, G.J.E.M., O'Donoghue, G.M., Anslow, P. et al. Can CT detect labyrinthine fistulae preopera-tively? *Acta Otolaryngol.* (Stockh.), 1988, 106, 40–45.
91. McCabe, B.F. Labyrinthine fistula in chronic mastoiditis. *Ann. Otol. Rhinol. Laryngol.,* 1984, 93 (Suppl. 112), 138–141.
92. Gacek, R. The surgical management of labyrinthine fistulae in chronic otitis media with cholesteatoma. *Ann. Otol. Rhinol. Laryngol.,* 1974, 83 (Suppl. 10), 1–19.
93. Sheehy, J. and Brackmann, D. Cholesteatoma surgery: management of the labyrinthine fistula — a report of 97 cases. *Laryngoscope,* 1979, 89, 78–87.
94. Quijano, M., Schuknecht, H.F., and Otte, J. Temporal bone pathology with intracranial abscess. *J. Otolaryngol. Relat. Spec.,* 1988, 50, 2–31.
95. Southwick, F.S., Richardson, E.P., Jr., and Swartz, M.N. Septic thrombosis of the dural venous sinuses. *Medicine,* 1986, 65, 82–106.
96. Karlin, R.J. and Robinson, W.A. Septic cavemous sinus thrombosis. *Ann. Emerg. Med.,* 1984, 13, 449–455.
97. Dawes, J.D.K., quoted in Alford, B.R. and Cohn, A.M. Complications of suppurative otitis media and mastoiditis. In Paparella, M.M. and Shumrick, D.A., Eds. *Otolaryngology,* 2nd ed. Philadelphia: W.B. Saunders, 1930, 1502.
98. Tveteras, K., Kristensen, S., and Dommerby, H. Septic cavernous and lateral sinus thrombosis — modern diagnostic and therapeutic principles. *J. Laryngol. Otol.,* 1988, 102, 877–882.
99. Teichgraeber, J.F., Per–Lee, J.H., and Turner, J.S., Jr. Lateral sinus thrombosis: a modern perspective. *Laryngoscope,* 1982, 92, 744–751.
100. Villringer, A., Seiderer, M., Bauer, W.M. et al. Diagnosis of superior sagittal sinus thrombosis by three dimensional magnetic resonance flow imaging. *Lancet,* 1989, 1(8646), 1086–1087.
101. Fritsch, M.H., Miyamoto, R.T., and Wood, T.L. Sigmoid sinus thrombosis diagnosis by contrasted MRI scanning. *Otolaryngol. Head Neck Surg.,* 1990, 103, 451–456.
102. Kelly, K.E., Jackler, R.K., and Dillon, W.P. Diagnosis of septic sigmoid sinus thrombosis with magnetic resonance imaging. *Otolaryngol. Head Neck Surg.,* 1991, 105, 617–624.

103. Holzmann, D., Huisman, T.A., and Linder, T.E. Lateral dural sinus thrombosis in childhood. *Laryngoscope*, 1999, 109, 645–651.
104. Seid, A.B. and Sellars, S.L. The management of otogenic lateral sinus disease at Groote Schuur Hospital. *Laryngoscope*, 1973, 83, 397–403.
105. Hawkins, D.B. Lateral sinus thrombosis: a sometimes unexpected diagnosis. *Laryngoscope*, 1985, 95, 674–677.
106. Bradley, P.J., Manning, K.P., and Shaw, M.D.M. Brain abscess secondary to otitis media. *J. Laryngol. Otol.*, 1984, 98, 1185–1191.
107. Yen, P.T., Chan, S.T., and Huang, T.S. Brain abscess: with special reference to otolaryngologic sources of infection. *Otolaryngol. Head Neck Surg.*, 1995, 113, 15–22.
108. Ayyagari, A., Pancholi, V.K., Kak, V.K. et al. Bacteriological spectrum of brain abscess with special reference to anaerobic bacteria. *Indian J. Med. Res.*, 1983, 77, 182–186.
109. Maurice-Williams, R.S. Open evacuation of pus: a satisfactory approach to the problem of brain abscess? *J. Neurol. Neurosurg. Psych.*, 1983, 46, 697–703.
110. Haines, S.J., Mampalam, T., Rosenblum, M.L. et al. Cranial and intracranial bacterial infections. In Youmans, J.R., Ed. *Neurological Surgery*. Philadelphia: W.B. Saunders, 1990, 3707–3735.
111. Britt, R.H. Brain abscess. In: Wilkins, R.H. and Rengachary, S.S., Eds. *Neurosurgery*. New York: McGraw–Hill, 1985, 1928–1956.
112. Glasscock, M.E., III and Shambaugh, G.E., Jr. Aural complications of otitis media. In Glasscock, M.E., III and Shambaugh, G.E., Jr., Eds. *Surgery of the Ear*, 4th ed. Philadelphia: W.B. Saunders, 1990, 277–292.
113. Haimes, A.B., Zimmerman, R.D., Morgello, S. et al. MR imaging of brain abscesses. *Roentgenology*, 1989, 152, 1073–1085.
114. Durack, D.T. and Perfect, J.R. Acute bacterial meningitis. In Wilkins, R.H. and Rengachary, S.S., Eds. *Neurosurgery*. New York: McGraw–Hill, 1983, 1921–1928.
115. Dodge, P.R., Davis, H., Feigin, R.D. et al. Prospective evaluation of hearing impairment as a sequela of acute bacterial meningitis. *New Engl. J. Med.*, 1984, 311, 869–874.
116. Lebel, M.H., Freij, B.J., Syrogiannopoulos, G.A. et al. Dexamethasone therapy for bacterial meningitis. Results of two double-blind placebo controlled trials. *New Engl. J. Med.*, 1988, 319, 964–971.
117. Francois, M., Laccourreye, L., Huy, E.T. et al. Hearing impairment in infants after meningitis: detection by transient evoked otoacoustic emissions. *J. Pediatr.*, 1997, 130, 712–717.
118. Renaudin, J.W. Cranial epidural abscess and subdural empyema. In Wilkins, R.H. and Rengachary, S.S., Eds. *Neurosurgery*. New York: McGraw–Hill, 1985, 1961–1963.
119. Symonds, C.P. Otitic hydrocephalus. *Brain*, 1931, 54, 55–71.
120. Quincke, H. Ueber meningitis serosa: Volkmann's Sammlung klinischer Vorträge. NF 1893, Nr 67, in Quincke, H. Ueber Meningitis serosa und verwandte Zustande. *Dtsch. Z. Nervenheilkd.*, 1897, 9, 149.
121. Isaacman, D.J. Otitic hydrocephalus: an uncommon complication of a common condition. *Ann. Emerg. Med.*, 1989, 18, 684–687.
122. Pfaltz, C.R. and Griesemer, C. Complications of acute middle ear infections. *Ann. Otol. Rhinol. Laryngol.*, 1984, 93 (Suppl. 112), 133–137.
123. Sennaroglu, L., Kaya, S., Gursel, B. et al. Role of MRI in the diagnosis of otitic hydrocephalus. *Am. J. Otol.*, 1996, 17, 784–786.
124. Tomkinson, A., Mills, R.G., and Cantrell, P.J. The pathophysiology of otitic hydrocephalus. *J. Laryngol. Otol.*, 1997, 111, 757–759.

29 Otologic Surgery

Daniel L. Wohl and Walter M. Belenky

Quality is never an accident. It is always the result of high intention, sincere effort, intelligent direction and skillful execution. It represents the wise choice of many alternatives.

Willa A. Foster

CONTENTS

INTRODUCTION

In the management of complications of pediatric otology, the initial focus should be on avoidance and recognition so that complications and their management will be minimized. To achieve this end, one must first recognize the uniqueness of the pediatric patient with regard to their otologic problems, especially in contrast with the adult patient. This uniqueness has a bearing on all aspects of their otologic care — the detection of a problem, its documentation, the treatment course, the timing of treatment, the postoperative care, and the long-term follow-up. If complications do occur, management may also vary from the adult patient with similar problems based on the age of the patient.

Factors in the pediatric patient which may influence avoidance, recognition, and management of complications include:

- Congenital malformation of the inner, middle and external ear, previously recognized or discovered at the time of surgery
- Congenital syndromes which may have a direct or indirect bearing upon otologic problems or may affect postoperative care.
- Congenital or acquired neurological problems that may influence or decrease the benefit of otologic surgery.
- Presence of laryngeal-pharyngeal acid reflux that may result in persistent symptoms and affect postoperative care.
- The propensity to develop acute otitis media influencing the timing of surgery and possibly complicating healing and recovery.
- The level of speech and language development in the patient.
- The ability of the patient and/or parents to handle postoperative care.
- The difficulty in young patients to accurately assess the type and degree of hearing loss preoperatively.

Whether the qualified surgeon is a general otolaryngologist, an otologist or pediatric otolaryngologist, awareness of these factors preoperatively can only enhance the outcome for the patient, fulfill the realistic expectations of the parents and minimize complications.

This chapter will cover surgical complications in managing tympanic membrane and middle ear pathology broadly characterized as chronic otitis media (COM):[1]

- Retraction and atelectasis — significant tympanic membrane attenuation with collapse into the middle ear space with or without contact to middle ear structures, and with or without a strong clinical history of acute otitis media
- Tympanic membrane perforation — nonintact tympanic membrane:
  - Secondary to an episode of acute otitis media with perforation
  - Following the extrusion or removal of a tympanostomy tube
  - Following tympanic membrane trauma, such as a cotton swab or other foreign body injury
  - Following prior tympanic membrane surgery
- Cholesteatoma — acquired (primary or secondary) or congenital
- Chronic mastoiditis — representing chronic suppurative otitis media (CSOM) with or without cholesteatoma

PERIOPERATIVE PLANNING

CLINICAL OBJECTIVES

- Establish or re-establish middle ear/mastoid aeration.
- Maintain or re-establish physiologic mucociliary flow.
- Maintain or re-establish sound conduction from the tympanic membrane to the inner ear.
- Create a "dry and safe" ear.
- Evaluate and make necessary accommodations for aural rehabilitation in educational and social settings.

INDICATIONS

Factors that should be taken into consideration when evaluating a child for major otologic surgical intervention include

- General clinical parameters: probability of continued eustachian tube dysfunction, status of contralateral ear, patient age, coexisting medical disease, and/or educational–psychosocial concerns potentially affecting surgery and/or recovery
- Specific current complications of middle ear/mastoid disease: persistent or refractory otorrhea, degree and persistence of otalgia, degree of conductive and/or sensorineural hearing loss, facial nerve weakness, balance issues, or acute neurological changes
- Goals and expectations of the patient and family: dry ear? improved hearing? elimination of current hearing aid? swimming? understanding of the limits and potential complications of the proposed surgical procedure?
- Complexity of the proposed surgery and the experience and skill of the proposed surgeon[2,3]

GENERAL CONSIDERATIONS

Establish reasonable expectations — in the patient and the family. This can sometimes be a difficult task for major ear surgery in children. Families may desire a second opinion to clarify surgical options and expected outcomes, which should be supported.

Patient age — no absolute technical contraindications to reparative tympanoplasty in very young children exist.[4,5] Most surgeons, however, prefer to wait until the child is older, typically between 5 and 8 years of age, when likelihood of more normal eustachian tube function is higher.

Although there are few strong guidelines, assessment of eustachian tube function or considering the clinical status of the contralateral ear may provide some guidance.[6]

Timing of procedure — no season of the year is the absolute "best" for school-age children. For relatively elective surgical procedures such as tympanoplasty in a dry ear or "second-look" cholesteatoma procedures, a discussion of the timing relative to school, sports, or summer activities is critical because of the potential 6 to 12 weeks to full recovery. The decision often depends on family priorities.

Major ear surgery may result in time off from school; restrictions from swimming, sports, or plane travel for a limited period of time; and a relatively brief but graduated return to regular daily activities. In some cases, full return to the most aggressive activities, such as contact sports, deep underwater events, and the playing of valsalva-inducing wind instruments, may be limited for a protracted period of time, particularly if eustachian tube function has not been established.[7] Furthermore, many surgeons prioritize avoidance of "cold" seasons, while others try to avoid swimming seasons. As a general rule, urgent case-specific priorities should take precedence over social priorities in almost all scenarios.

Anticipated hearing loss — tympanoplasty for perforations in otherwise uncomplicated ears usually results in a satisfactory improvement in hearing if a preoperative loss is identified.[8,9] If only short-term hearing loss is expected, the patient and family should be informed that preferential seating in school might be sufficient. Depending on the pathology, if a significant hearing loss for several months or more is at least a possibility, the patient and family should be provided with information on available options to maximize hearing and communication, especially in the school setting. If permanent hearing loss is anticipated, a full preoperative discussion of rehabilitative options is appropriate and necessary.

PREOPERATIVE CONSIDERATIONS

Most if not all of the potential variations within acceptable standards of care should be discussed with the patient and family prior to the proposed surgery date. Any discussion about what the family may perceive as a major deviation from acknowledged standards must be documented.

Preoperative computed tomographic (CT) scan — obtaining a preoperative CT scan of the temporal bones can be very helpful with chronic disease other than a stable, dry perforation. Additionally, even in the presence of a dry perforation, a CT may be helpful if the hearing loss is greater than expected or if a sensorineural component is present.[10]

Preoperative audiogram — a recent reliable preoperative audiogram with air and bone thresholds should be part of all preoperative planning. In the uncommon situation in which reliable thresholds are not obtainable (related to age or neurologic status), auditory brainstem evoked responses (ABR) and/or otoacoustic emissions should be strongly considered.

Preoperative adenoidectomy — in general, studies support no single conclusion about the usefulness of preoperative adenoidectomy for major ear surgery.[8,11,12] In younger children, at a minimum, it is reasonable to assess the potential interference with eustachian tube function by the history and a flexible fiberoptic nasopharyngeal examination or a soft-tissue lateral neck x-ray. If an adenoidectomy is reasonable by accepted indications, such as clinically significant obstructed breathing, chronic rhinosinusitis, or a long-standing history of otitis media with effusion or other chronic middle ear disease, the surgeon is provided an excellent opportunity to evaluate the diseased ear under general anesthesia at the time of adenoidectomy. If an adenoidectomy is first performed, it is reasonable to wait at least 4 to 6 weeks to allow resolution of postoperative inflammatory edema and to see if there are any positive benefits to the diseased ear (ears) as a result of adenoid removal.

POSTOPERATIVE CONSIDERATIONS

In-patient vs. out-patient surgery — whether an otherwise healthy child is discharged to home the same day often depends on his or her age and what time of day the surgery was completed. Several other factors should be considered, including the distance the family lives from the surgical facility, whether they have a telephone in case of emergency, whether the child has other medical issues, or concern over who takes off the dressing or removes the drain on the first postoperative day. Additionally, insurance may be more likely to cover out-patient procedures and can be a major consideration; however, it should not solely dictate whether a postoperative overnight stay is appropriate.

Short-term postsurgical follow-up — will the child be cooperative for a postoperative microscopic examination in the office to maintain adequate aural hygiene? In some children, this may be an unreasonable expectation. Therefore, discussion of the possibility of a short-term follow-up procedure under anesthesia may be appropriate.

Long-term follow-up — document discussion of the potential for "second-look" and/or staged reconstructive procedures. Potential advantages and disadvantages of serial follow-up imaging studies should also be discussed. Staged endoscopic second-look procedures are not routinely advocated in children, although they may be considered in selected cases.

Postoperative audiometric follow-up — an audiometric evaluation can be considered any time in the postoperative period, but a wait of 6 to 8 weeks after surgery allows for resolution of edema, dissolution of middle ear packing, and/or dissolution or removal of ear canal packing. Similarly, tympanometry testing should also be deferred for 6 to 8 weeks to allow completion of healing after tympanoplasty. If a significant or unanticipated change in hearing is suspected, an audiometric evaluation can be undertaken at any time.

SURGICAL TECHNIQUE CONSIDERATIONS

Surgical approach[13,14] — retroauricular vs. endaural: there is no one "best way." Safe and adequate exposure of key areas is the defining criteria. In general, young children's smaller anatomy often is more amenable to a retroauricular approach. Particularly with anterior pathology, a retroauricular approach affords the greatest visibility and access to the mastoid and the facial recess.[9]

External incision — "in the crease" vs. "behind the crease" — some surgeons prefer to make an incision a few millimeters behind the crease because they feel it is easier to approximate the skin at closure and that the incision site is less likely to interfere subsequently with wearing glasses. Other surgeons believe cosmesis is improved by "hiding" the incision in a ready-made crease. Either way, it is necessary to recognize that the developing mastoid tip does not always provide facial nerve protection in infants and very young children.

Hair shaving — most children and almost all parents appreciate minimizing external appearance changes. The use of an adhesive drape barrier with only minimal shaving, if necessary, is often a good compromise that eliminates hair from the surgical site.

Anesthetic considerations[15] — urine output monitoring in long cases is a reasonable consideration from the anesthesiologist's perspective if a lengthy surgical procedure is anticipated. Nitrous oxide can perfuse into the middle ear space and create positive pressure that may interfere with the intraoperative stability of packing, graft material, or prosthesis. Therefore, if appropriate, it is advisable to discuss turning off the nitrous oxide with the anesthesiologist well before the end of the surgical portion of the case.

Muscle relaxants — if monitoring of the facial nerve is anticipated, muscle relaxants should not be used for the surgical portion of the general anesthetic.

Intraoperative intravenous antibiotics — in pediatric surgery, antibiotic coverage is recommended for clean-contaminated, contaminated, and dirty cases; consensus for whether to recommend antimicrobial prophylaxis in clean cases, however, has not been established.[16] Although the benefit of intravenous antibiotics with repairs of dry perforations or in exploratory tympanotomy surgery for nonsuppurative pathology has not been demonstrated,[17] some surgeons consider antibiotic coverage beneficial if in circulation before the initial incision. In some cases, streptococcal bacterial endocarditis (SBE) prophylaxis may be indicated and should be discussed with the patient's cardiologist and the anesthesiologist before the beginning of the case.

Facial nerve monitoring — is one available or was one requested? What operative procedure is being performed? The key determinant of safety is knowledge of anatomy, recognition of landmarks, and experience. Nonetheless, in major ear surgery, even the most experienced otologic surgeon can benefit from the supplemental use of a facial nerve monitor.[18] This is particularly true in cases in which anatomic variations are more likely to be encountered, such as congenitally abnormal ears, revision tympanomastoidectomy surgery, or when using the facial recess approach.

Tympanostomy tube placement — the placement of a tympanostomy tube during major ear surgery is determined by the potential significance of tympanic membrane, middle ear, or eustachian tube pathology.[19]

Drains — in general, the location and significance of encountered intraoperative bleeding determines whether a drain is placed or not. Because the drain is usually left in place at least overnight, its use may be an impediment to same-day discharge.

Head dressing — the type of surgery performed generally determines the need for a head dressing.[20] The goal of a mastoid dressing is to provide pressure over the dissected postauricular tissue planes. It will also blot up any bleeding from the incision site. Hand-wrapped or commercial products are both effective, but care must be taken to avoid excessive tightness, which could result in pressure necrosis. In choosing a dressing, cost may be a factor; the commercially available ones generally are more expensive. If the patient is discharged from the hospital with the dressing in place, instructions should be provided for removal or loosening.

Instrumentation — A well-maintained array of otologic instrumentation is essential for any major procedure. A good binocular operating microscope with inclinable eyepieces will allow excellent visualization as well as surgeon comfort (especially important for long or complicated cases). Side ports for observation, "side arms," and a camera make teaching ear surgery easier and much safer. An organized instrument display and a knowledgeable scrub nurse will reduce the overall length of the operation. A good selection of angled instruments for removal of small areas of cholesteatoma, redundancy of all sizes of suction catheters and suction–irrigator catheters, several varieties and sizes of sharp knives, and a full complement of drill bits and diamond burrs are essential.

Use of rod-lens "telescopes" — Angled telescopes, especially the 20-cm, 2.8-mm diameter, 30° telescope, can be used to visualize anatomic regions that cannot be seen easily (or at all) using the single-plane axis of a surgical microscope. In the past, surgeons have used a small mirror, especially prior to the availability of telescopes, to see around corners, particularly into the sinus tympani and into the protympanum. Although this can be helpful, bleeding, fogging, and scratches on the mirror may make its use difficult.

TYMPANOPLASTY

Techniques for the surgical repair of tympanic membrane (TM) pathology span from limited myringoplasty procedures to complex operations whose success is as much a function of the pathology as it is dependent on the skill level of the surgeon. Failure to assess the pathology accurately may result in inadequate management. Failure to implement adequate intervention may result in progressively more serious pathology.[4,5,21–27] Small perforations are managed differently from clinically significant tympanic membrane retractions or large perforations. In the absence of ossicular chain pathology, the surgeon may often first consider simple measures before moving on to more complex procedures.

TYMPANIC MEMBRANE PATHOLOGY

Immediate perforations from tube removal[13,28] — indications for elective removal of a retained tympanostomy tube: the surgeon may choose to remove the tube if

- Otorrhea has been continuous refractory to office hygiene and medical management.
- A tympanostomy tube has been in far longer than the anticipated need.
- Evidence of early cholesteatoma formation is found.

These (usually) small, dry perforations may heal spontaneously or can be managed with a modest immediate myringoplasty procedure, creating "fresh edges" of outer epithelium and inner mucosa and placing a "patch" of Steri-Strip (or similar material) on top of or spanning the perforation. The ear canal should be kept dry postoperatively to avoid migration of the grafted material and to avoid infection due to water contamination. If associated drainage or cholesteatoma development is present, removal of the tube and any associated granulation tissue or migrating epithelium may be sufficient for the ear drum to heal with or without adjunctive use of absorbable packing (saturated with a medicated ear drop suspension)

Persistent, small, central perforations — these may be amenable to a myringoplasty procedure using fat surgical adhesive strip or tape, or "cigarette paper." In older children, in the office and under microscopic visualization, after application of a topical anesthetic, circumferential cauterization of the perforation edge or tissue manipulation of the perforation, with or without placement of a "patch," may prove successful. However, most repairs of persistent, small central perforation in children are performed under general anesthesia. If an adenoidectomy is planned, consider simultaneous myringoplasty, even with larger perforations, rather than directly moving on to formal reparative tympanoplasty at the same time — it may close.

Tympanic membrane retractions[13,29] — If the hearing is normal, or near normal, and stable; the area of retraction is clean and dry; the entire extent of the retracted area is clearly visible; and the patient can reliably follow up, watchful waiting may be adequate. However, if the retraction is deep or associated with middle ear fluid or with a conductive hearing loss, placement of a tympanostomy tube may arrest continued retraction. However, consider a limited myringectomy procedure in which the diseased, nonfunctional portion of TM is removed endaurally if

- The tympanic membrane is stretched beyond a critical threshold and significant conductive hearing loss is significant.
- A repeat tube fails to maintain adequate tympanic membrane elevation.
- A part of the tympanic membrane does not "come up" with a tube (i.e., an adhesive retraction) and conductive hearing is significant or progressive.
- There is continued retraction with accumulation of squamous debris within the retraction but the edges of the retraction can be seen and the retraction can be completely cleaned.

The mesotympanum can be layered with slowly absorbable packing, creating a framework for epithelial migration. Allow time for the strong regenerative forces to take effect.[9] A functional neotympanum may heal. Reassess for clinical significance as indicated earlier.

If all of the preceding fails and the resultant perforation does not close and conductive hearing loss is significant, or the extent of the retraction is not clearly visible and conductive hearing loss is significant, a formal reparative tympanoplasty procedure should be considered. Furthermore, when managing significant retractions, if the retraction is draining and/or filled with squamous debris, tympanoplasty with ossiculoplasty and possible mastoidectomy may need to be considered.

Persistent, large central, or marginal perforations — these require formal reparative tympanoplasty. With or without a history of recurrent otorrhea, these perforations are almost always associated with a clinically significant conductive hearing loss and/or significant or recurrent drainage with water exposure.

GENERAL PRINCIPLES

For graft material,[13,30] always measure anticipated size of the graft first and then add extra for shrinkage or trimming before taking the graft. Loose areolar tissue overlying the temporalis muscle fascia should be prepared adequately to assure serviceable thickness; this tissue may be better for modestly sized perforations. True temporalis muscle fascia[9] is most popular and more commonly used for revision cases or large perforations due to its more uniform thickness. Tragal cartilage is advocated for children with known long-standing eustachian tube dysfunction.[31,32] The attached perichondrium flap can be used as part of the graft. Cartilage grafts are often advocated for posterior/superior perforation in an attempt to avoid retraction into the attic postoperatively. Perichondrium or pericranium is useful in the absence of adequate temporalis fascia such as in revision cases.

To place the graft, assure 360° of good contact with epithelial edges, whether underlay or overlay. Check for malleus retraction; the graft may need to be cut to fit around a very retracted malleus. Consider placing absorbable "spacer" between promontory and graft material (underlay or overlay) to help maintain middle ear space.

During healing time, maintain good incision care with retroauricular or endaural approach. Buried absorbable subcuticular or subcutaneous sutures, as needed for skin closure, are easy to manage in children because stitches do not need to be removed. Maintain dry ear precautions until grafted tympanic membrane and the canal incision(s) are healed. Beware of the potential for children to remove canal packing prematurely.

SURGICAL TECHNIQUE

Overlay vs. Underlay vs. "Other"

The surgeon should perform what he or she knows best; however, it is important to be comfortable with more than one technique. Overlay and underlay techniques, as well as their variations, have more than adequate success rates as measured by repair stability and postoperative hearing.[2,4,8,13,14,30,33–36]

Overlay

Although lateral grafting (overlay) has a higher initial success rate in experienced hands, it has a lower initial success rate with the less experienced otologic surgeon. This method allows for independent healing of mucosa medially and skin laterally. It also provides better access to anterior pathology (more often seen in children than in adults) by providing easier access to remove bony anterior canal bulge.

The overlay approach makes it easier to address myringosclerotic plaques. If plaques are not adherent to the annulus and not inhibiting TM vibration, the surgeon may not need to remove them. If it is not possible to get a reasonable tympanic membrane repair without removing the plaques, then removal may be indicated. Removal of plaques, however, may significantly decrease the area of the residual TM with which the surgeon has to work.

Overlay has been advocated for revision cases. Because it is technically more difficult, the surgeon must be skilled in mobilizing various types of canal skin flaps and know how to "peel" outer epithelium from the fibrous layer and/or annulus. The epithelial separation is usually best started at the beginning of the fibrous annulus anterior to the pars flaccida.

This approach may limit view of the ossicles; if a posterior portion of healthy fibrous TM remains after removal of the lateral epithelium, the incudostapedial joint may not be visible. This may make it more difficult to assess the integrity of the ossicular chain prior to placing the lateral graft. An endoscopic evaluation may be useful in this situation.

The surgeon should beware of blunting potential and take steps to minimize it.[37] He or she can create a "pseudosulcus" immediately lateral to the annulus and "tuck in" the fascial graft and epithelium. Another option is to place the epithelium and fascial graft on the tympanic membrane remnant in contact with each other onto the annular sulcus anteriorly. If the malleus is exposed, the graft should be "locked in" around the manubrium if it is exposed. At a minimum, it is necessary to expose the short process of the malleus to the outer skin graft so that good contact is maintained between epithelium and the ossicular chain.

The surgeon needs to be aware of increased potential for disorganized canal skin migration. The mobilized canal skin graft should be oriented in anatomic alignment (i.e., the flaps put back in close to their original location within the ear canal) to promote natural epithelial migration and reduce the potential for accumulation of keratin debris and unremitting "chronic otitis externa." As much exposed bone of the ear canal as possible should be covered in order to cut down on possible sources of granulation tissue formation during the healing process.

Underlay

Medial grafting ("underlay") is easier to perform with endaural or retroauricular access (the most common approach used in residency training programs). It is necessary to "freshen" the edges of the perforation before raising the tympanomeatal flap and observe the medial surface of tympanic membrane, especially in the area of the perforation, to assure complete epithelial removal.

Postoperative retractive forces on the graft may result in its separation before healing is complete. The most common area of failure for a medial graft is anteriorly — it is more difficult to maneuver a graft into place with anterior perforations. It is important to develop techniques to maintain graft positioning, such as "overpacking" the middle ear anteriorly to limit potential for physiologic aeration via the eustachian tube to disrupt the graft. Other techniques used to fasten the graft anteriorly include placement of small metal clips or bringing the graft up onto the anterior canal wall between the annulus and the ear canal wall.[38]

Other Tympanoplasty Techniques

Cartilage "inlay"[35] is a technique newly described in children. Cartilage is durable and readily available and can be used with or without the attached perichondrium. The long-term success rate with widespread use is not known. Visualization of the middle ear medial to the cartilage is not possible from the ear canal. Growth factor and hyaluronic acid-impregnated disks are still experimental.[34,39] Their clinical utility may be modest when compared with expectant natural healing in small perforations.

Ossiculoplasty

Conductive hearing gain with a functional middle ear transformer mechanism is an integral component of tympanoplasty when coexisting ossicular chain pathology is present.[40–44] Reconstruction is preferable at the time of primary tympanoplasty because it may eliminate a second procedure if successful. It is appropriate and encouraged if the surgeon is confident of creating a "dry and safe" middle ear. In some cases — widespread cholesteatoma or significant middle ear mucosal edema or bleeding, for example — it would not be reasonable to reconstruct until a follow-up procedure assured no regrowth of cholesteatoma and/or more normal middle ear mucosa.

Reconstruction may not be advisable if the tympanic membrane perforation being repaired is large and the newly created ossicular chain would need to be wedged between the graft and stapes or oval window. The time of secondary tympanoplasty provides the surgeon with a less inflamed environment and often more easily defined pathology and anatomy. However, this means that more than one "big" procedure is required.

Choice of ossicular reconstruction material includes

- Autograft — cartilage: dampens vibrations if only connector; useful to diffuse contact of prosthesis with tympanic membrane
- Ossicle — incus or malleus available; needs to be reshaped, but the surgeon can customize appropriately for the pathology

- Calvarial bone — always available but uncommonly employed; beware bleeding at donor site; can be useful in ear canal reconstruction
- Prosthesis — wide array of commercial choices with excellent characteristics: must firmly establish continuity of ossicular chain from tympanic membrane to oval window; maintain knowledge and supply of appropriate partial and total ossicular prostheses (PORPs and TORPs) and incudostapedial join connectors; length may need to be customized for the pediatric mesotympanum; "head" may need to be customized to assure stable contact laterally with tympanic membrane

TORP vs. PORP. If it is certain that the stapes crurae are stable and have a normal position with regard to the oval window, a PORP is preferred. Hearing results are comparable with either prosthesis type if a functional oval window is present.

Stabilization of reconstruction depends on mucosal regrowth; a true diarthrodial joint cannot be replaced with current technology. With PORPS, the surgeon should consider a drop of (expensive) "tissue glue" or well-placed bone dust and a drop of blood (depending on the shape of the prosthesis, some may fit better than others and thus be more stable).

There is potential for separation of the prosthesis with (limited) growth of mesotympanum depth with age or from slippage with aggressive activity, especially early after reconstruction). Prothesis extrusion will occur in a small percentage over time; this may be due to retraction of the tympanic membrane secondary to healing or eustachian tube dysfunction or long-term incompatibility of graft material with surrounding tissue (the placement of a cartilage "spacer" may reduce extrusion potential).

MASTOIDECTOMY

Failure to perform an appropriate operation may result in progressive pathology. Failure to identify landmarks accurately may result in an intraoperative complication.[10,46–50]

TEMPORAL BONE PATHOLOGY

Chronic suppurative otitis media (CSOM) — represents chronic drainage through a nonintact tympanic membrane — through a tympanostomy tube or perforation unresponsive to aggressive medical management. Surgical techniques for the management of CSOM, with or without cholesteatoma, span from a "simple" cortical mastoidectomy to extensive canal-wall-down procedures. Accompanying tympanoplasty, with or without ossiculoplasty, may also be necessary.

Cholesteatoma — represents the presence of epithelial extension or ectopic epithelial growth within the middle ear; it is a surgical disease and can be very aggressive in children, with a high recurrence/persistence rate, up to 50% in some series. Therefore, every effort should be made to remove all visible disease at the time of each procedure. If extension is limited or fully accessible through the canal, a basic tympanoplasty technique may be sufficient. Otherwise, a combined mastoidectomy with tympanoplasty is usually most appropriate.

Congenital anatomic abnormalities — should be considered and prepared for, especially in children with syndromic features. These include abnormal ossicles (fused, missing, or misshapen); a facial nerve that is dehiscent, in an uncommon location (such as on/over the footplate), or divided; an anterior sigmoid sinus; low-lying tegmen; high-riding jugular bulb; or dehiscent carotid artery (usually at the entrance to the eustachian tube). If the patient has had prior surgery, it may be difficult or impossible to know whether the anatomical abnormality is congenital or acquired.

GENERAL PRINCIPLES

Procedure Selection

Chronic inflammatory changes, congenital otologic pathology, and distortion of landmarks from disease or previous surgery increase the potential for a surgical complication. A key initial step in avoiding complications is determining the correct procedure for the identified pathology. Even with preoperative, high-resolution, diagnostic imaging studies, however, the surgeon may not be able to make a final decision until he or she has looked directly into the mastoid and middle ear space in the operating room.

The main surgical technique used in the management of CSOM (with or without cholesteatoma) is tympanoplasty (see earlier discussion) with mastoidectomy. Mastoidectomy may be canal wall up (CWU), canal wall down (CWD), or much less commonly, a Bondy modified radical mastoidectomy (BMRM) that can be performed without tympanoplasty, or a radical mastoidectomy performed without tympanoplasty (see later discussion).

SURGICAL TECHNIQUES

The decision to use a canal wall up (CWU) or canal wall down (CWD) approach is related to[30,46,47,49]

- Location of disease
- Extent of disease
- Type and extent of prior surgical intervention
- Degree of residual hearing
- Whether existing or prior disease involves the canal wall
- Surgical experience

Canal Wall Up

Indications

The CWU approach should be considered if:

- Mastoid disease is accessible with a complete mastoidectomy
- Mastoid disease can be accessed using a complete mastoidectomy combined with tympanoplasty

The CWU mastoidectomy is most often considered for the first surgical intervention in children with cholesteatoma or when chronic and extensive mucosal disease is present. A CWU mastoidectomy can always be converted to a CWD mastoidectomy, intraoperatively, if disease or access to disease dictates. The usefulness of the CWU approach can be extended to include disease in the facial recess by adding a facial recess (posterior tympanotomy) dissection to the surgical approach. This will provide access to the incudostapedial joint area and, when combined with partial or complete removal of the incus buttress, access to disease in the epitympanum. An atticotomy can also be used to extend the visualization available in the CWU approach.

Advantages

- Maintaining a closed mastoid cavity, which eliminates a need for office cleaning and water precautions
- Possibly making it easier to maintain a reasonably sized middle ear space
- Possibly making it easier to reconstruct the middle ear conduction mechanism

- Possibly resulting in better hearing results
- Possibly making it easier to fit an ear mold for a hearing aid because of little distortion of the external auditory canal
- Having a shorter healing period

Disadvantages

- Possibly having a higher risk of residual/recurrent disease, including that secondary to attic retraction, because it is more difficult to access disease in the sinus tympani, infrapyramidal recess, epitympanum, and facial recess
- Not being possible if the external auditory canal has already been removed surgically or by disease
- The necessity to combine with a facial recess approach to access disease in the facial recess

Canal Wall Down

Indications

The canal wall down approach should be considered if

- The external auditory canal has already been removed by prior surgery or disease.
- The mastoid cavity is contracted and surgical access to disease is significantly limited — from a low-lying tegmen or anterior sigmoid sinus, for example.
- Refractory disease is present within the sinus tympani.
- Extensive disease is present around the facial nerve.
- Long-term ventilation will be difficult — from a small or obstructed aditus ad antrum, for example.
- Disease such as a lateral semicircular canal fistula in the mastoid needs to be exteriorized.

The CWD approach should also be strongly considered in an only hearing or significantly better hearing ear because there is less chance of recurrence of cholesteatoma reducing the possibility of the need for further surgery. Finally, CWD surgery can be considered if the surgeon is concerned about the family's ability to bring the child for long-term follow-up, or if the child has other medical issues that make adequate examination in the office problematic.

Advantages

- Visualization of the mastoid cavity from the EAC
- Primary option if EAC has been already removed by disease or prior surgery
- Usefulness if the mastoid cavity is very small and contracted
- Good visualization of vertical segment of the facial nerve

Disadvantages

- Need for cleaning of the mastoid cavity on a regular basis
- Narrower middle ear space
- Less favorable hearing results
- Need to create and maintain an adequate meatoplasty

Modified Radical, Bondy Modified Radical, Radical Mastoidectomy, and Mastoid Obliteration

CWU and CWD mastoidectomy procedures are frequently used with tympanoplasty so that the middle ear space is closed. Conversely, the modified radical and radical mastoidectomy procedures create an open mastoid cavity in continuity with the middle ear. The modified radical mastoidectomy and Bondy modified radical mastoidectomy can be used with tympanoplasty; the radical mastoidectomy cannot.

The CWD and modified radical mastoid terms are often confused. The Bondy modified radical mastoidectomy approach — sometimes referred to as an "inside out" approach — is used much less often than in the past. Indications for this technique are to exteriorize cholesteatomas of the attic or pars flaccida lateral to the ossicles in which cochlear reserve is good. The resultant conductive hearing loss may be minimal or conducive to tympanoplasty.

Indications for "open cavity" procedures include

- Unresectable disease
- Anticipation of poor follow-up
- Unreconstructable canal wall
- Disease in an only hearing ear or in a dead ear (where tympanoplasty for hearing improvement would not be contemplated)
- Nonfunctioning eustachian tube

Advantages of the Bondy modified radical mastoidectomy include

- Maintenance of tympanic membrane and middle ear space
- Allowance for possibility of tympanoplasty if indicated
- Smaller mastoid cavity than in a CWD procedure
- Endaural or posterior auricular incision may be used
- Frequent indication in an only hearing ear
- Completion in one setting that does not need to be staged

Disadvantages of the Bondy modified radical mastoidectomy include

- It cannot be used with large cholesteatomas that extend down behind the pars tensa or a large attic or other type of cholesteatoma.
- The cavity and entrance to the cavity are essentially through or adjacent to the posterior superior aspect of the tympanic membrane; it may therefore be difficult and painful to clean.
- Because the cavity and entrance to the created cavity are small, they may trap moisture, leading to recurrent otorrhea.
- If the cavity is difficult to clean, trapped squamous debris may lead to recurrence of cholesteatoma.

Radical mastoidectomy is performed to eradicate middle ear and mastoid disease in which the mastoid antrum, middle ear, and external auditory canal are converted into a common cavity. It involves removal of the tympanic membrane and any remaining ossicles (except the stapes, if still present) and does not involve any grafting or reconstruction. Although performed much less frequently than in the past, it still has a place in the contemporary management of pediatric cholesteatoma.

Indications for a radical mastoidectomy include

- When irreversible disease, such as cochlear fistula, is in the promontory area
- When osteitis cannot be removed
- When tympanoplasty would result in entrapment of unresectable cholesteatoma, such as cholesteatoma extending down the eustachian tube
- When chronic perilabyrinthine cholesteatoma is present

Advantages of radical mastoidectomy include

- Exteriorizing extensive disease
- Allowing for direct examination of the middle ear and mastoid spaces

Disadvantages of radical mastoidectomy are that

- The middle ear is rarely reconstructed to improve hearing because this might trap disease and middle ear space is limited.
- Water exposure often results in moist mucosa with resultant infection.
- The cavity needs to be cleaned for the life of the patient.
- It may be difficult to make an ear mold for a hearing aid due to the size and shape of the reconstructed ear canal.

Mastoid obliteration is used when there is a desire to make the cavity smaller and easier to clean. This can be accomplished using bone paté and/or a Palva flap (an anteriorly based posterior auricular subcutaneous flap). The lateral mastoid tip can also be amputated to allow soft tissue to fall into the cavity, thus decreasing it in size inferiorly.

REVISION SURGERY[30,51]

Surgical Considerations

Unfortunately, because of the high recurrence and persistence rates of CSOM (especially with cholesteatoma), revision surgery is common. Reasons for possible recurrence include[30,51]

- Persistent mucosal disease and/or cholesteatoma in unopened mastoid air cells, including the tegmen, mastoid tip, epitympanum, hypotympanum, sinus tympani, and facial recess, or behind a high facial ridge
- Persistent mucosal disease secondary to water exposure
- Too small an opening into a mastoid cavity, which is difficult to clean or can result in moisture or debris getting trapped
- Poor ventilation of the middle ear/mastoid
- Foreign body reaction to silastic sheeting or other foreign substance in the middle ear or mastoid
- Undiagnosed pathology (previously unsuspected cholesteatoma, Langerhans cell histiocytosis, tuberculosis, etc.)

Revision tympanomastoidectomy is challenging. The landmarks may be missing or buried in pathology or fibrotic scar tissue. Previous operative summaries may be missing or lacking in detail. Even if previous operative notes are available and accurate, ongoing pathology or scarring may have altered residual anatomy and landmarks since the patient's last operation.

Revision surgery is usually undertaken due to recurrent/residual disease. The surgeon, therefore, must be prepared to do a "bigger" operation than on previous occasions, including removing any remaining air cells opening into the sinus tympani, epitympanum, and other hard-to-reach (and see into) areas; removing ossicles; and performing an acceptable meatoplasty. At the time of revision surgery, the facial nerve, dura along the tegmen, lateral semicircular canal, and sigmoid sinus may be especially at risk because the bone over these areas may already be thinned (or missing) secondary to surgery or pathology or covered in granulation tissue or cholesteatoma, making identification difficult.

If tympanoplasty is performed at the time of revision surgery, the temporalis prefascia has usually been taken during previous surgery, so true temporalis fascia may need to be used. If temporalis fascia was already used, it may be necessary to extend the search for fascia anteriorly and superiorly over the temporalis muscle. Alternative sources of fascia include the contralateral side or alternatives to fascia such as perichondrium and pericranium.

CT of the temporal bones may be helpful in revision surgery to look for erosion of remaining structures or to identify thinning of such areas as the tegmen or basal turn of the cochlea. However, CT cannot often distinguish between granulation tissue and cholesteatoma unless bony erosion is present. Use of a facial nerve monitor does not substitute for direct knowledge of the anatomy, but is an additional tool that may provide early warning and can be used to stimulate structures in an attempt to help identify the facial nerve.

"Second-look" procedures — Most otolaryngologists advocate a second-look procedure after the initial operation to remove middle ear or mastoid cholesteatoma. Although the use of a temporal bone CT instead of a second surgical look is a consideration, the major indicator of cholesteatoma on a CT scan is bone erosion. Unfortunately, it is entirely possible for cholesteatoma to return or persist without signs of erosion on CT. The use of a rod-lens telescope to re-evaluate the middle ear after cholesteatoma surgery has also been discussed. The use of an endoscope, however, requires a nonmoving patient and excellent hemostasis — two things difficult to achieve in children in an office setting. Additionally, even though the optics in the rod-lens telescopes are good, it is still difficult to see all the areas of concern or interest, particularly with an intact canal wall or tympanic membrane, without a larger procedure. Postsurgical mastoid cavities are often filled with adhesions and/or congealed coagulum that needs to be evacuated, rendering a "mini-incision" second-look procedure impractical. For all of these reasons, in children, the second-look surgical procedure remains the current standard to detect the recurrence of cholesteatoma or other pathology.

AVOIDANCE AND RECOGNITION OF SURGICAL COMPLICATIONS IN OTOLOGIC SURGERY

AVOIDANCE

General Principles

Following the emergence of the antibiotic era, complications of chronic otitis media have decreased dramatically. Correspondingly, the overall incidence of surgical complications has decreased. However, the degree of difficulty with a difficult case has not dramatically changed. It is prudent, therefore, to remain mindful that the more complicated the disease process is, the more likely it is that the management may become complicated.[52]

There is no substitute for experience and good technique. Complications can happen to any surgeon. Paying attention to the details, however, will reduce the potential for iatrogenic injuries. The surgeon should

- Inject cleanly and under direct vision.
- Raise clean flaps, cutting from "behind" if necessary.

- Preplan and make the flaps appropriately long enough to cover anticipated canal deficits.
- When drilling, perform broad dissection first, working from level to level.
- Avoid making holes by cutting with the "side" of the bur.
- Accurately identify the tegmen, the lateral semicircular canal, and the fossa incudus.
- Identify the sigmoid sinus early in the mastoid dissection; it can have a widely variable presentation from case to case.
- Recognize the digastric ridge if mastoid dissection needs to extend inferiorly.
- If the integrity of the ossicles is undetermined (usually because of surrounding pathology), use exceptional caution when dissecting off disease, particularly around the stapes and oval window.
- Know where the eustachian tube enters the protympanum and its relationship to the cochleariform process.
- Recognize the round window and be able to identify the facial ridge; remember that the facial nerve courses increasingly laterally as it descends through the mastoid segment.
- In general, maximize exposure, removing pathology a portion at a time, if necessary, and consistently identifying landmarks proceeding from "known to unknown."
- Assiduously try to maintain a bloodless field.
- When possible, dissect parallel to vital anatomic structures to minimize potential torque and stress.
- Most importantly, limit dissection if the comfort limit is reached. Stop if an identified complication cannot be handled; it is acceptable to bring in another surgeon.

RECOGNITION

Complications of major otologic surgery, such as obvious disruption of the facial nerve, major hemorrhage, or visible disruption in tegmen integrity, may be recognized during surgery. An immediate management plan can then be considered. Other complications, such as facial palsy, conductive hearing loss, or sensorineural hearing loss, may not be recognized until after the procedure is concluded. Iatrogenic injury is always a possibility but can be minimized with the application of sound surgical principles with practical techniques.[8,9,45] Particularly in children, there is also the potential for complications from new acute otitis media episodes, sometimes necessitating the placement of a ventilation tube within a grafted and healed tympanic membrane, in addition to the potential for ongoing postoperative chronic infectious concerns.[53]

Possible Complications of Tympanoplasty

Possible complications of tympanoplasty can include

- Limited hearing gain
- Failure to heal or reperforation
- Cholestetoma development

Possible Complications of Mastoidectomy

Possible complications of mastoidectomy can include

- Brain herniation in the area of the tegmen in the area of the mastoid or epitympanum
- CSF leak
- Facial nerve injury
- Bleeding
- Ossicular disruption

- Bony ear canal defects
- Labyrinthine fistula
- Persistent middle ear/mastoid disease
- New onset of infection
- Hearing loss (conductive or sensorineural)
- Tinnitus
- Vertigo
- Taste disturbance due to damage of the chorda tympani
- Ear canal stenosis

All of these potential complications can also occur secondary to the disease, so it is important to document preoperatively facial nerve function; audiometric status; physical findings of the tympanic membrane, mastoid, and ear canal; and presence/absence of tinnitus or taste disturbance.[51]

MANAGEMENT OF SURGICAL COMPLICATIONS IN OTOLOGIC SURGERY

INTRAOPERATIVE COMPLICATIONS

Any major recognized intraoperative complication during otologic surgery can shake the confidence of even the most experienced surgeon. Correspondingly, even the most experienced surgeon recognizes the potential for major complications to occur. On these occasions, it may be appropriate for the primary surgeon to call in another otolaryngologist–head and neck surgeon for an emergent intraoperative consultation.

Major Bleeding

Catastrophic bleeding may be encountered with a tear into the sigmoid sinus, jugular bulb, or carotid artery.

The sigmoid sinus — is a low-pressure venous system. Small injuries can often be controlled with the application of gelatin sponge soaked in thrombin or other hemostatic agent, or with bipolar cautery. Larger lacerations can be controlled with application of tissue or surgical hemostatic agent and pressure intra- or extraluminally. In very severe hemorrhage, the internal jugular vein may need to be ligated to prevent embolization.

The jugular bulb — may be found lying above the level of the inferior tympanic annulus in 6 to 7% of ears. Bleeding from the jugular bulb may occur secondary to removal of cholesteatoma or other pathology from the hypotympanum, retrofacial air cells, or even elevation of a tympanomeatal flap. Bleeding from a small area of injury may be controlled with gelatin sponge or bone wax compressed by a cotton applicator or a neurosurgical cottonoid. Larger defects may be controlled using hemostatic gauze between the bulb and the bony defect. Overpacking, however, may result in unwanted pressure on cranial nerves IX, X, and XII. If bleeding results from the elevation of a tympanomeatal flap, the flap should be put back into place and the ear canal packed firmly with gauze. This should be left in place for a week and then slowly advanced. If bleeding from a high jugular bulb cannot be controlled in the preceding ways, the internal jugular vein may need to be ligated in the neck to prevent embolization; then, the proximal sigmoid and bulb lumen should be obliterated with packing.

The carotid artery system — may be injured resulting from catastrophic hemorrhage and should be addressed with packing and firm pressure followed by an emergent consult with a skull-base or vascular surgeon and/or neurosurgeon. Balloon occlusion or ligation of the artery, if appropriate, may be required.

Dural Tear

A dural tear with visible loss of tegmen integrity should be promptly assessed to minimize the potential for infectious spread from an infected mastoid cavity or for herniation of brain tissue. If the tear is small, the application of dural sutures, possibly with the use of a topical hemostatic agent approved for dural use, may be sufficient to stop the leak. If the tear is large or there is an obvious dural defect, a tissue "patch" should be fashioned from fascia, perichondrium, pericranium, or possibly cartilage. If intraoperative CSF leak persists — even with patching, suturing, or the application of a hemostatic agent — the placement of a lumbar drain may need to be considered. Finally, the operating otologic surgeon should not hesitate to consult a neurosurgeon intraoperatively if the tear cannot be easily managed and/or brain herniation or injury is suspected. If CSF drainage was observed, a change from the anticipated postoperative care needs to be considered because bed rest and observation are keys to successful healing; the health care team needs to remain vigilant for developing secondary complications.

Facial Nerve Injury

Immediate repair of facial nerve injuries is preferred to delayed repair in most cases when the site of injury is recognized intraoperatively. Although an extensive discussion about facial nerve injury cannot be held here, generally the type and degree of injury will dictate the options. If the nerve is merely uncovered (i.e., the bone is drilled away) and otherwise entirely intact, further intervention is generally not required. If the nerve is uncovered and there is concern about disruption of the perineurium, some surgeons would advocate removing more of the bone covering the nerve prox-imally and distally to allow the nerve to swell with less possibility of bony compression. If however, the nerve is disrupted for more than a third of its diameter, or is completely transected, then direct repair with removal of the damaged segment and reanastomosis or interposition grafting is warranted.

Primary repair without tension is the most successful technique to minimize postrepair sequelae and short segment mobilization can be considered. However, if the area of injury is greater than 1 cm, it is better to consider an interposition graft from an accessible nerve such as the sensory greater auricular nerve.

If the operating surgeon recognizes a partial or complete transection intraoperatively, but is unable to repair it at the same sitting due to uncertainly about the type of repair needed, patient stability at the time of the surgery, or other issues, the wound can be closed and the procedure terminated. However, if repair is to be considered, it should be undertaken as soon as the patient is stable and a surgeon with expertise in facial nerve repair is available, generally within 3 to 30 days (the sooner the better).

Labyrinthine Fistula and Perilymph Leak

Labyrinthine fistula, although very uncommon, usually occurs in one of three places: the lateral semicircular canal, the oval window, or the promontory. Fortunately, sensorineural hearing loss secondary to these fistulas is less common than originally thought. If a fistula is identified intra-operatively, the leak should be closed using tissue. If ossiculoplasty is being considered, it should be postponed until the next surgery. Creation of labyrinthine fistulas can often be avoided by very careful removal of cholesteatoma or granulation tissue from the above structures; incomplete removal should be considered over complete removal if creation of a fistula can be avoided by doing so. Residual cholesteatoma or granulation tissue may be able to be more easily removed at a subsequent surgery when inflammation may be less and any leak has healed.

Perilymph leakage may result from manipulation of the stapes and may sometimes seem quite brisk; this is often referred to as a "gusher." If the integrity of the footplate has been lost, it is usually safe to suction the excess overflowing clear fluid gently until the perilymph exiting pressure equilibrates and then repair the defect with a stabilized tissue patch. Placement of a lumbar drain may be needed if the perilymph leak does not stop on its own or with the application of tissue or other appropriate packing material.

Ossicular Dislocation or Disruption

Unplanned ossicular dislocation or disruption, in most cases, should be immediately repaired with a replacement prosthesis, a spanning prosthesis, or a fashioned ossicular autograft (see the previous subsection on ossiculoplasty for intraoperative considerations).

POSTOPERATIVE COMPLICATIONS

Some tympanoplasty repairs don't "take." Most reports indicate a least a 10% failure rate after one procedure regardless of technique or surgeon experience. Failure rate may be more likely to be higher if there is significant ongoing middle ear/mastoid disease, or ongoing eustachian tube dysfunction. Reassess the clinical situation and carefully consider a revision procedure if indicated.

Cholesteatoma may develop in what was an otherwise disease-free middle ear space or under external canal flaps from inadvertently trapped epithelium. Incomplete removal of cholesteatoma at the time of surgery will result in residual ectopic epithelial growth. Revision surgery is necessary in these cases. If identified early, "pearls" of cholesteatoma may be straightforwardly identified and removed. In other cases, more extensive regrowth requires resection using standard surgical techniques. Recurrence more often occurs in the difficult to dissect regions such as the sinus tympani, around the oval window and ossicles (if left intact), or attached to other middle ear structures such as the cochleariform process and muscle tendons.

Facial Nerve Injury

If facial palsy is recognized in the immediate postoperative period, the surgeon feels the nerve was intact, and local anesthetic came into contact with the middle ear (and therefore potentially the nerve), the patient should be observed for several hours, allowing time for local anesthetic-induced paralysis to wear off. If after several hours, however, no obvious return of function has taken place, then the facial nerve needs to be investigated for an unrecognized injury. Although CT or MRI may provide some information about the integrity of the nerve, direct visualization of the operative site by returning the patient to the operating room is usually indicated (see the earlier subsection on intraoperative complications about timing and type of repair).

Sensorineural Hearing Loss, Vertigo, and Tinnitus

If sensorineural hearing loss and/or vertigo from perilymph leakage is suspected in the immediate postoperative period, particularly in revision cases,[54] prompt return to the operating room is appropriate if the loss is progressive or moderate to severe, or the vertigo is significant.

Sensorineural hearing loss may also result from fistulation of the labyrinth (by disease or the operating surgeon), excessive manipulation of the ossicular chain (during tympanoplasty or direct removal of cholesteatoma or other disease from the chain), or possibly from transmitted instrumentation vibrations to the inner ear. The majority of these hearing losses are in the high-frequency range (4000 Hz and above), and some improvement may occur in the first few months after surgery.

Tinnitus may acutely result from middle ear structure instrumentation and is often associated with nausea and vomiting; it should resolve spontaneously. Prolonged postoperative tinnitus warrants consideration of injury to the inner ear structures from primary dissection or secondarily from ossicular chain manipulation.

Conductive Hearing Loss

Hearing gain is expected in most cases, but "best" results are postoperative thresholds within comfortable speech hearing range; the overall result is rarely as good as what nature originally created. Establish reasonable expectations preoperatively. There may be gradual improvement over several months if the graft attenuates.

If clinically significant hearing loss is identified at a follow-up audiogram and the type and degree of surgical intervention or patient disease at the time of surgery cannot explain the loss, then unsuspected loss of ossicular chain integrity needs to be investigated. If a mild or moderate conductive loss is identified, the possibility of a lateralized tympanoplasty graft, or that incomplete tympanic membrane contact with the ossicular chain has developed, needs to be investigated. If a progressive conductive hearing loss is noted over months or years, recurrent cholesteatoma must also be suspected, even if it cannot be visualized on physical examination.

Canal Granulation Tissue

Granulation tissue in the external auditory canal may be encountered when epithelial tissue edges are exposed. Careful placement of ear canal packing at the time of the initial surgery can minimize this occurrence; however, when identified, it should be addressed early, usually in the office, with local debridement and selective cautery. In uncooperative children, this may need to be done in the operating room. Topical eardrops with a steroid component can assist resolution of small areas of granulation tissue. On occasion, even when granulation tissue has resolved, normal external canal epithelial migration is altered and ongoing maintenance may be required.

Acquired Canal Stenosis

On a rare occasion, exuberant canal scarring may result in acquired canal stenosis. This unfortunate outcome almost always requires surgical revision using mobilized flaps or free skin grafts.

Canal Dehiscence

The temporomandibular joint may be inadvertently exposed during surgery[55] involving the medial and anterior portion or the external auditory canal. If a small portion of joint perichondrium is exposed but no joint prolapse is identified, conservative management may be all that is necessary. Larger defects, however, may result in joint prolapse or exposure; then intervention is usually recommended in consultation with a temporomandibular joint specialist.

Taste Changes

If the chorda tympani nerve is overly stretched or cut, disruption in taste sensation and appreciation may develop. This is often described as a "metallic sensation." Although care should be taken to preserve the nerve whenever possible, if access to middle ear disease requires significant chorda tympani mobilization, sharp transection is preferable to a random tearing or shearing injury. Although nerve regeneration is possible,[56] return of completely normal taste sensation is uncommon even when the nerve is still intact; gradual accommodation is the most reasonable management plan.

Neck Injury/Positioning

In general, care should always be taken not to rotate the head and neck overmuch during otologic surgery. Particularly in Down syndrome children,[57] extreme neck extension should be avoided in order to minimize the potential for vertebral body subluxation injury.

Other

An unusual anatomic anomaly, such as an aberrant carotid artery in the middle ear,[58] may present catastrophic complications if not recognized. Cross innervation of the chorda tympani and Arnold's nerves within the middle ear may result in postoperative "gustatory otalgia."[59] In one unusual case (personal communication, DLW), an otherwise normal patient with a previously unidentified arterial brachiocephalic trunk anomaly developed a case-delaying pulsatile head vibration and carotid bruit when the head was overly rotated during ear surgery; turning the bed and not the patient's head would have avoided this problem.

PATIENT COMPLIANCE AND FAMILY COMMUNICATION

Children are sometimes very uncooperative patients. On occasion, they cannot be reasoned with. They will prematurely pull out ear canal packing and may excessively tug at their ears, which results in an incisional dehiscence. Even modest intervention, such as the placement of medicated eardrops, may become an emotionally consuming process for their parents. It is up to the otologic surgeon to work with the parents to find ways to accommodate the needs of their children while still maintaining adequate care during the recovery phase.

ERGONOMICS AND OPERATOR COMFORT

Otologic surgery requires the ability to focus on fine motor movements for an extended period of time. It is critical, therefore, for the surgeon to develop comfortable techniques to limit upper extremity and shoulder girdle movement in an ergonomically efficient manner. Additionally, a fair amount of potential stress can permeate and stiffen the entire body when one is working near the facial nerve, drilling out the semicircular canals, or manipulating around the stapes crurae, for example. The laterality of the operative ear and the position of teaching side arms and video camera, if used, should be considered before the procedure begins. The neck and lower spine are especially vulnerable to such protracted "mind and body" forces. The use of an adjustable chair at the right height and an operating microscope with inclinable eye-pieces and well-balanced articulating arms, as well as an operating table that can be easily adjusted, can provide the surgeon with a comfortable posture in which to work.

CONCLUSION

REASONABLE EXPECTATIONS

Key to successful long-term results in pediatric otology is the establishment of reasonable expectations within the family and the patient. They should be counseled about the range of outcomes for hearing improvement after tympanoplasty, with or without ossicular reconstruction, as well as the potential lifestyle changes that may need to be instituted after tympanoplasty or mastoidectomy.

It is just as critical for the proposed surgeon first to establish realistic expectations in himself. He must be comfortable with multiple techniques so as to be adaptable when appropriate and needs to assure his maintenance of skills and knowledge of the pediatric ear. Although most temporal bone laboratories exist within academic settings, many universities welcome the use of these facilities by affiliated and qualified private practice staff. The ongoing need for surgeon access to temporal bone "practice" facilities has also been at least partially met with a wide range of postgraduate temporal bone courses available throughout the year. In addition to didactic education, it is reasonable for the occasional but determined otologic surgeon to take advantage of these technical continuing education forums.

REFERENCES

1. Bluestone, C.D. and Klein, J.O. Intratemporal complications and sequelae of otitis media. In Bluestone, C.D., Stool, S.E., Kenna, M.A., Eds. *Pediatric Otolaryngology,* 3rd ed., Philadelphia: W.B. Saunders, 1996, 583–635.

2. Rizer, F.M. Overlay versus underlay tympanoplasty. Part II: the study. *Laryngoscope* 1997, 107, 26–36.

3. Levenson, M.J. Methods of teaching stapedectomy. *Laryngoscope* 1999, 109, 1731–1739.

4. Tos, M., Orntoft, S., and Stangerup, S.E. Results of tympanoplasty in children after 15 to 27 years. *Ann. Otol., Rhinol. Laryngol.* 2000, 109, 17–23.

5. Lancaster. J.L., Makura, Z.G.G., Porter, G., and McCormic, M. Pediatric tympanoplasty. *J. Laryngol. Otol.* 1999, 113, 628–632.

6. Megerian, C.A. Pediatric tympanoplasty and the role of preoperative eustachian tube evaluation. *Arch. Otolaryngol. Head Neck Surg.* 2000, 126, 1039–1041.

7. House, J.W., Toh, E.H., and Perez, A. Los Angeles, California, and Zapopan, Mexico. Diving after stapedectomy: clinical experience and recommendations. *Otolaryngol. Head Neck Surg.* 2001, 125, 356–60.

8. Vrabec, J.T., Deskin, R.W., and Grady, J.J. Meta-analysis of pediatric tympanoplasty. *Arch. Otolaryngol. Head Neck Surg.* 1999, 125, 530–534.

9. Rizer, F.M. Tympanoplasty: a historical review and a comparison of techniques. *Laryngoscope* 1997, 107, 1–36.

10. Smyth, G.D. and Toner, J.G. Mastoidectomy: canal wall down techniques. In Brackmann, D., Ed. *Otologic Surgery.* Philadelphia: W.B. Saunders, 1994, 225–240.

11. Gianoli, G.J., Worley, N.K., and Guarisco, J.L. Pediatric tympanoplasty: the role of adenoidectomy. *Otolaryngol. Head Neck Surg.* 1995, 113, 380–386.

12. Vartiainen, E. and Vartiainen, J. Tympanoplasty in young patients: the role of adenoidectomy. *Otolaryngol. Head Neck Surg.* 1997, 117, 583–585.

13. Bluestone, C.D. Myringoplasty and tympanoplasty. In Bluestone, C.D. and Rosenfeld, R.M., Eds. *Surgical Atlas of Pediatric Otolaryngology.* Hamilton, Ontario: B.C. Decker Inc., 2002, 1–19.

14. Shea, M.C. Tympanoplasty: the undersurface graft technique. In Brackmann, D., Ed. *Otologic Surgery.* Philadelphia: W.B. Saunders, 1994, 133–140.

15. Mojdehi, K. Pediatric anesthesia. In Bluestone, C.D. and Rosenfeld, R.M., Eds. *Surgical Atlas of Pediatric Otolaryngology.* Hamilton, Ontario: B.C. Decker Inc., 2002, 823–828.

16. Ashcraft, K.W. Pediatric surgery: surgical infectious disease, *Antibiotic Prophylaxis.* 118–119.

17. Jackson, C.G. Antimicrobial prophylaxis in ear surgery. *Laryngoscope* 1988, 98, 1116–1123.

18. Noss, R.S., Lalwani, A.K., and Yingling, C.D. Facial nerve monitoring in middle ear and mastoid surgery. *Laryngoscope* 2001, 111, 831–836.

19. O'Hare, T. and Goebel, J.A. Anterior subannular T-tube for long-term middle ear ventilation during tympanoplasty. *Am. J. Otol.* 1999, 20, 304–308.

20. Castelli, M.L., DiLisi, D., Marcato, P., Tavormina, P., Cappellaro, E., and Sartoris, A. Is pressure dressing necessary after ear surgery? *Ann. Otol., Rhinol. Laryngol.* 2001, 110.

21. Caylan, R., Titis, A., Falcioni, M., DeDonato, G., Russo, A., Taibah, A., and Sanna, M. Myringoplasty in children: factors influencing surgical outcome. *Otolaryngol. Head Neck Surg.* 1998, 118, 709–713.

22. Denoyelle, F., Roger, G., Chauvin, P., and Garabedian, E.N. Myringoplasty in children: predictive factors of outcome. *Laryngoscope* 1999, 109, 47–51.

23. Hamans, E.P.P.M., Govaerts, P.J., Somers, T., and Offeciers, F.E. Allograft tympoplasty type 1 in the childhood population. *Ann. Otol., Rhinol. Laryngol.* 1996, 105, 871–876.

24. Mitchell, R.B., Pereira, K.D., and Lazar, R.H. Fat graft myringoplasty in children — a safe and successful day-stay procedure. *J. Laryngol. Otol.* 1997, 111, 106–108.

25. Podoshin, L., Fradis M., Malatskey, S., and Ben-David, J. Type I tympanoplasty in children. *Am. J. Otol.* 1996, 17, 293–296.

26. Srinizasan, V., Toynton, S.C., and Mangat, K.S. Transtympanic myringoplasty in children. *Int. J. Pediatr. Otorhinolaryngol.* 1997, 39, 199–204.

27. Wehrs, R.E. Grafting techniques. *Otolaryngol. Clin. North Am.* 1999, 32, 443–455.

28. Te, G.O., Rizer, F.M., and Sshuring, A.G. Pediatric tympanoplasty of iatrogenic perforations from ventilation tube therapy. *Am. J. Otol.* 1998, 19, 301–305.

29. Dornhoffer, J.L. Surgical management of the atelectatic ear. *Am. J. Otol.* 2000, 21, 315–321.
30. Kriskovich, M. and Shelton, C. Surgical treatment of chronic otitis media and cholesteatoma. In Canalis, R.F. and Lambert, P.R., Eds. *The Ear. Comprehensive Otology.* Philadelphia: Lippincott Williams and Wilkins, 2000, 447–465.
31. Dornhoffer, J.L. Hearing results with cartilage tympanoplasty. *Laryngoscope* 107, 1094–1099, 1997.
32. Gerber, M.J., Mason, J.C., and Lambert, P.R. Hearing results after primary cartilage tympanoplasty. *Laryngoscope* 2000, 110, 1994–1999.
33. Sheehy, J.L. Tympanoplasty: the undersurface grafting technique. In Brackmann, D., Ed. *Otologic Surgery.* Philadelphia: W.B. Saunders, 1994, 121–132.
34. Mondain, M. and Ryan, A. Histological study of the healing of traumatic tympanic membrane perforation after basic fibroblast growth factor application. *Laryngoscope* 1993, 103, 312–318.
35. Eavey, R.D. Inlay tympanoplasty: cartilage butterfly technique. *Laryngoscope* 1998, 108, 657–661.
36. Bajaj, Y., Bais, A.S., and Mukherjee, B. Tympanoplasy in children — a prospective study. *J. Laryngol. Otol.* 1998, 112, 1147–1149.
37. Sperling, N.M. and Kay, D. Diagnosis and management of the lateralized tympanic membrane. *Laryngoscope* 2000, 110, 1987–1993.
38. Scally, C.M., Allen, L., and Kerr, A.G. The anterior hitch method of tympanic membrane repair. *ENT — Ear, Nose Throat J.* 1996, 75, 244–247.
39. Krupala, J.L., Gianoli, G.J., and Smith, R.A. The efficacy of hyaluronic acid foam as a middle ear packing in experimental tympanoplasty. *Am. J. Otol.* 1998, 195, 46–50.
40. Daniels, R.L., Rizer, F.M., Schuring, A.G., and Lippy, W.L. Partial ossicular reconstruction in children: a review of 62 operations. *Laryngoscope* 1998, 108, 1674–1681.
41. Lippy, W.H., Burkey, J.M., Schuring, A.G., and Rizer, F.M. Short- and long-term results of stapedectomy in children. *Laryngoscope* 1998, 108, 569–572.
42. Maceri, D.R. Stabilization of total ossicular replacement prosthesis in ossiculoplasty. *Laryngoscope* 1999, 109, 1884–1885.
43. Murphy, T.P. Hearing results in pediatric patients with chronic otitis media after ossicular reconstruction with partial ossicular replacement prostheses and total ossicular replacement prostheses. *Laryngoscope* 2000, 110, 536–544.
44. Schwetschenau, E.L. and Isaacson, G. Ossiculoplasty in young children with the applebaum incudostapedial joint prosthesis. *Laryngoscope* 1999, 109, 1621–1625.
45. Attallah, M.S. and Zakzouk, S.M. Iatrogenic incudostapedial joint dislocation in transcanal tympanoplasty. *Am. J. Otol.* 1999, 20, 199–201.
46. Glasscock, M.E. and Shambaugh, G.E. The simple mastoid operation. In *Surgery of the Ear,* 4th ed. Philadelphia: W.B. Saunders, 1996, 217–227.
47. Glasscock, M.E. and Shambaugh, G.E. The open cavity operations. In *Surgery of the Ear,* 4th ed. Philadelphia: W.B. Saunders, 1996, 229–247.
48. Bluestone, C.D. Mastoidectomy and cholesteatoma. In Bluestone, C.D. and Rosenfeld, R.M., Eds. *Surgical Atlas of Pediatric Otolaryngology.* Hamilton, Ontario: B.C. Decker Inc., 2002, 91–122.
49. Bluestone, C.D. Approaches to the middle ear and mastoid. In Bluestone, C.D. and Rosenfeld, R.M., Eds. *Surgical Atlas of Pediatric Otolaryngology.* Hamilton, Ontario: B.C. Decker Inc., 2002, 21–37.
50. Sheehy, J.L. Mastoidectomy: the intact canal wall procedure. In Brackmann, D., Ed. *Otologic Surgery.* Philadelphia: W.B. Saunders, 1994, 211–224.
51. Hashisaki, GT. Complications of chronic otitis media. In Canalis, R.F. and P.R. Lambert, P.R., Eds. *The Ear. Comprehensive Otology.* Philadelphia; Lippincott Williams and Wilkins, 2000, 433–445.
52. Greenberg, J.S. and Manolidis, S. High incidence of complications encountered in chronic otitis media surgery in a U.S. metropolitan public hospital. *Otolaryngol. Head Neck Surg.* 2001, 125, 623–627.
53. Wiet, R.J., Harvey, S.A., and Bauer, G.P. Management of complications of chronic otitis media. In Brackmann, D., Ed. *Otologic Surgery.* Philadelphia: W.B. Saunders, 1994, 251–256.
54. Manolidis, S. Complications associated with labyrinthine fistula in surgery for chronic otitis media. *Otolaryngol. Head Neck Surg.* 2000, 123, 733–737.
55. Nunn, D.R. and Strasnick, B. Temporormandibular joint prolapse after tympanoplasty. *Otolaryngol. Head Neck Surg.* 1997, 117, 169–171.
56. Saito, T. Incidence of regeneration of the chorda tympani nerve after middle ear surgery. *Ann. Otol., Rhinol. Laryngol.* 2002, 111, 357–363.

57. Todd, N.W., Holt, P.J., and Allen, A.T. Safety of neck rotation for ear surgery in children with Down syndrome. *Laryngoscope* 2000, 110, 1442–1445.
58. Chang, C.Y.J. Aberrant carotid artery of the middle ear. *Otolaryngol. Head Neck Surg.*, 122, 154, 2000.
59. Saito, H. Gustatory otalgia and wet ear syndrome: a possible cross-innervation after ear surgery. *Laryngoscope* 1997, 107, 1–36.

30 Cochlear Implantation

Adrien A. Eshraghi, Audie L. Woolley, Thomas J. Balkany, and Judith M. Barnes

Persons with cochlear implants must still be considered at increased risk for meningitis.

T.J. Balkany, M.D., N.L. Cohen, M.D., and W.L. Luxford, M.D.

CONTENTS

INTRODUCTION

Cochlear implantation has been established as a medical treatment for children with profound or severe-to-profound hearing loss who do not derive benefit from hearing aids. Multichannel cochlear implants first received FDA approval for use in children in 1990. The implant consists of external components and a surgically implanted internal device. The external portion of the device includes a microphone, microprocessor-based speech processor, and a radio frequency transmitting coil. The implanted portion houses a radio frequency receiver coil, microprocessor-based stimulator, and multichannel electrode array. Cochlear implants (CI) do not restore normal hearing, but provide access to sound at a level similar to that of less hearing-impaired patients who are successful hearing aid users.

Devices currently used in children in the United States include those manufactured by Advanced Bionics Corporation (Sylmar, California), Cochlear Corporation (Sydney, Australia) and MedEl Corporation (Innsbruck, Austria). Rapid progress has occurred in the last 5 years in speech processing technology. Although feature extraction strategies, which proved successful during the mid-90s, are still in use, continuous sampler strategies are now available in all three current devices, and one device offers an analog option as well (Clarion, Advanced Bionics). Loudness continues to be transmitted by the intensity of the electrical current in all strategies.

Young hearing-impaired individuals differ from their adult counterparts in that they depend on their implants to develop spoken language and thus require more prolonged habilitation. Although the vast majority of pediatric CI recipients are successful users, results vary. However, congenitally deaf and peri- and postlingually deafened children using implants have demonstrated development of listening and oral language abilities with adequate follow-up therapy, education, and active family support.

SOCIAL AND EDUCATIONAL ISSUES

THE DEAF COMMUNITY

Although cochlear implantation is an effective treatment option for profound deafness, to many deaf activists it represents unwanted technology that demeans and threatens their way of life. The American deaf community sees its way of life as emotionally fulfilling, promising, and independent. Organized attempts to suppress the use of cochlear implants, particularly in children, occurred throughout the 1990s, due to the opinion that if a large number of deaf children received cochlear implants, they would become part of mainstream society, and the deaf society, as we know it, could be diminished.

The ethical questions regarding cochlear implantation are concerned with who should make the decision whether an individual child should receive an implant and what the basis of the decision should be. Parents or legal guardians have the right and responsibility to exercise free informed consent on behalf of their child and their decisions should be based only on the best interests of their child.[1] As experience continues to demonstrate the safety and effectiveness of cochlear implants, many deaf organizations are moderating their opposition to the implantation of children.

EDUCATIONAL APPROACHES AND COMMUNICATION MODE

A strong family commitment to aural (re)habilitation is important to successful outcome with a CI. Educational environments for hearing-impaired children traditionally have been based on mode of communication.[2] The educational approaches and techniques in deaf education that have been developed for children with hearing loss include auditory/verbal, auditory/oral, sign language of the deaf, total communication, and cued speech.

- *Auditory/verbal* is a (re)habilitation approach that de-emphasizes lip-reading skills with emphasis on the development of auditory perception for spoken communication. Most children using this habilitative method are schooled with their normal-hearing peers.
- *Auditory/oral* emphasizes the development of listening skills to facilitate spoken language. Visual cues through lip reading and tactile cues may be used. With early amplification, this strategy usually is selected for children with severe hearing losses and many children with cochlear implants.
- *Sign language of the deaf,* specific to each country, is a totally visual and gestural system that provides no auditory input. Sign language of the deaf does not match the syntactic structure of English, as well as most other spoken languages, and is not used simultaneously with spoken language. Reading and writing are secondary. Proponents of this system are aligned with the deaf community. A reduced reading comprehension level is the norm for those educated in this system.
- *Total communication* is a common educational system in the U.S. for deaf children. Total communication involves attempts to use the gestural, lip-reading, and auditory components of speech — by combining signed English with spoken English, for example. Users must match the morpheme of spoken English with a sign or finger-spelled marker. This strategy has been associated with poorer results for spoken language with cochlear implant recipients than have auditory/oral methods.
- *Cued speech* is a method that uses hand cues to inform the child visually of the presence of auditory information during spoken communication. Cued speech transliterators may be used in the classroom to facilitate comprehension.

If cochlear implantation is to be considered, the auditory/oral or auditory/verbal approach may be indicated. If the total communication approach is selected, a strong emphasis on oral communication and auditory training are thought to be essential.

SURGICAL INDICATIONS

Avoidance of complications begins with good patient selection. Criteria for cochlear implantation in children have evolved substantially in the past 5 years; the minimum age for implantation has decreased and the acceptable level of residual hearing in children allowing implantation has increased. Cochlear implants were once restricted to children who were essentially anacoustic; those with even minimal amounts of residual hearing were considered borderline, and those with any open-set word recognition were not considered for candidacy. Experience has shown that children with more residual hearing often perform better with implants, and those with some measurable open-set speech recognition ability prior to implantation perform better with implants than do children without residual open-set word recognition.

Medical and radiological criteria have been expanded to include children with significant cochlear abnormalities in addition to other substantial medical conditions. Given these expansions, it is perhaps more important than ever that each case be considered individually by an experienced cochlear implant team consisting of an otolaryngologist, audiologist, speech–language pathologist, rehabilitation and educational professionals, psychologists, social workers, and any others deemed necessary for a specific case.[3]

SELECTION CRITERIA (2002)

In 2002, the established selection criteria for cochlear implants included

- One year of age or older
- Profound or severe-to-profound bilateral sensorineural hearing loss

- Little or no benefit from hearing aids for speech information
- No known medical contraindications for surgery
- Family support, motivation, and appropriate expectations
- (Re)habilitation support for development of oral language, speech, and listening.

The only absolute contraindications are agenesis of the inner ear (Michel syndrome) and absence of cochlear nerve.

AUDIOLOGIC ASSESSMENT

The audiologic evaluation is an essential means of determining suitability for cochlear implantation and should be performed by trained and experienced implant team audiologists. By itself, audiometric testing helps determine the degree of hearing loss, but does not establish a diagnosis. To do so requires evaluation of the whole child because the ear is part of the respiratory, circulatory, endocrine, immunologic, skeletal, and central nervous systems. Genetic evaluation is now possible and may be helpful in determining long-term expectations.

It is important to be able to obtain ear-specific auditory information in aided and unaided conditions. Obtaining this information in children, however, often requires therapeutic intervention and repeat visits. Testing young children in a sound booth, even with hearing aids, is not adequate to determine candidacy. Young children should be enrolled in a program of habilitation using their hearing aids for a period of months to determine benefit from amplification and therapy.

Evaluation of the benefits provided by amplification must be completed and can be accomplished through evaluation of speech perception abilities in the best aided condition, using age-appropriate tests, open set as well as closed set. For older children, the following tests may be used:

- Early Speech Perception (ESP) Test, Standard Version
- Glendonald Auditory Screening Procedure (GASP)
- Multisyllabic Lexical Neighborhood Test (MLNT)
- Lexical Neighborhood Test (LNT)
- Meaningful Auditory Integration Scale (MAIS)

For older children with more speech and language skills, appropriate sentence tests or the Northwestern Phonetically Balanced Kindergarten Test (PBK) might be administered. For younger children under the age of 5 years, the Early Speech Perception (ESP) Test, Low Verbal; the Infant-Toddler Meaningful Auditory Integration Scale (IT-MAIS); the GASP; and the MLNT may be used. For infants and toddlers under age 2, the IT-MAIS and ongoing diagnostic therapy are, perhaps, the best tools for evaluation of aided speech perception benefit.

HISTORY AND PHYSICAL EXAMINATION

Evaluation of candidacy for implantation should include assessment of the patient's general health and ability to undergo general anesthesia. A complete medical history and physical examination should be performed along with appropriate laboratory tests and imaging studies. Otoscopic evaluation of the tympanic membrane is performed, with special attention given to the status of the middle ear and any congenital malformations that might be associated with abnormal facial nerve position.

Children with all types of concurrent medical conditions are now being considered for cochlear implantation, and implant surgeons often find it necessary to consult with other specialists involved with the child's medical management. Ophthalmological opinion should be sought on these children in view of the potential for visual disorders, such as Usher's syndrome. If family history includes sudden cardiac death, electrocardiography should be carried out in order to exclude cardiac abnormalities such as those seen with Jervell–Lange–Nielson syndrome. Renal and skeletal abnormalities should also be considered.

PARENTAL EXPECTATIONS

In addition to the medical and audiological evaluation, assessment of parental expectations and support, hearing aid history, and anticipated compliance with the therapy process are important aspects of the evaluation of the very young child in consideration of cochlear implantation.

PREOPERATIVE PLANNING

COMPUTERIZED TOMOGRAPHY

Assessment of the temporal bone CT includes completing the following checklist:[4]

- Mastoid pneumatization
- Thickness of parietal bone
- Facial nerve
- Facial recess
- Cochlear anatomy
- Round window
- Vascular anatomy (carotid artery, sigmoid sinus, emissary veins)
- Cochlea and vestibular aqueduct
- Internal auditory canal

Computed tomography of the temporal bone is vital in helping the surgeon assess the feasibility of implantation in a particular candidate. It assists in the decision of the ear in which to implant and allows the surgeon to ensure that the inner ear morphology is normal, including patency of the cochlea. Congenital cochlear abnormalities do not necessarily preclude implantation, but need to be identified preoperatively in order to assist in the surgical planning.

MAGNETIC RESONANCE IMAGING

MRI is useful when

- IACs are less than 1.5 mm, to demonstrate the presence of the cochlear nerve.
- The CT demonstrates questionable ossification of the cochlea.
- Sclerosing labyrinthitis with soft tissue obliteration may not be accurately imaged by CT scan (the T2-weighted MRI will demonstrate loss of the endolymph/perilymph signal).

MANAGEMENT OF MIDDLE EAR EFFUSION

During presurgical assessment, the conductive component of the overall hearing loss needs to be corrected in order to ensure that only the cochlear loss is being assessed. Otitis media should be managed aggressively so as not to delay implantation. A noninfected ear is a preoperative prerequisite. Treatment may require parenteral antibiotics, insertion of ventilation tubes, and rarely, mastoidectomy with or without obliteration. It has been suggested that ventilation tubes be placed preoperatively in children with unremitting otitis media with effusion and left in place for spontaneous extrusion.[5] Others have suggested that ventilation tubes should normally be removed prior to surgery in order to have an intact tympanic membrane, thereby reducing the chance of a secondary middle ear infection in the immediate postoperative period.

SURGICAL TECHNIQUE

Cochlear implantation in the pediatric age group requires particular attention to the delicate tissues and small dimensions that can provide a challenge for even the most experienced otologic surgeon. Experience with CI surgery has led to the evolution and development of surgical techniques that can simplify the procedure and avoid complications. The cochlear implant surgeon should be familiar with the specific physical characteristics of the implantable electronic package and electrode array as well as the device-specific surgical techniques recommended to minimize complications.

Variations to the skin incision may be used; the limiting criteria are access to the mastoid process, coverage of the external portion of the implant package, and preservation of the blood supply of the postauricular skin. A complete mastoidectomy is performed, the horizontal semicircular canal and incus are identified, and the facial recess is opened. To ensure sufficient working room, one must be able to pass a 5F suction easily through the fascial recess anteriorly and inferiorly. In some cases, it may be necessary to sacrifice the chorda tympani nerve by creating an extended fascial recess. Working through the fascial recess, the round window niche is identified approximately 2 mm inferior to the stapes.

The round window niche may be obscured by an overlying fascial nerve in the vertical segment, by a prominent pyramidal eminence, or in some cases, by ossification. It is very important for the surgeon to realize the relationship of the round window to the stapes and the oval window because this prevents the surgeon from being misdirected by prominent hypotympanic air cells. Entry into the cochlea is carried out with a small fenestration placed anteriorly and slightly inferiorly to the annulus of the round window membrane to bypass the hook area of the scala tympani, thus allowing direct insertion of the active electrode array.

Returning to the mastoid cortex, the site of the template is drilled through the cortex and down to the inner table of the skull, creating as deep a well as possible so that the implant is adequately recessed. In very young children, some surgeons remove the inner table of the skull and the implant is placed directly on the dura. The surgeon should attempt to preserve the inner table of the skull and thin it down so that bone is able to be "egg shelled" over the dura.

The electrode and as many retaining rings as possible are inserted into the scala tympani through the cochleostomy. Specifically engineered insertion tools are available with some implant devices. Excessive force must not be used, particularly when inserting the long channel electrodes, because this may lead to damage of intracochlear tissue and kinking of the electrode. Routine anterior and posterior skull films should be obtained in the operating room prior to extubation to document electrode position and lack of electrode compression.

The cochleostomy is packed and sealed with fascia, preventing electrode migration and perilymphatic fluid leakage. The implant is then secured within the circular well in the cortex of the skull. The skin is closed in two layers. A drain may or may not be used.

INTRAOPERATIVE CONSIDERATIONS

COCHLEA OSSIFICATION

Ossification of the labyrinth in the scala tympani is a common complication in bacterial meningitis. In an earlier report of cochlear implants in children who were deafened by meningitis, 80% were noted to have some degree of ossification.[6] The degree and location of the cochlea ossification defines the surgical approach that should be taken.

If obstruction is limited to the inferior segment of the cochlea (the category of ossification most frequently seen following meningitis), the obstruction may be removed, or a tunnel may be created through the obstruction to reach an open window within the cochlea.[7] This technique is successful if obstruction is limited to 8 to10 mm measured from the round window membrane. In those cases, the new bone formation will be recognized as less dense and a lighter color. Following this bone anteriorly leads the surgeon into a patent scala tympani if the obstructed inferior segment is short. Complete electrode insertion is possible if the obstruction is limited to the inferior segment. Results in these cases are equivalent to those for implanted patients with patent cochlea.[7]

If obstruction extends apically into the ascending segment, the scala vestibuli can be opened by widening the cochleostomy 1 to 2 mm superiorly. Steenerson et al. have reported successful electrode insertion in the scala vestibuli of patients with obstruction of the scala tympani.[8] It is thought that meningogenic osteoneogenesis occurs through the cochlear aqueduct, which opens into the scala tympani. In some cases, ossification may be limited to the scala tympani, sparing the scala vestibuli.[9]

If the scala vestibuli is also obstructed, the only way to achieve a complete electrode insertion in the cochlea is to drill an open trough around the modiolus as described by Gantz et al.[10] This technique is performed by beginning with a radical mastoidectomy. The skin and mucosa are removed from the middle ear, including the tympanic membrane, malleus, and incus. Drilling begins by locating the carotid artery in the middle ear so that it can be identified and avoided. An inferior tunnel approximately 8 to 10 mm in depth is created at the usual site of the cochleostomy. Next, a second trough of approximately 6 to 8 mm in length is created anteriorly from the oval window and then the two troughs are connected by carefully drilling around the modiolus. Great care must be taken not to drill into the modiolus. Once the trough has been drilled around the modiolus, the electrode is curled into the trough and held into place by fascia and tissue glue. Although experience with this surgery is limited, the results of patients implanted by the Gantz procedure have been encouraging. More recently, split electrodes are also used for totally ossified cochlea. These electrodes feature two separate electrode branches and are designed for insertion into two drilled channels — one located at the lower basal coil, and the other placed into the cochlea in front of the oval window (interior and superior cochleostomy). The spiral ganglion cells and the modiolus are thus surrounded by the electrode array.

Although CT is quite helpful in identifying osteoneogenesis within the cochlea, it can also be misleading. Jackler et al. reported that a normal preoperative CT does not exclude the possibility of compromised cochlear patency.[11] In their series, a 48% false negative rate existed because of subtle degrees of osseous or fibrous obliteration of the cochlea that were beyond the recognition of CT.[11] In any child with postmeningitic deafness, the cochlear implant surgeon must be prepared to encounter some degree of ossification, even when CT is normal. MRI scans may be helpful in identifying soft tissue obstruction within the cochlea.

CONGENITAL INNER EAR MALFORMATIONS

In cochlea malformations, the cribiform area between the modiolus and the internal auditory canal is often very thin and may actually be absent. In the ear with an enlarged vestibular aqueduct, the endolymphatic sac may be significantly dilated, thus allowing potential communication with the cerebrospinal fluid (CSF) and increasing the risk of CSF fluid leak during the cochleostomy.[12] Malpositions of the facial nerve are also more common in patients with congenital inner ear malformations.

A "gusher" may be encountered and is managed by allowing the cerebrospinal fluid reservoir to drain off. Once the CSF leak slows, the electrode may be inserted into the cochlea, followed by packing around the cochleostomy with fascia and muscle. Although this usually seals the leak, occasionally a lumbar drain may be used to reduce the CSF reservoir until a satisfactory seal has occurred.

COMPLICATIONS IN IMPLANTING THE ANOMALOUS EAR

Until recently, profoundly deaf children suffering from bilateral inner ear malformations have not been implanted in many cochlear implant centers because of the complex process of evaluation, surgery, and rehabilitation. The malformation of the inner ear is no longer considered an absolute contraindication, although abnormal anatomy of the cochlea and facial nerve still raises concerns regarding safe and effective electrode insertion, which may affect expected benefit. Surgical concepts have been developed and specific solutions to problems encountered described.

If a well-pneumatized mastoid is present, a standard posterior approach is chosen. If middle ear structures and an intact vestibular system exist, these landmarks must be exposed and a standard facial recess approach is performed. A combined posteroanterior approach can be helpful when the promontory is flat. Fixation of the electrode is an important consideration when the internal bony architecture is incomplete or absent and the split-bridge technique of electrode insertion can be used to prevent extrusion. The superstructure of the stapes should always be preserved for stapedius reflex measurement, which is helpful for the exact electrode positioning and postoperative C-level fitting.

The direction of insertion of the electrode array depends on the preoperative CT scan. The array should not be directed toward osseous defects in order to minimize the danger of electrode misplacement. The cochleostomy should be as small as possible to facilitate sealing in case of a gusher. If a cerebrospinal fluid gusher occurs, it can be controlled with routine packing of the cochleostomy. In some cases, it may be necessary to obliterate the vestibule and middle ear with muscle and apply temporary packing to the eustachian tube. The insertion of the cochlear implantation electrode must be completed without inserting a lumbar cerebrospinal fluid drain so as to ensure watertight closure.[13]

In malformations consisting of incomplete partition (Mondini malformation), enlarged vestibule, or dilated vestibular aqueduct, routine cochleostomy and insertion of the electrode may be performed. In cochlear dysplasia of a more severe degree, also known as hypoplasia or common cavity, the basal turn is wide and the modiolus is absent. Additionally, the facial nerve may run in the lateral wall of the presumptive cochlea and, in some cases, obstruct the facial recess. In these situations, the electrode array may be inserted into an opening created in the lateral recess of the common cavity, roughly corresponding to the expected position of the ampullated limb of the lateral semicircular canal. Insertion in this area avoids the abnormal fascial nerve. A large cochleostomy (3 to 4 mm) is created and a loop of electrode is inserted if the multichannel electrode will not track smoothly around the periphery of the cavity. Cochlear endoscopy can be used to confirm electrode position. The entire cavity then is packed with fascia and/or muscle.

Fascial nerve monitoring is used primarily for safety reasons because atypical routing and split fascial nerves need to be anticipated, particularly in hypoplastic cochleas. Intraoperative information of fascial nerve stimulation may be relevant for electrode array positioning and the stimulation strategy. Postoperative fascial nerve stimulation can occur because of an atypical course of the facial nerve. This problem can be managed by reprogramming and C-level reduction. The option of intraoperative CT scans or x-rays should be available in case of atypical reaction to stimulation and to ensure correct electrode positioning.

REVISION SURGERY

Although histopathologic studies of insertion trauma have shown iatrogenic damage to the stria, spiral ligament, and organ of Corti, corresponding severe loss of spiral ganglion cells did not occur.[14] Survival of these ganglion cells, which are thought to be stimulated by cochlear implants, may in part explain the overall good results of reimplantation. Other important factors include the ease of removal and reinsertion of complex electrode arrays and the risk of complications such as skin breakdown, infection, facial nerve injury, or cerebrospinal fluid leakage following reimplantation.

Although most prior reimplantations have involved upgrading a single-channel to a multichannel device, several authors have commented on the safety of reimplantation of multichannel devices and found that hearing outcomes were as good as or better than those with the initial CI. However, Miyamoto et al., in their series, found reduced reinsertion lengths and number of activated channels following reimplantation but did not comment on hearing results.[15] In contrast, it has been reported that reimplantation with advanced technology suggests that outcomes can be as good as or better than those following the initial procedure, with increased reinsertion lengths and somewhat increased mean active channels.[16] Furthermore, in comparative tests of auditory-only, open-set speech recognition, significant postreimplantation improvement occurred.

POSTOPERATIVE COMPLICATIONS

Fortunately, complications with cochlear implantation done by experienced surgeons have been infrequent. Pooled data on 255 operations divided the complications in adults into major and minor.[17] The major complications were further subdivided into three groups: failure of the implant electrode (1.6%); problems requiring revision surgery (4.3%); and all other major complications such as hemorrhage, long-lasting facial palsy, and persistent perilymph leak (5.9%). This gave a major overall complication rate of 10.2%, which is similar to the figure of 9.5% quoted by Cohen and Hoffman.[18] In addition to these major complications, Summerfield and Marshall report the rate of minor complications to be 24%.[19] A minor complication, by definition, is one that can be overcome by medical or audiological management, including wound infection, nonauditory electrode stimulation, etc.

Data compiled by Hoffman and Cohen on 1905 children indicated that direct surgical complications occurred in fewer than 2% of the cases.[20] The most common was skin-flap problem in 1.75% of the cases. Fascial nerve injury at surgery occurred in 0.58%, postsurgical electrode migration in 1.31%, and fascial nerve stimulation in 0.94% of cases. In children, although the potential for complications from surgery is similar to that for adults, the most likely complications to occur are from nonsurgical causes. The most serious of these is device failure.

FLAP COMPLICATIONS

Among the most frequently encountered complications are those associated with the incision and postauricular flap. They continue to be the most common complications, although their rates have fallen from 5.44% in 1988 to 2.79% in 1995. Flap necrosis, flap infections, and delayed healing are the major flap complications, 55% of which require revision surgery.[20]

Flap necrosis and implant exposure may require explantation of the device. However, when limited exposure of a device occurs as a result of flap breakdown, coverage may be accomplished by rotation of a local flap or by anterior rotation of the implant. One adjunctive measure advocated to increase the viability of the flap in cases of compromise has been hyperbaric oxygen.

FASCIAL NERVE PALSY

Postoperative fascial nerve paresis has decreased from 1.74% in 1988 to 0.56% in 1995.[19] The lowering of complication rates is likely the result of better training in cochlear implant surgery and more experience among surgeons.

The fascial nerve is at risk of direct trauma during the facial recess approach to the mesotympanum. This nerve can be visualized through the thinned bone overlying the fallopian canal without actually uncovering it. A thin shell of bone covering the fascial nerve also provides a measure of protection from any required instrumentation performed through the fascial recess and may be helpful if revision surgery is needed. Delayed fascial paresis may be attributed to heat generated by the burr shaft. It is managed by administering oral prednisone and is usually resolved by 1 to 3 months.[21]

INFECTION

Concern was expressed at the theoretical possibility that infection might extend along the active electrode into the inner ear resulting in such complications as labyrinthitis meningitis. Before 2000, only one case of meningitis as a result of CI has been reported.[22] The tissue seal packed around the cochleostomy site creates an adequate seal of the cochleostomy created for insertion of the electrode array.

Recently, several cases of meningitis following cochlear implant surgery have been reported. The cause of these attacks of meningitis remains uncertain, but the FDA cites that the design of the implants and the surgical technique to implant them may be contributing factors. After investigating this possibility, one type of implant (i.e., CLARION Hi Focus II) has been identified as a possible source for this complication and has been removed from the market. The FDA report also suggested several other possible predisposing factors, such as a congenital malformation of the inner ear, otitis media, and the presence of an immunodeficiency disorder. They noted that patients with inner ear malformations are predisposed to meningitis even in the absence of a cochlear implant. Vaccines against the bacterial pathogens causing meningitis, i.e., *Streptococcus pneumoniae* and *Haemophilus influenzae,* should be administered to all patients who have, or will undergo a cochlear implantation procedure.

Some surgeons have recently begun sealing the cochleostomy with foreign materials, such as bone wax or fibrine glue. A case of otitis meningitis has recently been reported under those circumstances. We would suggest that soft tissue closure remains the appropriate method of sealing the cochleostomy.

The incidence of acute otitis media actually drops 35 to 60% in the implanted ear after surgery.[23] When middle ear effusion occurs in an ear in which a cochlear implant device has been previously placed, it is not absolutely necessary to manage with myringotomy tube placement. However, some CI surgeons still prefer to do so to avoid the potential risk for the development of acute otitis media.

INFECTED IMPLANT

If there is any evidence of systemic infection, such as meningitis, an infected implant must be removed. Milder infections may be treated in a more limited manner. A functioning multichannel implant is a substantial financial and personal investment. It should not be removed if appropriate corrective surgery with vascularized flaps and intravenous antibiotics can solve the problem safely.[24] However, if these treatment options are unsuccessful, the implant should be removed.

If the infection is confined to the receiver or stimulator device, one may simply remove that portion of the device and cut the electrode as it enters into the cochleostomy and then close the skin incisions. Once the infection has resolved and the scalp flaps are well vascularized and well healed, the surgeon may choose to reimplant this ear at a later date in a staged procedure in which implantation would be carried out by following the electrode array into the cochlea and then removing the old array at that time and replacing the array with a new implant. By leaving the old array in place, the track into the cochleostomy will remain patent and not become fibrosed during the healing time.

ELECTRODE COMPLICATIONS

At switch-on (first postoperative stimulation of the implant) and during subsequent reprogramming, electrodes can, in some patients, be found to be nonfunctional or to be performing suboptimally. The offending or nonfunctioning electrodes may be turned off and the device programmed to take full advantage of the working electrodes. The most common reason for an electrode to require deactivation has been found to be facial nerve stimulation; poor sound quality and pain are also very common. Other reasons include absence of auditory stimulation, vibration, reduced dynamic range, throat sensations, absence of loudness growth, or dizziness.[25]

DEVICE FAILURE

Device failure has been seen in 4 to 10% of cases depending on device,[26] although manufacturer changes in implant design over the past few years have resulted in a decrease in device failure rates. Children may have an increased risk for device failure in part because of their high level of activity with the potential for traumatic injury to the internal receiver or stimulator. Device failure produces considerable psychological trauma to parents and child. In addition, it causes a period with decreased or absent auditory stimulation at a time when a child is learning to hear.

FOLLOW-UP CONSIDERATIONS

SURGICAL FOLLOW-UP

Surgery may take from 1.5 to 3.0 hours, and the patients are planned for discharge to home on the day following surgery. The first postoperative visit is at 1 week to check the wound. The next follow-up is approximately 4 to 6 weeks later, after flap edema has resolved, and the fitting and the mapping of the signal processor can begin. There is, then, considerable lag time before positive results can be identified. It is important, therefore, to establish reasonable expectations clearly with the patient and family before proceeding with surgery.

COMMITMENT TO REHABILITATION

Potential pitfalls over the long-term continue to exist. It can be argued that successful implantation depends on the ages of onset of deafness and implantation, innate intelligence of the child, the number of surviving ganglion cells, the commitment of the parents, and the socioeconomic status of the family unit.[26] However, lack of expected progress of a child may be an indication of partial device failure. In children with ossification or fibrosis of cochlea, delayed stimulation may occur. Aural rehabilitation is a life-long commitment. Some children, especially teenagers, may become nonusers of the implant due to incorrect educational placement or as a result of a change in their emotional disposition to having an implant. It is to the benefit of the child/adolescent patient to have an intact cochlear team throughout his or her educational years.

CONCLUSION

Cochlear implantation has become a recognized treatment option for severe to profound and profoundly deaf children and advances in technology will only increase the accessibility of this successful procedure. Complications, however, continue to occur following cochlear implantation. Methods of avoidance include good patient selection and radiological assessment, proper surgical and device-specific training, identification and protection of facial nerve during posterior tympanotomy, adequate cochleostomy, and gentle electrode insertion. Surgical management of the ossified cochlea and inner ear malformation demands expert knowledge and surgical technique for successful implantation. Device failure does occur and must be evaluated by the manufacturer so that prompt corrective action may be applied to future production. Nonsurgical difficulties may arise and present problematic circumstances for the nonsurgical members of the implant team. These include delayed stimulation, incorrect educational placement, and disruption of coordinated postcochlear implant therapeutic services throughout childhood and adolescence.

REFERENCES

1. Balkany, T., Hodges, A.V., and Goodman, K.W. Ethics of cochlear implantation in young children. *Otolaryngol. Head Neck Surg.* 1999, 121, 673–675.
2. Barker, E.J., Dettman, S.J., and Dowell, R.C. Habilitation: infants and young children. In Clark, G.M., Cowan, R.S.C., and Dowell, R.C., Eds. *Cochlear Implantation for Infants and Children: Advances.* San Diego: Singular Pulishing; 1997, 171–190.
3. Zwolen, T.A., Zimmerman-Phillips, S., Ashbaugh, C.J. et al. Cochlear implantation of children with minimal open set speech recognition skills. *Ear Hear* 1997, 18, 240–251.

4. Woolley, A.L., Orser, A.B., Lusk, R.P., and Bahadori, R.S. Preoperative temporal bone computed tomography scan and its use in evaluating the pediatric cochlear implant candidate. *Laryngoscope* 1999, 107, 1100–1106.

5. Papsin, B.C., Bailey, C.M., Albert, D.M. et al. Otitis media with effusion in pediatric cochlear implantees: the role of peri-implant grommet insertion. *Int. J. Pediatr. Otolaryngol.* 1996, 38, 13–19.

6. Eisenberg, L., Luxford, W., Becker, T., and House, W. Electrical stimulation of the auditory system in children deafened by meningitis. *Otolaryngol. Head Neck Surg.* 1984, 92, 700–705.

7. Balkany, T., Bird, P., Hodges, A.V. et al. Surgical technique for implanting the ossified cochlea. *Laryngoscope* 1998, 108, 988–992.

8. Steenerson, R., Gary, L., and Wynens, M. Scala vestibuli cochlear implantation for labyrinthine ossification. *Am. J. Otol.* 1990, 11, 360–363.

9. Green, J., Jr., Marion, M., and Hinojosa, R. Labyrinthitis ossificans: histiopathologic considerations for cochlear implantation. *Otolaryngol. Head Neck Surg.* 1991, 104, 320–326.

10. Gantz, B., McCabe, B., and Tyler, R. Use of multichannel cochlear implants in obstructed in obliterated cochlea. *Otolaryngol. Head Neck Surg.* 1997, 98, 72–81.

11. Jackler, R., Luxford, W., Schindler, R., and McKerrow, W. Cochlear patency problems in cochlear implantation. *Laryngoscope* 1987, 97, 801–805.

12. Hirsch, B.E., Weissman, J.L., Curtin, H.D., and Kamer, D.B. Magnetic resonance imaging of the large vestibular aqueduct. *Arch. Otolaryngol. Head Neck Surg.* 1992, 118, 1124–1127.

13. Luntz, M., Balkany, T.J., and Hodges, A.V. Cochlear implants in children with congenital inner ear malformations. *Arch. Otolaryngol. Head Neck Surg.* 1997, 123, 974–977.

14. Fayad, J., Linthicum, F.H., Jr., Otto, S.R., Galey, F.R., and House, W.F. Cochlear implants: histopathologic findings related to performance in 16 human temporal bones. *Ann. Otol. Rhinol. Laryngol.* 1991, 100, 807–811.

15. Miyamoto, R.T., Svirsky, M.A., Myres, W.A., Kirk, K.I., and Schulz, J. Cochlear implant reimplantation. *Am. J. Otol.* 1997, 18, 560–561.

16. Balkany, T.J., Hodges, A.V., Gomez-Marin, O. et al. Cochlear reimplantation. *Laryngoscope* 1999, 109, 351–355.

17. Proops, D.W., Stoddart, R.L., and Donaldson, I. Medical, surgical and audiological complications of the first 100 adult cochlear implant patients in Birmingham. *J. Laryngol. Otol.* 1999, 24, 14–17.

18. Cohen, N.L. and Hoffman, R.A. Surgical complications of multichannel cochlear implants in North America. In Fraysse, B. and Deguine. O., Eds. *Cochlear Implants: New Perspectives. Advances in Otolaryngology.* Karger Basel, Switzerland, 1993, 70–74.

19. Summerfield, A.Q. and Marshall, D. Cochlear implantation in the U.K. 1990–1994. Report by the MRC Institute of Hearing Research on the Evaluation of the National Cochlear Implant Programme. Main report. HMSO 1995, 191–198.

20. Hoffman, R.A. and Cohen, N.L. Complications of cochlear implant surgery. *Ann. Otol. Rhinol. Laryngol.* (Suppl.), 1995, 166, 420–422.

21. Miyamoto, R.T., Young, M., Myres, W.A., Kessler, W.K., and Kirk, K.I. Complications of pediatric cochlear implantation. *Eur. Arch. Otorhinolaryngol.* 1996, 253, 1–4.

22. Daspit, C.P. Meningitis as a result of a cochlear implant: case report. *Otolaryngol. Head Neck Surg.* 1991, 105, 115–116.

23. House, W., Luxford, W., and Courtney, B. Otitis media in children following cochlear implantation. *Ear Hear* 1985, 6, 24S–26S.

24. Rubinstein, J.T., Gantz, B.J., and Parkinson, W.S. Management of cochlear implant infections. *Am. J. Otol.* 1999, 20, 46–49.

25. Stoddart, R.L. and Cooper, H.R. Electrode complications in 100 adults with multichannel cochlear implants. *J. Laryngol. Otol.* 1999, 24, 18–20.

26. Luetje, C.M. and Jackson, K. Cochlear implants in children: what constitutes a complication. *Otolaryngol. Head Neck Surg.* 1997, 117, 243–247.

31 Microtia and Atretic Ear Surgery

Roland D. Eavey and Paul Lambert

The mere formulation of a problem is often far more essential than its solution. To raise new questions, new possibilities, to regard old problems from a new angle, requires creative imagination and marks real advances in science.

Albert Einstein

CONTENTS

GENERAL INTRODUCTION

Although they often occur together, microtia and canal atresia may occur independently. Therefore, the two topics are discussed individually within this chapter. Microtia reconstructive surgery will be discussed first, followed by aural atresia surgery because correction proceeds in that order.

INTRODUCTION TO MICROTIA RECONSTRUCTIVE SURGERY

The focus of this section is prospective considerations toward optimization of the eventual result. Unexpected outcomes can occur; however, preoperative and intraoperative anticipation will be emphasized.

Once the infant has undergone an ear examination and hearing measurement, counsel should be given to the parents regarding surgical reconstruction of the malformed ear. Part of the counsel should be to stress patience.[1,2] The parents may feel uncomfortable because well-intentioned friends and relatives might urge them to have this malformation repaired as soon as possible. For example, one could be tempted at least to start by elimination of seemingly extraneous tissue. The malformed ear should not be amputated as a "first stage" because this scars the area and removes invaluable tissue that will be used for eventual reconstructive purposes. Also, ideally, skin tags should not be removed except by the surgeon who will eventually perform the entire corrective procedure.

If classical rib reconstruction is elected, the timing for the surgery is approximately 6 years of age. Occasionally, a particularly large child can have an ear operated on by the age of 5 years. There is certainly no rush to correct the ear because (1) the surgeon needs to have sufficient cartilaginous rib in order to reconstruct an adult sized ear and (2) the contralateral normal ear does not usually reach near adult proportions until approximately the age of 6 years.

It is also unnecessary to get a CT scan to evaluate the middle and inner ear status because early acquisition of this information will not provide an accurate map for the later otologic effort. This will be discussed later in this chapter. For the exceptional situation of a child with only a moderate auricular malformation, earlier reconstruction might be able to be performed. However, a surgeon very experienced with this type of work should make the decision, rather than the occasional surgeon, because a moderate malformation will require unique reconstructive techniques customized for that particular child.

The external ear reconstruction effort should precede the aural atresia repair because the aural atresia effort will violate the skin, causing scarring that makes microtia reconstruction efforts more difficult and may necessitate a temporoparietal fascia graft procedure, which otherwise would not have been necessary. Another reason, more importantly for the aural atresia repair, is that maintenance of a patent meatus is assisted by having a circumferential cartilaginous rim from the earlier microtia repair rather than mere soft tissue, which can stenose with healing. Again, in rare circumstances with moderate microtia and a canal stenosis, one of the authors (R.D.E.) has performed the canal procedure and microtia procedures simultaneously, but that circumstance is truly the exception.

CLASSICAL RIB RECONSTRUCTION

Several illuminating works about details of reconstruction techniques are available.[3–10] Conventional microtia classification is labeled as type I, type II, and type III. Unfortunately, the system is vague on details for reconstruction efforts. For example, if the patient has hemifacial microsomia, the ear position will appear to rise as the mandible is vertically distracted. The presence of even a diminutive external auditory canal will limit auricular positioning. The level of the hairline, amount of rudimentary cartilage, and presence of skin tags will contribute to reconstructive decisions.[11]

To obtain the rib, a small incision should be used to decrease morbidity as well as improve cosmetic appearance of the chest. The incision is approximately 4 to 5 cm in length rather than the traditional 9 to 10 cm. The underlying rectus muscle should not be divided, but instead retracted, thus preventing later indentation from the divided muscle healing with a linear constriction at the division site. This also prevents the ipsilateral ribs from flaring months later, which can mimic the appearance of premature unilateral breast development. To avoid pneumothorax, care should be taken when dissecting the interior surface of the rib. Entry into the pleura is common because the tissue is tenuous and thin; nevertheless, pneumothorax is preventable. The opening into the pleura can be easily handled by a purse-string suture around a catheter withdrawn under a vacuum. A chest x-ray in the operating room indicates the absence of pneumothorax.

The rib is maintained in a bowl of sterile saline into which antibiotics have been placed as a prophylactic measure to prevent potential postoperative infection, which is rare, but may require intravenous antibiotics. Storing the rib in saline also prevents desiccation. Carving the rib to fabricate the ear framework should never be attempted unless the surgeon feels extremely comfortable with this procedure. Serious practice on various materials should occur before the surgeon ever tries live human rib. Materials such as supermarket rib from a bovine or a porcine source can be helpful, especially if cartilaginous rather than osseous rib is available. Soap can be carved. Vegetables such as potatoes and carrots can be used. Cadaveric rib, if available, can also be carved to provide a more realistic practice experience.

The process to reconstruct an ear is extremely complicated and the surgeon should not be in a situation in the operating room sitting with a textbook or an atlas trying to review the next steps. Because microtia reconstruction is an art form, hopefully the surgeon will have shifted somewhat from the left-brain type of surgery of basic training programs, which recapitulates work that has been done by others, to the right brain, which adds the dimension of creativity.

The skin pocket actually can be more challenging to create than the carving of the rib. The standard incision is placed anterior to the actual ear site. It is advisable first to demarcate the superficial temporalis artery in order to preserve this vessel. An alternative, less obvious incision can be made in the scalp; however, the dissection in the cephalad–caudad direction is more challenging because of the distance required. Skin thickness is best gauged by using the thickness of the skin over the malformed cartilaginous remnant. There is no automatic tissue plane, so dissecting initially to the cartilaginous remnant and continuing the thickness of the skin as one extends well beyond the remnant is a very helpful maneuver. If the skin covering is too thick, detail will be lost in the final result; if it turns out too thin, necrosis is a possibility. The pocket should be overly generous so that the skin can co-apt into the three-dimensional convolutions that have been carved into the rib because the previously two-dimensional skin will need sufficient laxity to cover three-dimensional contours.

Placement of the rib framework will require preoperative measurements. In most patients, the microtia is unilateral. Measurements from the other ear can be obtained for the overall dimensions. The position of the ear relative to the lateral canthus to the lobule as well as to the helical root should be obtained. The position on the side of the head relative to the eyebrow will have been noted (usually the cephalad position of the auricle corresponds to the lateral aspect of the eyebrow, but occasionally the ear can sit a bit more cephalad or a bit more caudad by a few millimeters). The auricular axis on the side of the head approximates the dorsum of the nose, although it is actually more vertical and should be noted preoperatively.

Ear placement relative to a symmetric jaw is an evolving process. Historically, when jaw reconstruction techniques were laborious and substantial, the family might have deferred on jaw reconstructive surgery. In that situation, the ear could not be placed by measurement but instead would need to be placed by aesthetics. Today, using contemporary distraction osseogenesis techniques, the jaw can be expanded dramatically in days with much less morbidity. Position of the ear now becomes dynamic because the auricle, in relation to the mandible, will seem to move on the side of the head as the jaw is expanded. Therefore, it is ideal for the oral surgeon to expand on the jaw as the ear surgeon reconstructs the pinna in order to attempt to optimize eventual placement. If ear placement later proves suboptimal, repositioning would be a substantial procedure.

Once the framework is placed in the skin pocket, drainage becomes important. Two vacuum butterfly drains are adequate to (1) evacuate blood and (2) maintain suction of the skin into the carved ear convolutions. If the skin appears blanched with the suctioning, the framework can be removed and shaved lower or the skin pocket can be enlarged to help avoid skin necrosis.

Pain medications can be provided by intravenous patient-controlled analgesia (PCA). We have used PCA on patients as young as 6 years without any difficulties. Early mobilization with attention to keeping compression against the lower chest helps to prevent pulmonary issues such as atelectasis and helps the patient with earlier and easier discharge.

Postoperatively, the ear can be examined easily and the dressing changed more comfortably if it is not a conventional gauze mastoid dressing. Instead, the gauze is held on with an external wrap of neoprene and Velcro design. This quick wrap makes it easier for the patient because dressing change does not involve cutting with bandage scissors and then extensive rewrapping with gauze requiring the patient to sit and be still for a considerable period. This can be uncomfortable when the patient has undergone chest surgery the day before.

Inspection of the ear is helpful to check the color and capillary refill of the skin. Usually, there will be expected color changes merely because the patient has undergone surgery in the area. Rarely, the ear can look slightly dusky. Hyperbaric oxygen is helpful to improve the color of the ear if the skin appearance is worrisome. Occasionally, the skin over the framework can break down, even after a considerable period of time. Usually, a small region (e.g., the size of a pencil diameter) need not be treated because the area will re-epithelize with minimal cosmetic alteration. If more extensive skin breakdown occurs, on a case-by-case basis, it may be necessary to consider whether a flap should be rotated to cover the exposed cartilage.

At the next operative stage, the goal is to create a rotation flap of soft tissue from the inferior aspect of the microtic ear into an earlobe. To avoid vascular compromise, the base should not be too narrow. The tissue must be tailored in order to fit nicely into the descending helix of the cartilage implant, which is already under the skin from the previous operation. Care must be taken that the new lobule does not angle out horizontally from the side of the head rather than hanging down. Care must also be taken that a space is available behind the lobe so that an earring can be placed as necessary; usually a hoop earring design is superior to a straight post style of earring for the reconstructed lobe. This can be placed after reconstruction has been completed.

Occasionally, the preauricular incision of stage 1 or the lobule rotation incisions of stage 2 can create hypertrophic scarring. Rather than early use of steroids or re-excision, the surgeon should strongly consider allowing the scar to fade over a couple of years before deciding if active management is necessary.

The skin graft necessary to create a postauricular sulcus will cause a scar from the donor site. Less donor skin will be necessary if the superior and lateral surfaces of the reconstructed ear have undergone laser treatment to remove scalp hair. Usually, a variable portion of the reconstructed ear is covered by hair-bearing scalp from the first stage because of the necessity to place a three-dimensional ear framework under two-dimensional skin. When skin grafting is done on the lateral aspect of the ear, the skin can look unnatural by color match and texture and has a tendency, perhaps, to look a bit shiny compared with the dull luster of natural auricular skin. The laser treatment may need to be repeated so that the skin on the lateral and superior surface of the ear will look natural.

For the sulcus creation, the skin graft site should be chosen with care; various surgeons have different preferences. Groin skin has been advocated. The advantage is that the incision site can fit more or less into the groin crease. However, pubic hair can grow later and the skin will need to be regrafted.

Conventionally, a dermatome can be used to shave skin from the buttock and upper thigh. If the donor site heals nicely, this technique can be an excellent way to obtain skin. However, if the patient heals with a hypertrophic scar or keloid, the donor site will appear unsightly. Ultra thin skin from the scalp has been used. The theory is that the hair follicles are deeper than the graft and will later regrow and there will be no visible donor site. However, the theoretical downside would be that a large, bald scar would be created if the graft were too deep. Someday artificial skin may be helpful. Currently, one of the authors (R.D.E.) uses full-thickness skin from over the lumbar spine area, which is closed in a vertical linear fashion. The patient cannot see the scar and the site is synonymous with the location expected for spinal surgery, so an observer is less likely to perceive the scar as a graft site. After surgery, prophylactic antibiotic ear drops are drizzled into the postauricular sulcus to assist with healing.

The construction of a tragus can be performed as an additional stage or, in older patients who have more cartilage with which to work, can be done at the first stage. Creation at the initial stage obviously reduces morbidity.

RELATED ISSUES

In patients who have only moderate microtia, use of the rib technique can be excessisve surgery. To minimize morbidity, one of the authors prefers to harvest contralateral conchal bowl cartilage and postauricular skin and then recreate a customized ear on a case-by-case basis. The procedure can be performed in only one or two stages, the ear feels very natural, and usually, no visible scars are left. Details of the surgery will not be described because each ear is an individual creation.

In the future, the tissue engineering of an auricle is a hopeful possibility to enhance results and to diminish morbidity further. Currently, this technique has been symbolized by the image of the "mouse with an ear on its back." The procedure would consist of obtaining a piece of the patient's cartilage, expanding the number of chondrocytes, placing those chondrocytes into a scaffold shaped like an ear, and implanting the ear into the patient.[12-16]

CONCLUSIONS TO MICROTIA SURGERY

Variables from patient to patient affect the final outcome. With microtia surgery, a major concept is the initial configuration of the malformed ear, which varies among individuals. Less available tissue makes the surgery more challenging and can adversely influence the outcome. Healing differences between individuals also can influence the result. Therefore, variations in outcome do not necessarily reflect skill fluctuations — especially when the same surgeon performs each case — and should not be considered a complication in the conventional sense. The situation in congenital microtia and aural atresia surgery differs from surgery for acquired conditions. With congenital absence, the surgeon tries to recreate anatomy that has never been present in order to provide a better result to the patient and his family, despite these difficulties.

INTRODUCTION TO ATRESIA SURGERY

Advances in radiographic imaging are improving selection of patients for congenital aural atresia surgery. Similarly, improved microsurgical techniques are optimizing the potential for hearing restoration. Despite these advances, however, the otologist's clinical acumen and surgical skills are frequently challenged. Intraoperative complications, such as facial nerve or labyrinthine injury, and postoperative complications, including canal stenosis, chronic infection, and recurrent conductive hearing loss, must be carefully considered relative to the potential benefits of surgery. This chapter will review the concepts and protocols of the preoperative evaluation, surgical procedure, and postoperative care of patients with congenital aural atresia that are helpful in minimizing the possibility of complications and maximizing the potential for hearing restoration.

EPIDEMIOLOGY AND CLASSIFICATION

Atresia of the ear canal with associated middle ear anomalies can occur in isolation or in association with microtia and/or craniofacial dysplasia. The reported incidence is 1 in 10,000 to 20,000 births.

Although genetic transmission occurs in many of the syndromes that include aural atresia, such as Treacher–Collins syndrome, it is rare in cases of isolated atresia. Aural atresia is bilateral in approximately one third of cases, and each side can vary in complexity.

Patients with congenital aural atresia are classified on the basis of auricular development and external canal/middle ear development. Deformity of the auricle is straightforward and is divided into three grades: grade I is a normal ear; grade II has some of the auricular framework present but an obvious deformity is noted; and grade III is the classic "peanut ear" deformity. Microtia has been discussed earlier in this chapter.

Ombredanne proposed dividing congenital aural atresia into major and minor malformations in which the primary difference is patency of the external canal in the minor group.[17] In the major malformation group, the membranous external canal is absent or ends in a pinpoint fistula-like opening. The bony canal is usually absent because the compact tympanic bone failed to recanalize; occasionally, a rudimentary bony canal is apparent. The tympanic membrane is absent and the middle ear space is reduced in size. The malleus and incus are deformed and fused, with the short process of the malleus typically attached to the atretic bone. In the most severe major cases, the middle ear cavity is represented only by a small cleft and no ossicles are discernable.

In the minor malformation category, the tympanic bone and eardrum are developed, but the external canal is usually smaller than normal, as is the tympanic membrane. Complex middle ear abnormalities may be present, including absence, deformity, or fixation of one or more of the ossicles.

PATIENT EVALUATION

Most cases of major congenital ear malformations are apparent at birth because of the microtia or other craniofacial deformity. Patients with normal or only slight microtia and a stenotic or blindly ending external canal may escape diagnosis for years. Unilateral minor congenital ear malformations with a relatively normal ear canal and tympanic membrane can be even more difficult to diagnose because they are discovered only with routine hearing screening in school. When the surgeon is initially confronted with an infant or young child with microtia and aural atresia, the principal objectives include

- Assessment of hearing status and the need for amplification
- Formulation of a treatment plan for the auricular malformation
- Acquisition of radiographic data necessary to determine candidacy for atresia repair
- Audiometric evaluation

Atresia of the external ear canal can be expected to cause a 50- to 60-dB conductive hearing loss. In most cases, sensorineural function is normal. In unilateral cases, routine behavioral audiometry can be used, although auditory brainstem response (ABR) testing may be necessary in young infants or children.

Patients with bilateral atresia present a masking dilemma. It is still possible, however, to obtain information on the cochlear function of each ear. This information is important in order to prevent operating on a patient's only hearing ear or, conversely, on an ear with little or no potential for hearing improvement. Wave I of the auditory brainstem response is generated by the distal portion of the auditory nerve and is best measured by a recording electrode ipsilateral to the stimulated ear. Because there is minimal crossover of the wave I response from the contralateral ear, it is possible to present a bone stimulus and obtain ear-specific information. When recording is conducted simultaneously from both ears with surface electrodes, the recorded wave I response represents primarily the activity from the underlying cochlea.

COMPUTED TOMOGRAPHY

High-resolution CT scans in the coronal and axial planes are the most important diagnostic test for determining surgical candidacy. Timing of the CT is dictated primarily by the timing of the surgical procedure. Radiographic studies on infants are not recommended because the information is rarely applicable to immediate rehabilitative plans. A CT is typically obtained at approximately 5 years of age. A grading system assessing CT anatomy has been developed.[18] Critical elements to be examined include the size of the middle ear space and the anatomy of the ossicles. In general, the risk for surgical complications is minimized, and the chances for successful hearing increased, if the size of the middle ear is at least two thirds of normal. A fused and malformed malleus–incus complex should be identified, and an intact stapes and patent oval window documented. Although normal development of the cochlea and vestibular labyrinth is anticipated, their appearance on the CT scans should be noted.

Rarely, a cholesteatoma can occur in association with congenital aural atresia. This occurs in cases in which sufficient canalization of the medial external canal has occurred, and the lateral end of the canal remains atretic or stenotic. Cholesteatoma formation typically does not develop in the first 3 or 4 years of life; thus, delaying the CT until age 5 in otherwise asymptomatic patients is reasonable.

HEARING AMPLIFICATION

Unilateral Atresia

No immediate intervention is necessary in a young child discovered to have unilateral atresia if hearing in the contralateral ear is normal. Little or no functional disability with regard to speech and language development is anticipated. A bone conduction hearing aid for the atretic ear is poorly accepted by most children and is thus not recommended. Preferential seating in school is advised.

Bilateral Atresia

Early amplification is essential in infants with bilateral atresia. Ideally, a bone conduction hearing aid is fitted within the first 3 to 4 months of life. For older children with bilateral atresia who do not meet the selection criteria for surgery, a bone-anchored hearing aid instead of the conventional bone-conduction aid can be considered.

SURGICAL MANAGEMENT

GENERAL CONSIDERATIONS

Controversy continues regarding operative intervention in patients with unilateral atresia. Reasons cited include difficulty in achieving consistent hearing improvement and the risks, especially to the facial nerve. The issue is not simply the unilateral hearing loss because there is little controversy involving middle ear exploration for a child with a maximum conductive hearing loss from other causes.

To place the preceding concerns in perspective, the following data should be kept in mind. Studies have shown that properly selected candidates for reconstruction can be expected to obtain an average gain in the pure-tone average (PTA) of 25 to 30 dB with 40% of patients achieving a postoperative PTA of ≤ 20 dB and 70% a PTA of ≤ 30 dB. Approximately 85% of these patients maintain these initial hearing results, although revision surgery may be needed in as many as one third of all cases.[2] For surgeons experienced with atresia surgery, the risks of facial nerve injury or sensorineural hearing loss is small, approximating that encountered during mastoid and middle ear surgery for cholesteatoma. It should be emphasized that the selection process is critical, and that approximately 40% of patients with unilateral atresia are not surgical candidates.

Selection criteria for patients with bilateral atresia are slightly less stringent than for unilateral cases. In contradistinction to ear selection for most otologic disorders, the better ear (as determined by CT evaluation) is selected for the initial surgical procedure.

Atresia surgery, whether the patient has a unilateral or bilateral problem, is performed near the time at which the child enters the first grade. At this age, accurate audiometric tests can be performed and most children are able to cooperate with the postoperative care. This timing also allows most of the multistaged microtia repair to be accomplished.

SURGICAL TECHNIQUE

Most atresia surgery is done using an anterior approach in which the middle ear is exposed directly through the atretic bone with limited opening into the mastoid ear cells. This approach prevents a mastoid cavity with its attendant problems of debris accumulation and infection.

Landmarks for drilling the external canal include the middle cranial fossa dural plate superiorly, the temporomandibular joint anteriorly, and the mastoid ear cells posteriorly. The bone removed is usually solid but may be cellular in areas. It is important to keep the posterior wall of the glenoid fossa (anterior wall of the new ear canal) as thin as possible to allow access to the anterior half of the middle ear space. It is also critical to enter the middle ear in the epitympanum, where the fused heads of the malleus and incus will be the first middle ear landmarks identified. This can be accomplished by following the middle fossa dural plate medially. The advantage of this technique is that the facial nerve is not put at jeopardy, because it always lies medial to the ossicular mass in the epitympanum. Care must be exercised in drilling the posterior inferior portion of the ear canal, however, because of the more anterior and lateral course of the vertical segment of the facial nerve in this area.

After the heads of the ossicles are exposed, the bone overlying the middle ear space is thinned, and then carefully removed with a small right-angle instrument. The malleus neck or the deformed manubrium is typically fused to the atretic bone, and it is usually necessary to excise the periosteal attachments sharply. To prevent bony refixation to the ossicular chain, it is important to remove sufficient bone around the ossicles so that a 2- to 3-mm space exists between these structures and the adjacent canal wall. The only exception is the area of the fossa incudis, which may be left intact. Once the middle ear is exposed, the integrity of the ossicular chain and particularly the mobility of the stapes are assessed. The contracted middle ear cavity and malformed lateral ossicular mass may limit access to the area of the oval window. Usually, however, enough of the stapes can be seen to determine mobility and the integrity of the incudostapedial joint.

If possible, the ossicular chain is maintained intact because long-term hearing results may be better among patients who do not require a prosthesis.[19] A thin fascia graft is placed over the mobilized ossicular chain. Lateralization of the graft is always a concern because the deformed or absent malleus manibrium prevents anchoring the fascia beneath this ossicle. To help maintain graft position, the fascia can be tucked beneath the superior and/or anterior bony ledge of the canal wall. It is also helpful to cover the fascia graft with the split-thickness skin graft from the canal and to place a Silastic button over the skin graft.

A meatoplasty approximately twice normal size is made, while present conchal cartilaginous support is maintained. Not infrequently, the bony external canal and the meatus are misaligned. In such cases, it is necessary to undermine the auricle so that it can be repositioned properly.

A split-thickness skin graft (0.008 in. thick) approximately 4 × 6 cm is harvested from the upper thigh or medial upper arm. If available, a short, anteriorly based "tragal" skin flap is created and used to line a portion of the anterior membranous canal. This flap creates a staggered "stair-step" suture line at the meatus, thus helping to prevent meatal stenosis. With the ear retracted forward, the split-thickness skin graft is positioned within the bony canal, with meticulous coverage of all surfaces in order to minimize postoperative granulations and stenosis. Once the skin graft is appropriately positioned, it is stabilized by packing the bony canal with Merocel ear wicks hydrated with Cortisporin suspension. After this packing, the auricle is returned to its normal position and working through the meatus, the lateral end of the split-thickness skin graft is grasped and pulled through the meatal opening. It is trimmed as necessary and sutured at the meatal edges. Additional Merocel packing is used to fill the lateral portion of the ear canal. All packing is removed 7 to 10 days postoperatively.

AVOIDING COMPLICATIONS

FACIAL NERVE

Facial nerve abnormalities are to be expected in atresia patients. Anticipated findings include dehiscence of the tympanic segment, inferior displacement of the tympanic segment with intrusion on the stapes, and anterior and lateral displacement of the mastoid segment. The mastoid segment will frequently obscure the round window, and its distal portion actually lies lateral to the middle ear space. A higher incidence of facial nerve abnormalities has been found among patients with more severe microtia.[20]

The facial nerve is particularly vulnerable to injury when the posterior and inferior portions of the external canal are drilled. Potential for injury can be minimized by adherence to several surgical guidelines. First, as the atretic bone is removed, the drilling should be concentrated superiorly, entering the middle ear first in the epitympanum. The predictable abnormality of the vertical segment of the facial nerve is anticipated, and the nerve sheath should be looked for in the posterior inferior portion of the canal — just as one identifies the vertical segment of the facial nerve when performing mastoid surgery for cholesteatoma. It should also be noted that the facial nerve could be injured when undermining the auricle to align the soft tissue meatus and the created bony canal. In a recent study of more than 1000 operations for congenital anomalies of the ear, facial nerve paresis or paralysis occurred in less than 1%.[21]

CANAL STENOSIS

Postoperative narrowing of the new external canal can occur in as many as 25% of patients. Secondary infections from trapped squamous debris and diminished hearing can result. Factors important in reducing stenosis include use of split-thickness vs. full-thickness skin grafts, meticulous coverage of all exposed soft tissue and bone, and a generous meatoplasty. As previously mentioned, using a short, anteriorly based, full-thickness skin flap at the anterior meatal edge prevents a circumferential suture line at this level and may decrease the incidence of stenosis. If early stenosis is identified, injection of small amounts (0.3 to 0.5 ml) of triamcinolone (40 mg/ml) suspension every 3 to 4 weeks can be used.

LABYRINTHINE INJURY

High-frequency sensorineural hearing loss has been noted in some patients postoperatively, although a significant loss in the speech frequencies occurs in fewer than 3% of patients.[2] It must be recognized that the ossicular mass is connected to the atretic bone, and energy from drilling is transmitted to the inner ear. Care in removing the final portion of the atretic bone from the ossicular chain is particularly important.

TREATING COMPLICATIONS

PERSISTENT/RECURRENT CONDUCTIVE HEARING LOSS

A patient's failure to achieve marked hearing improvement in the immediate postoperative period is suggestive of an unrecognized ossicular chain abnormality such as stapes fixation. Gradual onset of a conductive hearing loss over months or years implicates the healing process as the cause of the loss. Regrowth of bone with refixation of the ossicular chain, lateralization or thickening of the tympanic membrane due to chronic inflammation, or middle ear adhesions must all be considered. If an ossicular reconstruction was necessary using artificial or autologous materials, displacement of the prosthesis is possible. Revision surgery should be considered in these patients. In a recent study, the risk of complications was no greater than with primary surgery, and many patients achieved a good hearing result.[2]

CANAL STENOSIS

In most cases of significant canal stenosis, it is necessary to redo the canaloplasty and replace the split-thickness skin graft. As in the primary procedure, the bony external canal and soft tissue meatus are widened, and a thin split-thickness graft is harvested. It is reasonable to raise the tympanic membrane to access ossicular mobility. If there is any concern about thickness or lateralization of the tympanic membrane, it is appropriate to regraft a tympanic membrane.

CONCLUSIONS

Many otologists have acknowledged that primary and revision surgical repairs of congenital aural atresia are among the most difficult tasks in otology. Thorough knowledge of the anatomic variations that can occur with abnormal development of the temporal bone is essential to minimize intraoperative and postoperative complications. Consistently excellent, long-term hearing results cannot yet be achieved in operations for atresia; however, restoration of serviceable hearing is possible.

ACKNOWLEDGMENT

Excellent word processing was provided by Betty Treanor.

REFERENCES

1. Eavey, R.D. Management strategies for congenital ear malformations. *Pediatr. Clin. North Am.,* 1989, 36, 1521–1534.
2. Eavey, R.D. Ear malformations: what a pediatrician can do to assist with auricular reconstruction. *Pediatr. Clin. North Am.,* 1996, 43, 1233–1244.
3. Eavey, R.D. Surgical repair of the auricle for microtia. Chapter 2 in Bluestone, C.D. and Stool, S.E., Eds. *Atlas of Pediatric Otolaryngology.* Philadelphia: W.B. Saunders, 1994.
4. Brent, B. The correction of microtia with autogenous cartilage grafts. I. The classic deformity. *Plast. Reconstr. Surg.,* 1980, 66, 1–12.
5. Brent, B. Total auricular reconstruction with scupted costal cartilage. In *The Artistry of Reconstructive Surgery.* St. Lous: C.V. Mosby, 1987, 113–127.
6. Tanzer, R.C. Total reconstruction of the external ear. *Plast. Reconstr. Surg.,* 1959, 23, 1–15.
7. Eavey, R.D. Microtia and significant auricular malformation: 92 pediatric patients. *Arch. Otolaryngol. Head Neck Surg.,* 1995, 121, 557–562.
8. Nagata, S. New method of total reconstruction of the auricle for microtia. *Plast. Reconstr. Surg.,* 1993, 92, 187–200.
9. Davis, J., Ed. *Otoplasty: Aesthetic and Reconstruction Techniques.* New York: Thieme–Verlag, 1997.
10. Eavey, R.D. and Ryan, D.P. Refinements in microtia surgery. *Arch. Otolaryngol. Head Neck Surg.,* 1996, 122, 617–620.
11. Eavey, R. and Cheney, M. Reconstruction of congenital auricular malformation. Chapter 38 in Natol, J. and Schuknecht, H., Eds. *Surgery of the Ear and Temporal Bone.* New York: Raven Press, 1993.
12. Toufexis, A. An eary tale. *Time,* Nov. 6, 1995, 60.

13. Rodriguez, A., Cao, Y.L., Ibarra, C., Pap, S., Vacanti, M., Eavey, R.D., and Vacanti, C.A. Characteristics of cartilage engineered from human pediatric auricular cartilage. *Plast. Reconstr. Surg.,* 1999, 103, 1111–1119.

14. Arevalo–Silva, C.A., Cao, Y., Vacanti, M., Weng, Y., Vacanti, C.A., and Eavey, R.D. Influence of growth factors on tissue engineered pediatric elastic cartilage. *Arch. Otolaryngol. Head Neck Surg.,* 2000, 126, 1234–1238.

15. Arevalo–Silva, C.A., Eavey, R.D. Cao, Y., Vacanti, M., Weng, Y., and Vacanti, C.A. Internal support of tissue-engineered cartilage. *Arch. Otolaryngol. Head Neck Surg.,* 2000, 126, 1448–1452.

16. Saim, A.B., Cao, Y., Weng, Y., Chang, C.N., Vacanti, M.A., Vacanti, C.A., and Eavey, R.D. Engineering autogenous cartilage in the shape of a helix using an injectable hydrogel scaffold. *Laryngoscope,* 2000, 110, 1694–1697.

17. Ombredanne, M. Chirugie des surdites congenitales par malformation ossiculaires. *Acta Otorhinolaryngol. Belg.,* 1971, 25, 837–840.

18. Jahrsdoerfer, R.A., Yeakley, J.W., Aguilar, E.A., Cole, R.R., and Gray, L.C. Grading system for the selection of patients with congenital aural atresia. *Am. J. Otolaryngol.,* 1992, 13, 6.

19. Lambert, P.R. Congenital aural atresia: stability of surgical results. *Laryngoscope,* 1998, 108, 1801–1805.

20. Lambert, P.R. Major congenital ear malformations: surgical management and results. *Ann. Otol. Rhinol.,* 1988, 97, 641–649.

21. Jahrsdoerfer, R.A. and Lambert, P.R. Facial nerve injury in congenital aural atresia surgery. *Am. J. Otol.,* 1998, 19, 283–287.

Section IX

Facial Plastic and
Reconstructive Surgery

32 Wound Healing

Ian N. Jacobs, David W. Low, and Timothy M. Crombleholme

You must take care of the present in order to have an opportunity to accomplish what you want in the future.

Tiger Woods

CONTENTS

INTRODUCTION

Surgical wound healing is regulated on a cellular and molecular level. The wound-healing response will improve or worsen the original problem. In the practice of pediatric otolaryngology, optimal wound healing is important and may influence the severity of a cutaneous scar on the face or restenosis of a narrow tubular structure, such as the subglottic larynx. In fact, a poor response may severely worsen the original problem. Moreover, wound healing is influenced by multiple intrinsic and extrinsic factors such as age, general medical status, and nutrition. Although the intrinsic factors are not amenable to change, one can optimize the extrinsic factors and use ideal surgical techniques. In addition, a number of topical and systemic medications may improve wound healing. Basic science as well as clinical issues of pediatric otolaryngologic wound healing will be discussed in this chapter.

BASIC SCIENCE

CELLULAR EVENTS

In general, wound healing can be divided into three main phases: inflammatory, proliferative, and remodeling. During each of these phases, specific cellular and molecular processes take place.

- The *inflammatory phase* begins immediately after an injury and lasts from 24 to 48 hours. During this phase, platelets and acute inflammatory cells migrate into the wound area and form a temporary plug for the wound matrix as the clotting cascade is activated. The platelets release growth factors that are chemoattractants for macrophages and neutrophils.

- In the *proliferative phase* with lymphocytes and mononuclear inflammatory cells migrate. These cells secrete cytokines that stimulate angiogenesis. The new small vessels bridge the gap across wound edges. Next, fibroblastic proliferation is induced by platelet- and macrophage-derived cytokines (growth factors). This begins the formation of a connective tissue matrix. Growth factors in the wound matrix cause the basal epithelial cells to migrate and epithelialize to fill in the wound gaps.

- During the *remodeling phase,* chronic changes take place as a mature scar matrix forms. Fibroblasts secrete types III and IV collagen under the stimulation of certain growth factors. Over the first 4 weeks, almost all collagen synthesis and deposition takes place. Then extensive remodeling of the wound matrix occurs as myofibroblasts cause wound contracture and soluble collagenases result in collagen metabolism. Over the next 6 months, additional wound strength is achieved as collagen cross-linking takes place. The tensile strength of the wound gradually increases to about 80% at 10 weeks.[1] Multiple factors including age, systemic illness, infection nutrition, and pharmacologic manipulation may affect this process.

This chapter will discuss these factors and strategies to optimize wound healing in children.

ROLE AND REGULATION OF GROWTH FACTORS

After an acute injury, certain polypeptide cytokines, known as growth factors, that regulate wound healing are released. Growth factors are signal proteins that act in an autocrine or paracrine fashion to influence wound healing. These polpeptide molecules affect wound healing on a cellular and a molecular level.[2] Intense research is being carried out in the study of growth factors actions and interactions. Moreover, one may optimize the wound healing process by manipulating the actions of growth factors.

The growth factor nomenclature is complicated and often misleading because growth factors are inconsistently named after their target cell or their source. Basically, the six families of growth factors include epidermal growth factors (EGF, TGF-α); fibroblast growth factors (FGF); transforming growth factors (TGF-β-1, β-3); platelet-derived growth factors (PDGF, vascular endothelial growth factor [VEGF]); insulin-like growth factors (IGF-1, IGF-2); and interleukins (IL-1, IL-2).[2]

The epidermal growth factors (EGFs) affect the initial phases of wound healing. EGF and transforming growth factor alpha (TGF-α) promote epithelialization; TGF-α stimulates angiogenesis. Fibroblast growth factor (FGF) induces the proliferation of vascular endothelial cells and stimulates neovascularization and granulation tissue formation. The TGF-β is a primary regulatory growth factor for wound healing.[2] TGF-β also has multiple interactions with other growth factors, is a promoter of fibrosis, and promotes fibroblastic expression of collagen.[2,3] Platelet-derived growth factor (PDGF) is mitogenic for fibroblasts and smooth muscle cells. PDGF also stimulates fibroblasts to produce collagenase for tissue remodeling, while VEGF stimulates endothelial cells and promotes angiogenesis.[2,4] The insulin-like growth factors (IGF-1, IGF-2) stimulate the mitosis of fibroblasts and smooth muscle cells. IGF-1 also induces the synthesis of glycogen, protein, and glycosaminoglycans.[2] IGF-1 is chemotactic for endothelial cells and promotes vascularization.[5]

Although investigators have examined growth factors with *in-vitro* and *in-vivo* models, the simplistic *in-vitro* model may not be comparable to the *in-vivo* animal model. For instance, a specific growth factor may have an opposite effect *in vivo* because of many other complex and poorly understood factors and interactions. In addition, in order to be effective, growth factors require sustained release and continuous presence in the wound. Sustained release of polypeptide growth factors has been achieved with implantable devices such as polyvinyl sponges, collagen matrix, gelfoam, or polyacrilamide gels in *in-vivo* systems.[6] The problem with an implanted artificial device is the inflammatory reaction. Nevertheless, the timed release of growth factor during the critical stages of wound healing is important. Slow-release vehicles such as osmotic pumps may allow the growth factor to be present during the critical stages of wound healing.

In addition, specific growth factors are more optimal when delivered in combination because synergistic interactions may take place. For instance, in rats pretreated with doxorubicin, TGF-β in combination with EGF and PDGF leads to greater expression of collagen than TGF-β alone.[7] The interactions of growth factors and other cytokines are highly complex and not well understood.

Gene Therapy Research and Applications

Implantable devices, which achieve a sustained release of growth factors, lead to a detrimental inflammatory response. Therefore, endogenous production as mediated by direct gene transfer may be an ideal way to create sustained release of growth factors during the critical stages of wound healing. Virally mediated transduction of target cells in wounds for the expression of cytokines or growth factors may be an ideal method to alter wound healing. Many growth factors, such as EGF, TGF-β, FGF, and VEGF, may be expressed by viral vectors.

An adenoviral vector is an excellent vector for wound-healing applications for several reasons:

- The adenoviral vector can be produced in high quantities and is quite stable.
- The virus has a strong affinity for the airway and can be delivered by aerosol.
- The virus may have a transient existence in its host, making it ideal for wound healing work.

The disadvantages include the potential inflammatory response and the immune response that may severely limit the duration of action.[8]

The ideal vector for wound healing should be of a transient nature and should also lead to a minimal or noninflammatory reaction in the target tissues. Recombinant viruses may be designed to express transgene products that inhibit certain growth factors in wound healing. For instance, TGF-β-3 and decorin are two inhibitors of TGF-β-1 activity. By inhibiting fibrosis, they may act as "antiscarring" agents.

The feasibility of adenoviral gene transfer in the rat laryngotracheal airway in an *in-vivo* model of subglottic stenosis has been studied. A reporter gene (beta galactosidase) was used to evaluate the adenovirus as a suitable vector for the modulation of airway wound healing. A significant, but transient, gene transfer in the rat airway model was achieved. Maximal expression peaked at 2 days after injection with a rapid decline and essentially complete loss of expression at 1 week. There was a mild inflammatory reaction.[9] The host's immune response will limit the duration of viral expression. Newer generations of recombinant viruses and "gutted" vectors are less immunogenic and may persist longer.

FETAL WOUND HEALING AND CLINICAL APPLICATIONS

An empiric observation from the new field of fetal surgery is that the midgestational fetus heals without scarring.[10] This confirms a previous observation by Rowlatt that the human fetus heals by mesenchymal regeneration without scar formation.[11] These observations sparked experimental studies in fetal wound healing in animal models, ranging from rats to rhesus monkeys, which consistently demonstrated differences between fetal and adult wound healing.[12] These differences in the fetal environment, cells, extracellular matrix, and milieu lead to scarless healing.[13]

The cellular component of fetal tissues has few inflammatory cells and lymphocytes are rarely observed. The fetal serum is devoid of natural immunoglobulins.[14] The sterile environment in the womb and highly immature fetal immune system is responsible for this. Other differences occur on a molecular level as well. The fetal extracellular matrix (ECM), which provides the scaffold for wound healing and remodeling, is highly organized and has minimal collagen content. Instead, greater quantities of hylauronic acid (HA), a glycosaminoglycan, provide for a more fluid flexible matrix and permit the more orderly deposition of collagen.[15] Thus, normal dermal structure is easily restored after skin injury.[16,17]

The fetal wound fluid also differs from the adult's. The amniotic fluid is rich in nutritional substances such as glucose and amino acids, as well as in HA, which inhibits fibrosis and collagen deposition.[15] The two growth factors TGF-β and PDGF, which induce normal, adult-like scarring, are largely absent in fetuses. TGF-β, which promotes fibrosis and collagen expression, is virtually absent in fetal wounds. In addition, Sullivan and coworkers found that administration of TGF-β-1 to fetal wounds resulted in normal postnatal scarring.[18]

A more fundamental understanding of the mechanisms that control the fetal wound-healing response has broad clinical applications. Not only could postnatal wound healing be modulated to heal without scarring, but certain diseases characterized by excessive fibroplasia and abnormal scar formation, such as burn contracture, keloids, strictures pulmonary fibrosis, hepatic cirrhosis, and subglottic stenosis, might also be modulated to heal without scarring. Current research is being carried out in pediatric and adult wounds to recreate the fetal state of wound healing. Antiscarring strategies include the use of anti-TGF-β-1 agents such as neutralizing antibodies or the addition of other substances such as HA to postnatal wounds.

CLINICAL WOUND HEALING IN THE INFANT AND CHILD

CLINICAL WOUND REPAIR

In infants and small children, optimal wound healing is essential in most clinical situations involving the head and neck region. It is beneficial, but not always possible, to have the patient in optimal health status prior to surgery. All systemic illnesses should be corrected if possible. The patient should be in an anabolic metabolic state and the nutritional status optimized. Prophylactic antibiotics may be helpful in children and adults in clean-contaminated and contaminated wounds and similar guidelines are followed. Reduction of the bacterial flora may decrease the risk of wound infection. These will be discussed later.

It is also important to adhere to certain surgical principles during the surgical wound repair. Because wound tension induces collagen formation, tension-free closure is important to reduce scarring. One should use maximal tensile strength sutures in wounds so as to elicit a minimal inflammatory reaction. In situations such as facial lacerations, topical skin adhesives may be helpful to reduce scarring. In addition, it is also best to avoid the formation of hematomas because these may be detrimental to the healing process. When postoperative blood or fluid collection is expected, drains are helpful. Excessive tissue edema may act as a barrier for oxygen and nutrient diffusion and thus should be minimized.

Because wound infections, which are due to an overgrowth of physiological bacteria or pathological bacteria, will delay normal healing, antibiotics and debridement may be necessary to prevent such delays. Nevertheless, infants and small children show a remarkable ability to heal quickly and generally with minimal scarring.

EXTRINSIC FACTORS AFFECTING WOUND HEALING

Multiple extrinsic factors affect wound healing, including age, nutritional status, gastroesophageal reflux, systemic illness, certain genetic and immunological conditions, and medications.

Nutritional status is very important. There are numerous essential nutrients for wound healing, including amino acids, lipids, carbohydrates, vitamins, and trace elements such as iron. First, protein metabolism is essential. Certain catabolic states, such as those present after starvation, may delay wound healing by impairing protein metabolism.[19] Other cellular processes, such as angiogenesis, require optimal protein metabolism.[20] Carbohydrate metabolism may be negatively affected in diabetes mellitus or malnutrition. Lack of carbohydrate availability leads to the breakdown of amino acids and a general catabolic state that adversely affects wound healing.

Specific vitamins and trace elements are important in wound healing. Vitamin C is necessary for hydroxylation of lysine and proline.[20] Vitamin A is a cellular membrane stabilizer; deficiencies of this vitamin may lead to decreased collagen synthesis, epithelialization, and wound infection.[21] Optimal nutrition is essential for stable wound healing. Parenteral nutrition should be used whenever possible or enteral nutrition, if necessary.

Coexisting systemic illnesses are important cofactors in wound healing. Hypoxia, sepsis, and generalized cardiogenic shock lead to decreased peripheral perfusion and poorer healing. Children undergoing chemotherapy or bone marrow transplantation for aggressive malignancies may be neutropenic as well as catabolic and heal more poorly. Correction of the underlying illness, if possible, is important prior to elective surgery.

Inherited genetic diseases may be associated with suboptimal healing. The most significant are connective tissue disorders. An example is Ehlers–Danlos syndrome, a disorder characterized by hypermobile joints, hyperextensible skin, and connective tissue fragility. The syndrome is associated with defects in the synthesis, cross-linking, and structure of collagen. This defect results in a decrease in wound strength and poor wound healing. Patients with epidermolysis bullosa, another genetic disease, have problems with skin healing and bullae formation. This may have a great impact on skin wound healing, as well on as the selection and closure of skin incisions. Skin tape should be avoided and protective dressings are helpful.

Patient age is not a significant factor, although this is probably related to other associated systemic illnesses at extremely young ages. In addition, small premature neonates may have a predilection for wound-healing problems in certain regions, such as the subglottic airway, because of the small caliber of the subglottic airway or other systemic illness.

Gastroesophageal reflux (GER) may have a negative impact on wound healing by creating an inflammatory reaction. Small premature infants may have increased episodes of GER, which is considered a potential risk factor for the development of subglottic stenosis.[22] Therefore, GER should be controlled prior to surgery on the upper airway. Medications, such as H-2 blockers, prokinetic agents, and proton pump inhibitors, and dietary modifications may be utilized. Occasionally, fundoplication may be necessary to control refractory reflux. In general, control of GER is essential prior to surgery on the upper airway on any patient.

PHARMACOLOGIC MANIPULATIONS

Corticosteroids, which have many inhibitory effects, affect clinical wound healing in multiple ways:

- They inhibit the function of polymorphonuclear leukocytes and macrophages.[23]
- They reduce the number of lymphocytes and mast cells in wounds.
- They reduce fibroblast activity, including reduced mitosis, active transport, and protein synthesis.

The result will be reduced tensile strength of wound. Although corticosteroids may reduce postoperative edema, they can have detrimental effects on wound healing. On the other hand, in certain clinical situations, such as granulation tissue formation, an exuberant wound-healing process may need to be diminished.

Mitomycin-C's potential role as an inhibitor of scar tissue formation in subglottic and tracheal stenosis has been evaluated in animal and clinical studies. Mitomycin-C is an antibiotic isolated from the broth of streptomyces caespitosus, which can inhibit fibroblast activity. In an experimental canine study, topical mitomycin prevented the formation of subglottic stenosis after wounding the subglottic airway.[24] In addition, the antrostomy sites of rabbits treated with topical mitomycin-C at a concentration of 1 mg/ml stayed open longer than those of controls.[25] Moreover, clinical studies have also demonstrated the effectiveness of topical mitomycin-C for the prevention of restenosis of the larynx and trachea[26,27] and choanal atresia[28] at a concentration of 0.04 mg/kg for 5 minutes. Although its safety has not been established in the pediatric population, no adverse effects with topical use have been reported.[26-28]

Hylauronic acid (HA), found in high concentrations in fetal tissues, may modulate fetal wound healing and is believed to inhibit fibroplasia, collagen deposition, and neovascularization.[15] Hellsstrom et al. demonstrated that HA improved tympanic membrane healing and closure.[29] HA imbedded in nasal splints may optimize the wound-healing process and reduce granulation tissue formation.

Topical ointments and *antibiotic preparations* are often used for incisions and local wounds. These include Bacitracin® or Polysporin®, which reduce the skin bacterial count and prevent drying of the wound. Parents will often ask about topical vitamin E or cocoa butter to improve the appearance of cutaneous scars. Although there is no clear evidence of any biochemical wound-healing benefit from such substances, daily application ensures that the scars are massaged routinely. Collagen remodeling responds to pressure, and it is more likely that the action of the finger rubbing the scar, rather than the lubricant applied, is beneficial.

PROPHYLACTIC ANTIBIOTICS

Normal wounds contain a finite bacterial flora. Wounds in which the bacterial floral count exceeds 10^5 organisms per milliliter are considered infected.[30] Clinically, a wound infection manifests as abnormal erythema of the skin edges and purulent fluid under the incision. Because wound infections impede normal wound healing, prophylactic antibiotics may reduce infection rates and improve healing with certain types of wounds and certain procedures in the head and neck region.

Wounds are classified as clean, clean-contaminated, contaminated, and dirty. Clean wounds, such as in elective facial, thyroid, or (external) salivary gland surgery, carry an infection rate of 1 to 5%. Most otolaryngologic procedures, such as those in the oropharyngeal cavity, are clean contaminated. The infection rate is much higher with no antibiotics and ranges from 28 to 87%.[30] Contaminated wounds include those with spillage from the GI tract or a break in sterile technique. A dirty wound would include an abscess or an infected traumatic wound.

Clean wounds do not warrant antibiotics,[31,32] but contaminated, clean-contaminated, and dirty wounds require prophylaxis. Furthermore, many areas in the head and neck region, such as the oral cavity, are contaminated with bacteria. Theoretically, the infection rate should be 100%. A number of clinical studies and practice guidelines for the use of prophylactic antibiotics are available.

Prophylactic antibiotic use is imperative for head and neck surgery in the oropharyngeal airway where there is wound contamination with saliva. In this situation, infection rates range from 28 to

87% without coverage. Prophylaxis has been shown to be effective in preventing wound infections.[26] A short course, such as 24 hours, is as effective as a longer course (2 to 7 days), and the shorter course may be less likely to yield resistant organisms.[33] The current practice includes use of combinations of antibiotics such as clindamycin and gentamycin administered via IV at least 1 hour prior to skin incision.[34] It is essential that the antibiotic be available prior to the initial incision and that only a short course be necessary.

The use of prophylactic antibiotics is effective at reducing the infection rate for compound mandibular fractures but not other types of facial fractures. With the use of cefazolin, the infection rate was 8.9% compared with 42.2% in the placebo group.[35] Similar results were also found by Zallen and Curry.[36] Clean facial lacerations and other clean surgeries of the face do not require antibiotics; however, animal and human bites anywhere do require treatment. Meticulous cleaning and debridement is helpful.[37] The current antibiotic recommendation is oral amoxicillin-clavulante, dicloxacillin, parental cefoxitin, or parental penicillin-G with beta-lactamase resistant penicillin or ticarcillin-clavulanate potassium (UNASYN®) for animal bites. Oral amoxicillin plus clavulanate, dicloxacillin, parental cefoxitin, or a first-generation cephalosporin with a beta-lactamase stable penicillin or ticarcillin-clavulanate potassium should be administered for human bites.

Prophylaxis treatment for tonsillectomy is helpful at reducing pain, fever, and mouth odor. Intravenous ampicillin in the operating room with oral amoxicillin for 10 days was shown by Telian and coworkers to be effective.[38] Laryngotracheal surgery in a clean-contaminated field requires prophylaxis. Currently, there are no controlled clinical studies evaluating antibiotic coverage for laryngotracheal reconstruction. One common practice is coverage for oral anaerobes with clindamycin and pseudomonas aeriginosa, in the presence of pre-existing tracheotomy, with ceftazadime.

SURGICAL ASPECTS OF WOUND CARE

ELECTIVE INCISIONS

Parents must understand that incisions on the face and neck will leave permanent scars no matter how carefully the incisions are placed and how meticulously the layers are closed. They may erroneously believe that the scars will disappear with time, or that a scar placed in infancy will appear to shrink as the child grows. An incision that extends halfway across the forehead will leave a permanent scar that goes halfway across the forehead. All attempts should be made to make the scar as short as possible without compromising adequate exposure for a safe operation.

As with adults, elective incisions should follow the natural expression lines on the face and neck. Although these are commonly called "Langer's lines," they are more accurately described as the wrinkle lines of Kraissl and run perpendicular to the direction of muscle action. Even babies have neck wrinkles, which mandate roughly horizontal incisions, and a lateral upper-eyelid crease incision leaves a nearly imperceptible scar when excising brow dermoids. It is preferable to parallel the nasolabial fold when excising lesions of the medial cheek.

On otherwise smooth areas, one should anticipate the direction of future wrinkle lines to optimize the appearance of the final scar. When excising nevi in ambiguous areas such as the glabella or chin, it is useful to excise the lesion first, and then determine the best direction of closure by manipulating the skin edges. At that point, the site can be converted into an elliptical shape by excising the lateral dog ears.

INSTRUMENTATION

In a vast majority of cases, the initial incision is made with a standard scalpel blade to provide the least amount of tissue injury and, hopefully, to optimize rapid healing and minimize scar formation. However, in conditions of high vascularity such as hemangiomas and vascular malformations, or in areas that traditionally heal well, such as the intraoral mucosa, a fine point cautery or Colorado microdissection needle (Colorado Biomedical, Evergreen, CO) tip will decrease blood loss. A narrow zone of thermal injury will still permit healing by primary intention. The carbon dioxide laser with a focused 0.1-mm tip will also rapidly incise skin and cauterize small vessels, but practice and experience are necessary to avoid excessive thermal injury. Beware thermal injury in the scalp that may damage hair follicles and result in a zone of scarring alopecia along the incision.

WOUND CLOSURE

The method of wound closure largely depends upon the surgeon's personal preference. Most surgeons perform a layered closure with an absorbable suture such as Vicryl (Ethicon, Somerville, NJ); Polysorb (US Surgical, Norwalk, CT); or chromic gut in the deep layer, followed by a more superficial layer of absorbable or nonabsorbable suture material. External sutures that remain longer than 5 to 7 days may leave permanent suture marks as the epidermis begins to migrate along the suture tracks. This is not a concern in the scalp area, but on the face it is preferable to use a fast-absorbing suture that will dissolve within a week or a monofilament suture that can be removed within a week. Theoretically, monofilament sutures will create less inflammatory response; however, clinically, no difference may be observed and the younger child has a distinct advantage if absorbable sutures are used.

It is also the surgeon's preference as to whether a simple over-and-over suture is used vs. a running subcuticular stitch. Neck incisions lend well to a running subcuticular closure, and over-and-over sutures can better evert and approximate the skin edges on the face while providing better hemostasis. Steri-strips (3M Health Care, St. Paul, MN) are commonly used, regardless of the method of final skin closure. In addition to providing support to the wound closure, they will help to keep out contaminants and prying fingers. Often, a layer of benzoin or Mastisol (Ferndale Labs, Ferndale, MI) is applied to prolong the duration of adhesiveness for 1 to 2 weeks.

Collodion (Amend, Irvington, NJ), a viscous combination of ethyl alcohol, ethyl ether, and nitrocellulose, provides a watertight seal and closure reinforcement in lieu of Steri-strips and may be particularly useful in hair-bearing areas such as the scalp and eyebrow. It can be drawn into a 3-cc syringe using a large-bore needle, which then provides a convenient delivery system. The wound edges should be closely approximated and dry before applying the collodion.

Dermabond (Ethicon, Somerville, NJ), 2-octyl cyanoacrylate, has been promoted for closure of skin lacerations in lieu of sutures and is supplied in user-friendly applicator vials. This minimizes the number of sutures required and eliminates suture removal. However, the edges still must be well approximated with deep dermal sutures, and as with Collodion, the wound must be dry before applying the sealant. The cosmetic outcome is the same as that from sutures.[39]

POSTOPERATIVE CARE

Head and neck incisions require a minimum amount of postoperative care. If skin has not been grafted, operative sites can tolerate exposure to water after 24 hours, even if Steri-strips have been applied. Alternatively, antibiotic ointment can be applied lightly to an exposed suture line two or three times daily to soften any crusts and provide a thin antibacterial coating. If significant crusting that is resistant to ointment occurs, a few drops of hydrogen peroxide will rapidly soften the hard secretions and clotted blood. If significant oozing is anticipated, it may be necessary to use gauze dressings secured with tape, gauze roll, or an elastic wrap, depending upon the location and size of the closure. Large scalp incisions may benefit from a compression dressing similar to that used in neurosurgical or craniofacial procedures. A stent secured with tie-over sutures is commonly used to secure a skin graft. The stent can usually be removed in 4 days — sooner, if a hematoma or infection is a concern.

Exposure to sunlight may be deleterious to the final outcome of a scar because the fragile epidermis may be more likely to burn. Additionally, while bruising persists, the ultraviolet light may tattoo the blood pigment into the dermis layer, resulting in permanent brown pigmentation (hemosiderin) at the operative site. Sun exposure should be minimized for at least several months, using a combination of sun avoidance, sun blocks, protective clothing, and/or adhesive bandage strips and Steri-strips.

Pediatric scars will undergo a period of remodeling that may last at least a year; parents should understand that scars will often become increasingly pink and hypertrophic over the first 2 months and then gradually soften, flatten, and lighten over the subsequent 10 months. Many scars will often widen in response to skin tension, even when the incision follows the natural wrinkle lines, and parents should be forewarned to avoid disappointment. Long-term (several months) application of support strips may decrease the hypertrophic tendency of scars and, possibly, their tendency to widen.[40]

The topical application of silicone rubber sheeting such as Mepiform (Mercy Surgical Dressing Group, Canonsburg, PA) or silicone gel (e.g., Scarfade, Hanson Medical, Kingston, WA) is commonly used to assist with scar remodeling because it may suppress the formation of hypertrophic scars and decrease the pink pigmentation associated with such scars. The mechanism of action is unclear, but the rubber should be applied daily for at least 2 months. The manufacturer recommends continuous use except when washing the skin; however, usage can be limited to nighttime application on the face and if the skin becomes irritated.

SPECIAL PROBLEMS AND COMPLICATIONS

HYPERTROPHIC SCARRING AND KELOIDS

The vast majority of pediatric scars will go through an initial hypertrophic phase that peaks about 2 months post-operative and then gradually subsides over the subsequent year. Unfortunately, some scars will maintain their hypertrophic character indefinitely. Treatment options include allowing more time, massage, application of silicone rubber sheeting or gel, injection of a long-acting steroid such as Kenalog (triamcinolone acetonide; Apothecon, Bristol-Myers Squibb, Princeton, NJ), and more recently, laser photocoagulation with a pulsed yellow dye laser (Candela, Wayland, MA).

Steroid injections should not exceed 40 mg in a given day and usually are not given more frequently than once a month. Kenalog is available as 10 or 40 mg/cc and can be diluted with saline if it needs to be distributed over a large area. Yellow-dye laser light is absorbed by oxyhemoglobin. It is most often used for cutaneous vascular malformations such as port wine stains and telangiectasia; however, it appears to have some utility in reducing the vascular pigmentation of a hypertrophic scar as well as its thickness. Multiple laser treatments, spaced 1 to 2 months apart, may be necessary for optimal results.

Keloids remain an unsolved problem in wound healing and are characterized by bundles of collagen, which collectively may far exceed the mass and boundaries of the original wound. Keloids occur more frequently in more darkly pigmented patients such as Asians and African-Americans, but can occur even in Caucasians. For unclear reasons, keloids are distinctly uncommon in the central facial area, but tend to occur along the lateral cheeks, ears, scalp, and neck.

There is still no completely reliable treatment for keloids. In addition to the previously mentioned options for hypertrophic scars, nonsurgical treatments include pressure dressings such as facial masks for burn patients and compression earrings for ear keloids injections of calcium channel blockers such as Verapamil (American Regent Laboratories, Shirley, NY). On occasion, surgical excision is recommended in the hope that the new scar can be manipulated to decrease the keloid tendency. Adults with strong keloid tendencies may benefit from 3 days of low-dose irradiation immediately following keloid excision to try to suppress recurrence,[41] although this is probably not appropriate in children.

Patients and their families must fully understand that surgical excision carries a risk of keloid recurrence that may exceed the severity of the original condition. They must also understand the need for periodic follow-up and compliance with pressure dressings and steroid injections, if these are included with the postoperative regimen.

HEMATOMAS

Hematomas secondary to blunt trauma will usually resolve on their own. Aspiration may speed resolution of fresh hematomas but well-organized clots usually cannot be aspirated until they begin to liquefy. Septal hematomas must be drained when diagnosed following nasal trauma in order to prevent necrosis of the septal cartilage and saddle nose deformity. Expanding postoperative hematomas usually mandate a return to the operating room for evacuation, exploration, and hemostatic control to avoid potential skin flap necrosis, suture line dehiscence, and delayed wound healing.

HEALING BY SECONDARY INTENTION

Heavily contaminated or infected wounds, deep abrasions, skin avulsions, and other significant facial wounds may not be amenable to primary or delayed primary closure. These wounds can be left open to granulate and, when they are clean enough, may be suitable for skin grafting. Alternatively, smaller wounds may be allowed to re-epithelialize spontaneously. Parents should be reassured that the patients may be eligible for future scar revision; however, they must also understand that unfortunately, the result will be permanent scars that can never be completely removed.

CONCLUSION

Clinical wound healing is a highly complex and interactive process. Many factors play a role in the wound-healing process; nutrition, medical condition, and surgical technique influence the outcome. Fetal wound healing is ideal and one can strive to mimic the fetal healing state in infants and young children. Current research endeavors to optimize wound healing with the use of appropriate growth factors and gene transfer techniques as well as recreating the cellular and molecular characteristics of fetal wound healing. Certain surgical techniques and principles are important to follow with regard to the head and neck region in children; close adherence to these principles will result in a better outcome in that region.

REFERENCES

1. Levenson, S. and Demetriou, A. Metabolic factors. In Cohen, K., Dieglemann, R., and Lindblad, E., Eds. *Wound Healing: Biochemical and Clinical Aspects*. Philadelphia: Harcourt Brace Jovanovich, 1992, 248–273.
2. Hom, D.B. Growth factors in wound healing. *Otolaryngol. Clin. North Am.*, 1995, 28(5), 933–953.
3. Hsuan, J.J. Transforming growth factors beta. *Br. Med. Bull.*, 1989, 45, 425–437.
4. Lynch, S.E., Nixon, J.C., Colvin, R.B. et al. Role of platelet-derived growth factors in wound healing: synergistic effects with other growth factors. *Proc. Natl. Acad. Sci. USA,* 1987, 84, 7696–7700.
5. Grant, M., Jerdan, J., and Merimmee, T.J. Insulin-like growth factor-1 modulates endothelial cell chemotaxis. *J. Clin. Endocrinol. Metab.*, 1987, 65, 370–371.
6. Cooper, M.L., Hansbrough, J.F., Foreman, T.J. et al. The effect of epidermal growth factor and basic fibroblast growth factor on epithelialization of meshed skin graft interstices. In Barbul, A., Caldwell, M.D., Eaglstein, W.H. et al., Eds. *Clinical and Experimental Approaches to Dermal and Epidermal Repair: Normal and Chronic Wounds*. New York: Wiley–Liss Publishers, 1991, 429–442.
7. Lawrence, W., Sporn, M., Gorschboth, C. et al. The reversal of adriamycin induced healing impairment with chemoattractants and growth factors. *Ann. Surg.,* 1986, 2, 143–147.
8. Jain, K.K., Ed. *Textbook of Gene Therapy*. Chap. 4. Seattle, WA: Hogrefe and Huber Publishers, 1998.

9. Jacobs, I.N., Tufano, R., Walsh, D., Crombleholme, T., and Radu, A. The temporal course of adenovirus mediated gene transfer in the rat larynx. *Abstracts of AAO-HNS, Research Forum,* Sept, 1999.

10. Harrison, M. (Personal communication).

11. Rowlatt, U. Intrauterine wound healing in a 20-week human fetus. *Virchow's Arch. A. Pathol. Anat. Histol.,* 1979, 381, 353–361.

12. Adzick, N.S. and Harrison, M.R. The fetal surgery experience. In Adzick, N.S. and Longaker, M.T., Eds. *Fetal Wound Healing.* New York: Elsevier Scientific Press, 1992.

13. Lorenz, H.P. and Adzick, N.S. Scarless skin wound repair in the fetus. *West J. Med.,* 1993, 159, 350–355.

14. Dostal, G.H. and Gamelli, R.L. Fetal wound healing. *Surg. Gynecol. Obstet.,* 1993, 176, 299–306.

15. Mast, B.A., Diegelmann, R.F., Krummel, T.M., and Cohen, I.K. Scarless wound healing in the mammalian fetus. *Surg. Gynecol. Obstet.,* 1992, 174, 441–451.

16. Broker, B.J. and Reiter, D. Fetal wound healing. *Otolaryngol. Head Neck Surg.,* 1994, 110, 547–549.

17. Burrington, J.D. Wound healing in the fetal lamb. *J. Pediatr. Surg.,* 1971, 6, 523–528.

18. Sullivan, K.M., Lorenz, H.P., Meuli, M., Lin, R.Y., and Adzick, N.S. A model of scarless human fetal wound repair is deficient in transforming growth factor beta. *J. Pediatr. Surg.,* 1995, 30, 198–203.

19. Howes, E., Briggs, H., Shea, R. et al. Effect of complete and partial starvation in the rate of fibroplasia in the healing wound. *Arch. Surg.,* 1933, 27, 846–858.

20. Ondrey, F.G. and Hom, D.B. Effects of nutrition on wound healing. *Otolaryngol. Head Neck Surg.,* 1994, 110, 557–559.

21. Pollack, S.V. Wound healing: a review. Nutritional factors affecting wound healing. *J. Dermatol. Surg. Oncol.,* 1979, 5, 615–619.

22. Little, F.B., Koufman, J.A., Kohut, R.I., and Marshall, R.B. Effect of gastric acid on the pathogenesis of subglottic stenosis. *Ann. Otol. Rhinol. Laryngol.,* 1985, 94, 516–519.

23. Hom, D.B. Growth factors and wound healing in otolaryngology. *Otolaryngol. Head Neck Surg.,* 1994, 110, 560–564.

24. Eliashar, R., Eliacher, I., Esclamado, R., Gramlich, T., and Strome, M. Can topical mitomycin prevent laryngotracheal stenosis? *Laryngoscope,* 1999, 109, 1594–1600.

25. Ingrams, D.R., Volk, M.S., Biesman, B.S., Pankratov, M.M., and Shapshay, S. Sinus surgery: does mitomycin-C reduce stenosis? *Laryngoscope,* 1998, 108, 883–886.

26. Ward, R.F. and April, M.M. Mitomycin-C in the treatment of tracheal cicatrix after tracheal reconstruction. *Int. J. Pediatr. Otolaryngol.,* 1998, 44, 221–226.

27. Rahbar, R., Shapshay, S., and Healy, G.B. Single exposure to mitomycin-C: effects on laryngeal and tracheal stenosis — benefits and complication. *Abstr. Am. Laryngol. Assoc.,* April 1999.

28. Holland, B.W. Surgical management of choanal atresia: improved outcome using mitomycin. *Arch. Otolaryngol. Head Neck Surg.,* 2001, 127(11), 1375–1380.

29. Laurent, C., Hellstrom, S., and Fellenius, E. Hyaluronan improves the healing of experimental tympanic membranes perforations. *Arch. Otolaryngol. Head Neck Surg.,* 1988, 114, 1435–1441.

30. Pou, A.M. and Johnson, J.T. Use of prophylactic antibiotics in otolaryngology. In Weissler, M.C. and Pillsbury, H.C., Eds. *Complications of Head and Neck Surgery.* New York: Thieme Medical Publishers, 1995.

31. Johnson, J.T. and Wagner, R.L. Infection following uncontaminated head and neck surgery. *Arch. Otolaryngol. Head Neck Surg.,* 1987, 113, 368–369.

32. Carrau, R.L, Byzakis, J., Wagner, R.L., and Johnson, J.T. Role of prophylactic antibiotics in uncontaminated neck dissections. *Arch. Otolaryngol. Head Neck Surg.,* 1991, 115, 194–195.

33. Mombelli, G., Coppens, L., Dor, P., and Klastersky, J. Antibiotic prophylaxis in surgery for head and neck cancer: Comparative study of short and prolonged administration of carbencillin. *J. Antimicrob. Chemother.,* 1981, 7, 665–671.

34. Johnson, J.T., Yu, V.L., Myers, E.N., and Wagner, R.L. An assessment of the need for Gram-negative bacterial coverage in antibiotic prophylaxis for oncological head and neck surgery. *J. Infect. Dis.,* 1987, 155, 331–333.

35. Chole, R.A. and Yee, J. Antibiotic prophylaxis for facial fractures. *Arch. Otolaryngol. Head Neck Surg.,* 1987, 113, 1055–1057.

36. Zallen, R.D. and Curry, J.T. A study of antibiotic usage in compound mandibular fractures. *J. Oral Surg.,* 1975, 33, 431–434.

37. Brook, I. Human and animal bites. *J. Fam. Pract.,* 1989, 28, 713–718.
38. Telian, S.A., Handler, S.D., Fleisher, G.R., Baranak, C.C., Wetmore, R.F., and Potsic, W.P. The effect of antibiotic therapy in recovery after tonsillectomy in children. A controlled study. *Arch. Otolaryngol. Head Neck Surg.,* 1986, 112, 610–615.
39. Quinn, J., Wells, G., Sutcliffe, T., Jarmuske, M., Maw, J., Stiell, I., and Johns, P. A randomized trial comparing octylcyanoacrylate tissue adhesive and sutures in the management of lacerations. *JAMA,* 1997, 277, 1527–1530.
40. Reiffel, R.S. Prevention of hypertrophic scars by long-term paper tape application. *Plast. Reconstr. Surg.,* 1995, 96(7), 1715–1718.
41. Klumpar, D.I., Murray, J.C., and Anschar, M. Keloids treated with excision followed by radiation therapy. *J. Am. Acad. Dermatol.,* 1994, 31, 225–231.

33 Cleft Lip and Palate

Charles M. Bower, Robert W. Seibert, and Harlan R. Muntz

The physician must generalize the disease and individualize the patient.

Christoph Wilhelm Hufeland

CONTENTS

INTRODUCTION

Cleft palate, cleft lip, and velopharyngeal insufficiency will be covered in this chapter. Each topic is looked at individually for a more comprehensive review of its potential complications, although the reader is reminded that these disease processes often coexist.

CLEFT PALATE

Surgical correction of cleft palate is performed to normalize form and function of the palate. The procedure results in separation of the oral from the nasal cavity with normalization of swallowing and speaking in the majority of patients. Complications of cleft palate, such as feeding difficulties, may occur early in life as a consequence of the cleft. Later complications include frequent otitis media and speech and language deficiencies. Complications may occur as a result of technical errors (transection of the palatine artery) or errors in judgment (attempt to repair a wide cleft too early in life), or may be unavoidable even with appropriately performed surgery (maxillary growth disturbance).

EARLY COMPLICATIONS

Early complications in newborns with cleft lip and palate include feeding and airway problems. Most infants with a cleft palate will have some difficulty feeding due to the inability to generate an adequate negative intraoral pressure. The size of the cleft, associated retrognathia, and involvement of the lip are factors influencing the severity of dysphagia. Failure to thrive has been reported in 32% of infants with unilateral cleft lip and palate, 38% with bilateral cleft lip and palate, and up to 49% for cleft palate.[1] Infants with Robin sequence almost always manifest failure to thrive due to difficulty breathing while swallowing.

Feeding technique is important in optimizing the infant's ability to obtain adequate calories. A well-trained nurse or speech or occupational therapist can observe and instruct parents in an appropriate technique of feeding, providing the infant a small amount of formula at a time, allowing frequent rest periods, and adequate burping. The use of soft bottles and large bore nipples provides the ability to deliver a pulse of formula to the infant. Two commonly used bottles are the Habermann and Mead–Johnson cleft feeders. The pigeon nipple has recently become a popular alternative. Breast-feeding is only occasionally successful.[2]

Failure to thrive secondary to feeding difficulties can usually be managed with optimal oral feeding techniques in infants with isolated cleft anomalies. In syndromic children, insufficient oral caloric intake may obligate the use of nasogastric or gastrostomy tube feeding. Infants with a wide cleft of the palate and feeding difficulties can be fit with a palatal obturator form to occlude the cleft, which may improve the ability to suck and reduce nasal reflux. Early dental consultation to fit a palatal prosthesis can facilitate discharge from the hospital. Monitoring for appropriate growth is necessary, especially during the first year of life.

The association of cleft palate with retrognathia and glossoptosis (Pierre Robin sequence) results in airway difficulties in the majority of children. Airway obstruction and feeding difficulties are usually mild and improve with prone positioning and feeding techniques as noted earlier. Monitoring by trained nurses and continuous pulse oximetry looking for evidence of upper airway obstruction prior to discharge are important. Overnight polysomnography is needed to evaluate the extent of obstruction in some patients. About 10 to 15% of patients with Robin sequence have continued severe airway obstruction, difficulty feeding, or failure to thrive despite optimal nursing care. Tracheotomy is necessary in these infants to provide an adequate airway. Lip–tongue adhesion, subperiosteal dissection of the floor of mouth,[3] and mandibular distraction osteogenesis[4] are alternatives recommended by some authors. Tracheotomy is more likely to be necessary in patients with Robin sequence with associated syndromes or other anomalies. Nasogastric or gastrostomy tube feedings are occasionally required even when the airway has been secured.[5]

Otitis media is a common finding in children with cleft palate. Failure of development of the palate is associated with inappropriate insertion of the tensor veli palatini muscle into the posterior palatal shelves and abnormal eustachian tube structure and function. Otitis media may be more common in isolated cleft palate than in unilateral or bilateral complete cleft lip and palate.[6] Otitis media with effusion and recurrent otitis media usually require tympanostomy with tube insertion. Repeated tube insertion over several years is not uncommon. Tubes are usually inserted at the time of palatoplasty, but in infants with severe recurrent infections, earlier surgery is recommended. The type of palate repair probably does not influence the outcome of otitis media.[7] Improved hearing with resulting improvement in speech and language is routinely noted after tube insertion.[8]

Sinusitis may also be more common in children with clefts. The maxillary sinuses have been reported to be small in childhood, growing to normal size by adult age. This is associated with an increased risk of severe sinusitis in cleft children, which seems to improve beyond the age of 10 years.[9]

CLEFT PALATE REPAIR

The intent of cleft palate repair is to restore normal form and function. Normal speech, swallowing, and facial growth are the most important variables to assess regarding an optimal procedure. The initial goals of cleft repair are to close the defect, lengthen the palate to a normal configuration, and restore soft palate muscle function. This needs to be accomplished in a manner that does not impair respiration, mastication, or facial growth. Unfortunately, all techniques of repair have a risk of velopharyngeal insufficiency, residual palate defect, or facial growth retardation.

The optimal age for repair of the cleft palate continues to be debated. Early repair of the cleft optimizes speech development and reduces problematic feeding difficulties and nasal reflux. Some authors have reported soft palate repair as early as 3 months of age.[10] Later repair of the cleft reduces the risk of maxillary growth retardation from early dissection of the bony palatal shelves. Delaying hard palate closure until age 5 or later, when transverse facial growth is complete, may minimize the effect on facial growth, but significantly impairs speech development and is generally not recommended.[11] Early closure of the soft palate with delayed closure of the hard palate at 5 years of age is recommended in some centers.[12] Many centers now advocate cleft palate repair between 9 and 18 months of age. Some centers advocate presurgical gingivoperiosteoplasty and/or active or passive orthopedic manipulation of the palate.[13]

Appropriate preoperative evaluation can minimize complications. Airway complications are more common in children operated on before the age of 1 year and in those undergoing velopharyngeal closure procedures along with cleft palate repair.[14,15] Patients with Robin sequence and other defined craniofacial anomalies are also at increased risk for airway problems. Airway assessment and careful operative planning, especially in infants with Robin sequence, is crucial. Significant preoperative airway obstruction predicts postoperative airway obstruction. Delaying the procedure until the patient is 2 years of age is appropriate in high-risk cases. The use of perioperative steroids (dexamethasone: 0.5 to 1 mg/kg IV) has been reported to decrease the risk of postoperative airway distress; however, steroid use remains controversial.[16]

Failure to thrive (weight under the fifth percentile) should be assessed and corrected if possible.[17] Preoperative hematologic and coagulation studies may not be needed. Associated anomalies (e.g., congential heart disease) should be stable before surgery is performed.

Commonly performed procedures for cleft palate repair include the V–Y pushback palatoplasty (Wardill–Kilner–Veau operation), the two-flap palatoplasty, and the Furlow double opposing Z-plasty. The Von Langenbeck procedure has also been used for clefts of the secondary palate.

The V–Y pushback palatoplasty is used for closure of secondary palate clefts. Incisions are made along the free edge of the palate and extended onto the hard palate. Lateral relaxing incisions are made and connected to the medial incision anteriorly to allow posteriorly based mucoperiosteal flaps to be dissected free from the hard palate. Care is taken to preserve the neurovascular pedical. Soft palate musculature is dissected from the posterior hard palate and approximated in the midline after closure of the nasal mucosa. The two mucoperiosteal flaps are pushed posteriorly and closed in the midline. This procedure allows for closure of clefts of the secondary palate with some degree of lengthening of the palate.

The two-flap palatoplasty is used in unilateral complete cleft palate. The incisions are similar to the V–Y pushback design, but are extended to the anterior edge of the secondary palate defect. The flaps are closed in the midline after closure of the nasal mucosperiosteum and soft palate muscle approximation. The three-flap palatoplasty, which is used for bilateral complete cleft palate, includes lateral relaxing incisions that are extended anteriorly to connect with the cleft free edge incisions, creating a posteriorly based flap. The mucoperiosteal flaps are elevated, taking care to preserve the greater palatine vessels. Once the muscles are dissected from the hard palate, a layered closure is performed. In all of these procedures, an intravelar veloplasty, in which the soft palate muscles are completely dissected free and plicated in the midline, is recommended by some authors. These procedures allow for closure of even wide palate defects and for lengthening of the palate. However, aggressive dissection and resulting bone exposure may increase the risk of palate growth disturbance.

The Furlow double-opposing Z-plasty uses a Z-plasty technique to lengthen the soft palate and reapproximate the soft palate musculature.[18] A Z-plasty is performed on the oral and the nasal surface of the soft palate in opposite orientation, leaving muscle attached to the mucosa. The flaps are transposed and secured in position. The procedure may be performed in conjunction with hard palate mucoperiosteal flap closure as described earlier. The advantage of the Furlow procedure is in the excellent palate lengthening. The main disadvantage of this more cumbersome procedure is an increased risk of palatal fistula.

Postoperative care includes a soft diet and avoidance of manipulation of the surgical site for several weeks. Avoiding utensils in the mouth and drinking from a cup, not a bottle, are recommended. Arm restraints are recommended to prevent injury to the palate repair. Home care is appropriate when oral intake is adequate and airway obstruction has resolved.

PERIOPERATIVE COMPLICATIONS

Intraoperative complications are uncommon in palatoplasty. Intubation may be difficult, especially in patients with Robin sequence.[19] Experienced anesthesiologists should be available for these difficult airways. Standard intubation may not be possible, and intubation with a flexible or rigid bronchoscope, intubation with a Bullard laryngoscope, use of a laryngeal mask airway, or even tracheotomy may be necessary. Blood loss is minimized by the injection of local vasoconstrictors prior to incision. Bleeding is usually controlled by electrocautery or pressure. The relaxing incisions may be packed with an absorbable hemostatic agent such as Avitene at the end of the procedure to prevent bleeding, cover bone, and medialize the palate flaps.

Avulsion of the greater palatine vessels can occur from overzealous dissection of the mucoperiosteal flaps. Bleeding can be controlled by ligation, electrocautery, or bone wax. Fortunately, the flaps usually remain viable, although an increased risk of flap necrosis, fistula formation, or palatal growth retardation can be expected. Wide clefts may be difficult to close, and avoidance of surgery until adequate tissue exists for closure is the best option. The use of vomer flaps and more laterally placed cleft edge incisions allows closure of the nasal layer. Careful dissection of the neurovascular bundle and infracturing of the hamulus can free the mucoperiosteal flaps to allow more medial rotation for closure. Secondary procedures are rarely necessary.

Tooth buds may be exposed in the lateral relaxing incisions. Care should be taken to avoid teeth, but specific intervention is not usually necessary.

Early postoperative complications include bleeding, airway obstruction, and infection. Significant postoperative bleeding requires a return to the operating room for identification of the source and appropriate hemostasis. Slight bleeding after repair is expected. Significant bleeding requiring intervention occurs in only 1% of patients on the first postoperative day and is rarely seen up to a week later.

A tongue stitch is usually used to control the airway immediately on extubation. Overnight monitoring in the hospital with a pulse oximeter and observation for respiratory distress are important. Supplemental oxygen and a mist hood are helpful. Reintubation is occasionally required for marked airway distress and may be complicated by bleeding. The use of a nasal trumpet or oral airway may improve the airway at the risk of pressure disruption of the suture line. Death due to airway obstruction has been reported, attesting to the importance of admission for observation, careful monitoring, and intervention for airway problems.[20]

Significant infection in the surgical site is uncommon, but local inflammation is typical. The use of prophylactic antibiotics is recommended to decrease oral odor and the possibility of secondary infections. Postoperative pneumonia may occur from poor pulmonary toilet or aspiration of blood or saliva. Early palatal dehiscence can occur from inadequate closure, excess wound tension, poor blood supply (loss of the greater palatine artery), infection, or local trauma. Small dehiscences will often heal without intervention. For a persistent fistula, early observation with delayed repair when the scar is mature is recommended (see the next section).

Complete flap loss is quite uncommon and very difficult to repair. Careful dissection and avoidance of the neurovascular pedical is important to prevent devascularization. Ensuring adequate flap width to maintain a good blood supply is also important. Delayed repair or prosthetic palliation of the resulting defect is recommended.

Nonsurgical infections are not uncommon and range from simple respiratory infections to pneumonia and gastroenteritis. Surgery should be delayed if patients are acutely ill, to prevent complications of infection after surgery. Careful attention to pulmonary toilet is necessary to prevent pulmonary complications, especially in children with other congenital anomalies or developmental delays.

LATE COMPLICATIONS

Late complications of cleft palate repair include oronasal fistulae, velopharyngeal incompetence, and facial growth disturbance. Fistulas occur in as few as 3.4% and as many as 36% of palatoplasty procedures.[21] Fistulas may occur anywhere along the length of the palate cleft. Labionasal and oronasal clefts of the alveolus are often left intentionally at the time of two-flap palatoplasty. Fistulas may occur in the hard palate, at the junction of the hard and soft palate, or in the soft palate. Fistulas are most common at the junction of the hard and soft palate because this is usually the area under greatest tension at the time of closure. Fistulas may result from inadequate closure, infection, hematoma formation, or avascular necrosis of tissue.

Fistula formation was not related to the sex of the patient, severity of the cleft, or type of repair in one series.[22] However, fistula formation was noted to be less common in patients who had palatal closure at an age younger than 12 months. Fistula formation has also been correlated with underweight infants at the time of surgery[17] and with the experience level of the operating surgeon. In one series of cleft patients, fistula repair was deemed necessary in 11 of 13 patients, and 91% of these fistulas were healed with a single operation.[22] Most fistulas can be closed by using local flaps and two- or three-layered closures.

A small labionasal fistula at the alveolus in complete cleft lip and palate is common and is best repaired at the time of alveolar ridge bone grafting. This should be performed after maxillary expansion (if deemed necessary) to prevent recurrence of the fistula. Incisions are made along the edges of the fistula, and mucoperiosteum are elevated exposing the bony defect. The nasal floor is closed with absorbable suture and the bony defect filled with cancellous bone. Usually, primary closure can be achieved in narrow clefts. Local rotation or advancement flaps taken from the labial mucosa are used to fill larger defects.

A small soft palate fistula can often be closed by excision of the tract and three-layer closure without significant dissection. Large defects are best repaired by complete revision of the palatoplasty with incision of the fistula free edge, elevation of palatal flaps, dissection of the palate musculature, and closure of the defect. Rarely are local soft tissue flaps from lip or tongue needed in addition to local tissue for closure of the defect. Elevation of mucoperisoteal flaps and muscle dissection are complicated by scarring from prior procedures; very careful surgery is required in order to avoid traumatizing mucosa or disrupting the neurovascular pedicle.

Fistulas of the hard palate require more extensive procedures. A variety of local flaps have been described with the common recommendations of elevation of a full-thickness mucoperiosteal flap and rotation or advancement of the flap for a tension-free closure. Two-layer closure is preferred, with rotation of mucosa to close the nasal layer and flap closure of the oral mucosa. Complete revision palatoplasty is advised in long fistulas.

In fistulas that are difficult to close, a variety of options have been described. Free grafts of mucosa have been used as well as tongue flaps,[23] free cartilage grafts,[24,25] or pedicaled buccal mucosa flaps.[26] In large defects, the use of a microvascular free flap has been advocated.[27,28]

Obturators designed to cover palatal fistulas also result in significant improvement in speech quality and are an alternative to surgery.[29]

Orthodontic treatment is expected in children with cleft palate. Dental consultation is recommended at an early age and throughout treatment. Maxillary expansion is often needed to correct deficient lateral facial growth. Maxillary advancement by Le Fort I osteotomy is used to correct more severe midface retrusion.

Airway obstruction — particularly obstructive sleep apnea (OSA) — may develop in children with cleft lip and palate. OSA is more common in children with retrognathia and glossoptosis (Pierre Robin sequence). Hypertrophy of the tonsils and adenoids can occur as it can in otherwise healthy children. Tonsillectomy can be performed with minimal difficulty, but partial adenoidectomy is recommended after palatoplasty to reduce the probability of developing velopharyngeal insufficiency (VPI). Suction electrocautery or a powered suction debrider can be used to remove only the anterior two thirds of the adenoids, leaving the posterior one third intact. Nasal obstruction from cleft-associated septal deviation is common. Septoplasty is often deferred until full growth is obtained to reduce the risk of growth disturbance.

Although VPI is common in children with repaired clefts, other speech and language delays can be identified. Lower developmental performance in fine-motor, gross-motor, and expressive-language domains was noted at 36 months in a recently performed longitudinal evaluation of children and infants with cleft lip and palate.[30] At 5 months, lower motor and self-help developmental quotients were evident in infants with cleft lip and palate. The need to monitor development in cleft lip and palate children is apparent; early referral to intervention services is more likely to be necessary.

Impaired psychological outcomes are common in children with cleft lip and palate. In one series, 73% of thirty-eight 15- and 20-year-old subjects felt their self-confidence had been very much affected as a result of their cleft. Of 112 interviewed patients, 60% had been teased about speech or cleft-related features.[31] Many of the 15-year-old subjects felt excluded from treatment planning decisions. Psychological outcomes should be monitored in children and adults with clefts. Adolescents should be involved in treatment decisions often deferred to parental judgment. Referral for counseling for cleft-associated emotional problems should be considered in patients noted to be struggling to cope.

Optimal surgical correction of congenital cleft lip and palate deformities requires a combination of skill, judgment, and experience unmatched, perhaps, in the gamut of facial plastic operations. Aesthetic and functional goals are realized with varying degrees of success, depending not only on the surgeon's capabilities but also on factors such as the anatomic deformity, wound healing, care-giver compliance, and complications, which are the focus of this chapter.

CLEFT LIP

Lip Adhesion

The lip adhesion operation described by Randall and Millard in the late 1960s remains a useful operation in some patients with wide complete unilateral and bilateral clefts.[32,33] It is most helpful when a great deal of advancement of the lateral lip segments is required. Such advancement is required for achieving vertical (lip height) symmetry in unilateral clefts and orbicularis oris muscle continuity/repair in severe bilateral clefts in which the premaxilla is markedly protrusive.

Complications

Excessive tension on the adhesion results in complete separation in about 4 to 5% of unilateral cases. In superior, "nasal sill" adhesions, partial inferior separation is more frequent but does not affect the goal of the procedure. The risk of separation is reduced by careful deep sutures and placement of a nonabsorbable retention suture anchoring the lateral lip segment to the membranous septum.[34] Such a retention suture has permitted complete success in bilateral adhesions in the authors' experience.

Even though no landmarks or tissue for definitive lip repair is sacrificed, breakdowns may cause increased scarring and potentially compromise the outcome of definitive cheiloplasty. In some patients, additional scarring with the adhesion causes increased bleeding in definitive repair. The adhesion is an additional operation with attendant aesthetic risk, expense, and commitment of caregivers. Although soft tissue dissection from the maxilla is minimal, long-term inhibitive effects on facial growth have been described as greater than previously appreciated.[35]

DEFINITIVE UNILATERAL CLEFT LIP REPAIR/CHEILOPLASTY

The rotation advancement (RA) technique of Millard continues to take precedence as the most common method of unilateral cleft lip repair. The triangular flap method, single method (Randall, Tennison), and double method (Skoog, Bardach) play a reduced but still significant role.

Complications

Major wound infection and bleeding are extremely rare after unilateral cheiloplasty, and flap necrosis is almost unheard of. Late stitch granuloma/abscess, however, is more common (5 to 10%), especially if deep polyvinyl sutures are placed. The intranasal area in the RA technique seems to have a special predilection for suture granulomas. Local care — topical antibiotic ointment or moist compresses and occasionally removal of the offending suture — is adequate treatment.

Because the RA method is a free-hand, cut-as-you-go technique, best results occur with increasing experience. Lip repair should not be attempted by the occasional surgeon; this rule applies especially to the RA technique. When much lip advancement is necessary, as in a very wide unilateral cleft, an adhesion is of considerable benefit (see earlier discussion). There is the risk, however, of overadvancement of the cleft side of the nose producing nostril stenosis and hypoplastic nasal envelope, an acquired deformity difficult, if not impossible, to correct completely.[36] Underadvancement of the cleft side lip results in vertical shortening and asymmetry and is common in wide complete clefts. Cupid's bow asymmetry is the result of insufficient rotation, generally caused by absence of Millard's back cut through skin and muscle of the rotation flap, the advancement flap edge being too short for the rotation edge, or shortening of the lip when the orbicularis oris muscle is repaired.

A good general rule is to make the rotation incision long enough to level the Cupid's bow peak height and then make the back cut as a precaution. With muscle repair, constant vigilance is needed to avoid losing the rotation and shortening the lip. Muscle approximation to the vermilion edge and lip border is important to avoid notching as well as for normal function. Small flaps (white roll) placed at or just above the vermilion cutaneous junction may assist in breaking up the scar line and may achieve additional rotation in a lip that is very slightly short (<1 mm).

Some authors recommend correction of the unilateral cleft lip nasal deformity at the time of lip repair or in early childhood.[37,38] Dissection of the lower lateral cartilages requires special care in the younger child. Cartilages may be repositioned by internal or through-and-through sutures. Late complications include the possibility of cartilage loss and vestibular stenosis from excessive scarring and compromised blood supply. An advantage of lip adhesion is often the remodeling of the nasal tip cartilages with improvement in long-term nasal configuration.[39]

BILATERAL CLEFT LIP REPAIR

As with unilateral cleft lip, bilateral clefts constitute a spectrum of deformities with features unique to the type. In complete bilateral clefts, blood supply to the premaxilla-prolabium is via small-paired posterior septal vessels with some contributions from terminal branches of the anterior ethmoids. The premaxilla can be protruding. This is a challenge for the surgeon. Various approaches for retropositioning to the premaxilla have been employed: presurgical orthopedics, prosthetics, active and passive, and surgical (set back/lip adhesions) as well as staged definitive repairs.[40] Prosthetic methods require the highly specialized expertise of a prosthodontist or orthodontist in dealing with the premaxilla. Without a dedicated caregiver and compliance, success with prosthetic methods is unlikely.

Complications

Poor blood supply is probably responsible for the increased incidence of wound infection, especially in single-stage repairs. Risk of further maxillary growth is also increased. An extremely shortened columella is a characteristic feature of the bilateral cleft lip nasal deformity. Correction of this deformity varies from prosthetic stretching of the nasal tip[41] to surgical shifting of tissue into the columella from the nasal tip[42] or from the nasal sill or philtrum.[43,44] Prosthetic approaches appear to have the same limitations as described previously: expertise and compliance. Insufficient lengthening from flap shrinkage or contracture is a risk with all surgical techniques; overprojection and nostril eversion may be more likely in the banked forked flap method (Millard).

THE ALVEOLUS

A periosteoplasty closes the alveolar cleft by periosteal tissue flaps taken from the margins of the cleft. Ideally, sufficient bone is produced by the periosteum to avoid the need for later bone grafting as well as closing nasal oral and nasolabial fistulae. The alveolar ridge segments must be in close approximation, if not actual contact, so presurgical orthopedics is required in many cases. Primary bone grafting with a rib graft placed at the time of lip repair in infancy has been advocated, but has generally not been accepted because of concerns of facial growth.[45,46] Secondary grafting is timed before the eruption of the permanent canine teeth on the cleft side, performed between 8 and 11 years of age, and follows initial orthodontic treatment, usually expansion for correction of crossbite. Autologous cancellus bone chips are used and can be taken from various sites, including iliac crest, cranium, rib, and mentum.[47]

COMPLICATIONS

Possible late complications of periosteoplasty include the inhibition of maxillary growth and inadequate bone deposition so that secondary grafting is eventually required. Pain at the donor site, especially the ilium, often exceeds that of the alveolus. Other donor site complications are rare but may be serious. The lateral femoral cutaneous nerve is at risk in iliac crest sites and damage may result in transient or permanent numbness. Penetration to the underlying peritoneum, pleura, or dura is an obvious risk depending upon the site. Unilateral alveolar grafts have a high take rate: 95 to 99%.[48] Bilateral grafts, especially performed as a single stage, are less successful. This is probably the result of poor blood supply and especially occurs when the premaxilla is rudimentary — occasionally, only a bony shell around one or two incisor teeth.

VELOPHARYNGEAL INSUFFICIENCY

Although many of the children who have cleft palate or cleft lip and palate will have problems with nasal resonance, aggressive speech therapy addressing articulation and resonance issues usually will allow them to have normal or near normal speech patterns by time of entry into school. Appropriate attention must be placed into the prevention of maladaptive (compensatory) articulation to improve speech intelligibility.

Unfortunately, a small percentage will have persistent velopharyngeal dysfunction or insufficiency in spite of this aggressive speech therapy. In that instance, something other than speech therapy management is necessary; this usually requires surgical intervention. The results of the surgical intervention for resonance issues and velopharyngeal dysfunction vary; however, it is usually rather successful. The complications of this type of surgery are (1) persistent hypernasality, (2) hyponasality, and (3) airway obstruction. Each of these will be examined.

COMPLICATIONS

The attempt for surgical management for velopharyngeal dysfunction is typically to obturate the remaining gap in the velopharynx that is causing the velopharyngeal dysfunction. The most successful attempts try to tailor the surgical procedure to the child's remaining gap on appropriate articulation. If diagnosis or assessment is inappropriate, then the probability of failure to reduce the hypernasality of any surgical procedure will be higher.

Flexible fiberoptic nasopharyngoscopy or video fluoroscopy can be useful in assessing the closure pattern in velopharyngeal dysfunction.[49] Closure pattern is typically divided into four subsets:

- Sagittal — both lateral walls take the predominant role in the closure of the velopharynx with a resultant midline sagittal gap.
- Coronal — the velum is the predominant element of velopharyngeal closure with a resultant posterior gap in a coronal orientation.
- Circular — the lateral walls and the velum contribute to the closure with a resultant circular central gap
- Circular with Passavant's — not only do the lateral walls and velum contribute to the closure pattern but Passavant's ridge (the superior border of the superior constrictor) also contributes to the closure pattern with a resultant circular, central gap.

Given these closure patterns, the resulting gap will be best surgically obturated by different surgical techniques. Techniques currently available for use are (1) Furlow double opposing Z-plasty, (2) sphincter pharyngoplasty, (3) superiorly based pharyngeal flap, and (4) posterior wall augmentation.

The Furlow double opposing Z-plasty seeks to lengthen the palate and reorient the levator sling in an appropriate transverse orientation.[50] This would be exceptionally helpful in the coronal closure pattern when a midline palatal notch is causing velopharyngeal dysfunction or the palate is short but almost reaching the posterior wall.

The sphincter pharyngoplasty is exceptionally good for obturating the posterior and lateral pharyngeal walls.[51,52] This will be helpful when the gap is coronal or if a larger central, circular gap, whether Passavant's, is noted or not. The superiorly based pharyngeal flap obturates the central portion of the velopharyngeal area and is therefore optimum when the gap is in the sagittal plane or if it is a small, circular gap.[53] The posterior wall augmentation allows a ridge of tissue to be created on the posterior pharyngeal wall and will be ideal when a very small gap is at the posterior wall, typically in the circular or coronal orientations.[54,55] If the decision as to the technique for surgical obturating of the gap is inappropriate, there will be a higher risk of failure of obturation and, thus, residual hypernasality.[56]

Sometimes the appropriate surgery has been selected but technical or healing factors contribute to failure. In sphincter pharyngoplasty, the superiorly based lateral pharyngeal wall myomucosal flaps are crossed and inserted in the posterior pharyngeal wall. If the palatal motion is minimal and the flaps are not tightened appropriately, there may still be persistent air escape. If the flaps are placed too low in the velopharynx or if they are placed in the superior oropharynx, the palate may not come in contact with this ridge to allow appropriate speech. Attention to the preoperative assessment can assist in defining the optimum level of insertion for the sphincter pharyngoplasty and the degree of flap tightness.

In pharyngeal flap surgery, scarring on the pharyngeal flap may turn a moderate to wide pharyngeal flap into a small string-like connection between the posterior pharyngeal wall and the velum. This can be a result of not lining the flap at the time of surgery. The use of a palate-splitting operation allows the pharyngeal flap to be covered more adequately and little raw tissue to remain. This will typically improve the chances of the flap not scarring and thinning.

The posterior wall implant or rolled flap may suffer from drifting of the implanted material, reabsorption of the implanted material, or reabsorption of the rolled flap.[57] One must take great care in selecting patients for this surgery and avoid the use of materials that may drift into the hypopharynx, thus potentially causing upper airway obstruction.

If the patient has undergone a sphincter pharyngoplasty and hypernasal resonance or emission is present, one may attempt a tightening of the sphincter.[58] This is relatively easily done by removing the mucosa on the posterior surface of the sphincter pharyngoplasty and closing this on itself to tighten the sphincter port. Care must be taken not to obstruct the nose completely. Tightening often leads to a better functional result. If the sphincter pharyngoplasty is placed too low, one can take down the sphincter pharyngoplasty and reinsert it at a higher level or remove the current sphincter pharyngoplasty and create myomusocal flaps from the lateral pharyngeal wall to be inserted at a higher level. All of the surgical plans need to be made based on the preoperative endoscopic assessment.

Correction of the failed pharyngeal flap is somewhat more difficult. However the preoperative endoscopy can allow one to determine whether one or both of the ports need to be reduced in size.[10] Two major ways of reducing the size of the lateral ports would be to (1) do a small V–Y advancement placing additional posterior pharyngeal wall tissue into the posterior wall of the lateral port or (2) take an additional narrow pharyngeal flap from the posterior pharyngeal wall and suture it into place into the lateral aspect of the pharyngeal flap, thereby reducing the dimension of the lateral port medially.

Based on the postoperative endoscopic findings, it is occasionally necessary to suggest a complete change in approach to the velopharyngeal dysfunction. Sometimes the pharyngeal flap may need to be substituted for a sphincter pharyngoplasty or vice versa. If airway obstruction is significant in spite of persistent velopharyngeal dysfunction, then one may consider the use of prosthetic devices to reduce the risk of velopharyngeal dysfunction while at the same time protecting the nasal airway.

In general, there has been a lack of concern with hyponasality as a complication of velopharyngeal surgery. Because hypernasality and nasal emission are far more concerning and affect the intelligibility and acceptance of the child's speech, surgeons have typically allowed hyponasality to be an accepted, if not an expected, complication of velopharyngeal surgery. In the initial design of the surgical treatment, the area of the velopharyngeal space that needs to be obturated should be well defined and the surgical intervention tailored to meet this. One would then hope that the risk of hyponasality could be reduced.[59] Occasionally, scarring may result in hyponasality in spite of a well-designed and executed technique.

Hyponasality is a difficult process to reverse. One must constantly weigh the risk of reintroducing hypernasality at the time of correcting hyponasality. Because hyponasality may be a result of other nasal airway obstruction, it is important to evaluate the child for other issues that may contribute to the hyponasal or denasal speech. Included in this must be nasal anatomy. Frequently, children with cleft lip and palate have a significantly deviated nasal septum, which may contribute to a hyponasal resonance in spite of a normal functioning velopharynx. In a similar vein, mucosal disease and increased nasal mucous production caused by allergy or infection may contribute to hyponasal or denasal speech. Medical management of allergy, nasal mucous, and infection is important to maintain the appropriate nasal resonance in these children. Use of topical nasal steroid sprays, saline washes, and appropriate antibiotics is very important. Occasionally, the child who is significantly denasal or hyponasal may do well with nasal septal reconstruction even before puberty to improve this speech production. If the hyponasality or denasality is so severe that the patient would have preferred his initial hypernasality, taking down the pharyngeal flap or opening the sphincter pharyngoplasty may be appropriate.

Velopharyngeal insufficiency surgery always obstructs the nasopharynx to some degree. Though this may lead to hyponasality as described earlier, the nasal airway obstruction may contribute to more serious difficulties. The child may be a constant mouth breather. The child who has severe nasal airway obstruction may suffer from chronic nasal drainage with difficulty blowing his nose and constant sniffing. This may be an additional psychosocial issue to the child struggling for peer acceptance. There is some debate as to whether nasal obstruction may contribute to "adenoid facies" with facial elongation and characteristic dental complications of molar crossbite. In the child who has a cleft lip and palate with risk of midface growth problems, this may be a further risk factor.

The worst potential complication from the nasal airway obstruction is obstructive sleep apnea.[60] The family must be questioned as to the potential presence of this condition. Although obstructive sleep apnea may often be well defined just by an interview with the parent, a sleep study will help establish the degree to which this apnea is bothering the child and, in addition, allow a better idea of the risks and benefits of any surgical intervention.[61]

Airway obstruction may be caused by the sphincter being too tight, lack of lateral port control during a pharyngeal flap surgery, excessive scarring in the lateral ports, or increased tonsillar/adenoid tissue in the postoperative period. Increased risk is also seen with Robin sequence and midface retrusion, in which skeletal deformity reduces airway dimension. Occasionally, the airway obstruction may be contributed to by the other anatomical and mucosal factors described in the section on hyponasality. Preoperative tonsillectomy and/or adenoidectomy may be helpful in reducing the airway risk.

If the child is suffering from obstructive sleep apnea and tonsil or adenoid tissue is present, removing the obstructing lymphatic tissue may offer significant improvement. Adenoids may be assessed with flexible fiberoptic endoscopy at the time of speech evaluation. Given the presence of an obturating flap in the velopharynx, the adenoids will typically be above this flap and removal most probably will need to be done with either a take-down of the flap or a transnasal microdebridement; increased hypernasality may result. If the tonsils are at all obstructing, these should be removed. Typically, less resultant hypernasality is present after tonsil removal.

If the problem seems to be related only to the pharyngeal flap or the sphincter pharyngoplasty, there have been successful treatments of airway obstruction by the use of continuous positive airway pressure (CPAP).[12] CPAP may be introduced at night through a face mask allowing the child to have significant improvement in breathing while sleeping. In some instances, over a period of time, the sphincter of pharyngeal flap may "stretch" or the child grow to the point that this is no longer necessary.

If the obstruction is very severe or the CPAP is not tolerated by the child, a take-down of the flap or the sphincter pharyngoplasty will be necessary. Although some documents in the literature suggest that occasional take-down of the pharyngeal flap will not lead to recurrent hypernasality, this must always be considered in discussing the possibility with the family. Consideration of prosthetic management of the velopharyngeal dysfunction in this situation is a must.

CONCLUSION

The child born with a cleft lip and/or palate requires a multidisciplinary approach over many years to treat the functional and aesthetic components of the disease adequately. The astute physician can recognize the problems of the disease early so that therapy can begin avoiding airway, feeding, and speech problems. Even in the most experienced hands, the outcome from surgical management may not be as anticipated. The surgeon and family must communicate so that realistic expectations from surgical therapy result.

REFERENCES

1. Pandya, A.N. and Boorman, J.G. Failure to thrive in babies with cleft lip and palate. *Br. J. Plastic Surg.*, 2001, 54, 471–475.
2. Crossman, K. Breastfeeding a baby with cleft palate: a case report. *J. Hum. Lactation*, 1998, 14, 47–50.
3. Caouette-Laberge, L., Plamondon, C., and Larocque, Y. Subperiosteal release of the floor of the mouth in Pierre Robin sequence: experience with 12 cases. *Cleft Palate-Craniofac. J.*, 1996, 33, 468–472.
4. Sidman, J.D., Sampson, D., and Templeton, B. Distraction osteogenesis of the mandible for airway obstruction in children. *Laryngoscope*, 2001, 111, 1137–1146.
5. Cruz, M.J., Kerschner, J.E., Beste, D.J., and Conley, S.F. Pierre Robin sequences: secondary respiratory difficulties and intrinsic feeding abnormalities. *Laryngoscope*, 1999, 109, 1632–1636.
6. Handzic-Cuk, J., Cuk, V., Gluhinic, M., Risavi, R., and Stajner-Katusic, S. Tympanometric findings in cleft palate patients: influence of age and cleft type. *J. Laryngol. Otol.*, 2001, 115, 91–96.
7. Guneren, E., Ozsoy, Z., Ulay, M., Eryilmaz, E., Ozkul, H., and Geary, P.M. A comparison of the effects of Veau-Wardill-Kilner palatoplasty and furlow double-opposing Z-plasty operations on eustachian tube function. *Cleft Palate-Craniofac. J.*, 2000, 37, 266–270.
8. Greig, A.V., Papesch, M.E., and Rowsell, A.R. Parental perceptions of grommet insertion in children with cleft palate. *J. Laryngol. Otol.*, 1999, 113, 1068–1071.
9. Suzuki, H., Yamaguchi, T., and Furukawa, M. Maxillary sinus development and sinusitis in patients with cleft lip and palate. *Auris, Nasus, Larynx*, 2000, 27, 253–256.
10. Kirschner, R.E., Randall, P., Wang, P. et al. Cleft palate repair at 3 to 7 months of age. *Plastic Reconstr. Surg.*, 2000, 105, 2127–2132.
11. Rohrich, R.J., Rowsell, A.R., Johns, D.F. et al. Timing of hard palatal closure: a critical long-term analysis. *Plastic Reconstr. Surg.*, 1996, 98, 236–246.
12. Friede, H., Priede, D., Moller, M., Maulina, I., Lilja, J., and Barkane, B. Comparisons of facial growth in patients with unilateral cleft lip and palate treated by different regimens for two-stage palatal repair. *Scand. J. Plastic Reconstr. Surg. Hand Surg.*, 1999, 33, 73–81.
13. LaRossa, D. The state of the art in cleft palate surgery. *Cleft Palate-Craniofacial J.*, 2000, 37, 225–228.
14. Henriksson, T.G. and Skoog, V.T. Identification of children at high anaesthetic risk at the time of primary palatoplasty. *Scand. J. Plastic Reconstr. Surg. Hand Surg.*, 2001, 35, 177–182.
15. Lin, K.Y., Goldberg, D., Williams, C., Borowitz, K., Persing, J., and Edgerton, M. Long-term outcome analysis of two treatment methods for cleft palate: combined levator retropositioning and pharyngeal flap versus double-opposing Z-plasty. *Cleft Palate-Craniofac. J.*, 1999, 36, 73–78.
16. Senders, C.W., Di Mauro, S.M., Brodie, H.A., Emery, B.E., and Sykes, J.M. The efficacy of perioperative steroid therapy in pediatric primary palatoplasty. *Cleft Palate-Craniofac. J.*, 1999, 36, 340–344.
17. Lazarus, D.D., Hudson, D.A., Fleming, A.N., Goddard, E.A., and Fernandes, D.B. Are children with clefts underweight for age at the time of primary surgery? *Plastic Reconstr. Surg.*, 1999, 103, 1624–1629.
18. Furlow, J.J. Cleft palate repair by double opposing Z-plasty. *Plastic Reconstr. Surg.*, 1986, 78, 724–736.
19. Eriksson, M. and Henriksson, T.G. Risk factors in children having palatoplasty. *Scand. J. Plastic Reconstr. Surg. Hand Surg.*, 2001, 35, 279–283.
20. Kravath, R., Pollack, D., and Borowiecki, B. Obstructive sleep apnea and death associated with surgical correction of velopharyngeal incompetence. *J. Pediatr.*, 1980, 96, 645.
21. Wilhelmi, B.J., Appelt, E.A., Hill, L., and Blackwell, S.J. Palatal fistulas: rare with the two-flap palatoplasty repair. *Plastic Reconstr. Surg.*, 2001, 107, 315–318.
22. Emory, R.E., Jr., Clay, R.P., Bite, U., and Jackson, I.T. Fistula formation and repair after palatal closure: an institutional perspective. *Plastic Reconstr. Surg.*, 1997, 99, 1535–1538.
23. Guzel, M.Z. and Altintas, F. Repair of large, anterior palatal fistulas using thin tongue flaps: long-term follow-up of 10 patients. *Ann. Plastic Surg.*, 2000, 45, 109–114; discussion 114–117.
24. Jeffery, S.L., Boorman, J.G., and Dive, D.C. Use of cartilage grafts for closure of cleft palate fistulae. *Br. J. Plastic Surg.*, 2000, 53, 551–554.
25. Mohanna, P.N., Kangesu, L., and Sommerlad, B.C. The use of conchal-cartilage grafts in the closure of recurrent palatal fistulae. *Br. J. Plastic Surg.*, 2001, 54, 274.

26. Honnebier, M.B., Johnson, D.S., Parsa, A.A., Dorian, A., and Parsa, F.D. Closure of palatal fistula with a local mucoperiosteal flap lined with buccal mucosal graft. *Cleft Palate-Craniofacial J.*, 2000, 37, 127–129.
27. Ninkovi, C.M., Hubli, E.H., Schwabegger, A., and Anderl, H. Free flap closure of recurrent palatal fistula in the cleft lip and palate patient. *J. Craniofacial Surg.*, 1997, 8, 491–495; discussion 496.
28. Turk, A.E., Chang, J., Soroudi, A.E., Hui, K., and Lineaweaver, W.C. Free flap closure in complex congenital and acquired defects of the palate. *Ann. Plastic Surg.*, 2000, 45, 274–279.
29. Pinborough-Zimmerman, J., Canady, C., Yamashiro, D.K., and Morales, L., Jr. Articulation and nasality changes resulting from sustained palatal fistula obturation. *Cleft Palate-Craniofac. J.*, 1998, 35, 81–87.
30. Neiman, G.S. and Savage, H.E. Development of infants and toddlers with clefts from birth to three years of age. *Cleft Palate-Craniofacial J.*, 1997, 34, 218–225.
31. Turner, S.R., Thomas, P.W., Dowell, T., Rumsey, N., and Sandy, J.R. Psychological outcomes amongst cleft patients and their families. *Br. J. Plastic Surg.*, 1997, 50, 1–9.
32. Millard, D.R., Jr. Refinements in rotation-advancement cleft lip technique. *Plast. Roconstr. Surg.*, 1964, 33, 26.
33. Randall, P. A lip adhesion operation in cleft lip surgery. *Plast Reconstr. Surg.*, 1965, 35(4), 371–376.
34. Seibert, R.W. Management of unilateral cleft lip and palate. *Curr. Ther. Otolaryngol.*, 1990, 316–322.
35. Kapucu, M.R. et al. The effect of cleft lip repair on maxillary morphology in patients with unilateral complete cleft lip and palate. *Plast. Reconstr. Surg.*, 1996, 97, 1371.
36. Cutting, C.B., Bardach, J., and Pang, R. A comparative study of the skin envelope of the unilateral cleft lip nose subsequent to rotation-advancement and triangular flap lip repairs. *Plast. Reconstr. Surg.*, 1989, 84(3), 409–419.
37. Sugihara, T. et al. Primary correction of the unilateral cleft nose. *Cleft Palate-Craniofac J.*, 1993, 30, 231.
38. Cook, T.A., Davis, R.E., and Israel, J.M. The extended Skoog technique for repair of the unilateral cleft lip and nose deformity. *Facial Plast. Surg.*, 1993, 9, 195.
39. Seibert, R.W. Management of unilateral cleft lip and palate. *Curr. Ther. Otolaryngol.*, 1990, 316–322.
40. Millard, R. *Cleft Craft, The Evolution of its Surgery, Bilateral and Rare Deformities*, Vol. II 1st ed. Boston: Little Brown, 1977, 41–80.
41. Cutting, C., Grayson, B., Brecht, L., Santiago, P., Wood, R., and Kwon, S. Presurgical columellar elongation and primary retrograde nasal reconstruction in one-stage bilateral cleft lip and nose repair. *Plast. Reconstr. Surg.*, 1998, 102(5), 1761–1762.
42. McComb, H. Primary repair of the bilateral cleft lip nose: a 15 year review and a new treatment plan. *Plast. Reconstr. Surg.*, 1990, 86(5), 882–889.
43. Cronin, T. Lengthening columella by use of skin from the nasal floor and alae. *Plast. Reconstr. Surg.*, 1958, 21, 417.
44. Millard, R. *Cleft Craft, The Evolution of its Surgery, Bilateral and Rare Deformities,* Vol II, 1st ed. Boston: Little Brown, 1977, 40–80.
45. Rosenstein, S., Kernahan, D., Dado, D., Grasseschi, M., and Griffith, B.H. Orthognathic surgery in cleft patients treated by early bone grafting. *Plast. Reconstr. Surg.*, 1991, 87(5), 835–892.
46. Millard, D.R., Jr. and Latham, R.A. Improved primary surgical and dental treatment of clefts. *Plast. Reconstr. Surg.*, 1990, 86(5), 856–871.
47. Cohen, M., Figueroa, A., Haviv, Y., Schafer, M.E., and Aduss, H. Iliac versus cranial bone for secondary grafting of residual alveolar clefts. *Plast. Reconstr Surg.*, 1991, 87(3), 423–428.
48. Bergland, O., Semb, G., Abyholm, F., Borchgrevink, H., and Eskeland, G. Secondary bone grafting and orthodontic treatment in patients with bilateral complete clefts of the lip and palate. *Ann. Plast. Surg.*, 1986, 17(6), 460–474.
49. Croft, C.B., Shprintzen, R.J., and Rakoff, S.J. Patterns of velopharyngeal valving in normal and cleft palate subjects: a multi-view videofluoroscopic and nasoendoscopic study. *Laryngoscope*, 1981, 91(2), 265–271.
50. Kirschner, R.E., Wang, P., Jawad, A.F., Duran, M., Cohen, M., Solot, C., Randall, P., and LaRossa, D. Cleft-palate repair by modified Furlow double-opposing Z-plasty: the Children's Hospital of Philadelphia experience. *Plast. Reconstr. Surg.*, 1999, 104(7), 1998–2010; discussion 2011–2014.

51. DeSerres, L.M., Deleyiannis, F.W., Eblen, L.E., Gruss, R.S., Richardson, M.A., and Sie, K.C. Results with sphincter pharyngoplasty and pharyngeal flap. *Int. J. Pediatr. Otorhinolaryngol.*, 1999, 48(1), 17–25.

52. Witt, P., Cohen, D., Grames, L.M., and Marsh, J. Sphincter pharyngoplasty for the surgical management of speech dysfunction associated with velocardiofacial syndrome. *Br. J. Plast. Surg.*, 1999, 52(8), 613–618.

53. Sloan, G.M. Posterior pharyngeal flap and sphincter pharyngoplasty: the state of the art. *Cleft Palate Craniofacial J.*, 2000, 37(20), 112–122.

54. Gray, S.D., Pinborough-Zimmerman, J., and Catten, M. Posterior wall augmentation for treatment of velopharyngeal insufficiency. *Otolaryngol. Head Neck Surg.*, 1999, 121(1), 107–112.

55. Witt, P.D., O'Daniel, T.G., Marsh, J.L., Grames, L.M., Muntz, H.R., and Pilgram, T.K. Surgical management of velopharyngeal dysfunction: outcome analysis of autogenous posterior pharyngeal wall augmentation. *Plast. Reconstr. Surg.*, 1997, 99(5), 1287–1296; discussion 1297–1300.

56. Ma, L., James, D.R., and Sell, D.A. Failed pharyngoplasty and subsequent management. *Br. J. Pral. Maxillofac. Surg.*, 1996, 34(5), 348–356.

57. Dejonckere, P.H. and Van Wijngaarden, H.A. Retropharyngeal autologous fat transplantation for congenital short palate: a nasometric assessment of functional results. *Ann. Otol. Rhinol. Laryngol.*, 2001, 110, 168–172.

58. Witt, P.D., Myckatyn, T., and Marsh, J.L. Salvaging the failed pharyngoplasty: intervention outcome. *Cleft Palate-Craniofac. J.*, 1998, 35(5), 447–453.

59. Sie, K.C., Tampakopoulou, D.A., de Serres, L.M., Gruss, J.S., Eblen, L.E., and Yonick, T. Sphincter pharyngoplasty: speech outcome and complications. *Laryngoscope*, 1998, 108(8 Pt. 1), 1211–1217.

60. Witt, P.D., Marsh, J.L., Muntz, H.R., Marty-Grames, L., and Watchmaker, G.P. Acute obstructive sleep apnea as a complication of sphincter pharyngoplasty. *Cleft Palate-Craniofac. J.*, 1996, 33(3), 183–189.

61. Wells, M.D., Vu, T.A., and Lace, E.A. Incidence and sequelae of nocturnal respiratory obstruction following posterior pharyngeal flap operation. *Ann. Plast. Surg.*, 1999, 43(3), 252–257.

34 Pediatric Maxillofacial Trauma

Harlan R. Muntz and Andrew Shapiro

The one mark of maturity, especially in a physician, and perhaps it is even rarer in a scientist, is the capacity to deal with uncertainty.

William B. Bean

CONTENTS

INTRODUCTION

The management of complex pediatric maxillofacial injuries has evolved from a "watch and see" approach to a point at which opportunities abound to intervene and shape the outcome. Repair of these injuries demands technical dexterity, creativity, and a three-dimensional appreciation of the facial skeletal anatomy. Furthermore, management is complicated by anatomic and physiologic nuances that vary according to age and the nature of injury. With respect to internal fixation, a sound knowledge of rapidly evolving technology is required, often relegating these patients to tertiary care centers. Perhaps the most challenging facet in the care of injured patients is to know *when* to use the available techniques — a decision based upon a limited amount of "hard data," personal experience, and a generous helping of common sense. Errors of omission and commission are possible every step along the way. This chapter will attempt to provide an overview of the management of soft tissue and skeletal injuries in children with an emphasis on potential complications of these injuries and their therapy.

INITIAL EVALUATION AND MANAGEMENT

The most common pediatric facial injuries are isolated soft tissue lacerations and abrasions. Facial fractures are relatively rare in the pediatric population. The landmark series published by Rowe suggested that less than 1% occurred in children less than 5 years of age, and less than 5% in children 12 and under;[1] more recently, Gussick et al. suggested that nearly 15% of maxillofacial fractures occurred in children.[2]

Any injury that evades identification represents a missed opportunity for appropriate treatment and may result in long-term functional or aesthetic complications. Thus, a comprehensive evaluation is the first step in avoiding complications. As stated previously, the most common presentation is a fairly limited trauma resulting in a facial laceration or isolated minimally displaced fracture. In this setting, the head and neck surgeon is consulted to provide wound care and precise approximation of soft tissue to ensure the best long-term result. However, it is essential to maintain vigilance even for these relatively simple injuries. It is necessary to ensure that the cervical spine has been examined in injuries resulting from playground falls and athletics. One should carefully assess vision and maintain a low threshold for ophthalmologic consultation for periorbital trauma. The patient's tetanus status should be reviewed.

In contrast, injuries caused by vehicular trauma, penetrating trauma, or high-velocity projectiles demand a comprehensive approach from a trauma team. In these cases, an accepted trauma algorithm should be used. Approximately 75% of children with facial trauma have associated injuries, most commonly involving the central nervous system.[3]

The first priority is maintenance of the airway because airway obstruction is the second most common cause of death in trauma patients. The oral cavity should be suctioned to remove clots, avulsed dentition, and other foreign material. Endotracheal intubation may be necessary for patients with concurrent injuries. Only rarely is displacement of maxillary or mandibular fractures sufficient to compromise the airway. Tracheotomy can be treacherous in an unsecured pediatric airway; preemptive intervention with elective intubation is almost always preferable. Pulmonary complications are common and gastric contents should be routinely evacuated.

The abundant vasculature of the maxillofacial structures enhances wound healing and reduces the infection rate, but can result in hemodynamic compromise from blood loss. The control of bleeding should take place simultaneously with volume replacement through adequate peripheral IV access. One should avoid aggressively clamping vessels because this may result in injury to neurologic structures; direct pressure is usually sufficient. Ligation may be necessary for the larger "named" vessels.

SECONDARY SURVEY: DIAGNOSIS OF FACIAL INJURIES

After the initial systemic management of the traumatized patient, a comprehensive head and neck examination is a key part of the secondary survey. A justifiably terrified child makes for a difficult evaluation. The examiner's approach should be calm and compassionate, but firm; a forewarning before each step helps establish trust. Typically, only a limited history can be obtained from the patient, so eyewitness reports are valuable and a thorough physical examination with appropriate radiological studies is essential.

Several anatomic characteristics render examination difficult following pediatric facial trauma. Generous subcutaneous fat provides for profound edema, and fractures, which are typically limited in displacement, may be difficult to identify. Mixed dentition makes accurate assessment of occlusion difficult. Therefore, the examiner must search for clues of underlying injury. Proceeding in a step-wise approach, he or she should inspect for abrasions, ecchymosis, and asymmetry and elicit extraocular movements. Facial motor and sensory function should be assessed. Periorbital ("racoon eyes") or mastoid ecchymosis (Battle's sign) indicate injury to the cranial base. Otoscopy is performed to identify external canal disruption or hemotympanum. One should palpate bony prominences and gently inspect lacerations.

Radiologic imaging is a vital facet of the diagnostic process. Fine-cut axial and coronal CT scans help identify fractures that physical examination might fail to identify due to limited displacement. Furthermore, identification of orbital floor displacement and prolapse of orbital contents into the maxillary and ethmoid sinuses may indicate the need for surgical reduction in the absence of significant physical findings.

SOFT TISSUE INJURIES

SKIN AND SUBCUTANEOUS TISSUE

The most notable complications related to soft tissue injuries are suboptimal scarring, resulting in aesthetic and functional compromise, and wound infection. A thorough discussion with the parents regarding potential outcomes, augmented by photo documentation of the injury, establishes a foundation and provides reinforcement for reasonable expectations. Psychosocial dysfunction from scarring is certainly a potential complication and should be addressed initially and at follow-up. Meticulous wound care is the key to minimizing these complications. The overall rate of wound infection for lacerations is approximately 4%. For "clean" lacerations without underlying fractures and closed within 6 hours, systemic antibiotics are usually unnecessary. Hypertrophic scarring and keloid formation represent abnormal wound-healing processes and are reviewed in the chapter on wound healing.

Some children require sedation and local anesthesia before any attempt at laceration management. A combination of intranasal midazolam and a choice of several available topical anesthetics are ideal in this setting. Previously, a mixture of tetracaine/cocaine/adrenaline had been popular, but seizures have been reported after mucosal exposure. A variety of agents applied topically, including lidocaine with epinephrine for injection, provide a margin of anesthetic that allows careful inspection and cleaning and the opportunity to inject local anesthetics. Toxicity should be considered in patients with multiple lacerations.

Wounds should be irrigated briskly to remove necrotic debris and foreign material; a large syringe or a pressurized 500-cc bag of saline directed through an IV catheter provides adequate force. Retained material in the wound may provide a nidus for persistent inflammation and result in traumatic tattooing. The wound should be prepped with a sterilizing agent such as povidone iodine; although this agent may be toxic to nonepithelial tissue, the risks of infection are probably more significant. Minimal debridement is required for pediatric facial injuries because marginal tissue often survives due to a very adequate blood supply.

A wound can be closed in many ways, but certain tenets do apply. In general, primary closure should be used in the initial management of a pediatric laceration. Flap rotation or "random pattern" techniques are best reserved for secondary revision of suboptimal results. One should not sacrifice uninjured tissue to close lacerations that the surgeon did not have the "privilege" of creating. Alternatively, careful undermining and a layered closure reduce the tension on the skin and allow primary closure in most cases.

The choice of skin suture varies, but removal within approximately 5 days should be accomplished to minimize "suture tracts." A rapidly absorbable 6-0 plain gut suture in a running locking fashion provides the necessary duration to allow healing. Sutureless methods using adhesives for skin closure are gaining increasing acceptance in emergency rooms and primary care offices, with results comparable to suture closure.[4] Areas of abrasion should be covered with an antibiotic ointment and allowed to re-epithelialize, rather than being excised.

Nonhuman animal bites (dogbites accounting for 80%) can usually be treated similarly. The infection rate for closed dog bite wounds is comparable to nonbite wounds. Obviously, the direct inoculation of large quantities of bacteria into the wound makes careful preparation essential. The most common organisms are *Pastuerella multocida, Staphylococcus aureus*, and *Streptococcus*. If greater than 6 to 12 hours has transpired since the injury, cleaning and debridement followed by delayed closure may be most appropriate. Puncture wounds are best left open.

Wound checks in 24 and 72 hours are essential for follow-up of bite injuries. Tetanus toxoid and rabies inoculations should be considered based upon standard guidelines. Human bites have a much higher risk of infection, although for facial lacerations, primary closure is still reasonable, after careful wound prep. Systemic antibiotics are usually recommended to reduce the risk of postoperative infection.[5]

SITES REQUIRING SPECIAL ATTENTION

Lacerations through the lip must be approximated perfectly or a noticeable step-off occurs. It is worthwhile to begin with a skin stitch directly through the vermilion border to restore this margin before placing deep sutures. Trauma to the pinna with exposed cartilage can result in chondritis and long-term deformity. In extensive injuries, careful debridement followed by "burying" the cartilage in the postauricular skin "baby-sits" the cartilage and provides a delayed skin flap for secondary repair.

Lacerations through the cheek may result in injury to the parotid duct. Injury to Stenson's duct, evidenced by expression of saliva into the wound when the parotid gland is compressed, should be repaired with fine, permanent sutures over an appropriately sized silicone tube. Last, injuries to peripheral branches of the facial nerve result in notable motor dysfunction. Disruptions lateral to the lateral canthus should be repaired with fine nonabsorbable sutures using microsurgical techniques. In a grossly contaminated wound, the best results derive from delayed repair. In the acute phase, distal segments should be tagged while the nerve is still able to be stimulated (usually the first 72 hours).

FRACTURES OF THE FACIAL SKELETON

In order to facilitate decision making and minimize complications in the treatment of pediatric facial fractures, an appreciation of facial skeletal anatomy, physiology, and growth is required. These factors tend to have the greatest impact on the pattern of injuries and the treatment of infants and young children; however, their significance gradually diminishes with age.

ANATOMIC FEATURES

- *Increased craniofacial ratio.* The ratio of cranial vault to facial skeleton decreases from approximately 8:1 in the infant to 2.5:1 in the adult. As a consequence, the cranium and central nervous system are much more vulnerable to injury in young children.
- *Adiposity.* The generous subcutaneous fat protects the facial skeleton from blows, but provides for impressive edema, which may hide underlying fractures.
- *Diminished paranasal sinus pneumatization.* Solid bone has yet to be replaced with air spaces, rendering the facial skeleton much more resistant to fracture and displacement. However, the lack of a "buttress" structure found in the mature face alters the predictability of fracture patterns such as Le Fort fractures. Midfacial fractures may cross the midline and extend to the cranium.
- *Unerupted dentition.* This provides additional stability to the midface by providing a "lock and key" mechanism. These unerupted permanent teeth are vulnerable to injury from rigid fixation devices.
- *Increased elasticity.* This results from an increased cancellous to cortical bone ratio, unfused cartilaginous suture lines, and reduced mineralization of bone. These features contribute to the frequent greenstick fractures characteristic of pediatric facial fractures.

PHYSIOLOGIC FEATURES

- Increased osteogenic potential. Fractures in children heal quickly compared with adults, so in many cases stable reduction (facilitated by the anatomic features noted above) need not be followed by internal fixation.
- Facial growth. This type of growth occurs as the result of two processes. *Remodeling* refers to the change in the shape of the bone, while *displacement* refers to the change in the bone's relative position due to growth. For instance, the mandible gradually assumes a more vertical orientation and is displaced inferiorly and anteriorly with growth. The driving force for facial growth remains controversial, but it is clear that functional demands, translated through the pull of muscle and soft tissues on the periosteum, has a major impact on growth.[6] Therefore, disruption of these forces secondary to trauma as well as attempts to repair it, via periosteal disruption and scarring of soft tissues, can have a disruptive affect on growth.

MANDIBULO-MAXILLARY FIXATION IN CHILDREN

The reduction of maxillary and mandibular fractures in adults is based upon the restoration of normal occlusion. This is rendered difficult in children because of the evolving status of the pediatric dentition. Deciduous teeth can be used for wiring, but care is required to avoid avulsing the teeth. Mixed dentition between 6 and 12 years of age makes determination of occlusion difficult. In young children without adequate dentition, the fabrication of acrylic splints may be necessary.

RIGID INTERNAL FIXATION IN PEDIATRIC FRACTURES

In adults, the management of maxillofacial fractures is based on wide exposure through cosmetically advantageous incisions, followed by direct reduction and rigid fixation with plates. These techniques have been applied to children with craniofacial anomalies and maxillofacial trauma. However, experimental models and clinical experience provide evidence of postoperative growth disruption proportional to the extent of the intervention.[7] A second issue is migration or "burying" of the plates resulting from differential addition of bone to the outer cortex with resorption of the inner cortex, particularly in the cranium. Last, fixation hardware may be palpable or create a noticeable contour deformity.

These factors must be considered in deciding when to use rigid fixation, particularly in young children. Because stable closed reduction can often be achieved in this group of patients, a conservative approach is frequently warranted. When internal fixation is required, short-segment plating or wires, using the smallest possible profile and limited periosteal elevation, is recommended. Other considerations in these patients include early plate removal and plating systems manufactured from absorbable materials.

FRACTURES OF SPECIFIC SITES

NASAL FRACTURES

The nasal bones are the most commonly fractured in the facial skeleton — not surprising in light of their vulnerable position and relative fragility. The diagnosis is based on the mechanism of injury and the physical examination. Common signs are external deformity, periorital ecchymosis, and epistaxis. X-rays are often obtained but are infrequently helpful. In children, an unfused midline suture typically produces an "open book" pattern of splaying of the nasal bones, rather than the c-shaped deformities characteristic of adults. Immediate complications of nasal fractures include significant deformity, nasal obstruction, and septal hematoma. Closed reduction is indicated for most nasal fractures; however, significant nasoseptal fractures can result in a loss of support for the nasal dorsum and may require open repair. Septal hematoma can result in septal cartilage necrosis; drainage and reapproximation of the mucoperichondrium is indicated. Impaired nasal growth is a risk following nasal injury and repair.[8]

MANDIBLE FRACTURES

The mandible is the second most commonly fractured facial bone; the incidence of these fractures increases as the mandible assumes a more prominent anterior position with age. Young children most commonly fracture the soft, spongy bone of the condyle as a result of falls on the chin. These injuries are historically associated with ankylosis and cessation of growth at the condyle with shortening of mandibular height. Treatment of condylar fractures in young children is based upon short periods (1 to 2 weeks) of mandibulo-maxillary fixation (MMF), followed by opening therapy, because rapid return to range of motion is essential to minimize these complications. Displacement of the condylar head can usually be managed conservatively, unless occlusion cannot be obtained or cosmetic deformity results.

Injuries to the body and angle of the mandible are managed conservatively in young children; rigid fixation can be used later in childhood to minimize malunion and resultant malocclusion. In adults, rigid fixation of mandible fractures reduces the likelihood of nonunion; overall, nonunion occurs in approximately 1% of fractures and is a major risk factor for infection. Placement of fixation hardware on the inferior edge of the mandible reduces the likelihood of injury to unerupted teeth and the inferior alveolar nerve. Nondevitalized teeth within the fracture line can usually remain and, in fact, may aid in stabilization of the fracture.

Older children most commonly suffer segmental fractures of the alveolar ridge. These can be reduced and stabilized with arch bars. Single avulsed teeth can be replaced in the socket and stabilized with circumdental wiring, with loss of the tooth reduced by rapid replacement. Impaction of deciduous teeth is a common injury that may result in delayed eruption.

MIDFACIAL FRACTURES (MAXILLARY AND ZYGOMATIC)

These types of fractures are the least common injuries in young children. Most often, they are greenstick fractures involving the alveolus or a split palatal suture. The key to management of these injuries in children is recognition of the unusual patterns and important sequelae.[9] Maxillary fractures do not follow the classic Le Fort designation, but may cross the midline and extend through the cranium. In children, 40% of maxillary fractures are associated with central nervous system injury and 14% with cerebral spinal fluid (CSF) otorrhea. Maxillary hypoplasia with aesthetic and functional compromise has been reported following childhood fractures.[10]

Reduction of these fractures can be accomplished without fixation in young children, due to the stability provided by unerupted dention and the absence of sinus pneumatization. In older children, three-dimensional reconstruction and rigid fixation are essential to restoring vertical height and projection accurately; prior to rigid fixation, maxillary retrusion and malocclusion were common. Unerupted teeth are vulnerable to fixation hardware; monocortical microplates with small screws are usually adequate.

Zygomatic arch fractures are most commonly minimally displaced greenstick injuries. Displaced zygomatic fractures may result in depression of the malar eminence and noticeable displacement of the lateral canthus. The coronoid process of the mandible can become entrapped by depressed fractures. Closed reduction through a Gillies approach is usually adequate; careful dissection deep to the outer layer of the deep temporalis fascia helps to avoid injury to the zygomatic branches of the facial nerve. Two- or three-point fixation may be used in displaced fractures of the zygomatic complex in older children. Bone grafting to augment the zygomatic contour should generally be deferred until adulthood.

ORBITAL FLOOR AND RIM FRACTURES

Inferior orbital rim and floor fractures are rare prior to significant pneumatization of the maxillary sinus. Injuries to the orbit and globe should prompt ophthalmologic consultation. Severe eye injuries occur in 2.5% of facial trauma patients, but in approximately 25% of orbital fractures. Other complications include enophthalmos, from increased orbital volume in "blow-out" injuries to the medial or lateral orbit, or loss of orbital contents. Ocular dystopia can occur following significant displacement. Lacrimal injuries are common. Entrapment may result in gaze restriction and diplopia.

Surgery to restore the orbit may result in similar complications. Corneal abrasions should be avoided by temporary tarsorraphy or placement of a scleral shield. Blindness can result from aggressive retraction on the globe or orbital hematoma, and vision should be assessed as soon as possible after surgery. Ectropion may result from subciliary or transconjunctival incisions and is most common following disruption of the orbital septum. Postoperatively, a Frost stitch and massage of the lower eyelid are used for several days.[11] Significant inferior displacement or comminution of the orbital floor requires reconstruction with autogenous materials; there is little experience with long-term allografts in pediatric facial fractures.

NASOETHMOID FRACTURES

Again, prior to sufficient sinus maturation (5 to 6 years of age), these fractures are rarely diagnosed. Loss of nasal projection, medial canthal disruption with rounding of the medial commisure, and telocanthus are potential complications. Reconstruction of these injuries is complex, requiring accurate reduction of bony fragments and replacement of the medial canthal ligament to prevent traumatic telocanthus.[12] Nasolacrimal injuries should be explored and repaired to prevent epiphora. Central nervous system injuries are common and necessitate neurosurgical consultation.

FRONTAL AND ORBITAL ROOF FRACTURES

In contrast to other fractures, these injuries are relatively more common in childhood. Absence of frontal sinus pneumatization before 5 to 10 years of age is associated with extensive fractures, which may extend from the orbital roof to the vertex of the skull and are associated with a high risk of central nervous system injuries. Neurosurgical consultation is essential. Orbital roof fractures may also result in immediate or delayed exophthalmos or encephalocele. Primary bone grafting of displaced orbital roof fractures appears to reduce this risk significantly.[13]

Later in childhood, frontal fractures are managed as they are for their adult counterparts. Anterior table fractures may result in cosmetic deformity. Entrapment of sinus mucosa or disruption of the nasofrontal drainage system may result in mucocele formation with potential central nervous system complications. Posterior table injuries may be associated with CSF otorrhea and central nervous system injury. If restoration of nasofrontal function cannot be achieved or significant comminution of the posterior table is encountered, cranialization or obliteration is recommended.

TEMPORAL BONE FRACTURE

Temporal bone trauma is typically a result of massive injury to the head in childhood. Fractures of the temporal bone are divided into three major categories: longitudinal, transverse, and mixed. The longitudinal temporal bone fracture is much more common than the transverse and affects the tympanic ring, ossicular chain, and middle ear. The direction of the fracture tends to cause more conductive hearing loss but less likely risk of facial nerve injury (20%).[14] On the other hand, transverse fractures typically traverse the skull base and the parasagittal plane, giving a greater risk of sensorineural hearing loss and damage to the facial nerve in the labyrinthine segment. Sensorineural hearing loss is most common and about half of the transverse fractures affect the facial nerve. The mixed fracture does not follow the exact line of the transverse or longitudinal fracture and may have a mixture of these complications.

INITIAL EVALUATION

The initial evaluation of a child with a potential temporal bone fracture should be the evaluation of the external ear and ear canal for evidence of laceration, bleeding, or CSF otorrhea. This may require a microscopic evaluation, which is difficult to conduct in the injured child. The evaluation of the postauricular area for a Battle's sign may also suggest temporal bone fracture. Hemotympanum is an indication of a temporal bone fracture.

The evaluation of facial and eye function is imperative. This will allow the definition of timing of any facial paralysis. Unfortunately, it is frequently overlooked in the initial evaluation by many emergency departments. The evaluation of the eyes for any sign of nystagmus may be helpful to demonstrate vesibulopathy. If the child is awake and cooperative, tuning forks may be used to establish conductive or sensorineural hearing loss.

Typically, a child with a temporal bone fracture will have enough significant neurological injury that immediate care must be directed there. Early management must include care of the eye if a facial paralysis exists. Sometimes, if a severe temporal bone fracture has been diagnosed by CT scan and persistent high-volume cerebral spinal fluid leakage is present, lumbar drainage or prompt surgical management may be necessary.[15]

ANATOMIC FEATURES

- *Facial nerve.* The facial nerve is located within the temporal bone from the internal auditory canal through the mastoid tip. The nerve exits laterally in the infant and issues a more medial location as the mastoid develops.
- *Inner ear.* The inner ear is fully developed at birth. It is encased in the endocondral bone of the otic capsule (the hardest, densest bone in the body). The vestibular and auditory portions can be injured with trauma.
- *Mastoid development.* The mastoid develops during childhood. The bone is softer. The fracture can course through this portion of the bone.

- *Middle ear and ossicular chain.* The middle ear is the airspace between the tympanic membrane and inner ear. The fracture can course through this area and increase the risk of fracture to the ossicles.

PHYSIOLOGIC FEATURES

- *Otic capsule.* The endochondrial bone of the otic capsule does not heal.
- *Severity of trauma.* Often, trauma severe enough to fracture the otic capsule will cause massive intracranial injury.
- *Vestibular symptoms.* Because the child usually equilibrates more rapidly than the adult, less severe or no vertigo is seen.

FACIAL NERVE PARALYSIS

If facial paralysis is noted by day 3, one should begin electrophysiologic testing of the facial nerve using an electroneurography (EnoG).[16–19] This may be continued for up to 3 weeks to monitor the performance of the facial nerve and assist in prognostication. If the ENoG response remains greater than 10% of the opposite nerve's function over that period of time, facial function usually returns without intervention. If, however, the ENoG deteriorates to lower than 10% during that time, surgical intervention should be considered when the child is stable. Surgical intervention is typically delayed until 3 weeks after injury to allow maximal axonal growth. If transection of the nerve is noted and the ENoG is noted to be diminished at the time of initial evaluation, more immediate repair is appropriate when the patient is medically stabilized.[20]

If the nerve has been transected, exposure with facial nerve repair should be accomplished. Decompression in the area of transection is necessary. If the vertical segment is transected, a complete mastoidectomy with decompression may allow adequate closure, although the typical areas of injury are in the horizontal segment, the ganglion, or the middle cranial fossa. Complete exposure of the nerve with appropriate closure with end-to-end anastomasosis is important. If damage to the nerve is significant, a cable graft may be done. The nerve should be reapproximated without tension. Mobilization of the nerve may be necessary. If there is concern regarding facial function after 3 weeks, electromyography (EMG) may assist in prognosis. If EMG offers no evidence of nerve continuity to the muscle motor end plates, one may consider facial nerve surgery.

Care for the eye is very important in facial nerve paralysis. If there is evidence of early problems with eye dryness or exposure keratophaty, consideration of gold weight implantation may be given. One should not use an eye patch because this may cause injury to the cornea. A humidity chamber is often used to assist during the time for the decision of the gold weight.[21]

Delayed facial reanimation is possible but will not be discussed in this chapter.[22]

HEARING LOSS

Initial hearing loss is frequently noted with most temporal bone fractures. The most common finding in temporal bone fracture is a hemotympanum, which will typically cause a 25- to 30-dB hearing loss. Longitudinal fractures of the temporal bone, however, have a greater risk of ossicular discontinuty or fracture. There is some risk for sensoineral hearing loss secondary to cochlear injury, although this is far less common than in transverse fractures. Spinal fluid leakage in longitudinal fractures has been documented.

Transverse fractures are more likely to result in a sensorineural hearing loss. These fractures are typically due to an occipital blow or a direct frontal blow. Transverse fractures may directly traverse the cochlea, causing significant and immediate sensorineural hearing loss.[15] Occasionally, a small fracture of the cochlea may be less evident on CT scanning but will result in a perilymphatic fistula, which may also cause significant sensorineural hearing loss.

If conductive hearing loss is persistent, middle ear exploration with possible ossiculoplasty is important. It is important to remember that in most situations, the present hemotympanum or middle ear effusion will resolve and a more certain assessment of the resultant conductive hearing loss can be performed. Middle ear exploration, even in childhood, can often be done through a transcanal approach. Assessment of an intact ossicular chain with documentation of appropriate round window reflex may assure ossicular chain continuity. One will often see discontinuity at the incudomalleolar or incudostapedial joint, or fracture of the long process of the incus.[15]

In children with significant transverse fractures of the temporal bone, the sensorinerual hearing loss is typically profound and unlikely to be corrected. It is important, however, to watch for cerebral spinal fluid leakage.[15] If this is massive or if the concern is that this leak is leading to meningitis, a transmastoid obliteration using a muscle plug is an appropriate approach.

LARYNGEAL TRAUMA

Motor vehicle accidents and all-terrain accidents account for much of the laryngeal trauma noted in childhood. Occasionally, injuries from penetrating trauma, such as gunshot wounds, occur. The motor vehicle accident typically demonstrates blunt trauma to the neck causing injury to the larynx. A "clothesline" injury is often seen from all-terrain vehicle accidents in which the child hits a rope or fence with his neck.

ANATOMIC FEATURES

- *Thyroid and cricoid cartilage.* These are not ossified until later, so greenstick fractures are common.
- *Cricothyroid membrane.* This membrane is very small in the toddler and difficult to palpate. Cricothyroidotomy is therefore very difficult to perform in the child.

PHYSIOLOGIC FEATURES

- *Airway.* Grossly, the cross-sectional airway area is related to r^2. This means that, in the small child, a very small decrease in the "radius" will affect the area to a great extent. Therefore, minimal edema can cause great airway obstruction.
- *Voice.* Even mild edema of the vocal folds can cause dysphonia. This can be an initial clue to laryngeal trauma.
- *Swallowing.* The larynx rises in the neck with swallowing. Dysphagia or odynophagia can be early signs of laryngeal injury.

INITIAL EVALUATION

Initial evaluation of the child's larynx should focus on whether the child has hoarseness, airway compromise, or dysphagia. If any of these is present, a complete endoscopic evaluation is required. Initial stabilization of the child with airway trauma is best done in concert with direct laryngoscopy, bronchoscopy, and esophagoscopy.[23] The preferred method to secure the airway is a tracheotomy because many of the injuries involve the cricoid and a cricothyrotomy is very dangerous. If the airway is unable to be secured by a tracheotomy, endotracheal intubation may be tried, although it carries the risk of passing the endotracheal tube into a false passage and further destroying mucosa.

Computed tomography of the larynx often will demonstrate the presence or absence of fractures, allowing one to plan surgical intervention. This should be done with a stable airway. After

CT and endoscopic evaluation are performed, the game plan is made based on the extent of intralaryngeal injury.

MANAGEMENT

If fractures have occurred, early repair seems to give the best long-term outcome.[24,25] Repair of the fractures by suturing or wiring will provide stabilization to the fracture fragments. At that same time, if significant mucosal damage is significant, a laryngotomy with repair of the mucosal damage is indicated. Leaving raw, exposed submucosal areas or cartilage may cause intense granulation formation and subsequent scarring.[26] Appropriate attention to detail in the control of the airway, the initial evaluation, and early treatment will help reduce the risk of complication; however, complications may occur regardless of the expertise of treatment.[27]

HOARSENESS

Hoarseness after laryngeal trauma is very common. Scarring to the larynx and, in particular, the true vocal folds may be seen even in minor trauma. Subsequent scarring of the Reinke's space and the lamina propria reduce vocal fold vibration. This is usually documented by a harsh voice. A breathy voice may indicate persistent laryngeal opening during phonation.

If a child has significant dysphonia after laryngeal trauma, repeated microlaryngoscopy is indicated. This may demonstrate areas of glottic scarring. If the child is cooperative, videostroboscopy can be done to define the areas of laryngeal scarring more specifically.

New microlaryngeal techniques to reverse some of the scarring process have been proposed, including the elevation of microflaps with the use of alternative substances to attempt to recreate Reinke's space.[28,29] If areas of lateral scarring have tethered portions of the cord so that a persistent chink and breathiness remains, injections of Gel Foam® or collagen may reduce the persistent glottic chink allowing for improved phonation. If successful, more permanent solutions may be advised.

VOCAL FOLD PARALYSIS

Vocal cord paralysis may happen with the initial direct blunt trauma or by severance of the nerve. If no regeneration occurs after 6 months, one may consider intervention at that time. Reanastamosis of a severed nerve causes synkinesis. The resultant dysphonia has a worse outcome than paralysis. If unilateral vocal fold paralysis causes a breathy voice or aspiration, a thyroidplasty[30,31] with medialization of the vocal cord may be done.[32–37] Gel foam or collagen injection is a reasonable alternative.[38] Occasionally, the child with a unilateral vocal cord paralysis will have compensation from the opposite cord, which will preclude the need for further intervention. Reinnervation techniques have rarely been done in children.[39–41]

If bilateral vocal cord paralysis persists, the child may have an adequate voice; however, he or she may have significant airway compromise. This airway compromise may require a tracheotomy or a vocal cord lateralization procedure. Arytenoidectomy or cordotomy have been tried with reasonable success, although postoperative vocal quality may be compromised.[42,43]

LARYNGEAL STENOSIS

A stenotic larynx after laryngotracheal trauma can result from granulation in the soft tissue or chondritis, which progresses to further stenosis. Chronic infection may also lead to this. Destruction of the cartilage may lead to malacia instead of stenosis, causing significant collapse of the airway and requiring intervention.

Appropriate attention to the immediate care of the child with laryngotracheal trauma may help preclude the chain of events leading to scar formation. If the contaminated wound causes infection or if loss of mucosal surface is significant, all of the preceding activities may happen.

The use of intralaryngeal stents at the initial repair may help reduce the risk of scarring. Though similar to a long-standing endotracheal tube, they do carry some risk of stenosis secondary to pressure-induced vascular compromise. If, after healing of the initial insult, one finds progressive or stable laryngeal scarring with subsequent airway compromise, surgical intervention may be necessary. The airway is typically controlled with a tracheotomy, although if the stenosis is mild enough, primary laryngotracheal reconstruction may be accomplished similarly to the repair of subglottic stenosis for prolonged intubation.[44–49] Laryngeal framework surgery should be considered and is often successful. If the airway is compromised by an anterior glottic web, a laryngotomy can often be successful.

Supraglottic scarring from injury to the false cords and/or epiglottis can cause supraglottic stenosis. This is a very difficult problem to correct; after excision of scar and forward placement of the epiglottis, prolonged stenting may allow airway stabilization.

A posterior glottic web may occur. If persistent posterior fistula is present, lysis of the posterior glottic web will often improve airway and vocal cord mobility.[50] If persistent posterior fistula does not occur, the posterior glottic airway may be opened using a posterior cricoid graft or scar removal allowing remucosalization of the posterior glottic area.

CONCLUSIONS

Trauma to the maxillo-facial skeleton, temporal bone, and larynx can and does occur in the pediatric patient. The ABCs (airway, breathing, and circulation) and neck stabilization are of primary importance. A complete history of the incident and thorough physical examination may make injuries obvious that may otherwise be unrecognized by the subtle findings. The astute clinician will use these clues and obtain appropriate ancillary tests such as x-rays or CT scans to ascertain the diagnosis, thus allowing appropriate treatment while avoiding complications.

REFERENCES

1. Rowe, N.L. Fractures of the facial skeleton in children. *J. Oral Surg.*, 1968, 26, 505–515.
2. Gussick, G., Luteman, A., Rodgers, K. et al. Pediatric maxillofacial trauma: unique features in diagnosis and treatment. *Laryngoscope*, 1987, 97, 925.
3. McGraw, B. and Cole, R. Pediatric maxillofaical trauma: age related variations in injury. *Arch. Otolaryngol. Head Neck Surg.*, 1990, 116, 41.
4. Quinn, J., Wells, G., Sutcliffe, T. et al. Tissue adhesive vs. suture wound repair at 1 year: randomized clinical trial correlating early, 3 month, and 1 year cosmetic outcomes. *Ann. Emerg. Med.*, 1998, 32, 645–649.
5. Stucker, F.J., Shaw, G.Y., Boyd, S., and Shockley, W.W. Management of animal and human bites in the head and neck. *Arch. Otolaryngol. Head Neck Surg.*, 1990, 116, 789–793.
6. Enlow, D.H. *Facial Growth*. Philadelphia: W.B. Saunders, 1990.
7. Bartlett, S.P. and De Lozier, J.B. Controversies in the management of pediatric facial fractures. *Clin. Plastic Surg.*, 1992, 19, 245–258.
8. Rock, W.P. and Brain, D.J. Effects of nasal trauma during childhood upon growth of the nose and midface. *Br. J. Orthodont.*, 1983, 10, 38–41.
9. Iuzuka, T., Thoren, H., Annino, D.J. et al. Midfacial fractures in pediatric patients; frequency, characteristics, and causes. *Arch. Otolaryngol. Head Neck Surg.*, 1995, 121, 1366–1371.
10. Ousterhout, D.K. and Vargervik, K. Maxillary hypoplasia secondary to midfacial trauma in childhood. *Plastic Reconstr. Surg.*, 1987, 80, 491–499.

11. Losken, H.W. Complications of pediatric craniofacial surgery. In Eisele, D.W., Ed. *Complications of Head and Neck Surgery*. Chicago: C.V. Mosby, 1993, 505–516.

12. Crocket, D.M. and Funk, G.F. Management of complicated fractures involving the orbits and naso-ethmoid complex in young children. *Otolaryngol. Clin. North Am.*, 1991, 24, 119.

13. Messinger, A., Radkowski, M., Greenwald, M.J., and Pensler, J.M. Orbital roof fractures in the pediatric population. *Plastic Reconstr. Surg.*, 1989, 84, 213–216.

14. Mattox, D.E. Temporal bone trauma. In Pillsbury, H.C., Ed. *Operative Challenges in Otolaryngology–Head and Neck Surgery*. Chicago: C.V. Mosby Year Book, 1990, 71–76.

15. Caniff, J.P. Otorrhea in head injuries. *Br. J. Oral Surg.*, 1971, 8, 203.

16. Gates, G. Nerve excitability testing: technical pitfalls and threshold norms using absolute values. *Laryngoscope*, 1993, 103, 379–385.

17. Sillman, J.S., Niparko, J.K., Lee, S.S., and Kileng, P.R. Prognostic value of evoked and standard electromyography in acute facial paralysis. *Otolaryngol. Head Neck Surg.*, 1992, 107, 377–381.

18. Halvorson, D.J., Coker, N.J., and Wang-Bennett, L.T. Histologic corrleation of the degenerating facial nerve with electroneurography. *Laryngoscope*, 1993, 103, 178–184.

19. Coker, J.N. Facial electroneurography: analysis of techinques and correlation with degenerating motor neurons. *Laryngoscope*, 1992, 102, 747–759.

20. Davis, R.K. and Pillsbury, H.C. Would healing: nerve grafts. In Myers, A., Ed. *Biological Basis of Plastic Surgery*. New York: Thieme Medical Publishers, Inc., 1993, 145, 153.

21. Gilberd, S.M. and Daspit, C.P. Reanimation of the paretic eyelid using gold weight implantation: a new approach and perspective evaluation. *Ophthalmol. Plastic Reconstr. Surg.*, 1991, 7, 93–103.

22. May, M., Sobol, S., and Mester, S. Hypoglossal-facial nerve interpositional implant graft for facial reanimation without tongue atrophy. *Otolaryngol. Head Neck Surg.*, 1994, 111, 446–449.

23. Link, D.T. and Cotton, R.T. The laryngotracheal complex in pediatric head and neck trauma. Securing the airway and management of external laryngeal injury. *Facial Plast. Surg.*, 1999, 2(2), 133–144.

24. Bent, J.P. and Porubsky, E.S. The management of blunt fractures of the thyroid cartilage. *Otolaryngol. Head Neck Surg.*, 1994, 110(2), 195–202.

25. Leopald, D.A. Laryngeal trauma. A historical comparison of treatment methods. *Arch. Otolaryngol.*, 1983, 109, 106–111.

26. Schild, J.A. and Denneny, E.C. Evaluation and treatment of acute laryngeal fractures. *Head Neck*, 1989, 11, 491–496.

27. Myer, C.M., Orobello, P., Cotton, R.T., and Bratcher, G.O. Blunt laryngeal trauma in children. *Laryngoscope*, 1987, 97, 1043–1048.

28. Benninger, M.S., Alessi, D., Archer, S., Bastian, R., Ford, C., Koufman, J., Sataloff, R., Spiegel, J., and Woo, P. Vocal fold scarring: current concepts and management. *Otolaryngol. Head Neck Surg.*, 1996, 115, 474–482.

29. Woo, P., Rahbar, R., and Wang, Z. Fat implantation into Reinke's space: a histologic and stroboscopic study in the canine. *Ann. Otol. Rhinol. Laryngol.*, 1999, 108, 738–744.

30. Tucker, H.M. Combined laryngeal framework medialization and reinnervation for unilateral vocal fold paralysis. *Ann. Otol. Rhinol. Laryngol.*, 1990, 99, 778–781.

31. Gardner, G.M., Altman, J.S., and Balakrishnan, G. Pediatric vocal fold medialization with silastic implant: intraoperative airway management. *Int. J. Pediatr. Otorhinolaryngol.*, 2000, 52, 37–44.

32. Levine, B.A., Jacobs, I.N., Wetmore, R.F., and Handler, S.D. Vocal cord injection in children with unilateral vocal cord paralysis. *Arch. Otolaryngol. Head Neck Surg.*, 1995, 121, 116–119.

33. Spiegel, J.R., Sataloff, R.T., and Gould, W.J. The treatment of vocal fold paralysis with injectable collagen: clinical concerns. *J. Voice*, 1987, 1(1), 119–121.

34. Ellis, J.C., McCaffrey, T.V., DeSanto, L.W., and Reiman, H.V. Migration of Teflon after vocal cord injection. *Otolaryngol. Head Neck Surg.*, 1987, 96, 63–66.

35. Ford, C.N., Gilchrist, K.W., and Bartell, T.E. Persistence of injectable collagen in the human larynx: a histopathologic study. *Laryngoscope*, 1987, 97, 724–727.

36. Ford, C.N. and Bless, D.M. Collagen injection in the scarred vocal fold. *J. Voice*, 1987, 1(1), 116–118.

37. Wexler, D.B., Jiang, J., Gray, S.D., and Titze, I.R. Phonosurgical studies: fat-graft reconstruction of injured canine vocal cords. *Ann. Otol. Rhinol. Laryngol.*, 1989, 98, 668–673.

38. Schramm, V.L., May, M., and Lavorato, A.S. Gelfoam paste injection for vocal cord paralysis: temporary rehabilitation of glottic incompetence. *Laryngoscope*, 1978, 88, 1268–1273.

39. Nunez, D.A. and Hanson, D.R. Laryngeal reinnervation in children: the Leeds experience. *ENT J.*, 1993, 72(8), 542–543.

40. Green, D.C., Berke, G.S., and Graves, M.C. A functional evaluation of ansa cervicalis nerve transfer for unilateral vocal cord paralysis: future directions for laryngeal reinnervation. *Otolaryngol. Head Neck Surg.*, 1991, 104, 453–466.

41. Crumley, R.L. Muscle transfer for laryngeal paralysis. *Arch. Otolaryngol. Head Neck Surg.*, 1991, 117, 1113–1117.

42. Crumley, R.L. Endoscopic laser medial arytenoidectomy for airway management in bilateral laryngeal paralysis. *Ann. Otol. Rhinol. Laryngol.*, 1993, 102, 81–84.

43. Bower, C.M., Choi, S.S., and Cotton, R.T. Arytenoidectomy in children. *Ann. Otol. Rhinol. Laryngol.*, 1994, 103, 271–278.

44. Narcy, P., Contencin, P., Fligny, I., and Francois, M. Surgical treatment for laryngotracheal stenosis in the pediatric patient. *Arch. Otolaryngol. Head Neck Surg.*, Sep, 1990, 116, 1047–1050.

45. Zalzal, G.H. Stentin for pediatric laryngotracheal stenosis. *Ann. Otol. Rhinol. Laryngol.*, 1922, 101, 651–655.

46. Zalzal, G.H. Rib cartilage grafts for the treatment of posterior glottic and subglottic stenosis in children. *Ann. Otol. Rhinol. Laryngol.*, 1988, 97, 506–510.

47. Seid, A.B., Pransky, S.M., and Kearns, D.B. One-stage laryngotracheoplasty. *Arch. Otolaryngol. Head Neck Surg.*, 1991, 117, 408–410.

48. Monnier, P., Savary, M., and Chapuis, G. Partial cricoid resection with primary tracheal anastomosis for subglottic stenosis in infants and children. *Laryngoscope*, 1993, 103, 1273–1283.

49. Myer, C.M. and Cotton, R.T. Historical development of surgery for pediatric laryngeal stenosis. *Ear Nose Throat J.*, 1995, 74(8), 560–564.

50. Goldberg, A.N. Endoscopic postcricoid advancement flap for posterior glottic stenosis. *Laryngoscope*, 2000, 110, 482–485.

35 Pediatric Facial Plastic and Reconstructive Surgery

William C. Giles and W. Scott McDonald

CONTENTS

INTRODUCTION

The practice of pediatric facial plastic and reconstructive surgery has changed dramatically over the last 40 years. The boundary between reconstructive and aesthetic surgery has and continues to narrow. With this natural progression of reconstruction, an acceptable aesthetic result is now demanded by society. Consequently, the facial plastic surgeon is charged with a tremendous responsibility.

The technical aspects of facial plastic surgery are learned as an integral part of the otolaryngologist's and plastic surgeon's training. The reasonable indications and expectations for performing the more elective procedures on children and adolescents, however, are not well studied. The psychological state of a patient and the impact of facial altering surgery must be considered. Helpful rules are to postpone surgery if concern over what appears to be a major deformity is minimal or if there is major concern over minor deformities. The patient must understand that he cannot expect the surgery to improve his psyche. In other words, the amount of improvement expected by the patient should be similar to the results anticipated by the surgeon. The demanding, indecisive, or immature patient will often have a troublesome perioperative and postoperative course.[1]

One should be aware that as early as preschool, children have a preference to interact with children that they think appear normal.[2] Research has found that even adults treat unattractive children more harshly and view them as less developmentally competent.[3,4] Unattractive children and adults are found to demonstrate more behavior problems and are at increased risk of psychological pathology.[5,6] The extent of negative correlations that accompany a less than normal appearance seems to be decreased if family and peers are supportive.[7,8] When contemplating surgery on a younger child (ages 0 to 9 years), the parents must have a clear understanding of the nature of the disfigurement as well as realistic goals for surgery. As the child grows into preadolescence, it is imperative that he be mature and have a complete understanding of the surgery and the hopeful outcome. He should also be allowed to participate in decision making.[9]

No procedure should be performed unless the patient, parents, and surgeon agree on the nature of the deformity, the degree of the deviation from the norm, and the hopeful outcome of the surgery. Severe psychiatric reaction, such as depression, psychosis, regression, and paranoia, following facial plastic surgery is prevented by identifying behavior abnormalities prior to surgery and has little to do with the actual surgical outcome.[10] Also, the surgeon must be aware of the patient who undergoes a substantial improvement in his body image and is no longer inhibited, self-conscious, or socially withdrawn, but is emotionally immature and naive. Thankfully, most studies show that correction of a facial deformity leads to improved self-esteem, social skills, and ability to adjust.[11–13]

OTOPLASTY

Plastic surgery of the ear is usually contemplated beginning at age 5. Anthropomorphic studies of the ear show that at the age of 7 in males and 6 in females, the ear has reached its mature size and 98% of its width as measured at 18 years of age.[14] The length of the ear at the age of 5 is 86% of that observed in an adult. Tanzer classified ear defects into five categories:[15]

- Stage 1: anotia
- Stage 2: classic microtia with or without atresia of the external canal
- Stage 3: hypoplasia of the middle one third of the auricle
- Stage 4: hypoplasia of the superior one third of the auricle (includes cup ear, constricted ear cryptotia, or lop ear)
- Stage 5: large or prominent ears

Most otolaryngologists currently use Weerda's three-stage system:[16]

- Stage 1: hypoplasia of the auricle
- Stage 2: minimal normal auricle structures
- Stage 3 (or third degree): no normal auricular structures; requires total reconstruction.

The surgeon must have a full understanding of the embryology and anatomy of the normal ear so that the correct procedure can be applied to the defect, and the proper outcome can be more likely achieved.[17] Surgical complications of otoplasty can occur during surgery or in the postoperative period. Most complications are related to technique.[18]

The complication of bleeding usually occurs 3 to 6 hours after surgery, when all surgical vasoconstriction has dissipated. Hematomas can be avoided by drain placement if one suspects bleeding will be a problem. Failure to deal with a hematoma will lead to irregular fibrous tissue that will result in a cauliflower ear. Overly constrictive head bandages can lead to necrosis of parts of the external ear. Hematomas and vascular compromised tissue present with extreme pain, so painful ears in the immediate postoperative period of 1 to 2 days must be examined. Head bandages should remain in place 24 to 48 hours after surgery.[19]

In the days following surgery, pain, tenderness, or itching could be signs of infection or inflammation. The surgeon should be quick to examine and treat problematic ears, especially during the first postoperative week, to prevent loss of contour, cartilage, or soft tissue. Tissue reaction, loss of normal cartilage spring, and visible sutures in the subcutaneous postauricular area are complications secondary to creating antihelical fold with permanent sutures. These complications can be reduced by good skin coverage of the sutures and minimizing the amount of skin excision.

Most late complications of otoplasty are related to overzealous cutting of the postauricular soft tissue or cartilage of the antihelical fold. The classic telephone deformity is caused by excising a wide ellipse of postauricular skin and placing mustarde sutures in the easily assessable middle one third of the ear with less attention to the top or lobe of the ear. This results in an outwardly displaced superior helix and lobe and "pinned back" middle external ear (Figure 35.1). The deformity can be prevented by an even strip of soft tissue excision in the postauricular area and placing a mustarde suture in the superior and inferior aspect of the antihelical fold as well as the middle, easily assessable portion of the ear. The defect is repaired by securing the most superior and most inferior

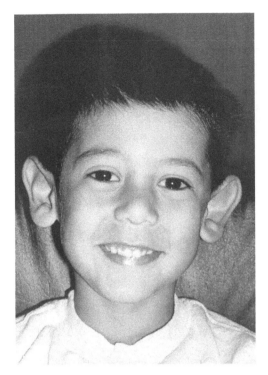
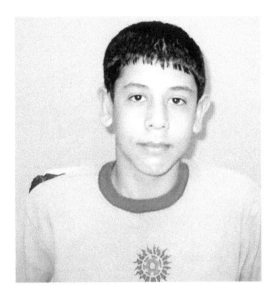

FIGURE 35.1 Preoperative and postoperative otoplasty patient. Note that superior and inferior thirds of the ear extend laterally beyond the middle third of the ear.

portion of the choncal bowl to the mastoid periosteum. Also, any soft tissue excision during this correction surgery should be limited to the superior and inferior aspect of the ear.

When cartilage scoring or excision techniques are performed, overexcision of the cartilage results in a very sharp, obvious fold. The conchal bowl must be carefully placed posteriorly and laterally or the external auditory canal will be occluded, leading to chronic external otitis secondary to poor drainage of moisture and cerumen.[20] Auricular keloids can also occur following otoplasty and can be treated early with injections of steroids; otherwise, the keloid will need to be excised and the skin closed without tension followed by regular steroid injections. Occasionally, a small dose of radiation therapy will greatly reduce the chances of recurrences.[21]

NASALPLASTY

The proper timing for nasal surgery in the pediatric population is a topic of great debate. Nasal height becomes fully developed in males at 15 years and at 12 years for females.[22] The protrusion of the nasal tip matures several years later. Septoplasty in young children does not greatly affect most aspects of facial growth; however, it may negatively influence the growth of the nasal dorsum[23] (Figure 35.2). The current trend is to limit the extent of nasal surgery on a developing child to cases in which the deformity is obvious or the airway is significantly occluded.

The surgeon must have a very conservative approach, especially toward cartilage excision and osteotomies. When a septoplasty is performed, surgery should be limited only to the area of the obstruction, thus minimizing perichondrium elevation. It appears that the most active areas of the nasal septum relating to nasal and facial growth are in the regions of the interface of the septum and the maxilla, vomer, and dorsum.[24] One must be careful if a complete transfixion incision is used; this can result in the loss of tip projection, tip ptosis, and a decrease in the nasal labial angle. If the condition warrants a transfixion incision, securing the lower lateral cartilages to the

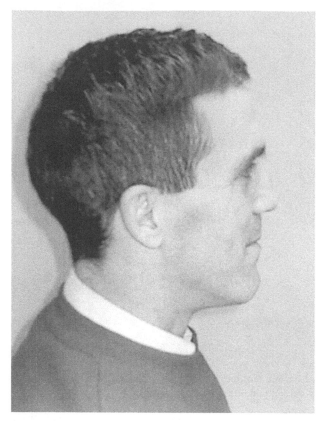

FIGURE 35.2 Adult who had a septoplasty at age 12. Note lack of growth and projection of the cartilaginous dorsum and nasal tip. (From Mulliken, Figure 3 and Figure 4, p. 25.)

septum in the correct anatomical location will be necessary to minimize the risk of loss of tip height and rotation.[25]

Postoperative complications include septal hematoma, which usually can be diagnosed by severe pain for several days following the procedure. The hematoma must be evacuated to prevent cartilage necrosis. Using a whipstitch across the septum will alleviate the need for packing and will usually prevent a hematoma. Symptomatic deflections of the septum can persist if the cartilage was too conservatively resected or not secured to the nasal floor. Revision surgery should not be undertaken for at least 6 to 9 months following the initial procedure. If growth disturbance does occur following surgery, augmentation of the cartilaginous skeleton using choncal bowl cartilage is the most common technique for correction.[26]

Rhinoplasty is a very popular procedure in the adolescent age group. Traumatic nasal defects are extremely challenging. Treatment of the twisted nose requires proper positioning of the bony dorsum using multiple osteotomies.[27] Deviation of the lower half of the nose is more difficult because this is a cartilage deformity. This deformity is often due to incomplete articulation of the septum with the nasal floor or upper lateral cartilage being too tall, pushing the septum and ipsilateral upper lateral cartilage to the side of the deviation. The crooked nose may be close to impossible to straighten. Correction of the deformity requires proper evaluation of the cause of the twisting and careful trimming of the upper lateral cartilage or septum, and then securing the septum to the floor of the nose and securing the lower lateral cartilages to each other to ensure symmetry.1

---

1 Small dorsum midline onlay grafts can greatly help correct a twisted nose.

Aesthetic surgery of the adolescent nose usually consists of decreasing the size of the tip or decreasing the nasal dorsum. One must not "overoperate" when performing a pediatric rhinoplasty. Incising, reshaping, and resecting tissue are only done as a last resort. It is easier to correct errors of omission than those of commission — repositioning cartilage and bone is preferable to reshaping and incising. The bony profile of an adolescent can usually be remodeled using a rasp because the tissue is immature and responds readily to rasping; thus, overresection can be avoided.[28]

The most common surgical fault of rhinoplasty is resection of the nasal skeleton without reconstruction of important structural elements of the nose. This can lead to defects of the lower third of the nose, including a blunted, ptotic, or pinched nasal tip; nasal tip asymmetry; flaring nostrils; retracted alae; hanging columella; or a polly beak deformity. In anticipation of this loss of projection of the lower third of the nose, a surgeon may resect the nasal dorsum to the tip, leading to the classic scooped nose that has the "operated" look.[29]

The lower third of the nose is most vulnerable to overresection. Complications can be avoided by symmetrical and conservative resection of the lower lateral cartilages. A columellar strut graft best corrects loss of projection of the tip. Tip deformities, including overrotation, asymmetry, and pinched appearance, are usually best corrected by a shield-shaped tip graft. Alar cartilage reinforcement of the lower lateral cartilage can be used to correct alar collapse and irregularities of the lateral tip. Care must be taken to ensure symmetrical positioning of the tip and lateral cartilages prior to suturing the cartilages and cartilage grafts.

The middle third of the nose is cartilaginous and overreduction leads to a pinched appearance and alteration of the nasal valve. Spreader grafts are used to stent upper lateral cartilage away from the dorsal edge of the septum and correct the defect.

The upper third of the nose is bony and comprises the nasal bones and nasal process of the maxilla. Overresection leads to a flat infantile appearance that lacks a discernible nasal starting point at the nasofrontal angle. Lateral osteotomies are performed to infracture the remaining bone of the dorsum to prevent a wide dorsum. If the dorsum has been overresected, the bones will not meet in the midline at the septum and the lateral bones will collapse and further drop the level of the dorsum, thus making the dorsum wider. This can be avoided by carefully extending hump removal into the nasofrontal angle to set the proper nasal starting point at the level of the superior palpebral fold. Due to the very thin skin in the area of the rhinion, the surgeon should leave a very small hump in the area of the bony and cartilage dorsum, thus leading to a proper profile. Cartilage onlay grafts or alloplastic material can be used to correct these defects.[30,31]

Airway difficulty following rhinoplasty can be due to collapse of the upper lateral cartilage. Excessive reduction of the lateral crura leading to collapse of the valve area is also a common defect. Synechiae and webs secondary to surgery often lead to obstruction. The cause of the obstruction needs to be identified and correction includes lysis of the adhesion, reinforcement of the soft triangle area with cartilage, increasing projection of the tip with a bolster, or decreasing turbinate size.[32]

In the immediate postoperative period, complications are fairly unusual. Septal hematoma or tight constricting dressings must be suspected if pain is excessive; nasal packing may be necessary for excessive bleeding. Soft tissue infection is unusual but should be suspected if a fever is noted 3 to 6 days after surgery. Ecymosis and periorbital edema can be expected if osteotomies were utilized; using steroids interoperatively may reduce this.[33] Skin breakdown is usually secondary to very tight taping of the nose or placing a hot cast on the nose following surgery. This defect should be treated conservatively by using antibiotic ointment or wet-to-dry dressing.

CRANIOFACIAL SURGERY

The highly specialized area of craniofacial surgery continues to grow and accept new challenges for correcting skull and facial abnormalities. To develop a proper treatment plan for correction of these abnormalities, knowledge of the classical deformities and their relationship to vital structures is necessary. The goal should be to have results approach the facial proportions and subunits described by Farkas and Ricketts.[34,35] Notable soft tissue relationships such as the nose, lip, and chin are necessary for harmony of the face.[36] In addition, complete understanding of the underlying bone through cephalometric analysis is necessary prior to embarking on a reconstructive plan.[37] One final critical aspect is planning for postoperative facial bone growth.[38]

The concept of a team approach to craniofacial anomalies was incorporated early in craniofacial surgery.[39,40] By design, each member of the team brings expertise usually gained through fellowship training and research in that specific specialty as it relates to craniofacial anomalies. Because of the complex nature of craniofacial deformity, this specialized team requires knowledgeable reconstructive surgeons, otolaryngologists, neurosurgeons, ophthalmologists, audiologists, speech pathologists and therapists, oral surgeons, prosthodontists, pediatric dentists, orthodontists, pediatricians, geneticists, psychiatrists, radiologists, psychologists, and social workers.

It is an accepted notion that patients enrolled in these teams will benefit from academic, technical, and social advances.

Preoperative preparation should include a comprehensive examination by a pediatrician and focused examination by the plastic surgeon and, if needed, a neurosurgeon. Pediatric anesthesiologists with experience in craniofacial surgery should examine the child and prepare for complications such as airway obstruction from edema, hemorrhage, or foreign bodies. Close fluid and blood-volume monitoring is an absolute and requires ready availability of blood products. Access to an intensive care unit with well-trained staff is also critical to prevent unnecessary morbidity. If these guidelines are followed, complications with craniofacial surgery will be few.

A review of several craniofacial programs' complications reveals overall complication rates of 15 to 20%. Infection rates occurred in 4 to 6% of cases; however, the rate appears to be lower in children.[41–44] Mortality rates of 1 to 2% are related to several consequences. Airway complications are a common cause, and every precaution should be taken to prevent this unneeded event. Hypovolemia or shock should be prevented by close monitoring of the urine output as well as the vital signs and central venous pressure.

Overwhelming, infection-like meningitis can be lethal and vigilance is necessary to prevent this grave complication. Soft tissue infections are also an important cause of morbidity, and antibiotic coverage for aerobic and anaerobic bacteria as well as good oral hygiene can be preventative. It also appears that, as experience with craniofacial surgery has grown, operative times have lowered, thus decreasing infection rates. Bone infections are a serious complication and must be dealt with aggressively with repeated sequestrectomy until control is achieved.

Blindness is always a concern when dissection of the periorbita is performed. Vision should be checked in the early postoperative period; decompression of the periorbita is indicated if high pressure is suspected. Careful dissection adjacent to the optic nerve is always indicated, particularly when power tools are used. Traction-induced hypotension and bradycardia are not uncommon, but they are usually transient and can be treated with atropine.

Bone grafting is frequently necessary for craniofacial surgery and a potential area for complications. Although donor site morbidity after bone grafts of the ileum can cause prolonged gait disturbances, these are usually short term in children. Inadvertent opening of the parietal pleura while harvesting rib grafts can be managed by placing a suction catheter and removal after the incision is closed. Of course, chest x-ray confirmation of a fully expanded lung is necessary in the postoperative period.

Cerebral spinal fluid (CSF) leaks are not uncommon after craniofacial procedures. In a large series of 507 intracranial procedures, a 4.5% rate of CSF leaks was reported.[42] Early management by attempting to decrease intracranial pressure with lowering the PACO2 or by using mannitol may obviate the need for lumbar drainage. However, if leaks persist, lumbar subarachnoid drainage may help or, if needed, ventriculoperitoneal or lumbar peritoneal shunts.

Hypertelorism correction presents some particular challenges for preventing complications. The nasal mucosa can be injured and a communication between the nasal cavity and cranium can occur.

TABLE 35.1
Causes of Congenital Anomalies in Humans

Cause	Percentage
Known genetic transmission	20
Chromosomal abberation	3–5
Environmental causes	
Radiations	1
Infections	2–3
Maternal metabolic imbalance	2
Drugs, vitamins, and chemicals	3–4
Unknown	65

Source: Whitaker, L.A. and Bartlett, S.P. In Jurkiecwicz, M.J., Krizek, T.J., Mathes, S.J., and Ariyan, S., Eds. *Plastic Surgery. Principles and Practice*, Vol. 1, St. Louis: C.V. Mosby, 1990, Chap. 7.

These injuries should be repaired if possible and pericranial flaps can be very helpful. Persistent CSF leaks in this region can lead to infections and, ultimately, to meningitis.

Intracranial edema or hemorrhage can occur after extensive cranial vault remodeling. Seizures may be an indication of cerebral damage and increased intracranial pressure. If acutely elevated intracranial pressure occurs in the postoperative setting, a release of bandages or the scalp closure may be necessary to allow adequate cerebral expansion. Consequently, documentation of the mental status in the early postoperative period is critical to prevent severe complications. Other complications of craniofacial surgery include pulmonary edema secondary to overhydration, bone graft resorption including the frontal bone flap, eyelid ptosis, ectropion, nasolacrimal duct obstructions, and fibrinolysis.[41]

CRANIOFACIAL DISORDERS

Craniofacial anomalies can have generic as well as environmental factors. Up to 20% of congenital deformities have been related to genetic transmission. Recently, discoveries in craniofacial genetics have exposed certain chromosomes that are related to craniofacial syndromes. Mutations in the gene that codes for fibroblast growth factor 2 have been related to Crouzan's, Apert's and other craniosynostosis syndromes,[45] other chromosomal anomalies have also been implicated in about 5% craniofascial disorders. Environmental factors such as radiation, infections, maternal metabolic conditions, and drugs are also associated causes, while the causes of most deformities, however, remain unknown (see Table 35.1).[46–48]

Facial clefts were best classified by Tessier in 1976 (Figure 35.3).[49] This classification is still widely used for accuracy and ease of communication. Craniosynostosis is best classified by describing the suture involved. These include the coronal, sagittal, metopic, and very occasionally, lambdoid sutures. The restricted growth perpendicular to the suture and a compensating overgrowth parallel to the suture cause the deformity (Figure 35.4).

Besides the obvious visible deformities and increased intracranial pressure, neurological and visual disturbances are important functional problems secondary to craniosynostosis. Intracranial hypertension may manifest as headaches, irritability, and sleeplessness. Skull x-rays might demonstrate a thin cortex and a "beaten metal" appearance of the inner cortex if intracranial pressure is significantly high. Even so, Marchac and Renier found an increased ICP in only 13% of patients with a single stenosed suture vs. 42% if multiple sutures were involved.[50]

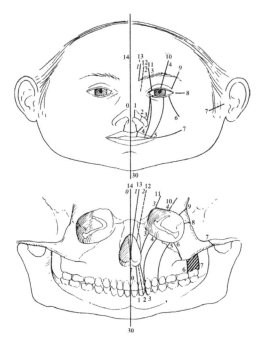

FIGURE 35.3 Tessier classification of facial clefts. (From Tessier, P., *J. Maxillofac. Surg.*, 4, 69, 1976. With permission.)

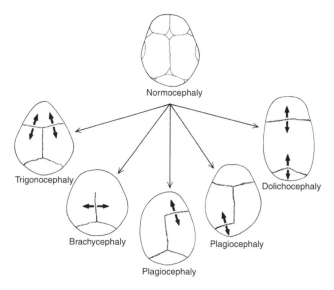

FIGURE 35.4 Unilateral coronal suture synostosis.

Metopic suture synostosis, which results in the unmistakable deformity of trigonocephaly, occurs in approximately 5% of patients with craniosynostosis. One may typically find a palpable and visible midline frontal ridge that usually extends from the anterior fontanelle to the glabella. It can present as severely as a forehead that is "keel" shaped. Orbital hypotelerisim, ethmoid hypoplasia, and a narrow bitemporal diameter are common findings. The correction of metopic synostosis usually requires a frontal craniotomy and cranial vault remodeling. A frontal and orbital osteotomy is created and the metopic suture is released. The lateral orbital rims are usually advanced and the midline osteomy may be widened with a bone graft or step cuts to correct the hypoteleorism.[49]

Sagittal synostosis, the most common form of craniosynostosis, presents with a characteristic oblong calvarial shape called scaphocephaly. There may also be a bitemporal narrowing and frontal bossing. Correction of isolated sagittal suture synostosis can be approached in two fashions that depend on the extent of deformity. If a mild deformity is present, a sagittal or parasagittal strip craniectomy may suffice, particularly in children less than 4 months of age.[50,51] In more significant deformities, a more extensive craniectomy and remodeling of the cranial vault may be necessary, including anterior and posterior shortening.[52]

Coronal suture synostosis may be unilateral or bilateral. Unilateral synostosis causes regional growth constriction and a compensated overexpansion of the opposite side that results in the classic shape of plagiocephaly. This should be differentiated from deformational plagiocephaly — a deformity that can usually be treated nonoperatively.[53]

In synostosic frontal plagiocephaly, the orbits and forehead are the center of attention. Correction of unilateral coronal synostosis can be achieved by a unilateral or bilateral frontorbital remodeling.[51] In one recent study, a comparison of frontal plagiocephaly anthropometric measurements after unilateral orbit and forehead corrections vs. bilateral orbit and forehead correction with nasal osteotomy revealed that a bilateral correction with a nasal osteotomy produced superior results.[54] Although unilateral coronal synostosis is a challenging reconstruction, complete coronal synostosis may produce a very significant deformity. One typically sees a shortened anterior–posterior diameter in the calvarium called "brachycephaly." The orbital rims may be hypoplastic and the temple and frontal bones protuberant. Correction should be achieved successfully with a complete frontal advancement.[55]

Several craniofacial syndromes are associated with craniosynostosis. Most of these involve a coronal synostosis along with other synoptic sutures. The facial deformity usually includes an excess in skull height with a tall forehead, exorbitism, midfacial retrusion, and brachycephaly.

More important are the possible functional conditions associated with these syndromes, including increased intracranial pressure, hydrocephalus, visual abnormalities, and mental retardation. A general guideline for treatment of these craniofacial syndromes would be an early surgery at less than 1 year of age to improve the craniofacial form and reduce any possible increased intracranial pressure. This would usually include an orbital advancement with a cranial bone remodeling procedure. At approximately 3 to 6 years a midface or frontofacial advancement procedure can be performed to correct the midface retrusion. After these initial surgeries, a secondary jaw surgery or other refinement surgery may be necessary. Complications associated with syndromic craniosynostosis vs. isolated synostosis are more common and include airway obstructions, seizures, and continued maldevelopment in the cranial vault.[56] Significant complications for monobloc frontofacial advancements have been reported, most notably epidural abscess, frontal bone necrosis, and CSF leaks.[57,58] Patients who have been shunted appear to have a higher complication rate.[59–61]

Craniofacial microsomia refers to the syndrome that affects the first two branchial arches. The clinical findings include underdevelopment of the mandible, zygoma, maxilla, temporal bone, muscles of mastication, face, palate, parotid gland, and external and middle ear. Cranial nerve deficits may also be present. Surgical correction of the mandibular deficiency can be performed by using free bone grafts or by distraction osteogenesis. Bone grafts require a donor site with subsequent morbidity.[62] Also, absorption of the grafts or relapse is possible, as well as infection. Distraction osteogenesis, an exciting technique recently applied to craniofacial surgery, still has many challenges to overcome.[63] The accuracy of distraction is still unpredictable and also reports of unacceptable external scars are still common.

Treacher–Collins syndrome involving multiple facial structures is inherited as a dominant trait with variable phenotypic expression. Consequently, it is of utmost importance to counsel persons with any expression of this syndrome about the possibilities of severely affected children. The primary goals of the reconstructive surgeon are to close the coloboma of the lower lid, reconstruct the zygoma, correct the dental occlusion, repair the macrostomia, and reconstruct the absence of the external ear. Final reconstruction might include reducing the nasal dorsum by reduction rhinoplasty. Vascularized or nonvascularized bone grafts can be used with success for zygoma recon-struction. A special consideration should be given to the possibility of a narrow airway because this can result in obstructive sleep apnea and neonatal death.[64]

REFERENCES

1. Garry, M. Malpractice. In Courtiss, E., Ed. *Aesthetic Surgery, Trouble, How to Avoid and How to Treat it.* St. Louis: C.V. Mosby Co., 1978, 1–13.
2. Nabors, L. and Keyes, A. Brief report: preschoolers' social preferences for interacting with peers with physical differences. *J. Pediatr. Psychol.*, 1977, 22, 113–122.
3. Berkowitz, L. and Frodi, A. Reactions to a child's mistakes as affected by his\her looks and speech. *School Psychol. Q.*, 1979, 42, 420–425.
4. Ritter, J., Casey, R., and Langlois, J. Adults' response to infants varying in appearance of age and attractiveness. *Child Dev.*, 1991, 62, 68–82.
5. Schneiderman, C. and Harding, J. Social ratings of children with cleft lip by school peers. *Cleft Palate Crainiofacial J.*, 1984, 21, 219.
6. Tobiasen, J. Social judgments of facial deformity. *Cleft Palate Crainiofacial J.*, 24, 323–327, 1987.
7. Perry, B. et. al. Neuropsychologic impact of facial deformities in children. *Clin. Plastic Surg.*, 1998, 25, 587–597.
8. Harrison, A. Facial plastic and reconstructive surgery in children: its impact on the psychological development of the child and recommendations for surgery. In Smith, J. and Bumsted, R., Eds., *Pediatric Facial Plastic and Reconstructive Surgery.* New York: Raven Press, 1993, 387–396.
9. Stal, S., Peterson, R., and Spira, M. Aesthetic considerations and the pediatric population. *Clin. Plastic Surg.*, 1998, 25, 631–649.
10. Goin, M. Psychiatric considerations. In Couctiss, E., Ed. *Aesthetic Surgery, Trouble How to Avoid and How to Treat It.* St. Louis: C.V. Mosby Co., 1978, 17–24.
11. Dinis, P. and Dinis, M. Pshcological consequences of nasal aesthetic and funtional surgery: a controlled prospective study in an ENT setting. *Rhinology*, 1998, 36, 32–36.
12. Kapp-Simon, K. and Simon, D., Self-perception, social skills, adjustment, and inhibition in young adolescents with craniofacial anomalies. *Cleft Palate Craniofacial J.*, 1992, 29, 352–356.
13. Goin, M. and Ewws, T. A. prospective study of patients psychological reactions to rhinoplasty. *Ann. Plast. Surg.*, 1991, 27, 210–213.
14. Farkas, L. and Posnick, J. Anthropometric growth study of the ear. *Cleft Palate Craniofacial J.*, 1992, 29, 324–327.
15. Tanzer, R. Congenital deformities. In Converse, J., Ed. *Reconstructive Plastic Surgery*, Vol. 3, 2nd ed. Philadelphia: W.B. Saunders, 1977, 1671–1719.
16. Weeda, H. Classification of congenital deformities of the auricle. *Facial Plastic Surg.*, 1988, 5, 385–388.
17. Farkas, L. Otoplastic architecture. In Davis, J., Ed. *Aesthetic and Reconstructive Otoplasty.* New York: Springer–Verlag, 1987, 13–52.
18. Davis, J. Prominent ear. In Davis, J., Ed. *Aesthetic and Reconstructive Otoplasty.* New York: Springer–Verlag, 1987, 129–185.
19. Bartley, J., How long should ears be bandaged after otoplasty? *J. Laryngol. Otol.*, 1998, 112, 531–532.
20. Calder, J. and Naasam, A. Morbidity of otoplasty: a review of 562 consecutive cases. *Br. J. Plastic Surg.*, 1994, 47, 170–174.
21. Davis, J. Aesthetic otoplasty. In Davis, J., Ed. *Otoplasty: Aesthetic and Reconstructive Techniques.* New York: Springer–Verlag, 1997, 3–23.
22. Farkas, L. and Posnick, J., Growth patterns of the nasolabial region: a morphometric study. *Cleft Palate Craniofacial J.*, 1992, 29, 318–325.
23. Bejar, I. and Farkas, L. Nasal growth after septoplasty in children. *Arch. Otolaryngol. Head Neck Surg.*, 1996, 122, 816–821.
24. Enlow, D. Introductory concepts of the growth process. In Enlow, D., Ed. *Facial Growth*, 3rd ed. Philadelphia: W.B. Saunders Co., 1990, 25–55.

25. McCollough, E. and Robertson, J. Nasal tip asymmetries. *Facial Plastic Clin. North Am.*, 1995, 3, 353–366.
26. Johnson, C. and Toriumi, D. Revision rhinoplasty case studies. In Johnson, C. and Toriumi, D., Eds. *Open Structure Rhinoplasty.* Philadelphia: W.B. Saunders Co., 1990, 411–513.
27. Ellis, D. and Shaikh, A., The twisted nose. In: Krause, C., Ed. *Aesthetic Facial Surgery.* Philadelphia: J.B. Lippincott, 1991, 313–327.
28. Gross, C. and Boyle, T. Nasal surgery for congenital and acquired disease. In: Smith, J.D. and Bumsted, R., Eds. *Pediatric Facial Plastic and Reconstructive Surgery.* New York: Raven Press, 1993, 31–41.
29. Toriumi, D. and Johnson, C. Revision rhinoplasty. In: Krause, C., Ed. *Aesthetic Facial Surgery.* Philadelphia: J.B. Lippincott, 1991, 411–456.
30. Silver, W., Augmentation of the Nasal Dorsum. In Krause, C., Ed. *Aesthetic Facial Surgery.* Philadelphia: J.B. Lippincott, 1991, 321–340.
31. Adamson, P. The over-resected nasal dorsum. *Facial Plastic Surg. Clin. North Am.*, 1995, 3, Nov., 407–419.
32. Bernstein, L. Airway problems after rhinoplasty. *Facial Plastic Surg. Clin. North Am.*, 1995, 3, Nov., 449–457.
33. Berinstein, T. and Bane, S., Steroid use in rhinoplasty: an objective assessment of postoperative edema. *Ear Nose Throat J.*, 1998, Jan., 40–43.
34. Farkas, L.G. et al. Vertical and horizontal proportions of the face in young adult North American Caucasians: revision of neoclassical canons. *Plastic Reconstr. Surg.*, 1985, 75, 328.
35. Ricketts, R.M. Divine proportion in facial esthetics. *Clin. Plastic Surg.*, 1982, 9, 401.
36. Patterson C.N. and Powell D.G. Facial analysis in patient evaluation for physiologic and cosmetic surgery. *Laryngoscope*, 1974, 84, 1004.
37. Grayson, B.H. Cephalometric analysis for the surgeon, *Clin. Plastic Surg.*, 1989, 16, 633.
38. Riolo, M.L. et al. *An Atlas of Craniofacial Growth.* Ann Arbor: Michigan Center for Human Growth and Development, 1974.
39. Munro, I.R. Orbito-cranio-facial surgery: the team approach. *Plastic Reconstr. Surg.*, 1975, 55, 170.
40. McCarthy, J.G. The concept of a craniofacial anomalies center. *Clin. Plastic Surg.*, 1976, 3, 611.
41. Whitaker, L.A. et al. Combined report of problems and complications in 793 craniofacial operations. *Plastic Reconstr. Surg.*, 1979, 64, 198.
42. Munro, I.R. and Sabatier, R.E. An analysis of 12 years of craniomaxillofacial surgery in Toronto. *Plastic Reconstr. Surg.*, 1985, 76, 29.
43. David, D.J. and Cooter, R.D. Craniofacial infection in 10 years of transcranial surgery. *Plastic Reconstr. Surg.*, 1987, 80, 213.
44. Poole, M.D. Complications in craniofacial surgery. *Br. J. Plastic Surg.*, 1988, 41, 608.
45. Kazanjian, V. Bone transplanting to the mandible. *Am. J. Surg.*, 1952, 83, 633.
46. Scheuerle, A.E. Recent advances in craniofacial genetics. *J. Craniofacial Surgeon*, 1995, 6, 440.
47. Slavkin, H.C. *Developmental Craniofacial Biology.* Philadelphia: Lea and Febiger, 1979.
48. Scheuerle, A.E. Recent advances in craniofacial genetics [editorial]. *J. Craniofacial Surgeon*, 1995, 6, 440.
49. Tessier, P. Anatomical classification of facial, craniofacial and lateral-facial clefts *J. Maxilofacial Surgeon*, 1976, 4, 69.
50. Marchac, D. and Renier, D. Intracranial pressure in craniosynostosis. *J. Neurosurgery*, 1982, 57, 370.
51. Posnick, J.C., Linkly, C.P., and Armstrong, D. Metopic synostosis: quantitative assessment of presenting deformity and surgical results based on CT scans. *Plastic Reconstr. Surg.*, 1994, 93, 16–24.
52. Shillito, J., Jr. and Matson, D.D. Craniostenosis: a review of 519 surgical patients. *Pediatrics*, 1968, 41, 829.
53. McCarthy, J.G. *Plastic Surgery.* Philadelphia: W.B. Saunders Company, 1990.
54. Marchac, D., Renier, D., and Broumard, S. Timing of treatment for craniosynostosis and facio-craniosynostosis: A 20 year experience. *Br. J. Plastic Surg.*, 1994, 47, 211.
55. Bruneteau, R.J. and Mulliken, J.B. Frontal plagiocephaly. Synostosis, compensational, or deformational. *Plastic Reconstr. Surg.*, 1992, 89, 21.
56. Hansen, M., Padwa, B.L., Scott, M., Stica, P.E., and Mulliken, J.B. Synostotic frontal plagiocephaly: anthoropometric comparison of three techniques for surgical correction. *Plastic Reconstr. Surg.*, 1995, 100, 1387.

57. McCarthy, J.G., Glasberg, S.B., Cutting, C.B., Epstein, F.J., Grayson, B.H., Ruff, G., Thorne, C.H., Wisoff, J., and Zide, B.M. Twenty year experience with early surgery for craniosynostosis: I. Isolated craniofacial synostosis — results and unsolved problems. *Plastic Reconstr. Surg.*, 1995, 96, 272–283.

58. Whitaker, L.A. and Bartlett, S.P. Craniofacial anomalies. In: Jurkiecwicz, M.J., Krizek, T.J., Mathes, S.J., and Ariyan, S., Eds. *Plastic Surgery. Principles and Practice*, Vol. 1. St. Louis: C.V. Mosby, 1990, Chap. 7.

59. McCarthy, J.G., Glasberg, S.B., Cutting, C.B., Epstein, F.J., Grayson, B.H., Ruff, G., Thorne, C.H., Wisoff, J., and Zide, B.M. Twenty year experience with early surgery for craniosynostosis: II. The craniofacial synostosis syndromes and pan synostosis — results and unsolved problems. *Plastic Reconstr. Surg.*, 1995, 96, 284–295.

60. Schaefer, M. Complications of the monobloc frontofacial advancement. Presented at the American Cleft Palate Association Conference on Long Term Results in Craniofacial Surgery, New York, May 17, 1986.

61. Wolfe, S.A., Morrison, G., Page, L.K., and Berkowitz, S. The monobloc frontofacial advancement. Do the pluses outweigh the minuses? *Plastic Reconstr. Surg.*, 1993, 91, 977–987.

62. Kawamoto, H.K., Jr. Complications associated with the monobloc frontofacial advancement. Presented at the American Association of Plastic Surgeons Meeting, Palm Beach, FL. May 3, 1998.

63. McCarthy, J.G., Stelnick, E.J., and Grayson, B.H. Distraction osteogenesis of the mandible: a ten year experience. *Semin. Orthod.*, 1999, 5, 3–8.

64. Shprintzen, R.J. et al. Phalyngeal hypoplasia in Treacher–Collins syndrome. *Arch. Otalyngol.*, 1979, 105, 127.

Section X

Epilogue

Epilogue: Beyond the Blame

Paul A. Gluck

There can be no justice so long as laws are absolute.

Jean Luc Picard

CONTENTS

INTRODUCTION

The Institute of Medicine (IOM) report "To Err Is Human: Building a Safer Health System"[1] thrust concerns about medical errors from the confidentiality of the deliberative peer review process onto front-page headlines and the network evening news. Released in November 1999, this report gave high visibility to the previous estimates of patient deaths from medical error of 44,000 from the Utah–Colorado Medical Practice Study[2] and 98,000 from the Harvard Medical Practice Study.[3,4]

With headlines such as "Medical Errors, Major Killer" (NBC Evening News, November 29, 1999) and "Doctors' Deadly Mistakes" (*Time,* November 12, 1999), it is understandable that the public lost confidence in the safety of their medical care. According to a report from the Commonwealth Fund (April 2002) in interviews of 6700 adults, researchers found that almost half claimed a medical error caused significant injury to them or to their immediate family.

The initial reaction in the medical community was outrage and defensiveness. The validity of the numbers was attacked from the perspective of hindsight bias. Reviewers, aware of the outcomes, were accused of being overly critical.[5,6] These results were replicated, however, in prospective observational studies. Others contended that these estimates were just the tip of the iceberg because many errors are concealed for fear of reprisals.[1] Another criticism was precisely how to define a medical error or adverse event. There is now consensus in the taxonomy of medical error. *Overuse* concerns a health care service that has more potential harm than benefit, *underuse* is the failure to provide an appropriate health care service, and *misuse* means the appropriate health care service is not executed properly, thus resulting in a preventable complication.[7]

Quibbling about the numbers is in one sense irrelevant and nonproductive. Should we accept any injury or death caused by medical care and not the underlying disease process? In order to make health care safer, we must understand (1) the evolution of patient safety principles; (2) the "system" of medical care; (3) error theory; and, from that, we can propose (4) safety solutions.

THE EVOLUTION OF PATIENT SAFETY

Patient safety, a vital dimension of medical quality, has its roots in risk management; however, there are several important differences. Traditional risk management is retrospective, focused on the individual outlier and outcome oriented, and seeks to remediate sentinel events with discipline and punishment. Aside from weeding out a very few substandard practitioners, this approach has done little to decrease the rate of medical errors, which are often rooted in the system of care. Patient safety, however, is prospective, interdisciplinary, process and outcome driven, nonpunitive, applicable to all health care workers, and recognizes that most adverse outcomes are due to system deficiencies and not to individual incompetence. Furthermore, we must admit that no matter how safe a system is developed, we can only reduce, not eliminate, all error. Therefore, system design must be resilient and provide for identification and mitigation of errors that we cannot prevent.

Because of public concern and outrage arising from headlines generated from the Institute of Medicine report, the patient safety movement has gathered momentum; considerable activity is occurring in Washington. As President, Mr. Clinton established the Quality Interagency Coordinating Council to coordinate the efforts of all federal agencies concerned with quality and safety. The Bush Administration recommendation that future Medicare reimbursements be linked to improvements in quality and safety has further advanced the executive branch's initiative on patient safety. Secretary of Health and Human Services Tommy Thompson established a taskforce to develop a confidential, easy-to-use, uniform system for error reporting. Currently, there are several bills working their way through Congress that address specific improvements in patient safety.

The Joint Commission for the Accreditation of Healthcare Organizations (JCAHO) has also made the transition to a patient-safety perspective. Initially, JCAHO required that bad outcomes, known as sentinel events, be reported and remediated. Realizing that most adverse events have multiple predisposing factors, the JCAHO now requires a root cause analysis to investigate all contributing factors and subsequent system solutions.[8] Finally, beginning January 2003, JCAHO promulgated specific explicit safety survey goals that will become a part of their survey process. The JCAHO safety goals are intended to be explicit, evidence based, derived from Sentinel Alerts, and measurable. Each year additional goals will be proposed and published for comment before being added to the surveys. Examples of current National Patient Safety Goals include improving the accuracy of patient identification before any intervention, improving the safety of infusion pumps, and improving communication effectiveness.

The Leapfrog Group from the National Business Roundtable is advancing the business case for safety. Representing more than 20 million insured lives, this coalition of major U.S. corporations will preferentially purchase insurance from health care organizations that can deliver three components shown to improve patient safety measurably: (1) 24-hour intensivist in house, (2) computerized physician order entry, and (3) centers of excellence that have experience for specific high-risk procedures.

SYSTEM OF MEDICAL CARE

WORKING AT THE "SHARP" END

Medicine is a disparate "system" consisting of "teams of caregivers who have widely differing professional backgrounds and who operate with unclear lines of authority."[9] Nurses, physicians, and other health care providers work at the "sharp" end of the medical system. They directly interact with the patient to provide care. Enabling these individuals to carry out their tasks is a large infrastructure at the "blunt" end of medical care, which includes administration, hospitals, engineering, laboratories, pharmacists, offices, and clinics.[10]

Two types of errors can occur within this system. Most adverse events are the result of latent errors embedded in the blunt end of the system.[10] These are hazards that have the potential to harm patients under the wrong circumstances but, for the most part, go undetected. An example is the current nursing shortage and staffing problems in hospitals. These dedicated individuals have learned to do more with less and, for the most part, perform their duties very well. However, this shortage has led to increased risks of errors measured by six specific clinical outcomes: urinary tract infection, skin pressure ulcers, increased length of stay, upper gastrointestinal bleeding, shock, and failed resuscitation. The patient can be harmed — not from a single cause, but more likely when several of these latent errors come together in the wrong way. There are many opportunities to detect and then correct these hazards before they result in an error.

Active errors, on the other hand, are unsafe acts committed by practitioners at the sharp end of care. Such errors are less common, sporadic, unpredictable, and more difficult to prevent. Their potential to cause harm is immediate. Examples of active errors would include technical surgical errors and administration of the wrong medication or wrong medication dosages. These errors must be addressed by having redundant systems (equipment and processes) at that point of care, as well as "alarms" to alert the individual before the patient is harmed.

ERROR THEORY

SWISS CHEESE THEORY OF ERROR

According to the concept developed by James Reason, an English psychologist, safe systems incorporate a variety of defensive barriers to prevent errors from harming the patient.[11] Each layer of defense has potential "holes" through which a hazard might pass undetected en route to harming the patient. A system can be made safer by creating more defensive barriers and by closing the potential holes in each layer. One example of this "Swiss cheese" theory follows.

> A patient was admitted as an emergency; although the ER nurse was aware of her penicillin allergy, in her haste to admit the patient, it was never recorded on the chart (a latent error was created). Upon admission to the floor, the attending physician ordered IV amoxicillin because he was unaware of the allergy (a hazard was created, but has not yet harmed the patient). The ward secretary, now with the history of the patient's allergy but unaware of the relationship to amoxicillin, transmitted the order to pharmacy, where it was dispensed before the allergy was known. On the floor, the nurse, caring for six patients because of decreased staffing, instructed the aide to administer the antibiotic. The patient was asleep, so the IV amoxicillin was hung without inquiring about allergies or checking patient's chart and she suffered an anaphylactic reaction. The hazard created by the physician passed through several potential barriers (secretary, pharmacist, nurse, aide, and even the patient) that could have recognized the error before the drug was administered and the patient harmed. In this case, a "perfect storm" of hazards and holes in the defensive barriers has aligned in just the wrong way to harm the patient.

MAKING HEALTH CARE SAFER

REDUCING MEDICAL ERRORS

Realizing that most medical errors are the result of system deficiencies, it follows that system changes are needed to reduce medical errors. High-reliability organizations can provide examples of system and cultural changes that have measurably improved safety. One such example is the remarkable changes in anesthesia practice.

In the past, the risk of death or serious injury as a direct result of anesthesia varied from 1/5000 to 1/10,000 procedures. Now the risk is 1/200,000 to 1/400,000. This dramatic improvement was achieved through the work of the Anesthesia Safety Foundation and by adopting strategies from the aviation industry. New technology designed for safety, such as the pulse oximeter and CO_2 monitors, has played an important role. A pin insertion safety system has replaced the universal gas coupling on anesthesia machines. This system has significantly reduced the thousands of deaths that occurred every year when the nitrous oxide line was inadvertently attached to the oxygen connection. Simulators recreate uncommon, high-risk conditions for training and protocol improvement. Confidential reporting of anesthesia mishaps and near misses captures valuable information for analysis and continuous improvement of equipment and procedures. Groups in different disciplines, who routinely work together, also train together, thereby breaking down the usual hierarchy. Team training, derived from aviation crew resource management, teaches that the individual best able to intervene is empowered to correct the problem regardless of their "rank."

Five principles can be applied to health care systems to improve safety:[12]

- Provide leadership for safety.
- Respect human limitations.
- Train in teams.
- Anticipate the unexpected.
- Create a learning environment.

First, leadership for a safe institution must begin in the boardroom with safety identified as a prime corporate objective. A culture of blame and retribution must be replaced with a nonpunitive culture of shared responsibility. Organizational goals, mission, processes, and structure must be aligned with improving patient safety. Lines of executive responsibility for safety must be clear, with adequate human and financial resources.

Second, system design must respect human limitations. Irrespective of individual training and dedication, any system that relies solely on human vigilance for safety is doomed to fail. Key processes must be simplified and standardized to reduce variation and the chance for error. Allowing for individual physician preferences as well as unusual clinical situations, standardized orders can still be developed for most patients and procedures. Computer physician order entry (CPOE) can further enhance this process. In the operating room, equipment and suture choices can vary tremendously; this variability introduces a greater chance for error and reduces the efficiency of the operating room.

Forcing functions must be embedded in critical processes. In automobiles, for example, it is impossible to start a car unless the gear is in park or neutral and impossible to shift into reverse unless the brake pedal is depressed. Similar constraints should be engineered into medical equipment such as infusion pumps. Memory is inadequate to keep track of medication, protocols, and patient-specific information. CPOE or other aids are needed. We cannot change the human condition, but we can change the conditions under which humans work.

Third, those expected to work in teams should train in teams. We work in multidisciplinary environments and rely on individuals with a variety of clinical skills. Training in teams will help break down some of the hierarchal barriers. The individual with the most knowledge to address a given critical situation should feel empowered to respond, irrespective of his or her position on the team. When possible, simulators and mock drills should be used for unusual emergencies. The patient should be incorporated as a valuable asset on the team and should understand his or her illness and treatment. The patient should be encouraged to challenge any perceived irregularities in his or her care.

Fourth, we must anticipate the unexpected. Equipment and care processes must be constantly examined and redesigned to detect and eliminate latent errors (failure mode and effects analysis).[13] Redundancy for certain critical functions is important. Provisions should be made to mitigate potentially serious errors before the patient is harmed. Information needed to make critical decisions must be timely, accurate, and readily available to those expected to make the decisions. For medication safety, CPOE is one such example.

Fifth, we must establish a learning environment to evaluate and improve patient safety continually. Information about hazards to patient safety should be open and flow easily among all members of the health care team. Information about safety problems and near misses should be exchanged openly within and between institutions without fear of litigation or punishment. At the same time, the privacy of the individual patient and confidential nature of the information must be respected. Health care must be transparent to the patient. In the event of adverse outcomes due to medical error, the patient deserves a truthful and compassionate explanation, remedies to ameliorate the problem, and assurances that system changes will be instituted to minimize the risk of others suffering from the same error.

CONCLUSIONS

The application of safety principles to medical care is a natural evolution of the continuous quality improvement efforts adapted from industry and already accepted by health care institutions. The IOM report, *To Err is Human: Building a Safer Health System*, has given this transition a new urgency. This cultural change has been further stimulated by regulatory scrutiny (JCAHO) and economic incentives (Leapfrog). It is most important to remember, however, that medicine should be not only about treating disease but also about protecting patients from harm incurred during medical care. A long-term commitment from all segments of the health care system to improve continually patient safety by minimizing system deficiencies is paramount if medicine is to continue to take a leadership role in its own management.

REFERENCES

1. Kohn, L., Corrigan, J., and Donaldson, M. *To Err Is Human: Building a Safer Health System.* Washington, D.C.: National Academy Press, 2000.
2. Gawande, A., Thomas, E., Zinner, M., and Brennan, T. The incidence and nature of surgical adverse events in Colorado and Utah in 1992. *Surgery,* 126, 66–75.
3. Harvard Medical Practice Study. *Patients, Doctors, and Lawyers: Medical Injury, Malpractice Litigation, and Patient Compensation in New York.* Cambridge, MA: Presidents and Fellows of Harvard College, 1990.
4. Brennan, T., Leape, L., Laird, N. et al. Incidence of adverse events and negligence in hospitalized patients: results of the Harvard Medical Practice Study. *New Engl. J. Med.,* 1991, 324, 370–376.
5. Thomas, E., Studdert, D., and Brennan, T. The reliability of medical record review for estimating adverse event rates. *Ann. Intern. Med.,* 2002, 136(11), 812-816.
6. Hayward, R. and Hofer, T. Estimating hospital deaths due to medical errors: preventability is in the eye of the reviewer. *JAMA,* 2001, 286, 415-420.
7. Chassin, M. and Galvin, R. The urgent need to improve health care quality. *JAMA,* 1998, 280, 1000–1005.
8. Bates, D. and Gawande, A. Error in medicine: what have we learned? *Ann. Intern. Med.,* 2000, 132, 763–767.
9. Kizer, K. Gen. Med., *Medscape* at www.medscape.com (accessed 3/21/02).
10. Cook, R., Woods, D., and Miller, C. *A Tale of Two Stories. Contrasting Views of Patient Safety.* Chicago: National Patient Safety Foundation, 1998. Available at: www.NPSF.org/exec/NPSF_rpt.po (accessed 2/28/2002).
11. Reason, J. *Managing the Risks of Organizational Accidents.* Aldershot, UK: Ashgate, 1997.
12. Kizer, K. Ten steps you can take to improve patient safety in your facility. *Briefings Patient Saf.,* 2000, 1(9), 1–4.
13. DeRosier, J., Stalhandske, E., Bagian, J., and Nudell, T. Using health care failure mode and effect analysis: the VA National Center for Patient Safety's prospective risk system. *J Qual. Improv.,* 2002, 28(5), 248–267.

Index

A

Abnormalities
  airway
    in craniofacial anomalies, 234
    in Down syndrome, 234
    in mucopolysaccaridoses, 234
    in Pierre Robin syndrome, 234
  congenital (*See also* Anomalies)
    external ear, 121
    internal ear, 121–122
    middle ear, 121–122
Abscess(es)
  Bezold's, 455, 458
  brain
    diagnosis, 466–467
      imaging in, 467
    FESS and, 436
    management, 467–468
    otitis media and, 455, 465–468
    pathophysiology, 465–466
    signs and symptoms, 466–467
    venous thrombophlebitis and, retrograde, 466
  deep neck, 257
  deep space, 264–267
  dysphagia and, 304
  extradural, 455, 463–464
    diagnosis, 463
    management, 463–464
    otitis media and, 455, 463–464
    pathophysiology, 463
  neck, 257
  orbital, 111, 429
  otitis media and, 455, 465–468
  parapharyngeal, 257, 266–267
  peritonsillar, 86, 257, 264–265
  retropharyngeal, 86, 115, 265–266
    adenotonsillectomy and, 248
    carotid artery narrowing and, 115–116
    as foreign body complication, 341
  sinusitis and, 111, 420, 421
  subperiosteal, 111
    diagnosis, 458–459
    management, 459
    otitis media and, 455, 458–459
    pathophysiology, 458
  thrombophlebitis and, 116, 117
Accreditation Council for Continuing Medical Education (ACCME), 14
Achalasia, 306
Achondroplasia, OSAS and, 222
Acidosis, respiratory, 64
Acne, skin infections and, 269

Acoustic stapedial reflex threshold test, 147
Acrochordon, surgical management of, 276–277
Acromegaly, laryngeal stenosis and, 352
Acute respiratory distress syndrome, 88
Adenitis, cervical, 257, 261–264
Adenoidectomy. *See also* Adenotonsillectomy
  before and after otologic surgery, 480, 481
  airway considerations, 234
  Down syndrome and, 238
  fluid intake following, 237–238
  hematologic preoperative evaluation, 234–235
  hemorrhage during, 232–234
  ketorolac administration during, 237
  velocardiofacial syndrome and, 116
Adenoiditis, 258
Adenotonsillar hyperplasia, swallowing disorders and, 305
Adenotonsillectomy, 72. *See also* Adenoidectomy;
      Tonsillectomy
  antibiotic therapy following, 247
  atlantoaxial subluxation and, 247
  depression and, 248
  Eagle stylohyoid syndrome and, 246–247
  fever and, 241–242
  identification of high-risk child for, 224
  intraoperative complications, 240–241
  meningitis and, 248
  mucopolysaccharidosis and, 239
  nasopharyngeal stenosis and, 246
  necrotizing fasciitis and, 248
  neuromuscular disease and, 239
  oropharyngeal stenosis and, 246
  for OSAS, 222, 223
  osteomyelitis and, 248
  otalgia and, 244
  perioperative precautions, 224–225
  phenylephrine during, 240
  pneumomediastinum with subcutaneous emphysema and, 248
  pneumoperitoneum and, 248
  postoperative complications, 241–248
    long-term, 244–247
    short-term, 241–244
    unusual, 247–248
  pulmonary edema and, 241
  retropharyngeal abscess and, 248
  sickle cell disease and, 239–2240
  throat pain and, 242–244
  tracheitis and, 248
  trismus secondary to mandible condyle fracture and, 248
  velopharyngeal insufficiency and, 244–245
Adolescent(s)
  development, 32

M

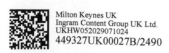

9 780367 392680